MUSIC, LANGUAGE, AND THE BRAIN

MUSIC, LANGUAGE, AND THE BRAIN

Aniruddh D. Patel

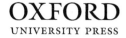

OXFORD

UNIVERSITY PRESS

OXFORD
UNIVERSITY PRESS

Oxford University Press, Inc., publishes works that further
Oxford University's objective of excellence
in research, scholarship, and education.

Oxford   New York
Auckland   Cape Town   Dar es Salaam   Hong Kong   Karachi
Kuala Lumpur   Madrid   Melbourne   Mexico City   Nairobi
New Delhi   Shanghai   Taipei   Toronto

With offices in
Argentina   Austria   Brazil   Chile   Czech Republic   France   Greece
Guatemala   Hungary   Italy   Japan   Poland   Portugal   Singapore
South Korea   Switzerland   Thailand   Turkey   Ukraine   Vietnam

Copyright © 2008 by Oxford University Press, Inc.

Published by Oxford University Press, Inc.
198 Madison Avenue, New York, New York 10016

www.oup.com

First issued as an Oxford University Press paperback, 2010

Oxford is a registered trademark of Oxford University Press

For sound and video examples referenced in this book, visit www.oup.com/us/patel.

Library of Congress Cataloging-in-Publication Data

Patel, Aniruddh D.
Music, language, and the brain / Aniruddh D. Patel.
    p. ; cm.
Includes bibliographical references.
ISBN 978-0-19-975530-1
1. Music—Psychological aspects. 2. Music—Physiological aspects. 3. Auditory perception—Physiological
aspects. 4. Language acquisition—Physiological aspects. 5. Cognitive neuroscience. 6. Neurobiology.
I. Title.
[DNLM: 1. Brain—physiology. 2. Music—psychology. 3. Auditory Perception—physiology.
4. Cognition—physiology. 5. Language. WL 300 P295m 2007]
ML3830.P33 2007
781'.11—dc22   2007014189

Printed in the United States of America
on acid-free paper

For my family

Preface

The existence of this book reflects the support and vision of two of the twentieth century's great natural scientists: Edward O. Wilson and Gerald M. Edelman. At Harvard University, Wilson gave me the freedom to pursue a Ph.D. on the biology of human music at a time when the topic was still in the academic hinterland. With his support, my graduate experiences ranged from field expeditions to Papua New Guinea, to collaborative work with specialists on music and brain (including leading figures such as Isabelle Peretz in Montreal), to training at the Max Planck Institute for Psycholinguistics (where Claus Heeschen introduced me to the world of language science). I spoke with Wilson while I was formulating this book, and his support helped launch the project. His own scientific writings inspired me to believe in the importance of synthesizing a broad variety of information when exploring an emerging research area.

After completing my degree I was fortunate to be hired at The Neurosciences Institute (NSI), where Gerald Edelman, with the help of W. Einar Gall, has created an unusual environment that encourages a small and interactive group of neuroscientists to pursue basic questions about the brain, taking their research in whatever directions those questions lead. Edelman's broad vision of neuroscience and of its relationship to humanistic knowledge has shaped this project and my own approach to science. As a consequence of Edelman and Gall's support of music research, I have once again had the freedom to work on a wide variety of issues, ranging from human brain imaging to the study of music perception in aphasia to the drumming abilities of elephants in Thailand. Equally importantly, I have had the benefit of extremely bright and talented colleagues, whose work has greatly enriched my knowledge of neuroscience. Edelman, who has remarked that science is imagination in the service of the verifiable truth, has created a community where imagination is encouraged while empirical research is held to the highest standard. The salutary effect of such an environment on a young scientist cannot be overestimated.

At NSI I have also had the privilege to be the Esther J. Burnham Senior Fellow. Esther Burnham's adventurous life and her passion for both the sciences and the arts continue to be an inspiration for me and my work. I am also grateful to the Neurosciences Research Foundation, the Institute's parent organization, for its continuing support of my work.

One person who spanned my last few years at Harvard and my first few years at NSI was Evan Balaban. Evan introduced me to the world of auditory neuroscience and to a creative and critical approach to interdisciplinary scientific research. Another person who has been a particularly close colleague is John Iversen, a deeply insightful scientist with whom I'm pleased to work on a daily basis.

This book has benefited from the expertise and constructive criticism of numerous outstanding scholars. John Sloboda, Carol Krumhansl, and D. Robert Ladd read the entire manuscript and provided comments that improved the book in important ways. I am also grateful to Bruno Repp, John Iversen, the late Peter Ladefoged, Jeff Elman, Sun-Ah Jun, Emmanuel Bigand, Stephen Davies, Bob Slevc, Erin Hannon, Lauren Stewart, Sarah Hawkins, Florian Jaeger, Benjamin Carson, and Amy Schafer for insightful comments on individual chapters, and to Oliver Sacks for sharing with me his observations and eloquent writings on music and the brain. Heidi Moomaw provided valuable assistance in organizing the index and references. I would also like to thank Joan Bossert at Oxford University Press for her energetic commitment to this project from its outset. Joan and Abby Gross in the editorial department and Christi Stanforth in production have been an outstanding publishing team.

On a personal note, my family has been essential in bringing this project to completion. My mother, Jyotsna Pandit Patel, has been an unending source of encouragement and inspiration. Kiran and Neelima Pandit, my late grandmother Indira Pandit, and Shirish and Rajani Patel have given their support in essential ways. Jennifer Burton has been a key part of this project from the beginning, as a fellow writer and scholar, as my wife, and as the mother of our two children, Roger and Lilia Burtonpatel.

As I intimated at the start of this preface, the past decade has seen a transformation in the study of music and the brain. A loose affiliation of researchers has developed into a dynamic research community whose numbers are growing steadily each year. I have been fortunate to be part of this community during this formative time. If this book can contribute to the growing excitement and promise of our field, I will have more than accomplished my goal.

Contents

MUSIC, LANGUAGE, AND THE BRAIN

1

Introduction

Language and music define us as human. These traits appear in every human society, no matter what other aspects of culture are absent (Nettl, 2000). Consider, for example, the Pirahã, a small tribe from the Brazilian Amazon. Members of this culture speak a language without numbers or a concept of counting. Their language has no fixed terms for colors. They have no creation myths, and they do not draw, aside from simple stick figures. Yet they have music in abundance, in the form of songs (Everett, 2005).

The central role of music and language in human existence and the fact that both involve complex and meaningful sound sequences naturally invite comparison between the two domains. Yet from the standpoint of modern cognitive science, music-language relations have barely begun to be explored. This situation appears to be poised to change rapidly, as researchers from diverse fields are increasingly drawn to this interdisciplinary enterprise. The appeal of such research is easy to understand. Humans are unparalleled in their ability to make sense out of sound. In many other branches of our experience (e.g., visual perception, touch), we can learn much from studying the behavior and brains of other animals because our experience is not that different from theirs. When it comes to language and music, however, our species is unique (cf. Chapter 7, on evolution). This makes it difficult to gain insight into language or music as a cognitive system by comparing humans to other organisms. Yet within our own minds are two systems that perform remarkably similar interpretive feats, converting complex acoustic sequences into perceptually discrete elements (such as words or chords) organized into hierarchical structures that convey rich meanings. This provides a special opportunity for cognitive science. Specifically, exploring both the similarities and the differences between music and language can deepen our understanding of the mechanisms that underlie our species' uniquely powerful communicative abilities.

Of course, interest in music-language relations does not originate with modern cognitive science. The topic has long drawn interest from a wide range of thinkers, including philosophers, biologists, poets, composers, linguists, and musicologists. Over 2,000 years ago, Plato claimed that the power of certain musical modes to uplift the spirit stemmed from their resemblance to the sounds of noble speech (Neubauer, 1986). Much later, Darwin (1871) considered how a form of communication intermediate between modern language and music may have been the origin of our species' communicative abilities. Many other historical figures have contemplated music-language relations, including Vincenzo Galilei (father of Galileo), Jean-Jacques Rousseau, and Ludwig Wittgenstein. This long line of speculative thinking has continued down to the modern era (e.g., Bernstein, 1976). In the era of cognitive science, however, research into this topic is undergoing a dramatic shift, using new concepts and tools to advance from suggestions and analogies to empirical research.

Part of what animates comparative research is a tension between two perspectives: one that emphasizes the differences between music and language, and one that seeks commonalities. Important differences do, of course, exist. To take a few examples, music organizes pitch and rhythm in ways that speech does not, and lacks the specificity of language in terms of semantic meaning. Language grammar is built from categories that are absent in music (such as nouns and verbs), whereas music appears to have much deeper power over our emotions than does ordinary speech. Furthermore, there is a long history in neuropsychology of documenting cases in which brain damage or brain abnormality impairs one domain but spares the other (e.g., amusia and aphasia). Considerations such as these have led to the suggestion that music and language have minimal cognitive overlap (e.g., Marin & Perry, 1999; Peretz, 2006).

This book promotes the alternative perspective, which emphasizes commonalities over differences. This perspective claims that these two domains, although having specialized representations (such as pitch intervals in music, and nouns and verbs in language), share a number of basic processing mechanisms, and that the comparative study of music and language provides a powerful way to explore these mechanisms. These mechanisms include the ability to form learned sound categories (Chapter 2), to extract statistical regularities from rhythmic and melodic sequences (Chapters 3 and 4), to integrate incoming elements (such as words and musical tones) into syntactic structures (Chapter 5), and to extract nuanced emotional meanings from acoustic signals (Chapter 6). The evidence supporting this perspective comes from diverse strands of research within cognitive science and neuroscience, strands that heretofore have not been unified in a common framework. The final chapter of the book (Chapter 7) takes an evolutionary perspective, and uses music-language comparisons to address the persistent question of whether music is an evolutionary adaptation.

Throughout the book the focus is on the relationship between ordinary spoken language and purely instrumental music. It is worth explaining the motivation for this choice, because initially it may seem more appropriate to compare instrumental music to an artistic form of language such as poetry, or to focus on vocal music, where music and language intertwine. The basic motivation is a cognitive one: To what extent does the making and perceiving of instrumental music draw on cognitive and neural mechanisms used in our everyday communication system? Comparing ordinary language to instrumental music forces us to search for the hidden connections that unify obviously different phenomena.

In taking such an approach, of course, it is vital to sift real connections from spurious ones, to avoid the distraction of superficial analogies between music and language. This requires a solid understanding of the structure of musical and linguistic systems. In consequence, each chapter discusses in detail the structure of music and/or language with regard to the chapter's topic, for example, rhythm or melody. These sections (sections 2 and 3 of each chapter) provide the context for the final section of the chapter, which explores a key cognitive link between music and language, providing empirical evidence and pointing the way to future studies.

Because music-language relations are of interest to researchers from diverse fields, this book is written to be accessible to individuals with primary training in either in music or language studies. In addition, each chapter can stand largely on its own, for readers who are primarily interested in a selected topic (e.g., syntax, evolution). Because each chapter covers a good deal of material, there is a sectional organization within each chapter. Each chapter also begins with a detailed table of contents, which can be used as a roadmap when reading.

My hope is that this book will help provide a framework for those interested in exploring music-language relations from a cognitive perspective. Whether one's theoretical perspective favors the search for differences or commonalities, one thing is certain: The comparative approach is opening up entirely new avenues of research, and we have just started the journey.

Chapter 2
Sound Elements

Appendixes

2

Sound Elements: Pitch and Timbre

2.1 Introduction

Every human infant is born into a world with two distinct sound systems. The first is linguistic and includes the vowels, consonants, and pitch contrasts of the native language. The second is musical and includes the timbres and pitches of the culture's music. Even without explicit instruction, most infants develop into adults who are proficient in their native language and who enjoy their culture's music. These traits come at a price, however; skill in one language can result in difficulty in hearing or producing certain sound distinctions in another, and a music lover from one culture may find another culture's music out of tune and annoying.[1] Why is this so? The simple answer is that our native sound system leaves an imprint on our minds. That is, learning a sound system leads to a mental framework of sound categories for our native language or music. This framework helps us extract distinctive units from physical signals rich in acoustic variation. Such frameworks are highly adaptive in our native sonic milieu, but can be liabilities when hearing another culture's language or music, because we "hear with an accent" based on our native sound system.

Of course, music and speech have one very obvious difference in their sound category systems. Although pitch is the primary basis for sound categories in music (such as intervals and chords), timbre is the primary basis sound for categories of speech (e.g., vowels and consonants). This chapter compares music and speech in terms of the way they organize pitch and timbre. Section 2.2 focuses on music, with an emphasis on musical scales and on pitch

---

[1] Indeed, one need not leave one's culture to have this experience. One of the difficulties of appreciating Western European music composed with microtonal scales, such as certain music by Charles Ives or Easley Blackwood, is that it can sound like an out-of-tune version of music composed using familiar scale systems. For those unfamiliar with the concept of a musical scale, see section 2.2.2, subsection "Introduction to Musical Scales."

intervals as learned sound categories in music. This section also discusses musical timbre, and explores why timbral contrasts are rarely the basis for musical sound systems. Section 2.3 then turns to language, and discusses how linguistic pitch and timbral organization compare to music. As we shall see, comparing "like to like" in this way (e.g., comparing musical and linguistic pitch systems, or musical and linguistic timbral systems) highlights the differences between music and speech. If, however, one focuses on cognitive processes of sound categorization, then similarities begin to emerge. In fact, there is growing evidence that speech and music share mechanisms for sound category learning, even though the two domains build their primary sound categories from different features of sound. The empirical comparative work supporting this idea will be reviewed in section 2.4. The implication of this work is that although the end *products* of sound category learning in music and speech are quite different (e.g., mental representations of pitch intervals vs. consonants), the *processes* that create sound categories have an important degree of overlap.

Before embarking on a comparison of speech and music, it is worth stepping back and viewing these sound systems in a broader biological perspective. What, if anything, distinguishes them from the great diversity of acoustic communication systems used by other animals? It is often noted that speech and music are "particulate" systems, in which a set of discrete elements of little inherent meaning (such as tones or phonemes) are combined to form structures with a great diversity of meanings (Hockett & Altmann, 1968; Merker, 2002). This property distinguishes speech and music from the holistic sound systems used by many animals, in which each sound is associated with a particular meaning but sounds are not recombined to form new meanings (a celebrated example of such a system is that of the Vervet monkey, *Cercopithecus aethiops,* an African primate with distinct alarm calls for different predators; Cheney & Seyfarth, 1982).

One might nevertheless argue that particulate sound systems are not unique to humans. Male humpback whales, for example, sing complex songs consisting of discrete elements organized into phrases and themes. Furthermore, individuals within a group converge on a very similar song, which changes incrementally throughout each breeding season, providing evidence that the elements and their patterning are learned (Payne, 2000; cf. Noad et al., 2000). Crucially, however, there is no evidence for a rich relationship between the order of elements and the meaning of the song. Instead, the songs always seem to mean the same thing, in other words, a combination of a sexual advertisement to females and an inter-male dominance display (Tyack & Clark, 2000). A similar point has been made about bird songs, which can have a particulate structure with discrete elements recombined to form novel sequences (e.g., in mockingbirds). Despite this structural feature, however, the songs appear to always convey the same small set of meanings, including readiness to mate, territorial display (Marler, 2000), and in some cases, an individual's identity (Gentner & Hulse, 1998).

Thus the particulate nature of speech and music is unique among biological sound systems. This fact alone, however, cannot be taken as evidence for some deep commonality between speech and music in terms of cognitive processing. Rather, both could have independently become particulate systems because such a system is a good solution to a certain kind of problem: namely, how to communicate a wide range of meanings in an economical way. For example, DNA, which is certainly not a product of the human mind, is a particulate system that transmits a great diversity of meanings (genetic information) using a finite set of discrete elements: the four chemical bases adenine, cytosine, guanine, and thymine. Thus, whether any significant cognitive similarities exist between spoken and musical sound systems is a question that requires empirical investigation.

One reason to suspect that there may be such similarities concerns an important difference between speech and music on the one hand and the particulate system of DNA on the other. Each chemical base in a DNA strand has an invariant physical structure. In contrast, any given building block of a spoken or musical sound system (such as a particular vowel or musical pitch interval) may vary in physical structure from token to token and as a function of context (Burns, 1999; Stevens, 1998). The mind must find some way to cope with this variability, separating variation within a category from variation that constitutes a change in category. Furthermore, the mapping between sounds and categories depends on the native language or music. One well-known example from language concerns the English phonemes /l/ and /r/. Although it may seem obvious that these are two distinct sound categories to an English speaker, to a Japanese speaker these sounds are merely two versions of the same speech sound and can be quite difficult to discriminate acoustically (Iverson et al., 2003). Analogously in music, the distinction between melodic pitch intervals of a major and minor third in Western European music may be irrelevant for the music of some cultures from New Guinea, where these are treated as variants of a single sound category (Chenoweth, 1980). Both of these examples illustrate that the "particles" of speech and music are not physical entities like a chemical base: They are psychological entities derived from a mental framework of learned sound categories.

2.2 Musical Sound Systems

2.2.1 Introduction to Musical Sound Systems

The 19th and 20th centuries saw a great expansion of research on the diversity of human musical systems. (For accessible introductions, see Pantaleoni, 1985; Reck, 1997; and Titon, 1996.) This research has led to one clear conclusion: There are very few universals in music (Nettl, 2000). Indeed, if "music" is defined as "sound organized in time, intended for, or perceived as, aesthetic experience" (Rodriguez, 1995, cited in Dowling, 2001:470) and "universal" is defined as a feature that appears in every musical system, it is quite clear that there are no sonic universals in music, other than the trivial one that music must involve sound in some way. For example, it is quite possible to have a modern piece of electronic music with no variation in pitch and no salient rhythmic patterning, consisting of a succession of noises distinguished by subtle differences in timbre. As long as the composer and audience consider this music, then it is music. Or consider John Cage's famous piece 4'33", in which a musician simply sits in front of a piano and does nothing while the audience listens in silence. In this case, the music is the ambient sound of the environment (such as the breathing sounds of the audience, or the horn of a passing car) filtered through the audience's intent to perceive whatever they hear in an aesthetic frame. These cases serve to illustrate that what is considered music by some individuals may have virtually nothing in common with what counts as music for others.

Nevertheless, if we restrict our attention to musical systems that are widely disseminated in their native culture, we begin to see certain patterns that emerge repeatedly. For example, two common properties of human music are the use of an organized system of pitch contrasts and the importance of musical timbre. The following two sections give an overview of pitch and timbral contrasts in music. When examining pitch contrasts, I focus on intervals rather than chords because the former are much more widespread in musical systems than are the latter.

2.2.2 Pitch Contrasts in Music

Pitch is one of the most salient perceptual aspects of a sound, defined as "that property of a sound that enables it to be ordered on a scale going from low to high" (Acoustical Society of America Standard Acoustical Terminology, cf. Randel, 1978).[2] The physical correlate of pitch is frequency (in cycles per second, or Hertz), and in a constant-frequency pure tone the pitch is essentially equal to the frequency of the tone (those desiring further introductory material on pitch may consult this chapter's appendix 1). Of course, every sound has several perceptual aspects other than pitch, notably loudness, length, timbre, and location. Each of these properties can vary independently of the other, and the human mind is capable of distinguishing several categories along any

---

[2] Pitch differences are commonly described using metaphor of height, but a cross-cultural perspective reveals that this is not the only metaphor for pitch. For example, instead of "high" and "low" the Havasupai native Americans (California) use "hard" and "soft" (Hinton, 1984:92), whereas the Kpelle of Liberia use "small" and "large" (Stone, 1982:65; cf. Herzog, 1945:230–231).

of these dimensions (Miller, 1956). Yet pitch is the most common dimension for creating an organized system of musical elements. For example, all cultures have some form of song, and songs almost always feature a stable system of pitch contrasts. Why is pitch a privileged dimension in building musical systems? Why do we not find numerous cultures in which loudness is the basis of musical contrast, and pitch variation is incidental or even suppressed? In such hypothetical (but perfectly possible) cultures, music would have minimal pitch variation but would vary in loudness across several distinct levels, perhaps from note to note, and this variation would be the basis for structural organization and aesthetic response.

Perhaps the most basic reason that pitch is favored as the basis for musical sound categories is that musical pitch perception is multidimensional.[3] For example, pitches separated by an octave (a doubling in frequency) are heard as very similar and are typically given the same name, referred to as the pitches' *pitch class* or *chroma* (e.g., all the notes called "C" on a piano keyboard). Such octave equivalence is one of the few aspects of music that is virtually universal: Most cultures recognize the similarity of musical pitches separated by an octave, and even novice listeners show sensitivity to this relationship (Dowling & Harwood, 1986). For example, men and women asked to sing the "same tune" in unison often sing an octave interval without realizing it, and young infants and monkeys treat octave transpositions of tunes as more similar than other transpositions (Demany & Armand, 1984; Wright et al., 2000). It is likely that this aspect of music reflects the neurophysiology of the auditory system.[4]

Thus the perceived similarity of pitches is governed not only by proximity in terms of pitch height but also by identity in terms of pitch chroma. One way to represent these two types of similarity in a single geometric diagram is via a helix in which pitch height increases in the vertical direction while pitch chroma changes in a circular fashion (Shepard, 1982). In such a diagram, pitches that are separated by an octave are near each other (Figure 2.1).

In contrast to this two-dimensional perceptual topology for pitch, there is no evidence for a second perceptual dimension linking sounds of different loudness, suggesting one reason why pitch is favored over loudness as a basis for structuring musical sound. Furthermore, individual pitches can be combined simultaneously to create new sonic entities (such as intervals and chords) that have distinctive perceptual qualities. For example, a pitch interval of six semitones (a tritone) has a distinctively rough perceptual quality compared to the smoother sound of intervals of five or seven semitones (a musical fourth

---

[3] Timbre perception is also multidimensional. Reasons why it seldom serves as the basis for an organized system of sound categories are discussed later, in section 2.2.4.

[4] It should be noted that as frequency increases, listeners prefer a frequency ratio slightly greater than 2:1 in making octave judgments. This "octave stretch" may have a neurophysiological basis (McKinney & Delgutte, 1999).

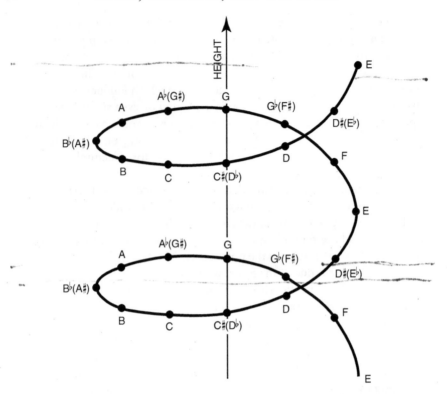

Figure 2.1 The pitch helix. Pitches are arranged along a line that spirals upward, indicating increasing pitch height, and that curves in a circular way so that pitches with the same chroma are aligned vertically, indicating octave equivalence. Adapted from Shepard, 1982.

and fifth, respectively). In contrast, there is no evidence that combining sounds of differing degrees of loudness leads to a perceptually diverse palette of new sounds. This difference between pitch and loudness is likely due to the nature of the auditory system, which is skilled at separating sound sources based on their pitch but not on their amplitude, thus providing a basis for greater sensitivity to pitch relations than to loudness relations.

Introduction to Musical Scales

One of the striking commonalities of musical pitch systems around the world is the organization of pitch contrasts in terms of a musical scale, in other words, a set of distinct pitches and intervals within the octave that serve as reference points in the creation of musical patterns. Because pitch intervals will be the primary focus of our examination of sound categories in music, it important to have a grasp of musical scale structure. In this section, I introduce some basic aspects of scale structure, focusing on Western European music because of its familiarity. To truly appreciate the cognitive significance of scale structure, however, it is necessary to examine scales cross-culturally, which is the topic of the next section.

In Western European "equal-tempered" music (the basis of most of Western music today), each octave is divided into 12 equal-sized intervals such that each note is approximately 6% higher in frequency than the note below.[5] This ratio is referred to as a "semitone." (See this chapter's appendix 2 for equations relating frequency ratios to semitones. Note that precise interval measurements are often reported in "cents," in which 1 semitone = 100 cents.) The 12 semitones of the octave are the "tonal material" of Western music (Dowling, 1978): They provide the raw materials from which different scales are constructed. A musical scale consists of a particular choice of intervals within the octave: Typically this choice repeats cyclically in each octave. For example, the set of ascending intervals (in semitones) [2 2 1 2 2 2 1] defines a "major scale" in Western music, a scale of seven pitches per octave (hence the term "octave," which is the eighth note of the scale). For example, starting on note C results in a C major scale, consisting of the notes [C D E F G A B C′], in which C′ designates the C an octave above the original.

One notable feature of the major scale is that it contains several intervals whose frequency ratios approximate small, whole-number ratios. For example, the intervals between the fifth, fourth, and third note of the scale and the first note are 7, 5, and 4 semitones. By converting semitones to frequency ratios, one can compute the frequency ratios of these intervals as 1.498, 1.335, and 1.260, respectively, values that are quite close to the ratios 3/2, 4/3, and 5/4. This is no coincidence: Western music theory has long valued intervals with simple, small-number frequency ratios, and these intervals play an important role in Western musical structure.[6] The Western fascination with such ratios in music dates back to Pythagoras, who noted that when strings with these ratio lengths were plucked simultaneously, the resulting sound was harmonious. Pythagoras had no real explanation for this, other than to appeal to the mystical power of numbers in governing the order of the universe (Walker, 1990, Ch. 3).

[5] Note that the similarity of pitches separated by an octave (a 2:1 ratio in pitch) lays the foundation for forming pitch intervals on a logarithmic basis, in other words, on the basis of frequency *ratios* rather than frequency *differences* (Dowling, 1978). For possible cases of musical pitch relations organized on a linear rather than a logarithmic basis, see Haeberli's (1979) discussion of ancient Peruvian panpipes and Will and Ellis's (1994, 1996) analysis of Australian aboriginal singing.

[6] Note that intervals of 7, 5, and 4 semitones do not yield the exact frequency ratios of 3:2, 4:3, and 5:4, respectively, because the equal-tempered scale is a compromise between an attempt to produce such ratios and the desire to move easily between different musical keys (Sethares, 1999).

As science has progressed, there have been increasingly plausible theories for the special status of certain musical intervals in perception, based on what is known about the structure and function of the auditory system. We will not delve into these theories here (interested readers may consult this chapter's appendix 3). The relevant point is that the desire to demonstrate a natural basis for scale structure has been a refrain in the study of Western music. Sometimes this desire has amusing consequences, as when Athanasius Kircher, in the influential *Musurgia Universalis* of 1650, reported that the natural laws that shaped European music applied even in the exotic jungles of the Americas, where sloths sang in the major scale (Clark & Rehding, 2001). There has also been a more serious consequence of this view, however, namely to focus scientific studies of scale structure on the auditory *properties* of musical intervals rather than the cognitive *processes* that underlie the acquisition and maintenance of pitch intervals as learned sound categories in the mind. That is, the Western perspective has tended to emphasize scales as natural systems rather than as phonological systems. To gain an appreciation of the latter view, it is necessary to look beyond Western culture.

Cultural Diversity and Commonality in Musical Scale Systems

If the structure of the auditory system provided a strong constraint on musical scales, one would expect scales to show little cultural variability. It is true that certain intervals appear in the scales of many cultures. For example, the fifth (which is the most important interval in Western music after the octave) is also important in a wide range of other musical traditions, ranging from large musical cultures in India and China to the music of small tribes in the islands of Oceania (Jairazbhoy, 1995; Koon, 1979, Zemp, 1981). A number of lines of empirical research suggest that this interval does have a special perceptual status, due to the nature of the auditory system (cf. this chapter's appendix 3).

A cross-cultural perspective reveals, however, that the auditory system provides a rather weak set of constraints on scale structure. In the late 19th century, Alexander Ellis conducted experiments on instruments that had arrived in Europe from all over the globe, and found a great diversity in musical scales (Ellis, 1885). Hermann von Helmholtz, one of the founders of music psychology, was well aware of such variation. In *On the Sensations of Tone* (1877:236), he wrote, "Just as little as the gothic painted arch, should our diatonic major scale be regarded as a natural product." He went on to note that although virtually all music used fixed pitches and intervals in building melodies, "In selecting the particular degrees of pitch, deviations of national taste become immediately apparent. The number of scales used by different nations is by no means small" (p. 253). The research of Ellis and his successors in the field of ethnomusicology has shown that although certain intervals are widespread in musical scales, such as the octave and fifth, it is certainly not the case that the scales used in Western music (or any music, for that matter) reflect a mandate of nature.

To appreciate the cognitive significance of this diversity, we will need to delve into some of the key differences and similarities among musical scales. Before doing this, it is worth noting that the concept of a scale (as a set of ordered intervals spanning the octave, from which melodies are made) does not exist in all musical cultures, even though the music may use an organized set of intervals. For example, Will and Ellis (1994) spliced the most commonly sounded frequencies out of a Western Australian aboriginal song and organized them as a scale, and then played them back to the original singer. "He commented that he could make nothing of this. . . . He pointed out through a new performance that a song was only well sung when it contained the connections (glides) between the peak frequencies as well as the ornamentations that characterized . . . the melody" (p. 12). Thus singers in a culture can organize their melodies in terms of stable pitch contrasts without having any explicit concept of a musical scale: Indeed, this is likely to be the case for many people in Western culture who enjoy singing but who have never studied music. When I speak of scales, then, I am speaking not of theoretical constructs within a culture, but of the patterning of intervals based on empirical measurements made from songs or from the sounds of musical instruments (cf. Meyer, 1956:216–217).

DIFFERENCES AMONG SCALE SYSTEMS   Widely used scale systems have been shown to differ in at least four ways. First, they differ in the amount of "tonal material" within each octave available for choosing pitches (Dowling, 1978). In Western music, there are 12 available pitches per octave, out of which 7 are typically chosen to make a musical scale such as the diatonic major scale. (The first 7 notes of "Joy to the World" contain the pitches of this scale in descending order.) In contrast, scales in Indian classical music typically choose 7 pitches from among 22 possible pitches in each octave, separated by approximately 1/2 semitone.[7] Thus in Indian music, two scales can differ only in terms of "microtones," as in Figure 2.2a (cf. Ayari & McAdams, 2003, for a discussion of microtones in Arabic music).

Second, scales differ in the number of pitches chosen per octave, ranging from 2 in some Native American musical systems to 7 tones per octave in a variety of cultures, including cultures in Europe, India, and Africa (Clough et al., 1993;

[7] The American composer Harry Partch (1901–1974) is well known for making scales from even finer subdivisions, and for building beautiful instruments with which to play this music. Toward the end of his life, Partch composed using scales based on a 43-fold division of the octave (Blackburn, 1997; Partch, 1974). The iconoclastic Partch once wryly referred to Western keyboards as "12 black and white bars in front of musical freedom" (Partch, 1991:12).

Rag Multani

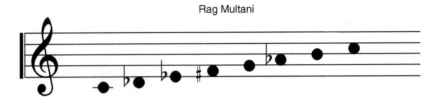

Rag Todi

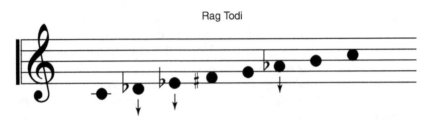

Figure 2.2a The ascending scales of two North Indian ragas. A raga is a musical form that includes a specific scale, particular melodic movements, and other features (Bor, 1999). In Rag Todi, three tones (d♭, e♭, and a♭) are slightly flatter (about 1/4 semitone) than their counterparts in Rag Multani (indicated by arrows). Courtesy of Dr. Arun Dravid and Michael Zarky.

Nettl, 1954; Nketia, 1974), with the most common number of tones per octave being 5 (Van Khê, 1977).

Third, scales differ in interval patterns. Thus two scales may both use 7 pitches per octave, but arrange the spacing of these pitches in very different ways. This is illustrated in Figure 2.2b, which shows the intervals of the Western major scale in comparison to pitch intervals of the 7-tone Javanese pelog scale used in Gamelan music. (Another Javanese scale, with 5 tones per octave, is also shown for comparison.) The Javanese scales are notable for their lack of intervals which correspond to small-whole number frequency ratios (Perlman & Krumhansl, 1996).

Finally, scale systems vary dramatically in how standardized the tunings are across different instruments. For example, in a study of 22 Javanese gamelans tuned using the slendro scale, Perlman found that no interval varied less than 30 cents, with some intervals varying as much as 75 cents (cited in Perlman & Krumhansl, 1996; cf. Arom et al., 1997, for data on interval variability in African xylophones). Does such variability imply that intervals are not important to people who listen to such music? Not necessarily: The lack of standardization between instruments may simply mean that listeners develop rather broad interval standards (Arom et al., 1997; Cooke, 1992).

Collectively, these four types of variation argue against the notion that the primary force in shaping musical scales is the pursuit of intervals with simple,

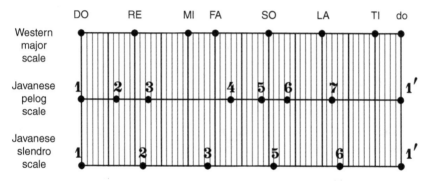

Figure 2.2b Frequency spacing between tones in the Western major scale and in two Javanese scales (pelog and slendro). The thin vertical lines mark 20-cent intervals. The tones of the Western scale are labeled with their solfège names. By convention, the five notes of the slendro scale are notated 1, 2, 3, 5, 6. Adapted from Sutton, 2001.

small-number ratios. Outside of Western culture, the dream of Pythagoras is not in accord with the facts.

COMMONALITIES AMONG SCALE SYSTEMS   Does the diversity of scale systems mean that the search for universal influences on scale systems should be discarded? Not at all. Indeed, the very fact of such diversity makes any widespread commonalities all the more significant in terms of suggesting common auditory and/or cognitive predispositions, as was observed earlier with the octave and musical fifth. Three such commonalities can be noted.

The first and most obvious commonality concerns the number of tones per octave, which typically ranges between 5 and 7. Even in cultures with microtonal divisions of the octave, such as India, any given scale typically involves between 5 and 7 pitches. Importantly, this limit is not predicted by human frequency discrimination, which is capable of distinguishing many more tones per octave. Instead, the limit is almost certainly due to the compromise between the desire for aesthetic variety and universal constraints on the number of distinct categories the human mind can reliably keep track of along a single physical continuum (Clough et al., 1993; Miller, 1956).

The second commonality concerns the size distribution of intervals in scales. Intervals between adjacent tones in a scale tend to be between 1 and 3 semitones in size (Nettl, 1954; Voisin, 1994). Nettl (2000) has observed that almost all cultures rely heavily on an interval of about 2 semitones in size in the construction of melodies. Even cultures with only two tones (1 interval) in their scale, such as certain native American tribes (Nettl, 1954:15), choose an interval in this range, though in principle they could opt for a single large interval. The reason large intervals are avoided may simply be ergonomic: Such scales would be associated with melodies that are awkward to sing because of the large pitch leaps. More interesting is the avoidance of intervals less than a semitone ("microintervals"), especially in circumstances in which there is an opportunity for them to occur. For example, in Indian classical music one could construct a scale in which two adjacent tones are separated by 1/2 semitone, but such scales do not occur in practice. The one exception to this pattern of which I am aware comes from Melanesian panpipes, in which Zemp (1981) recorded two tubes from a single set of pipes that differed by only 33 cents. However, this turned out to be an exception that proved the rule, as the tubes were placed on opposite ends of the panpipes and were never played in succession. Thus the auditory system seems to favor intervals of at least a semitone between adjacent notes of a scale. The reason for this is suggested by research by Burns and Ward (1978), who examined the ability of musical novices to discriminate between two intervals on the basis of their size. In their study, the absolute frequency of the lower tone of the interval was allowed to vary. In such a context, which prevents a strategy of using a fixed lower pitch as a reference and forces true interval comparison, the threshold for discrimination was about 80 cents. This suggests that in musical contexts intervals should differ by at least a semitone if they are to be reliably discriminated in size. This is precisely what is ensured when the smallest interval in the scale is about 1 semitone.

The third commonality, and perhaps the most interesting from a cognitive standpoint, concerns the patterning of interval sizes within musical scales. It is far more common for scales to have intervals of different sizes (e.g., 1 and 2 semitones in the case of the Western major scale) than to have all intervals of approximately the same size.[8] Put more succinctly, asymmetric scales are far more common than symmetric ones. Examples of symmetric scales include Javanese slendro, with 5 intervals of almost equal size, and in the Western whole-tone scale, with 6 intervals of equal size, which was used by Claude Debussy. What might account for the dominance of asymmetric scales? Balzano (1980) and others have noted that a pattern of unequal intervals serves to make each tone in the scale unique in terms of its pattern of intervals with respect to other scale tones.

This property of *uniqueness* may help listeners maintain a sense of where they are in relation to the first tone of the scale, a property that would help the first tone to act as a perceptual anchor point or tonal center. In symmetric scales, it may be more difficult to sense one's position with respect to the tonal center on the basis of pitch intervals alone, so that tonal orientation would have to be provided by other cues, such as the clearly defined melodic and rhythmic cycles of Gamelan music. One interesting line of evidence with respect to this issue is a study of the perception of asymmetric versus symmetric scale

---

[8] It has been further claimed that when scales have intervals of different sizes, they tend to clump into two distinct size classes, though I am not aware of any empirical evidence on this issue.

structure by infants and adults. Trehub et al. (1999) constructed unfamiliar asymmetric and symmetric scales based on 7 intervals per octave, and tested the ability of infants and adults to detect subtle pitch changes in repetitions of these scales. Infants were better at detecting such changes in the asymmetric scales, even though both scales were unfamiliar, suggesting that the asymmetry conferred some processing advantage. Interestingly, however, adults showed poor performance on both types of unfamiliar scales, and performed well only when a familiar, major scale was used. In other words, any inherent processing advantage of the asymmetric scales was overwhelmed by the effect of cultural familiarity. Nevertheless, Trehub et al.'s results may be relevant to the origin of musical scale structure in diverse cultures, because in contexts in which there is no "familiar" scale, the cognitive system may be biased toward choosing an asymmetric scale structure over a symmetric one because of a predisposition for music with a clear tonal center.[9]

CULTURAL DIVERSITY AND COMMONALITY: CONCLUSIONS What is the cognitive significance of the similarities and differences among scale systems? Treating similarities first, it appears that some commonalities (number of tones per octave and their spacing) can be explained by basic forces that shape communicative systems. These commonalities emerge because there are limits on the number of sound categories that can be discerned along a given physical continuum, and because of inherent tradeoffs between ergonomics and perceptual discriminability in sound systems. More interesting from a cognitive standpoint is the predominance of asymmetric scales. This suggests that most cultures favor scale patterns that promote a sense of orientation with respect to a tonal center, and raises the deeper question of why this should be. One possibility is that having a tonal center provides a cognitive reference point for pitch perception, which in turn makes it easier to learn and remember complex melodic sequences (Rosch, 1973, 1975; cf. Krumhansl, 1990).

Turning to the differences among scales, the great variability in scale structure suggests that the search for a "natural basis" for musical pitch intervals is an inherently limited endeavor. A broader field of enquiry emerges if one shifts the emphasis from scales as natural systems to scales as phonological systems, in other words, to an interest in how pitch categories are created and maintained in the context of an organized system of pitch contrasts. In this light, the natural basis of certain intervals (such as the fifth; cf. this chapter's appendix 3)

---

[9] Debussy's use of a symmetric scale is an interesting case study in cognitive musicology. It is known that Debussy heard Javanese music at the Paris Exposition of 1889. In his case, the appeal of the whole-tone scales may have been their tonal ambiguity, which fit with his own tendency to use a shifting harmonic palette that resisted clear tonal centers.

simply illustrates that there is a link between auditory predispositions and category formation. Such a link is not unique to music: Speech also exploits inherent aspects of the auditory system in forming organized sound contrasts. For example, the difference between voiced and voiceless consonants (such as /b/ and /p/) appears to exploit a natural auditory boundary that is independent of culture (Pisoni, 1977; Holt et al., 2004, Steinschneider et al., 2005). Thus it is likely that in both music and speech the inherent properties of the auditory system influence the "learnability" of certain categories and contrasts. In terms of understanding the broader question of how the mind makes and maintains sound categories, however, this is simply one piece of the puzzle.

2.2.3 Pitch Intervals as Learned Sound Categories in Music

Having described some fundamental aspects of musical scales and intervals, it is now time to take a cognitive perspective and examine pitch intervals as learned sound categories rather than as fixed frequency ratios between tones. The motivation for this is that in the real world, intervals are seldom realized in a precise, Platonic fashion. The "same" pitch interval can vary in size both due to chance variation and to the influence of local melodic context (Jairazbhoy & Stone, 1963; Levy, 1982; Morton, 1974; Rakowski, 1990). This is why listeners require mechanisms that help them recognize the structural equivalence of different tokens and map acoustic variability on to stable mental categories. The four subsections below provide evidence for intervals as learned sound categories by demonstrating that the processing of pitch relations is influenced by the structure of a culture's interval system.

Pitch Intervals and a Perceptual Illusion

Shepard and Jordan (1984) provided early and compelling evidence for pitch intervals as learned sound categories. They had participants listen to an ascending sequence of tones that divided the octave into 7 equal-sized intervals (meaning that the ratio of successive pitches in the scale was $2^{1/7}$ or about 1.1, so that each pitch was about 10% higher in frequency than the one below it). Listeners were asked to judge the size of each interval in relation to the preceding one, and indicate whether the current interval was larger, smaller, or the same size. The listeners varied widely in their degree of musical training, and had just learned about the physical measure of log frequency in a college class. They were explicitly asked to base their judgments on the *physical sizes of intervals* and not their musical relations (they were not told that the scale had equal-sized steps). The interesting result was that participants judged the 3rd and 7th intervals to be larger than the others. These are precisely the intervals that are small (1 semitone) in a Western major scale, suggesting that listeners had assimilated the novel scale to a set of internal sound categories. It is especially notable that these learned internal interval standards were applied automatically, even when instructions did not encourage musical listening.

Pitch Intervals and Melody Perception

Although memory for highly familiar melodies includes some information about absolute pitch (Levitin, 1994; Schellenberg & Trehub, 2003), melody recognition clearly involves the perception of pitch relations because listeners can recognize the same melody in different registers (e.g., played on a tuba or a piccolo) or when played by the same instrument in different keys. One factor involved in melody recognition is the melodic contour: the patterns of ups and downs without regard to precise interval size. For example, the contour of the melody in Figure 2.3a can be represented as +,+,−,−,−,+.

Another factor is the sequence of precise intervals. The relative importance of these two factors has been explored in studies by Dowling and others over many years (e.g., Dowling, 1978; Edworthy, 1985a,b; Dowling et al., 1995). In a typical experiment, a listener hears a novel melody (e.g., Figure 2.3a), and then later hears a target melody (Figure 2.3b–d). The target melody can be a transposition that preserves the precise pattern of intervals between tones (an exact transposition, which amounts to a change of key, Figure 2.3b). In other cases, the target can be slightly altered from an exact transposition so that it has the same contour but a different pattern of intervals (a "same contour lure," as in Figure 2.3c). Finally, the target can have an entirely different contour from the original (a "different contour lure," in Figure 2.3d; cf. Sound Example 2.1).

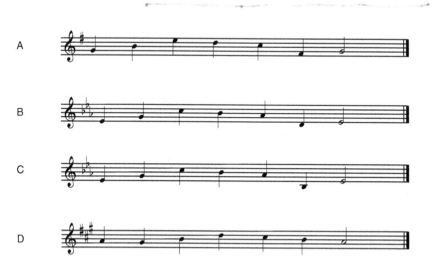

Figure 2.3 Tone sequences B, C, and D have different relations to tone sequence A. (B = exact transposition, C = same contour but different intervals, D = different contour.) After Dowling, Kwak, & Andrews, 1995. Cf. sound example 2.1a–d.

Listeners are instructed about the difference between exact transpositions and the two different kind of lures using a familiar melody as an example (such as "Twinkle, Twinkle, Little Star"), and told that during the experiment they should respond "yes" only to targets that are an exact transposition of the first melody.

When the delay between the two melodies is brief, listeners often confuse exact transpositions with same contour lures, indicating that their response is dominated by contour similarity (Dowling, 1978). If, however, a longer delay is used (which can be filled with other melodies or with some distracting task), this discrimination ability *improves,* indicating that contour declines in importance in favor of exact pitch intervals, as if the mental representation of pitch relations was being consolidated in terms of a sequence of interval categories (Dowling & Bartlett, 1981; Dewitt & Crowder, 1986).

Pitch Intervals and Categorical Perception

The two approaches outlined above provide indirect evidence that intervals act as learned sound categories in perception, and are notable for finding effects in individuals who were not selected for their musical expertise. We now turn to studies of categorical perception (CP), a particular type of perception that has been widely explored in speech.

CP refers to two related phenomena. First, sounds that lie along a physical continuum are perceived as belonging to distinct categories, rather than gradually changing from one category to another. Second, sounds of a given degree of physical difference are much easier to discriminate if they straddle a category boundary than if they fall within the same category. CP is thus studied using both identification and discrimination tasks. Strong evidence for CP consists of identification functions with steep transitions between categories combined with discrimination functions that have pronounced maxima near category boundaries (Figure 2.4).

Early demonstrations of CP for certain speech contrasts in infants (such as /p/ vs. /b/) were taken as evidence that speech relied on special neural mechanisms to transform continuous sound into discrete mental categories (Eimas et al., 1971). Subsequent research showed that CP for speech contrasts could be observed in animals (Kuhl & Miller, 1975), indicating that CP is not a special mechanism evolved for human speech. Instead, speech perception may in some cases take advantage of natural auditory boundaries (Handel, 1989; Holt et al., 2004). Furthermore, many important speech sounds, such as vowels and the lexical tones of tone languages, show little or no evidence of CP, despite the fact that they act as stable sound categories in perception (Fry et al., 1962; Stevens et al., 1969; Repp, 1984; Repp & Williams, 1987; Francis et al., 2003). This is an important point that bears repetition: The perception of vowels and lexical tones shows that the mind can map acoustic variation onto stable internal sound categories without CP. (I will return to this point later in this chapter, when comparing vowel perception in speech to chord perception in music.) For the moment the relevant point is this: Although evidence of CP proves that sounds are perceived in terms of discrete categories, lack of evidence of CP does not prove the converse. That is, sounds can be "categorically interpreted" without being categorically perceived (cf. Ladd & Morton, 1997). Thus lack of evidence of CP for musical intervals cannot really help us decide if pitch intervals act as learned sound categories or not.

Nevertheless, studies of CP in music are worth discussing because they highlight an issue that runs through the music cognition literature, namely cognitive differences between musicians and nonmusicians. Burns and Ward (1978) found evidence for CP of intervals by musicians, and suggested that musicians' CP for interval size was as sharp as phonetic CP in speech (cf. Zatorre & Halpern, 1979; Howard et al., 1992). Nonmusicians, however, showed no convincing evidence of CP.[10] Smith et al. (1994) conducted more extensive tests of nonmusicians, and tried to eliminate some of the task-related factors that might have obscured their performance in the Burns and Ward study. For example, listeners were given a thorough introduction to the concept of an interval, including many musical examples. One subgroup was trained on standard category labels (e.g., "major third"), whereas the other was given labels corresponding to familiar tunes, to encourage them to use their memory of these tunes in the interval identification task (e.g., the label "perfect fourth" was replaced with the label "Here comes the bride" because this familiar melody begins with this interval). Smith et al. found that the use of familiar tunes did make listener's identification functions steeper and more categorical, but listeners in both groups performed poorly on the discrimination tasks, with the category boundary having only a weak effect on discrimination. Thus nonmusicians did not show strong evidence of categorical perception of intervals.

---

[10] The methodology of musical CP studies is simple: The size of an interval is varied in small increments between two endpoints. For example, intervals might range from a minor third to a perfect fourth (3 to 5 semitones) in steps of 12.5 cents. Listeners are presented with intervals in a random order and asked to give each one a label from a set of N labels, in which N = the number of interval categories under investigation (3 in the above example: minor third, major third, and perfect fourth). Then, pairs of intervals that differ by a fixed amount in size are presented for same-different discrimination. The resulting identification and discrimination functions are then examined for evidence of CP. (In assessing such studies, it is important to discern whether the authors used intervals whose first tones were allowed to vary, or if the first tone was always kept at a fixed frequency. Only the former method forces the use of abstract interval categories and prevents pitch-matching strategies, and is thus a strong test of CP.)

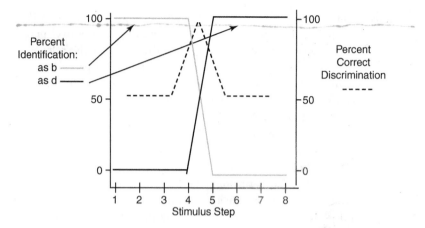

Figure 2.4 An idealized categorical perception function. A speech sound is changed from /b/ to /d/ via small acoustic steps of equal in size. Perception of the stimuli shifts dramatically from one category to the other at a particular point in the stimulus continuum, and discrimination between stimuli separated by one step along the continuum is best at this perceptual boundary. Courtesy of Louis Goldstein.

The issue of CP in nonmusicians has received little attention recently, but is worth discussing because it reflects a larger debate between those who see musicians and nonmusicians as having largely similar mental representations for music, differing only in skill at certain explicit procedures for which musicians have been trained (Bigand, 2003; Bigand & Poulin-Charronnat, 2006) and those who entertain the possibility that the mental representations for music in musicians and nonmusicians may be quite different (e.g., Dowling, 1986; Smith, 1997). For the current purposes, the lesson of this research is that one should remain open to the idea that the framework of learned interval standards may show substantial variability, not only between musicians and nonmusicians, but even among trained musicians (Cooke, 1992; Perlman & Krumhansl, 1996). In the end, the question of individual differences in sound category structure can be resolved only by empirical research. In the meantime, it is important not to think of variability among individuals as "bad." In fact, from the standpoint of cognitive neuroscience, it is good because it creates the opportunity to study how the brain changes with experience.

Pitch Intervals and Neuroscience

In recent years, a novel approach to the study of musical sound categories has arisen thanks to research on a brain response called the mismatch negativity, or MMN (Näätänen, 1992). The MMN is an event-related potential (ERP) associated with automatic change detection in a repetitive auditory signal, and has neural generators in the auditory cortex. It is typically studied in an "odd-ball" paradigm in which a standard sound or sound pattern (e.g., a tone or a short sequence of tones) is presented repeatedly, with an occasional deviant introduced in a pseudorandom fashion. For example, in a simple version of this paradigm, the standard could be a short pure tone of 400 Hz that occurs with 85% probability, with the remaining tones being deviants of 420 Hz. A listener is typically instructed to ignore the tones (e.g., to read a book) while electrical (EEG) or magnetic (MEG) brain wave responses are recorded continuously from the scalp. Segments of the brain wave signal time-locked to the stimulus onset are averaged to produce ERPs to the standard and deviant tones. The MMN is the difference between the ERP to the standard and the deviant, and consists of a negative-going wave that peaks between 80 and 200 ms after the onset of the deviant tone (for one review, see Näätänen & Winkler, 1999; for a possible single-neuron correlate of the MMN, see Ulanovsky et al., 2003)

If the MMN were sensitive only to physical differences between stimuli, it would be of little interest to cognitive science. There is evidence, however, that the MMN is sensitive to learned sound categories. For example, Brattico et al. (2001) used a sequence of 5 short tones ascending in pitch as the standard stimulus. The deviant stimulus was the same sequence with the third tone raised in pitch above all the other tones, creating a salient change in the melodic contour. In one condition, the standard sequence conformed to the first 5 tones of a major scale, with semitone intervals of 2, 2, 1, and 2 between successive tones. In a second condition, the ascending tones of the standard sequence had unfamiliar intervals (0.8, 1.15, 1.59, and 2.22 st). The deviant in both conditions produced an MMN, as expected. The result of interest was that the MMN was significantly larger in the first condition, which used culturally familiar intervals. Importantly, both musicians and nonmusicians showed this effect (though the musicians showed a shorter latency of onset for the MMN).

Trainor, McDonald, and Alain (2002; cf. Fujioka et al., 2004) also conducted an MMN study in which nonmusicians showed sensitivity to musical intervals. Listeners heard a repeating 5-note sequence that was transposed on every repetition (i.e., the starting pitch was different but the pattern of intervals was the same). On some repetitions, the final interval was changed in size in a manner such that the overall contour of the sequence was preserved. Thus the interval pattern was the only thing that distinguished the sequences. The nonmusicians produced a robust MMN to the altered final interval, even though they were ignoring the sounds, suggesting that their auditory systems were sensitive to interval structure in music, presumably due to years of exposure to music.

Although the above studies are consistent with the notion that the brain represents culturally familiar musical intervals as learned sound categories, it would be desirable to use the MMN to test this idea in a more direct fashion. Specifically, one could conduct studies in which the standard was a musical interval (e.g., a minor third, 300 cents) and the deviant was an interval of different size. The size of the deviant could be altered in small steps across different blocks of the experiment, so that at some point it crosses an interval category (e.g., 350 to 450 cents in steps of 20 cents). One could then measure the MMN as a function of frequency distance. The question of interest is if the size of the MMN simply grows linearly with frequency difference, or if there is a jump in MMN size as the interval crosses into a new category. If so, this would be neural evidence that pitch intervals were acting as sound categories in perception.[11] MMN studies using musical intervals have already been conducted that suggest the feasibility of such a study (Paavilainen et al., 1999).

2.2.4 Timbral Contrasts in Music

We turn now from pitch to timbre. From an aesthetic standpoint, timbre is arguably as important as pitch as a perceptual feature of music. (Imagine, for example, the difference in the aesthetic and emotional impact of a jazz ballad expertly played on a real saxophone vs. on a cheap keyboard synthesizer.) From a cognitive standpoint however, timbre differs sharply from pitch in that the former is rarely the basis for organized sound contrasts produced by individual instruments. Of course, timbral contrasts *between* instruments are quite organized, and are used in systematic ways by composers from numerous cultures, for example, in Western, Javanese, and African instrument ensembles. A notable study in this regard is that of Cogan (1984), who conducted spectral analyses of symphonic music and proposed a theory of timbral contrasts inspired by linguistic phonetics (cf. Cogan & Escot, 1976).[12] However, the salient point is that organized systems of timbral contrasts *within* instruments of a culture are rare. Why is this so? Before addressing this question, it is important to review some basic information about musical timbre.

Timbre, or sound quality, is usually defined as that aspect of a sound that distinguishes it from other sounds of the same pitch, duration, and loudness. For example, timbre is what distinguishes the sound of a trumpet from the sound of a flute playing the same tone, when pitch, loudness, and duration are identical. This definition is not very satisfying, as it does not address what timbre is, only

[11] Another way to do this study is to have a single deviant and vary the presence of a category boundary by varying the cultural background of the listeners. Thus the deviant would cross into a new category for some listeners but not for others. This approach has been used successfully in the study of native language vowel categories using the MMN (Näätänen et al., 1997).

[12] Enriching the timbral diversity of ensembles has long been a concern of modern music. In an early modernist manifesto promoting the use of noise in music, Luigi Russolo (1913/1986) inveighed against the traditional orchestra's limited timbral palette, calling the concert hall a "hospital for anemic sounds."

what it is not. To make an analogy, imagine describing human faces in terms of four qualities: height, width, and complexion, and "looks," in which "looks" is meant to capture "what makes one person's face different from another, when faces are matched for height, width, and complexion." "Looks" clearly does not refer to a unitary physical dimension, but is a label for an overall quality created by the interplay of a number of different features (in a face, this might include the shape of the nose, the thickness of the eyebrows, etc.).

A review of the many features that influence musical timbre is beyond the scope of this book (for one such review, see Hajda et al., 1997). Here I focus on two prominent factors that are relevant for comparing music and speech: the temporal and spectral profile of a sound. The temporal profile refers to the temporal evolution of the amplitude of a sound, whereas the spectral profile refers to the distribution of frequencies that make up a sound, as well as their relative amplitudes (commonly referred to as the spectrum of a sound). For example, the temporal profile of a piano tone has a sharp attack and a rapid decay, giving it a percussive quality. In contrast, the onset and offset of a tone played in a legato manner by a violin are much more gradual (Figure 2.5).

The importance of the temporal envelope in the perception of a sound's timbre can easily be demonstrated by playing a short passage of piano music backward in time, as in Sound Example 2.2: The result sounds like a different

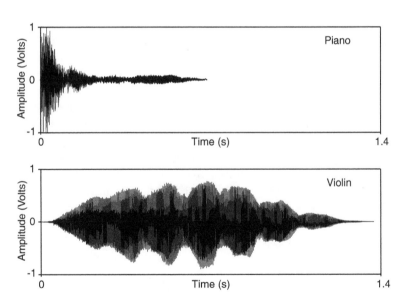

Figure 2.5 Acoustic waveform of a piano tone (top panel) and a violin tone (bottom panel). Note the sharp attack and rapid decay of the piano tone vs. the gradual attack and decay of the violin tone.

instrument. To illustrate the spectral profile of a sound, consider Figure 2.6, which shows the spectrum of a clarinet and a trumpet playing a single note.

A salient difference between these spectra is that in the case of the clarinet, the spectrum is dominated by partials that are odd number multiples of the fundamental (i.e., partials 1,3,5, etc., in which 1 is the fundamental). In contrast, the trumpet spectrum does not have this asymmetric frequency structure.

There is one respect in which pictures of spectra, such as in Figure 2.6, can be misleading with regard to timbre. Such pictures are static, and might be taken to imply that each instrument has a spectrum that yields its characteristic timbre. In fact, the spectral profile of an instrument depends on the note being played and how loudly it is being produced. Furthermore, the spectral profile of a given note can vary at different points in a room because of acoustic reflections. Yet humans do not perceive dramatic changes in timbre because of these spectral changes (Risset & Wessel, 1999). This has led to a growing interest in dynamic and relational aspects of spectra, in the hope that more invariant features will emerge. For example, two dynamic features that underlie the characteristic timbre of a brass trumpet are the faster buildup of amplitude in lower versus higher harmonics as a note starts, and an increase in the number of harmonics as intensity increases within a note (Risset & Wessel, 1999, cf. McAdams et al., 1999; Figure 2.7).

Turning to the issue of musical timbre perception, empirical research in this area has relied heavily on similarity judgments. Typically, studies of this sort present the sounds of instruments in pairs (e.g., a French horn playing a note followed by a clarinet playing the same note), and ask listeners to rate how similar the two sounds are. After rating many such pairs, the similarity data are transformed using statistical techniques such as multidimensional scaling in an attempt to reveal the listener's perceptual dimensions for judging timbral contrasts between instruments (Grey, 1977). One notable finding of such studies is that relatively few dimensions are needed to capture most of the variance in the data, at least when instruments from Western orchestras are used. For example, in a study by McAdams et al. (1995), three primary dimensions emerged, relating to the rise time of the amplitude envelope, the spectral centroid (i.e., the amplitude-weighted mean of the frequency components), and the spectral flux (a measure of how much the shape of the spectral profile changes over time within a single tone). Thus perceptual research confirms the point that there is more to timbre than a static snapshot of a spectral profile (cf. Caclin et al., 2005).

The Rarity of Timbral Contrasts as a Basis for Musical Sound Systems

Why do timbral contrasts rarely serve as the basis for musical sound systems? In section 2.2.2, I argued that pitch had an advantage (over loudness) as the basis for sound categories because it was perceptually multidimensional. Yet as

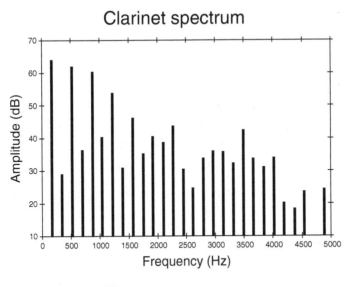

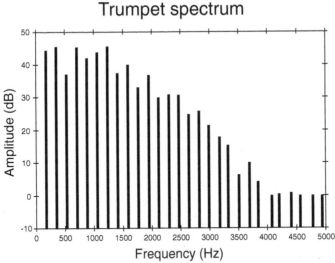

Figure 2.6 Spectrum of a clarinet (top) and a trumpet (bottom) playing the tone F3 (fundamental frequency ≈ 175 Hz). Note the dominance of the odd-numbered partials among the first 10 partials of the clarinet spectrum. (Note: y axis is logarithmic). Courtesy of James Beauchamp.

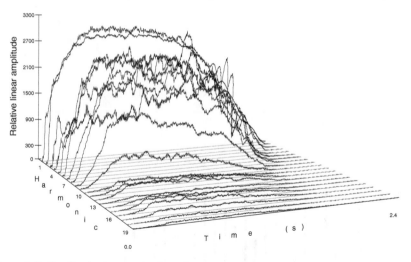

Figure 2.7 Amplitude dynamics of the first 20 partials of a trumpet tone (i.e., the fundamental and 19 harmonics). Note the faster buildup of amplitude in partials 1 and 2 versus 3–10 early in the tone, and the lack of energy in the partials 11–20 until ~200 ms. Courtesy of James Beauchamp.

noted at the end of the preceding section, timbre also has this quality. Furthermore, many musical instruments can produce salient timbral contrasts. A cello, for example, can produce a variety of timbres depending on how it is bowed. Specifically, a brighter sound quality results from bowing close to the bridge (*sul ponticello*) and a darker, mellower quality from bowing near the fingerboard (*sul tasto*). Both of these timbres are distinct from the sound produced by striking the strings with the wooden part of the bow instead of the hair (*col legno*). Further timbral possibilities are provided by playing harmonics, or by plucking instead of bowing. A talented cello player would likely be able to demonstrate several other distinct timbres based on different manners of bowing (cf. Randel, 1978; "bowing"). Despite this range of possible timbres, however, normal cello music is not organized primarily around timbral contrasts. This observation is true for most musical instruments, despite a few notable exceptions. For example, the music of the simple Jew's harp emphasizes rapid timbral contrasts, and the Australian didgeridoo is renowned as an instrument in which timbre is the primary principle of sonic organization.

I believe that there are both physical and cognitive reasons why timbre is rarely used as the basis for organized sound contrasts in music. The physical reason is that dramatic changes in timbre usually require some change in the way the instrument is excited (e.g., how it is struck or blown) or in the geometry and resonance properties of the instrument itself. For many instruments, rapid changes in either of these parameters are difficult or simply impossible. (Note that the Jew's harp uses the mouth cavity as a resonator, which can change its resonant properties quickly by changing shape.) The cognitive reason is that timbral contrasts are not organized in a system of orderly perceptual distances from one another, for example, in terms of "timbre intervals" (cf. Krumhansl, 1989). In pitch, having a system of intervals allows higher-level relations to emerge. For example, a move from C and G can be recognized as similar in size as a move from A to E: The pitches are different but the interval is the same.

Ehresman and Wessel (1978) and McAdams and Cunibile (1992) have investigated whether listeners are capable of hearing "timbre intervals." The latter study is discussed here. McAdams and Cunibile defined a timbre interval as a vector between two points in a two-dimensional perceptual space in which attack time and spectral centroid were the two dimensions (this space is derived from perceptual research on timbral similarities between instruments, as discussed in the previous section; see Figure 2.8).

The vector indicates the degree of change along each underlying perceptual dimension. Thus in Figure 2.8, the difference between the timbres of a trombone and a "guitarnet" (a hybrid of guitar and clarinet) defines one tim-

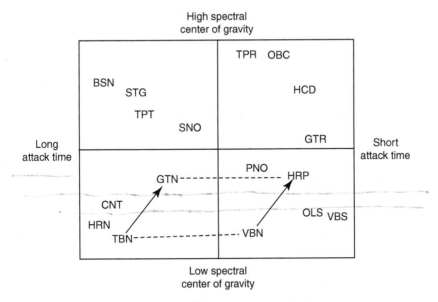

Figure 2.8 Timbre intervals. Acronyms refer to real or synthetic instruments studied by McAdams and Cunibile (1992), arrayed in a two-dimensional timbre space. A timbre interval consists of a move of a particular direction and magnitude (i.e., a vector) in this space, as between TBN and GTN (trombone and guitarnet) or between VBN and HRP (vibrone and harp). From McAdams, 1996.

bre interval. Starting at another sound and moving through a similar interval requires a move in this timbre space of the same direction and magnitude as the original vector. This is illustrated in Figure 2.8 by a move from a "vibrone" (a hybrid of a vibraphone and a trombone) to a harp. McAdams and Cunibile presented listeners with successive pairs of sounds (e.g., AB, followed by CD, in which each letter represents a sound), and asked in which case the change from A to B most resembled the change from C to D. They found some evidence for their proposed timbre intervals, but also found a good deal of variation among listeners, as well as context sensitivity (i.e., a dependence on the particular sounds that formed the interval rather than just on their vector distance). Their research raises the possibility that timbre relations are not perceived with enough uniformity to provide a basis for a shared category system among composers and listeners akin to the interval system provided by musical pitch (cf. Krumhansl, 1989).

Example of a Timbre-Based Musical System

Arnold Schoenberg (1911:470–471) once articulated a desideratum for a timbre-based music:

> If it is possible to make compositional structures from sounds which differ according to pitch, structures which we call melodies . . . then it must also be possible to create such sequences from . . . timbre. Such sequences would work with an inherent logic, equivalent to the kind of logic which is effective in the melodies based on pitch. . . . All this seems a fantasy of the future, which it probably is. Yet I am firmly convinced that it can be realized.

Given the many innovations in music since Schoenberg's time (including computer music, which eliminates the constraints of physical instruments), it is a curious fact that "timbre melody" (*Klangfarbenmelodie*) has not become a common feature on the musical landscape in Western culture. As discussed above, it may be that timbre-based music has not succeeded in the West because of the difficulty of organizing timbre in terms of intervals or scales.

There are, however, other ways to organize timbral systems. After all, the existence of speech shows that rich sound systems can be based on timbral contrasts that have nothing to do with intervals or scales. Thus it likely no coincidence that one successful musical tradition based on timbral contrasts uses a system with strong parallels to the organization of timbre in speech. This is a drumming tradition of North India based on the tabla (Figure 2.9).

The tabla consists of a pair of hand drums used to provide the rhythmic accompaniment to instrumentalists and singers in classical and popular music (Courtney, 1998; Kippen, 1988). The player, seated on the ground, plays the smaller, high-pitched drum with the right hand and the larger low-pitched drum

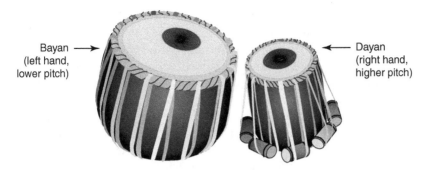

Figure 2.9 North Indian tabla drums. The pitch of the dayan is tuned to the basic note of the scale being played on the melodic instrument that it accompanies. The pitch of the bayan is tuned lower, and can be modulated by applying pressure with the heel of the palm to the drum head.

with the left hand. Drum strokes are distinguished in several ways: by which fingers hit the drum, the region of the membrane struck, whether other fingers damp the membrane while striking it, whether the striking finger bounces off the membrane (open stroke) or is kept pressed to the membrane after the strike (closed stroke), and whether just one drum is struck or both are struck (see Figure 2.10). Each particular combination gives rise to a distinct timbre. Table 2.1 provides details on 8 tabla strokes, which can be heard in Sound Examples 2.3a–h. The number of timbrally distinct drum strokes is about 12. (This is fewer than the

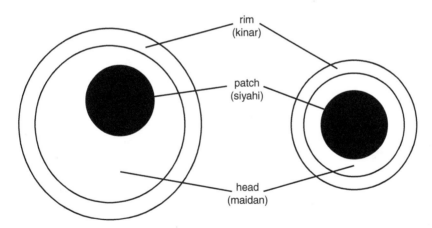

Figure 2.10 Top view of dayan (right) and bayan (left). Each drum surface is divided into three regions: a rim, a head, and a central circular patch of iron fillings and paste. Indian names of the regions are also given. Surface diameters: dayan ~14 cm, bayan ~22 cm.

number of different vocables because different vocables are sometimes used to name the same stroke depending on context.)

Parallels between the timbral organization of tabla drumming and speech take two forms. First, the different ways of striking the drum can be represented in terms of matrix of "place and manner of articulation," akin to the organization of speech sounds (cf. Section 2.3.3, Table 2.3; cf. Chandola, 1988). For example, the sound produced by striking the right drum with the index finger differs dramatically depending where the drum is struck ("place of articulation," e.g., edge vs. center) and how it is struck ("manner of articulation," e.g., with a bouncing stroke or with a closed stroke that results in damping). The second parallel between musical and spoken timbre is more explicit. Each kind of drum stroke is associated with a particular verbal label (a nonsense syllable or "vocable") that is used in teaching and composition, as this is an oral tradition. Players have an intuition that there is an acoustic and perceptual resemblance between each stroke and its associated vocable (called a "bol," from the Hindi word for speech sound). Empirical research has confirmed this link, which is interesting given that the drum and the voice produce sounds in very different ways (Patel & Iversen, 2003). This research will be described in more detail (in section 2.3.3, subsection "Mapping Linguistic

Table 2.1 Details of 8 Tabla Strokes and Vocables (Bols)

Bol	Manner of Playing
Tin /ʈin/	*Dayan:* Index finger strikes head. Third finger damps fundamental by resting on head.
Tun /ʈun/	*Dayan:* Index finger strikes patch; no damping.
Kat /kət/	*Bayan:* Damped stroke played with flat hand across rim, head, and patch.
Ghe /gʰe/	*Bayan:* Index finger strikes head at far edge of patch. Heel of hand, on head, can alter pitch.
Tra /ʈrə/	*Dayan:* Damped stroke: middle and index fingers strike patch in rapid succession, and remain on drum.
Kra /krə/	*Bayan:* Damped flat-hand stroke similar to Kat. *Dayan:* Index finger strikes rim. Third finger damps fundamental by resting on head.
Ta /ʈa/	*Dayan:* Index finger strikes rim. Third finger damps fundamental by resting on head.
Dha /ɖʰa/	Simultaneous striking of Ta and Ghe.

Note that fingers bounce off drum (open stroke) unless the stroke is damped (closed). IPA symbols are between slashes.

Timbral Contrasts Onto Musical Sounds") after discussing timbral contrasts in speech.

The tabla is but one of several drumming traditions that feature parallels to speech in terms of the organization of timbral patterning (for an example from Africa, see Tsukada, 1997). To my knowledge, however, tabla drumming is unsurpassed among widespread musical traditions in terms of the diversity and speed of timbral contrasts produced by a single player. A sense of the rhythmic virtuosity of a talented tabla player is given in Sound/Video Example 2.4.

2.3 Linguistic Sound Systems

2.3.1 Introduction to Linguistic Sound Systems

The purpose of this part of the chapter is to discuss organized sound contrasts in language in terms of their similarities and differences to musical sound systems. Before embarking, it is worth reviewing a few basic concepts concerning the study of speech sounds.

The study of linguistic sound systems is divided into two broad and overlapping fields: phonetics and phonology. Phonetics is the science of speech sounds, and includes the study of the acoustic structure of speech and the mechanisms by which speech is produced and perceived (acoustic, articulatory, and auditory phonetics). Phonology is the study of the sound patterns of language, and includes the study of how speech sounds are organized into higher level units such as syllables and words, how sounds vary as a function of context, and how knowledge of the sound patterns of language is represented in the mind of a speaker or listener.

To illustrate the difference between these two approaches to sound systems, consider the phenomenon of syllable stress in English. Syllables in English speech vary in their perceptual prominence, even in sentences spoken without any special emphasis on a particular word or phrase. For example, if a listener is asked to mark the prominent syllables in "the committee will meet for a special debate," most listeners will perceive the following syllables as stressed: The com*mit*tee will *meet* for a *spe*cial de*bate*. A study that focused on the acoustic differences between stressed and unstressed syllables in English (e.g., quantifying the extent to which perceived stress corresponds to parameters such as increased duration or intensity) would be a study in phonetics. In contrast, a study that focused on the patterning of stress in English words and sentences (e.g., the location of stress in English words, whether there is a tendency for stressed and unstressed syllables to alternate in an utterance) would be a study in phonology. This example illustrates the fact that in practice, phonetics usually deals with the measurement of continuous acoustic or articulatory parameters, whereas phonology usually deals with the organization of categorically defined elements.[13]

A fundamental concept in the study of linguistic sound systems is the *phoneme*. A phoneme is the minimal speech unit that can distinguish two different words in a language. For example, in American English, the vowel in the word "bit" and the vowel in the word "beet" are different phonemes, because these words mean different things. In a different language, however, the English pronunciation of these two syllables might mean the same thing, indicating that the two sounds are variants (allophones) of a single phoneme. Thus the definition of a phoneme relies on the meaning of words. Linguists have developed efficient ways to represent phonemes in writing, using a standardized system known as the International Phonetic Alphabet, or IPA.[14]

Another key linguistic concept is that sound structure in speech is hierarchically organized, and that the phoneme is just one level in this hierarchy. Going down one level, phonemes are often analyzed as bundles of *distinctive features* (Jakobson et al., 1952; Chomsky & Halle, 1968). One motivation for this lower level of analysis is that the phonemes of a language are not simply an unordered set of items, but have relationships of similarity and difference in terms of the way they are produced. For example, the two phonemes /p/ and /b/ are similar in many respects, both involving a closure of the lips followed by a rapid release and the onset of vocal fold vibration (though the interval between release and the onset of vocal fold vibration, referred to as voice onset time, is much shorter in /b/ than in /p/). Thus the two phonemes can be analyzed as sharing a number of articulatory features, and differing in a few others. Analysis in terms of features has proved useful in linguistics because it can help shed light on certain sound patterns in speech, such as why certain phonemes are replaced by others in historical language change.[15] Going one level up, phonemes are organized into syllables, which play an important role in many aspects of a language,

---

[13] Of course, the line between phonetics and phonology is not always clear cut, and there are a growing number of studies that combine these two approaches (e.g., see the LabPhon series of conferences and books). To take just one example, the study of speech rhythm was long the province of phonology, which divided languages into distinct rhythmic classes based on the patterning of syllables and stress. However, recent approaches to speech rhythm have combined the insights of phonology (in terms of the factors underlying speech rhythm) with phonetic measurements of speech, as discussed in Chapter 3.

[14] A Web-based resource for IPA symbols and their corresponding sounds is provided by the UCLA phonetics laboratory: http://hctv.humnet.ucla.edu/departments/linguistics/VowelsandConsonants/course/chapter1/chapter1.html.

[15] Analysis of phoneme features can also be based on the acoustics of sounds, leading to the concept of "auditory distinctive features" (Jakobson, Fant, & Halle, 1952/1961). For example, the feature "grave" refers to speech sounds with predominantly low frequency energy, no matter how they are produced. Thus it groups together sounds independently

including speech rhythm. Syllables are organized around vowels: A syllable is minimally a vowel and is typically a vowel plus preceding and/or following consonants, bound into a coherent unit in both speech production and speech perception (syllables are discussed in greater detail in Chapter 3).[16]

A final important point concerns linguistic diversity. There are almost 7,000 languages in the world[17] (cf. Comrie et al., 1996). Some are spoken by a handful of individuals and one, Mandarin Chinese, by over a billion. The search for general patterns in linguistic sound systems requires a genetically diverse sample of languages, not simply a sample of languages that are widely spoken today (Maddieson, 1984). This point is analogous to the point that generalizations about musical sound systems require a cross-cultural perspective, not just a focus on widely disseminated musics. To take just one example, in the cognitive science literature, the language that is most commonly used to illustrate a tone language is Mandarin. (For those who do not know what a tone language is, see the following section.) Mandarin has four tones: Tone 1 is a level tone of fixed pitch, whereas tones 2–4 are contour tones involving salient pitch movement. A survey of diverse tone languages reveals, however, that having only 1 level tone is typologically very unusual (Maddieson, 1999). This fact is relevant to the comparative study of language and music, because linguistic systems with level tones are the logical place to look for a close comparison between pitch contrasts in speech and music. This is the topic of the next section.

2.3.2 Pitch Contrasts in Language

How do the organized pitch contrasts of language compare to the organized pitch contrasts of music? To address this question, it is first necessary to give some background on the use of pitch in speech.

---

of their mode of articulation. Hyman (1973) gives examples of how this feature affects the patterning of speech sounds.

[16] Although the syllable is an intuitive linguistic concept, there is debate among linguists over its precise definition. I have used a simplified definition here, based on the idea that a syllable must contain a vowel. In fact, one can have "syllabic consonants," such as the /n/ of "button" when pronounced as "butn," and syllables in which the nucleus is a voiced consonant rather than a vowel, for example, /tkznt/ in the Berber language (Coleman, 1999). For the purposes of this book, these subtleties are not important. What *is* worth noting is that although it is normally assumed that the phoneme is the elementary unit of speech perception, there are a number of speech scientists who argue that this role is actually played by the syllable, a debate that is unfortunately beyond the scope of this book (Greenberg, 2006).

[17] This estimate, which is generally accepted by linguists, is based on information from *Ethnologue: Languages of the World* (see http://www.ethnologue.org).

Although humans are capable of speaking on a monotone, they rarely do so. Instead, speech features salient modulation of voice pitch, whose most important physical correlate is the fundamental frequency of vocal fold vibration (abbreviated F0 ["F-zero" or "F-nought"]; see Chapter 4 for more details). This modulation is far from random: It is richly structured and conveys a variety of linguistic, attitudinal, and emotional information ('t Hart et al., 1990). Certain aspects of pitch variation due to emotion are universal. For example, happiness is associated with a wide pitch range and sadness with a narrow pitch range, reflecting the greater degree of arousal in the former state. This is an example of a gradient pitch contrast: Pitch range due to emotion is not produced or perceived in a discrete fashion, but varies continuously to reflect a continuously variable affective state.

Of primary interest here are linguistic pitch contrasts that are organized and perceived in terms of discrete categories. Such organization reaches its pinnacle in tone languages. A tone language is a language in which pitch is as much a part of a word's identity as are the vowels and consonants, so that changing the pitch can completely change the meaning of the word. Figure 2.11 shows a plot of the pitch of the voice as a speaker says four words in Mambila, a language from the Nigeria-Cameroon border in West Africa (Connell, 2000). These tones were produced by speaking words that were matched for segmental content but differed in tone.

Tone languages may seem exotic to a speaker of a European language, but in fact over half of the world's languages are tonal, including the majority of languages in Africa and southeast Asia (Fromkin, 1978). Such languages are

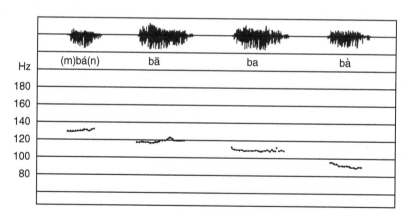

Figure 2.11 Examples of words with 4 different level tones from Mambila, a language from the Nigeria-Cameroon border. The four words illustrating these tones are as follows: T1 = mbán (breast), T2 = bā (bag), T3 = ba (palm of hand), T4 = bà (wing). The top panels shows the acoustic waveforms of the words, and the bottom panel shows voice pitch as recorded from one speaker. From Connell, 2000.

a logical place to look if one is interested in asking how close linguistic pitch systems can come to musical ones. Examination of such languages can help isolate the essential differences between music and speech in terms of how pitch contrasts are structured.

Pitch Contrasts Between Level Tones in Language: General Features

In seeking tone languages to compare to music, the researcher is naturally drawn to languages that use level tones (such as Mambila) rather than contour tones. As mentioned previously, a contour tone is a pitch trajectory that cannot be broken down into more basic units, as illustrated by tones 2–4 of Mandarin Chinese. In contrast, a level tone represents a level pitch target. A focus on Mandarin might lead one to think that level tones are unusual in language. Maddieson (1978, cf. Maddieson 2005) has conducted a cross-linguistic survey that reveals that the truth is in fact the reverse: The great majority of tone language have *only* level tones, with the most common number of levels being 2, though 3 tones is not uncommon. Maddieson also found that the large majority of languages with 2 or 3 tones have only level tones, and that the step from 3 to 4 tones represents a break point in the organization of tone languages. Specifically, this is the point at which contour tones begin to become important: Such tones are rare in 3-tone systems, but quite common in 4-tone systems. Thus there are no languages with only contour tones, and languages with large tonal inventories typically contrast no more than 3 level tones and use contour tones for the rest of their inventory. The generalization that emerges from these studies is that languages with level tones generally do not contrast more than 3 pitch levels.

What is known about level tones in language and their pitch contrasts? First, the maximum number of level tones in a language is 5, and languages with this many levels are very rare (Maddieson, 1978; Edmondson & Gregerson, 1992). Table 2.2 lists some languages with 5 level tones, whereas Figure 2.12 shows a phonological analysis of the tones of one such language. Figure 2.13 shows the geographic distribution of African languages with 5 level tones, showing their relative rarity (Wedekind, 1985).

Table 2.2 Languages With 5 Level Tones

Language	Location	Source
Miao	China	Anderson, 1978
Trique	Mexico	Longacre, 1952
Dan	Ivory Coast, Africa	Bearth & Zemp, 1967
Wobé	Ivory Coast, Africa	Filk, 1977
Benčnon	Ethiopia	Wedekind, 1983

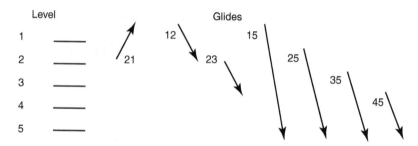

Figure 2.12 The linguistic tones of Ticuna, a tone language spoken by a small group of people from the Amazon regions of Peru, Columbia, and Brazil. This language has been analyzed as having 5 level tones and 7 glides. The numerals represent relative pitch levels in a speaker's voice. From Anderson, 1959, cited in Edmondson & Gregerson, 1992.

Second, level tones divide up frequency space in a particular way. This topic was investigated by Maddieson (1991), who contrasted two different hypotheses about how frequency space was allocated to level tones as the number of level tones in a language increased. The first hypothesis is that based on the idea of maximal dispersion, tones will be as far apart as they can be in the pitch range of a speaker. Thus a system with 2 level tones has a wide spacing between them, and additional tones subdivide the fixed pitch space in a manner that maximized intertone distance. The second hypothesis proposes that there is a "more-or-less fixed interval, relative to a speaker's range, which serves as a satisfactory degree of contrast between levels" (Maddieson, 1991, p. 150), and thus a larger number of tones will occupy a larger pitch range than a smaller number.

The available data favor the second hypothesis: As the number of tones in a language grows, so does the pitch range, suggesting that there is a basic minimal interval between level tones that languages attempt to attain. Although there is not a great deal of empirical data on tone spacing between level tones, the available data suggest that the minimum interval is between 1 and 2 semitones, the maximum is about 4 semitones, and an intertone spacing of 2–3 semitones is common (Maddieson 1991; Connell, 2000; Hogan & Manyeh, 1996). This suggests why the maximum number of level tones in human languages is 5. Because pitch range increases with the number of tones, 5 level tones may correspond to the maximum range that can be both comfortably produced and clearly subdivided in terms of perception.

A Closer Look at Pitch Contrasts Between Level Tones in Tone Languages

In order to make a close comparison between pitch contrasts in a level tone language and pitch contrasts in music, it is necessary to analyze speech from level tone languages in detail. Which languages should be analyzed? Among

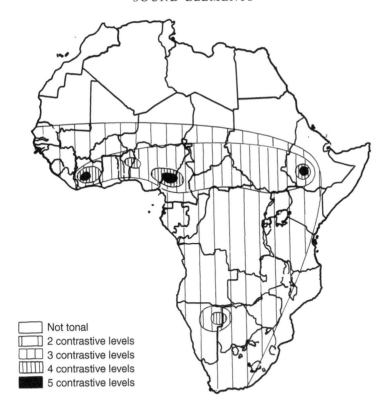

Figure 2.13 The geographic distribution of African tone languages according to their number of level tones. Note the pattern whereby 2-tone languages surround 3-tone languages, which in turn surround 4-tone languages, which in turn surround 5-tone languages. This may suggest a historical process of increasing or decreasing tonal differentiation. From Wedekind, 1985.

level tone languages (also called register tone languages), there are two subcategories. In one, the overall pitch of the voice lowers as a sentence progresses ("downtrend") due to various linguistic factors (Connell, 1999). In such languages a tone is high or low only in relation to its immediate neighbors, so that a "high" tone near the end of a sentence may actually be lower in pitch than a "low" tone near its beginning (Hyman, 2001). Clearly, pitch contrasts in such languages are not suitable for comparison with music. However, there are other tone languages that do not have downtrend. Such "discrete level" tone languages are the best languages for comparing pitch contrasts in language and music. An early description of discrete level tone languages is offered by Welmers (1973:81):

In many such languages, each level tone is restricted to a relatively narrow range of absolute pitch (absolute for a given speaker under given environmental conditions) within a phrase, and these tonemic ranges are discrete—never over-lapping, and separated by pitch ranges which are not used—throughout the phrase, though they may all tilt downward at the very end of the phrase in a brief final contour. Thus, in a three-level system, high tone near the end of the phrase has virtually the same absolute pitch as a high tone at the beginning of the phrase, and is higher than any mid tone in the phrase. Usually there are few restrictions in tone sequences. These phenomena may be illustrated by the following sentence in Jukun (Nigeria):

> áku pèrè ní zè budyi à syi ní bi kéré
> h m l l h l m m l m h m h h   (h = high, m = medium, l = low)
> "That person brought this food here"

Every possible sequence of two successive tones occurs in this sentence. The three levels are discrete throughout the sentence, and so precisely limited that playing them on three notes on a piano (a major triad does very well) does not appreciably distort the pitches of normal speech.

(NB: A "major triad" consists of three tones, the upper two of which are 4 and 7 semitones above the lowest tone, e.g., C-E-G on a piano.) Welmers' report is provocative, particularly because he implies stable pitch intervals. He also notes that Jukun is not an isolated case, but one of many West and Central African languages with discrete level tone systems of 2 to 4 tones. It should be noted, though, that Welmers wrote in the days before easy F0 extraction, and that his descriptions have yet to be verified by empirical data.

The study of languages such as Jukun would allow us to see how close speech can come to music in terms of pitch contrasts. In particular, by labeling tones in sentences of such languages and examining the frequency distances between them, one could ask if there is any evidence for stable intervals. (Of course, it should be kept in mind that intervals in music are subject to contextual varia-tion; cf. Rakowski, 1990. Thus in comparing interval stability in music vs. speech, the comparison of interest would be the *degree* of contextual variation.) There is reason to suspect that there will be a great deal of flexibility in tone spacing in speech. Recall that pitch in speech does double duty, carrying both affective signals and linguistic ones. Thus it would be adaptive to make pitch contrasts in speech flexible in terms of the physical distances between tones. This way, tonal contrasts could accommodate to elastic changes in the overall pitch range due to affective factors, or due to other factors that change pitch range in a gradient way, such as the loudness with which one speaks (Ladd, 1996:35).

The flexibility of pitch spacing in speech is supported by a research on pitch range by Ladd and a number of his students (Ladd, forthcoming). Based on this work, Ladd suggests that speech tones are scaled relative to two reference fre-quencies corresponding to the top and bottom of an individual's speaking range. This range can vary between speakers, and can be elastic within a speaker, for example, growing when speaking loudly or with strong positive affect. Ladd argues that what stays relatively constant across contexts and speakers is pitch level as a *proportion* of the current range. (See this chapter's appendix 4 for the relevant equation; this idea was also articulated by Earle, 1975.) Figure 2.14 illustrates this idea using a hypothetical example based on language with four level tones: low, low-mid, high-mid, and high.

In Figure 2.14, the same tones are spoken by Speakers A, B, and C. Speaker A's frequencies range from 100 to 200 Hz. (These frequencies might have been measured from the speaker saying words in citation form, as in Figure 2.11). Speaker B is, say, a male with a deep voice (range 60 to 120 Hz), whereas Speaker C has a narrow range, between 100 and 133 Hz. (A narrow range can be due to affective factors, such as sadness; Scherer, 1986.) Note that in each case, the level of a tone as a proportion of the speaker's range is the same: The low and high tones are at the bottom/top of the range, whereas the mid and mid-high tones are 20% and 50% of the way from the bottom to the top.

For the present discussion, what is notable about this scheme is that both the absolute frequency of tones *and the pitch intervals between tones* (in semitones) vary between speakers. Thus Speakers A and B have identical pitch intervals, but this is only because they have the same pitch range when measured in semitones (in this case, 1 octave). For both of these speakers, tones are separated by approximately 3, 4, and 5 semitones as one goes between tones in ascending order. However, for Speaker C, who has a narrow pitch range (about 5 semitones) the ascending intervals are about 1, 1.5, and 2 semitones.

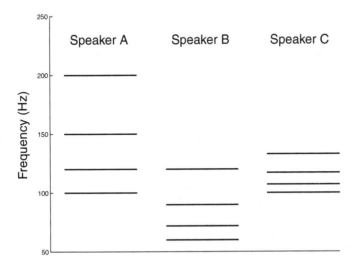

Figure 2.14 Examples of linguistic tone spacing illustrating the notion of range-based proportional scaling. See text for details.

Ladd argues that this range-based scaling of linguistic pitch levels applies within utterances as well, when pitch range changes over the course of an utterance. In fact, it is quite common for pitch range to shrink over the course of an utterance as part of F0 declination (cf. Vaissiere, 1983). Thus, for example, a speaker may start a long sentence with a range of about 1 octave but end it with a range of only 11 semitones. According to Ladd's scheme, the intervals between tones will shrink over the course of the utterance. Although Welmers' description suggests that discrete level tone languages may be immune from this sort of declination, empirical work is needed to show if this is in fact the case. However, even if such languages do not show declination, it seems very likely that measurements will show that discrete level tone languages do not use fixed pitch intervals. One reason for this is the elasticity of the pitch range, which is in turn driven by factors such as affect and the loudness with which one speaks. Another is that in connected discourse, lexical tones are subject to contextual forces (such as articulatory sluggishness) that can change their surface form (Xu, 2006).

Before closing this section, it might interest the reader to hear a sample of Jukun. Sound Example 2.5 presents a short spoken passage in Jukun (Wukari dialect, the dialect probably referred to by Welmers).[18] This passage is from a translation of a story called "The North Wind and the Sun," which has been recorded in many languages for the purpose of comparative phonetic analysis. Of course, this simply represents a single speaker, and is provided simply as an illustration.

Absolute Pitch in Speech?

The preceding section introduced the idea that a key to a linguistic tone's identity as a sound category is its position as a percent of a speaker's pitch range. This suggests that linguistic tone production and perception is a relative matter: A tone's identity depends on its position in a pitch range, a range that can change from speaker to speaker or even within the utterances of a single speaker (cf. Wong & Diehl, 2003, for relevant empirical data). If this view is correct, a listener must have some way of getting a relatively rapid and accurate estimate of where a given tone falls in the pitch range of a speaker. Interestingly, it may be possible for a listener to make such judgments even on isolated syllables, due to voice-quality factors that vary depending on location in the speaker's pitch range (Honorof & Whalen, 2005).

In contrast to the view that linguistic tone is a relative matter, Deutsch et al. (2004) have articulated the idea that a linguistic tone's absolute frequency can

---

[18] I am grateful to Neelima K. Pandit for organizing a field trip to make this recording in Nigeria in 2000.

be part of its identity as a sound category. In support of this idea, they report a study in which speakers of Vietnamese and Mandarin were asked to read a word list in their native language on 2 separate days. The words used the different linguistic tones of each language. For each speaker, the mean pitch of each word was quantified on Day 1 and Day 2. The main finding was a high degree of within-speaker consistency in the pitch of a given word across the two recordings. For most speakers, the difference in the pitch of a word on Day 1 and Day 2 was quite small: a 1/2 semitone or less. English speakers, in contrast, showed less pitch consistency on the same task.

Based on these results, Deutsch et al. suggest that tone-language speakers have a precise and stable absolute pitch template that they use for speech purposes. They argue that such a template is acquired as a normal part of early development, in the same way that infants acquire other aspects of their native phonology. In support of this notion, they point to research in music perception suggesting that infants can use absolute pitch cues when learning about the structure of nonlinguistic tone sequences (e.g., Saffran & Griepentrog, 2001; Saffran, 2003; Saffran et al., 2005; but see Trainor, 2005, for a critique). Deutsch et al. argue that absolute pitch originated as a feature of speech, with musical absolute pitch—the rare ability to classify pitches into well-defined musical categories without using any reference note—piggybacking on this ability (musical absolute pitch is discussed in more detail in Chapter 7, in sections 7.3.4 and 7.3.5).

As one might expect, the ideas of Deutsch et al. (2004) are proving quite controversial. In response to Deutsch et al.'s ideas, one issue being examined by speech scientists is the claim that tone-language and nontone-language speakers are really different in terms of the pitch consistency with which they read words on separate days. Burnham et al. (2004) addressed this issue in a study that used Mandarin, Vietnamese, and English speakers. A novel aspect of their study was that they tested whether a fixed word order in the reading list (as used by Deutsch et al.) might influence the results. They found that even when the order of words was changed from Day 1 and Day 2, Mandarin and Vietnamese speakers showed higher intraword pitch consistency than English speakers. However, the difference was small: around 3/4 semitone for tone language speakers versus about 1 semitone for English speakers. Thus there does not appear to be a huge difference between tone-language and nontone-language speakers in this regard.

It is clear that the debate over absolute pitch in speech is not over. For the moment, the idea that absolute pitch plays a role in speech is best regarded as tentative. A more compelling link between language and music with regard to absolute pitch is the finding by Deutsch and colleagues (2006) that musicians who are native speakers of a tone language are substantially more likely to have musical absolute pitch than are musicians who do not speak a tone language. The researchers tested a large number of musicians in the Central Conservatory of Music in Beijing and in the Eastman School of Music in New York, respectively. Participants were given a musical AP test involving naming the pitch class of isolated tones spanning a 3-octave range. Differences between the Chinese and American groups on this test were dramatic. For example, for students who had begun musical training between ages 4 and 5, approximately 60% of Chinese musicians showed AP, compared to 14% of the English speakers. This finding raises the interesting question of whether developing a framework for the categorical interpretation of pitch in speech facilitates the acquisition of musical pitch categories.[19]

Mapping Linguistic Tone Contrasts Onto Musical Instruments

The current review of pitch contrasts in language suggests that pitch relations in speech and music are fundamentally incommensurate, with the most salient difference being the lack of stable intervals in speech. It may come as a surprise, then, that there are cases in which musical instruments with fixed pitches are used to convey linguistic messages. One famous example of such a "speech surrogate" is the talking drum of West Africa (Herzog, 1945; Locke & Agbeli, 1980; Cloarec-Heiss, 1999). A talking drum communicates messages by mimicking the tones and syllabic rhythms of utterances in a tone language. Some talking drums allow the player to adjust the tension of the drum membrane (and thus its pitch) by pressing on thongs connected to the drumheads: These drums can mimic gliding tones in speech. Other drums have no membranes and are made entirely of wood: These drums produce fixed pitches that reflect the resonance properties of the instrument. Wooden instruments can reach a considerable size and are capable of conveying messages over long distances, up to several miles. For example, Carrington (1949a, 1949b) described a cylindrical log used by the Lokele of the upper Congo. The log is hollowed out via a simple rectangular slit (Figure 2.15a).

The hollowing is asymmetrical, so that there is a deeper pocket under one lip of the drum than the other (Figure 2.15b). The drum produces two tones: a

---

[19] Independent of the putative link between tone languages and musical absolute pitch, it may be that learning a tone language shapes the perception of nonlinguistic pitch more generally. For example, Bent, Bradlow, and Wright (2006) showed that speakers of Mandarin and English differ in a nonspeech pitch contour identification task. Mandarin speakers showed a tendency to judge low flat contours as falling in pitch, and high flat contours as rising in pitch, which may reflect listening strategies associated with accurate categorization of linguistic tones in Mandarin. Interestingly, the Mandarin and English listeners showed no difference in contour discrimination tasks, suggesting that the influence of language on nonlinguistic pitch perception entered at the more abstract stage of categorization (vs. raw discrimination).

A   B

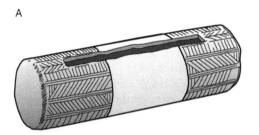
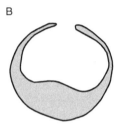

Figure 2.15 A talking drum of the Lokele people of the upper Congo in central Africa. A side view of the drum is shown in (A). The two tones are produced by striking the drum lips on either side of the central slit. A cross section of the drum is shown in (B), revealing the asymmetric degree of hollowing under the two lips of the drum. From Carrington, 1949b.

lower tone when the lip over the hollower side is struck, and a higher pitched tone when the other side is struck. These two tones are meant to mimic the two linguistic tones of spoken Lokele. Carrington noted that one such drum had an interval of approximately a minor third between the tones (3 semitones), but that other drums had other intervals, and there was no fixed tuning scheme. This suggests that relations between linguistic tones are not conceived (or perceived) in terms of standardized intervals.[20]

Another example of a pitch-based speech surrogate is whistled speech (Cowan, 1948; Stern, 1957; Sebeok & Umiker-Sebeok, 1976; Thierry, 2002, Rialland, 2005). In tone languages, the pitch of the whistle acts as a surrogate for linguistic tones ("tonal whistled speech").[21] A description of the efficacy of this communication system is provided by Foris (2000), a linguist who spent many years studying the Mexican tone language Chinantec. Chinantec whistled

[20] A key principle in the organization of talking drum messages is redundancy. Because many words have the same tonal pattern, it is necessary to disambiguate the words by placing them in longer phrases. These tend to be stereotyped, poetic phrases that form part of the oral tradition of a tribe. For example, the word "moon" may be embedded in the longer phrase "the moon looks down at the earth." Carrington (1971) estimated that approximately eight syllables of drum language were needed for each syllable of ordinary language in order to convey unambiguous messages.

[21] There is a basic distinction between "articulated" and "tonal" whistled speech. In the former, vowels and consonants have whistled counterparts, with vowels being indicated by differences in relative pitch, and consonants by pitch transitions and amplitude envelope cues (Busnel & Classe, 1976; Thierry, 2002; Rialland, 2003, 2005; Meyer, 2004). This allows the communication of virtually any message that can be spoken. The best-studied case occurs in the Canary Islands, though articulated whistled speech is also known from other regions, including the French Pyrenees and Turkey.

speech uses a combination of tone and stress distinctions to communicate messages with minimal ambiguity. Foris writes:

> Virtually anything that can be expressed by speech can be communicated by whistling. The most complex example that I had interpreted for me was on the occasion that the supply plane was due to come in. Because of heavy rains, I checked the dirt airstrip for erosion and saw that it needed extensive repairs. I went to the town president and explained the need for immediate repairs, a job that was the responsibility of the town police in those days. The town is set in a horseshoe-shaped hillside; his house is at one end of the "arm," with the town hall at the centre, about 1/2 a kilometre away. He put his fingers in his mouth and whistled to get their attention. They responded that they were listening, and he whistled a long message. I asked for the interpretation, which he gave as the following: "The plane will be here soon. The airstrip needs to be repaired. Get the picks, shovels, and wheelbarrows and fix it right away." (pp. 30–31)

If verified, this is indeed a remarkable finding. Quite apart from this example, there are well-documented accounts of tonal whistled speech from other cultures in which whistling is used to exchange simpler and more stereotyped messages. For the current purpose, the relevant question is whether these systems use fixed pitch intervals. Unfortunately, there are no good empirical data to address this issue. Because tonal whistled speech is usually produced by mouth rather than by an instrument with fixed pitches, it seems unlikely that there is a tuning scheme that relies on standardized pitch intervals.

Perhaps the closest that a speech surrogate comes to using a fixed tuning scheme is the "krar speech" of southwest Ethiopia. The krar is a 5-string instrument resembling a guitar, which is used to imitate the 5 discrete level tones of the language Benčnon. Wedekind (1983) describes a game in which an object is hidden, and then the seeker is asked to find it. The only clues the seeker receives come from the krar player, who "tells" the seeker where the object is hidden using the musical instrument to imitate the linguistic tones of utterances. Krar speech merits study, because the intervals between tones are fixed, at least for a given krar. How important are the particular intervals to the communication of linguistic messages? One could test this by studying how much one could alter the exact tuning of a given krar and still communicate messages with a given efficacy. If standardized pitch intervals are not important for linguistic tones, one would predict that a good deal of mistuning would be tolerable before communication efficacy dropped below a predetermined threshold.

2.3.3 Timbral Contrasts in Language

Although pitch contrasts can be quite organized in language, as demonstrated by discrete level tone languages, there is no question that the primary dimension for organized sound contrasts in language is timbre. This can be shown by a thought experiment. Imagine asking a speaker of a language to listen to computer-synthesized monologue in which all sentences are rendered on a monotone. For speakers of nontone languages such as English, such speech would still be highly intelligible, if artificial. For speakers of tone languages, there may be a loss of intelligibility, but it is unlikely that intelligibility would drop to zero, especially in languages such as Mandarin, in which a syllable's tone may be correlated with other cues (such as duration and amplitude; Whalen & Xu, 1992).[22] Now conduct the converse experiment: Allow the pitch of the synthesized sentences to vary normally but replace all phonemes with one timbre, say the vowel /a/. Intelligibility would be reduced to zero for all languages, irrespective of whether they were tone languages or not (except perhaps in rare cases such as Chinantec, in which it is claimed that the combination of tone and stress results in over 30 distinctions that can be communicated with minimal ambiguity; cf. the previous section).

Speech is thus fundamentally a system of organized timbral contrasts. (One might argue that durational patterning is also fundamental to speech, but without timbral contrasts there would be no basis for defining distinct phonemes or syllables, and hence no basis for making durational contrasts.) The human voice is the supreme instrument of timbral contrast. A survey of languages reveals that the human voice is capable of producing timbres corresponding to ~800 distinct phonemes, and this represents only phonemes known from extant languages (Maddieson, 1984). Of course, no single speaker or language uses this many contrasts: Phoneme inventories range in size from 11 (5 vowels and 6 consonants in Rotokas, a language of Papua New Guinea) to 156 (28 vowels and 128 consonants in !Xóõ, a Khoisan language from South Africa), with the average inventory size being 27 phonemes (Trail, 1994; Maddieson, 1999).

As noted in section 2.2.4, musical systems based on sequences of organized timbral contrasts are rare. In terms of comparing music and language, why then delve into the organization of timbre in speech? There are two principal reasons for doing so. First, timbre is the primary basis for linguistic sound categories. Because the focus of the next section (section 2.4) is on comparing sound categorization mechanisms in speech and music, understanding the physical basis of speech sound categories is essential. The second reason is an understanding of timbre in language provides the basis for examining the relationship between the musical and linguistic timbres of a culture. For these reasons, the remainder of this section (2.3.3) provides a brief overview of timbral contrasts in language. Readers already knowledgeable about speech acoustics may wish

---

[22] Indeed, when all F0 variation is removed from sentences of Mandarin, native speakers still understand the sentences with nearly 100% intelligibility, likely due to semantic and pragmatic constraints that result from having the words in sentence context (Patel & Xu, in preparation).

to skip ahead to the subsection "Mapping Linguistic Timbral Contrasts Onto Musical Sounds" below.

Timbral Contrasts in Language: Overview

The timbral contrasts of speech result from continuous changes in the shape of the vocal tract as sound is produced from a variety of sources. Consider the English word "sleepy," which is written in IPA symbols as /slipi/. The /s/ is produced by shaping the tongue into a groove so that a jet of air is forced across the teeth, resulting in acoustic turbulence that produces a hissing sound (a fricative). The /l/ and /i/, on the other hand, rely on the harmonically rich sound of vocal fold vibration (by lightly touching the fingers to the "Adam's apple" one can feel the onset of vocal fold vibration associated with the transition from the /s/ to the /l/). This harmonically rich spectrum is sculpted in different ways for the /l/ and the /i/ by differing positions of the tongue in the vocal tract. Specifically, during the /l/, the tip of the tongue makes contact with the alveolar ridge (just behind the teeth), forming a pocket of air over the tongue. This air pocket acts to attenuate the spectrum of the sound source in a particular frequency region (Johnson, 1997:155). After the release of the /l/, the tongue body moves to a position high and forward in the mouth, where it serves to shape the voice spectrum in such a way such that an /i/ sound is produced (cf. the following section, on vowels). During the /p/, vocal fold vibration stops as the mouth closes and pressure builds up in preparation for a burst of air. Soon after the burst,[23] the vocal folds begin vibrating again as the mouth opens, completing the /p/ sound as the tongue moves into position for the final /i/.

This example illustrates two general properties of speech. First, the succession of timbral contrasts is extremely rapid: It takes about 500 milliseconds to utter the word "sleepy," yielding an average of 1 phoneme every 100 ms, or 10 phonemes/sec. In connected speech, a rate of 10 phonemes per second is not at all unusual. The second property of speech illustrated by the above example is the rough alternation of consonants and vowels. This ensures a rapid succession of timbral contrasts, as consonants and vowels tend to have very different articulations, and consequently, distinct timbres. This occurs because consonants are typically produced via a narrowing or closure of the vocal tract, whereas vowels are associated with an unimpeded flow of air from the lungs through the vocal tract. X-ray movies of the vocal tract during speech show this

---

[23] To be precise, the burst of a /p/ can involve three sources of sound with partial temporal overlap, all in the course of approximately 30 milliseconds: a transient burst at the lips, a brief turbulence (frication) in the narrow region between the lips just after the closure is released, and a brief aspiration noise at the vocal folds before they resume vibrating (Stevens, 1997:492–494).

succession of narrowings and openings as part of a remarkable choreography of moving articulators during speech.[24]

How are the timbres of a language organized with respect to each other? As the above example suggests, timbral contrasts in speech are intimately linked to the articulations that give rise to speech sounds. In fact, the most widely used modern taxonomy of speech sounds (the IPA) is based on articulatory features. For example, consonants are classified in terms of their manner of articulation and their place of their primary constriction. Manner refers to the kind of constriction made by the articulators when producing the consonant, and place refers to the location of this constriction in the vocal tract. The organization of some English consonants by manner and place is shown in Table 2.3. The table uses IPA symbols,[25] and a schematic diagram showing some places of articulation used in the world's languages is shown in Figure 2.16.

In Table 2.3, consonants that appear in pairs are distinguished by voicing (for example, /f/ and /v/ are both fricatives in which the frication noise is produced in exactly the same way, but the vocal folds vibrate during a /v/).

Both the degree of timbral contrast in speech and the rate at which such contrast occurs are far in excess of anything produced by a nonvocal musical instrument. However, the organization of timbral contrasts in speech is not irrelevant to music. In fact, it may help explain why certain musical traditions with organized timbral contrasts are successful. One such tradition is North Indian tabla drumming, described earlier in section 2.2.4 (subsection "Example of a Timbre-Based Musical System"). As noted in that section, in tabla music the contrasting timbres are organized in terms of distinctive places and manners of articulation. The places are regions of the drum heads that are struck, the manners are the ways in which the drum heads are struck, and the articulators are the different fingers that do the striking. This example illustrates how a successful "timbre music" can be built from a speech-like system of organization. Another long-lived musical tradition which emphasizes timbral contrast is Tibetan tantric chanting. In this music, timbral contrasts slowly unfold while pitch maintains a drone-like pattern (Cogan, 1984:28–35). A key to the aesthetic success of this tradition may be that it takes an aspect of human experience that is normally experienced extremely rapidly (timbral speech contrast) and slows it down to a completely different timescale, thus giving the opportunity to experience something familiar a new way.

---

[24] An X-ray database of speech (with some online clips) is available courtesy of Kevin Munhall: http://psyc.queensu.ca/~munhallk/05_database.htm.

[25] For those unfamiliar with IPA, some symbols used in table 2.3 are: ŋ (ng) is the final consonant in "sing," θ is the initial consonant in "thin," ð is the initial consonant in "the," ʃ is the initial consonant in "she," and ʒ is the second consonant in "unusual." For the full IPA chart of sounds with audio examples, visit the website listed in footnote 14.

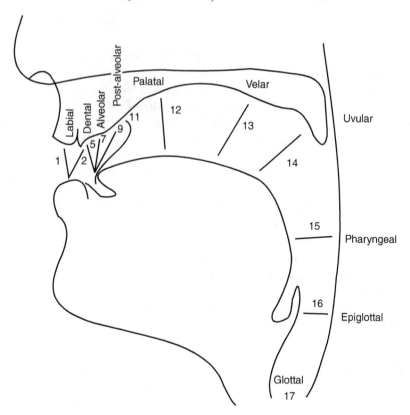

Figure 2.16 Places of articulation in a cross-sectional view of the vocal tract. Numbered lines indicate some of the 17 named articulatory gestures (e.g., 2 is a labiodental maneuver in which the lower lip touches the upper teeth). Note the concentration of places of articulation near the front of the vocal tract. From Ladefoged & Madiesson, 1996.

Timbral Contrasts Among Vowels

A basic understanding of vowel production and acoustics is essential for those interested in comparing speech and music, because vowels are the most musical of speech sounds, having a clear pitch and a rich harmonic structure. The primary way that the vowels of a language differ from each is in their timbre, and each language has a distinctive palette of vocalic timbres. The number of vowels in a language ranges from 3 in a small number of languages, including Arrernte (Australia), Pirahã (Amazonian rain forest), and Aleut (Alaska), to 24 in Germanic dialects, such as the Dutch dialect of Weert (P. Ladefoged, personal communication). A genetically diverse sample of languages reveals that the modal number of vowels in a human language is 5 (Maddieson, 1999).

Table 2.3 Manner Versus Place Classification for Some English Consonants

	Place					
Manner	Bilabial	Labiodental	Dental	Alveolar	Post-alveolar	Velar
Plosive: Total closure in the vocal tract, followed by a sudden release	p b			t d		k g
Nasal: Complete closure of the vocal tract, with lowering of soft palate so air is forced through the nose	m			n		ŋ
Fricative: Narrowing of the vocal tract, causing air turbulence as a jet of air hits the teeth.		f v	θ ð	s z	ʃ ʒ	

American English has 15 vowels, and is thus on the rich end of the vowel spectrum.[26]

Vowel production has two main features. The first is *voicing,* referring to the vibration of the tensed vocal folds as air rushes past them, resulting in a buzzy sound source. This sound source has a frequency spectrum that consists of a fundamental frequency (F0, corresponding to the perceived pitch) and a large number of harmonics. The strongest harmonics are in the bass, typically being the first 5 or 6 multiples of the fundamental. Vowels spoken in isolation almost always have some F0 movement, and this is part of what gives a vowel its "speechy" quality (Sundberg, 1987).

---

[26] One way that languages can increase their inventory of vowels by making phonemic contrasts between vowels based on length or voice quality. Thus in Japanese and Estonian, vowel duration is contrastive, so that a word can change its meaning if a short versus long version of the same vowel is used. In Jalapa Mazatec, a word can mean three entirely different things if the vowel is spoken in a normal ("modal") voice, in a breathy voice, or a creaky voice (Ladefoged & Maddieson, 1996).

The second key feature for vowels is the tongue's position in the vocal tract, which results in acoustic resonances that filter the underlying source spectrum via the emphasis of certain frequency bands (Figure 2.17).

The position and sharpness of these resonances, called *formants,* provide the vowel with its characteristic timbre, which in turn determines its linguistic identity. The position of the first two formants (F1 and F2) are the most important cue for vowel identity, and the vowels of any language can be represented by placing them on a graph whose axes are the center frequencies of the first and second formant (Figure 2.18).[27]

As Figure 2.18 implies, changing either F1 or F2 can change a vowel's timbre and eventually move it far enough so that it changes linguistic identity. Of course, where the boundaries between vowel phonemes are depends on the language in question. Note that even within a language, the acoustic boundaries between vowels are not sharp. Vowels seem to be organized into acoustic regions with better or more prototypical exemplars in the middle of the regions and poorer exemplars toward the boundaries of regions (cf. Kuhl, 1991). Of course, the precise location of these regions (and hence of the best exemplars) depends on the voice being analyzed. For example, /i/ vowels produced by adult males occupy a somewhat different region in F1–F2 space from those produced by an adult females or children due to differences in vocal tract length (shorter vocal tracts produce higher resonant frequencies). Listeners normalize for these differences in judging how good an exemplar a vowel is (Nearey, 1978; Most et al., 2000).

Because there is a strong relationship between articulatory configuration and the acoustics of a vowel, vowel relations are often described in articulatory terms. Thus linguists frequently speak of front vowels, high vowels, mid vowels, and so on. These terms refer to the position of the tongue body during vowel production. Articulatory vowel space thus has 4 distinct corners (high front, high back, low front, and low back), corresponding to the "cardinal" vowels i, u, a, *a* (as in "beet," "boot," "father," and "awful"). Figure 2.19 shows the full IPA vowel chart: a two-dimensional grid of tongue body position, in which the vertical dimension is tongue *height* and the horizontal dimension is tongue *backness.* (Note that most languages have only 5 vowels: No language has all the vowels shown in the IPA chart; cf. Maddieson, 1984.)

Vowel systems and vowel perception have many interesting features (Liljencrants & Lindblom, 1972; Stevens, 1989, 1998; Ladefoged, 2001; Diehl et al., 2003), which unfortunately cannot be discussed here because our focus is on comparison with music. (One aspect of vowel perception, the "perceptual

---

[27] F3 is important in some vowel distinctions, for example, in the *r*-colored vowel in "bird."

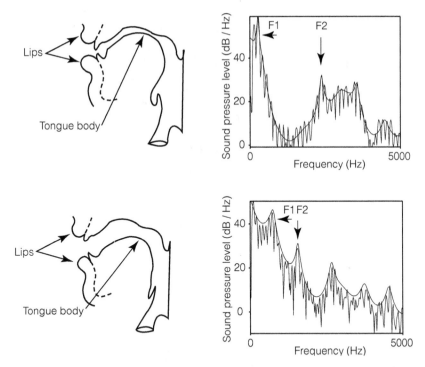

Figure 2.17 Examples of vocal tract configurations and frequency spectra for the vowels /i/ (in "beat") and /æ/ (in "bat") are shown in the top and bottom row, respectively. In the frequency spectra, the jagged lines show the harmonics of the voice, and the smooth curves shows mathematical estimates of vocal tract resonances. The formants are the peaks in the resonance curves. The first two formant peaks are indicated by arrows. The vowel /i/ has a low F1 and high F2, and /æ/ has a high F1 and low F2. These resonances result from differing positions of the tongue in the vocal tract. Vocal tract drawings courtesy of Kenneth Stevens. Spectra courtesy of Laura Dilley.

magnet effect," is discussed later in section 2.4.3.) Here I simply mention one other aspect of vowel production relevant to comparative issues. This is the fact that the acoustic structure of a vowel can vary a great deal depending on context. For example, if one measures the formant frequencies of an English vowel spoken in a word produced in isolation (e.g., from an individual's reading of a word list in a laboratory) and then measures the formants of that same vowel in rapid and informal speech, the formants in the latter case may undershoot their laboratory values by a substantial amount (i.e., by hundreds of Hz). At the other extreme, if the same word is spoken in the context of infant-directed speech, a form of very clear speech, the formant values may substantially overshoot their values in clear adult-directed speech (Kuhl et al., 1997). Thus part of normal speech includes variation between hypo- and hyperarticulation of

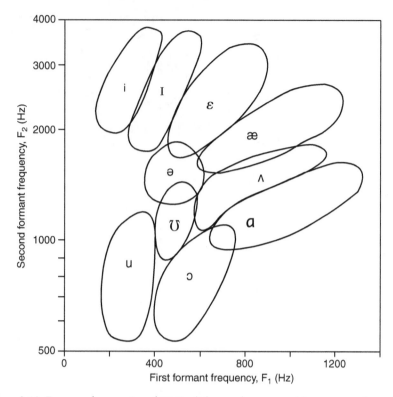

Figure 2.18 Formant frequencies of 10 English vowels as uttered by a range of speakers (*x* axis = F1, *y* axis = F2). The ovals enclose the majority of tokens of vowels in a single perceptual category. Symbols follow IPA conventions. Adapted from Peterson & Barney, 1952.

vowels depending on speech context (Lindblom, 1990). The amount of acoustic variation is likely to far exceed the contextual variation of musical sounds (e.g., variation in the size of a pitch interval or in the spectrum of a given note produced by one instrument over the course of a piece).

Spectrum, Timbre, and Phoneme

Up till this point, I have been purposefully vague about the relationship between acoustic spectrum, perceived timbre, and phonemic identity in speech, in order to introduce basic concepts. However, it is time to be more specific. The key point is that a snapshot of a static spectrum, such as those of the vowels in the previous section, should not be confused with "a timbre," and a single timbre should not be confused with "a phoneme."

The idea that a spectrum should not be confused with a timbre has already been introduced in the discussion of musical timbre in section 2.2.4. For

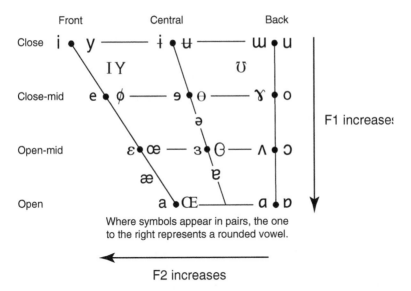

Where symbols appear in pairs, the one to the right represents a rounded vowel.

Figure 2.19 The IPA vowel chart. "Front," "back," "close," and "open" refer to the position of the tongue body in the mouth (close = high, open = low). From Ladefoged, 2006. To hear the sounds in this figure, visit: http://hctv.humnet.ucla.edu/departments/linguistics/VowelsandConsonants/course/chapter1/vowels.html

example, the spectrum of a musical note may change (e.g., as a function of the loudness with which it is played) but the timbre may remain the same. Furthermore, the characteristic timbre of a sound may rely on dynamic *changes* in the spectrum. For vowels, this is illustrated by diphthongs such as /ai/ (the vowel in the English word "I"), in which the tongue moves from a low central to a high front position, with a corresponding decrease in F1 and increase in F2. For consonants, this is illustrated by stop consonants such as /b/ and /d/, in which spectral change is a vital part of creating their characteristic timbre. Such consonants are always coproduced with a vowel, and are acoustically characterized by a period of silence (corresponding to the vocal tract closure), followed by a sudden broadband burst of energy (as the vocal tract constriction is released), followed by formant transitions that typically last about 50 ms. These transitions occur because the acoustic resonance properties of the vocal tract change rapidly as the mouth opens and the tongue moves toward its target position (Stevens, 1998).

The second point, that a timbre should not be confused with a phoneme, can easily be demonstrated by synthesizing different versions of a vowel that differ slightly in F1 and F2 and that are noticeably different in sound quality, but nevertheless are still perceived as the same vowel (Kuhl, 1991).

Given these points, what does it mean to say that speech is an organized system of timbral contrasts? All that is intended by this statement is that phonemes have different timbres, and that because speech can be analyzed as a succession of phonemes, it can also be considered a succession of timbres.

A Brief Introduction to the Spectrogram

Because spectrograms are fundamental in speech research and are used in a comparative study of spoken and musical timbre described in the next section, a brief introduction to them is given here. A spectrogram is a series of spectra taken at successive points in time that allows a scientist to view the temporal evolution of the frequency structure of a signal. In a spectrogram, time is plotted on the horizontal axis, frequency on the vertical axis, and spectral amplitude is plotted using a gray scale, so that higher amplitudes are darker. Spectrograms of a voice saying the vowels /i/ and /æ/ are shown in Figure 2.20.

When compared to the static spectra in Figure 2.17 above, one salient difference is obvious: The individual harmonics can no longer be seen. Instead, one simply sees broad energy bands that correspond to the formants, as well as thin vertical striations corresponding to the fundamental period of the vocal fold vibration (F0 is the inverse of this period). This is due to the fact that these spectrograms were made with a coarse frequency resolution, in order to obtain a good time resolution: There is a fundamental tradeoff between these two types of resolution in spectral analysis (Rosen & Howell, 1991).

Of course, if speech consisted of a succession of static vowels with little formant movement, there would be no need for spectrograms. One could simply

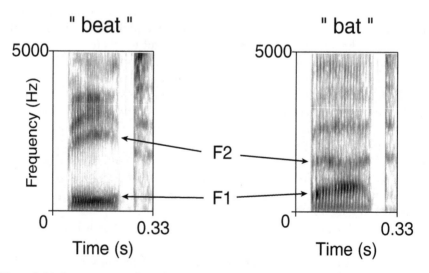

Figure 2.20 Spectrograms of a male speaker saying the words "beat" and "bat," to illustrate the vowels /i/ and /æ/. Arrows point to the first and second formants of the vowels. Note the low F1 and high F2 in /i/, and the inverse pattern in /æ/.

plot a succession of static spectra (as in Figure 2.17) with a record of when one changed to another. However, one of the defining features of speech is that spectral structure changes rapidly over time. Figure 2.21a shows a spectrogram of a speaker saying a sentence of British English, together with the acoustic waveform of the sentence (cf. Sound Example 2.6).

The position of all the vowels in this utterance are marked in Figure 2.21b, and word onsets in Figure 2.21c. Three important points about speech are obvious from these plots. First, the formants of speech, visible as the dark undulating lines, are in almost constant motion. For example, notice the dramatic formant movement in vowels 9 and 16 of Figure 2.21b (the first vowel of "opera" and of "success," respectively), due to coarticulation with the following consonant (/p/ and /k/, respectively). Second, vowels are not the only phonemes with formants (also evident from Figure 2.21b). Formants figure prominently in the spectrum of many speech sounds, because every vocal tract configuration is associated with acoustic resonances that shape the spectrum of the sound source. (This will be important for a subsequent discussion of the perception of /l/ and /r/ by English vs. Japanese speakers.) Third, as seen in Figure 2.21c, the boundaries of words do not necessarily correspond to obvious acoustic discontinuities in the waveform or spectrogram, which is one reason why in listening to a foreign language we may have no idea where one word ends and the next begins. This "segmentation problem" is particularly keen for infants, who cannot rely on a preexisting vocabulary to help them extract words from the flow of sound. As

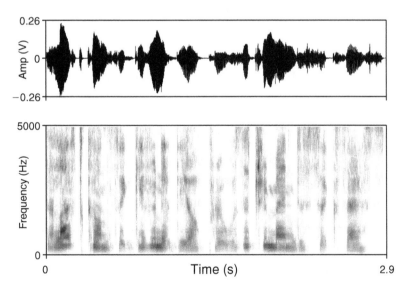

Figure 2.21a Acoustic waveform and spectrogram of a female British English speaker saying the sentence, "The last concert given at the opera was a tremendous success."

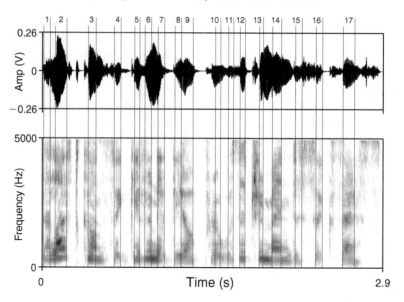

Figure 2.21b Spectrogram of the same sentence as in 2.21a with the onset and offset of each of the 17 successive vowels marked. (Note that "opera" is pronounced "opra").

we shall see in Chapter 3, speech rhythm is thought to play a role in helping infants and adults segment words from connected speech (Cutler, 1994).

Mapping Linguistic Timbral Contrasts Onto Musical Sounds

All human cultures have two distinct repertoires of timbres: linguistic and musical. In any given culture one can ask, "What relationship exists between these two sound systems?" One approach to this question is to examine cases in which nonsense syllables or "vocables" are used in systematic ways to represent musical sounds. Vocables are typically shared by members of a musical community and are used for oral teaching of musical patterns. Such traditions are found in many parts of the world, including Africa, India, Japan, and China (Locke & Agbeli, 1980; Kippen, 1988; Hughes, 2000; Li, 2001). (For a study of the informal use of vocables by Western orchestral musicians when singing melodies without text, see Sundberg, 1994.) A familiar Western example is solfège, in which the notes of the scale are represented by the syllables *do, re, mi,* and so forth. Of course, in Solfège there is no systematic mapping between vocable sounds and the musical sounds they represent. More interesting are cases in which there seems to be some acoustic and perceptual resemblance between speech sounds and musical sounds, especially if this resemblance lies in the domain of timbre. Such cases of timbral "sound symbolism" (Hinton et al., 1994)

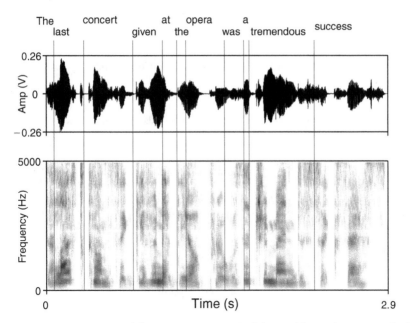

The last concert given at the opera was a tremendous success

Figure 2.21c Spectrogram of the same sentence as in 2.21a, with word onsets marked.

allow one to ask what cues humans find salient in musical timbres, and how they go about imitating these cues using linguistic mechanisms.

The North Indian tabla, described earlier in section 2.2.4 (subsection "Example of a Timbre-Based Musical System") is a prime candidate for a study of timbral sound symbolism. Players of tabla have an intuition that the vocables in this tradition resemble the drum sounds. However, a voice and a drum make sounds in very different ways, presenting an excellent opportunity to compare corresponding speech and drum sounds and ask what makes them sound similar despite radically different production mechanisms. Patel and Iversen (2003) conducted one such study, examining eight vocables and their corresponding drums sounds as spoken and drummed by six professional tabla players. (Examples of each drum sound can be heard in Sound Examples 2.3a–h, and the corresponding vocables can be heard in Sound Examples 2.7a–h. For a description of how the drum is struck for each of the sounds, refer back to Table 2.1.)

We organized the vocables into four pairs to focus on distinctive timbral contrasts between similar vocables. (For example, the vocables "Tin" and "Tun" differed only by the identity of the vowel in each syllable.) For each vocable pair, we examined acoustic differences between the vocables, as well as acoustic differences between the corresponding drum sounds. The question of interest was how timbral differences between drum sounds were mapped onto linguistic cues. We found a different kind of mapping for each pair of vocables and drum sounds we examined. Table 2.4 shows some of these mappings. (Quantitative data can

Table 2.4 Mapping Between Drum Sounds and Their Corresponding Vocables in North Indian Tabla Drumming

Vocable Pair	Drum Struck(right = dayan, left = bayan; cf. Figure 2.9)	Acoustic Difference Between Drum Sounds	Linguistic Cue Mapped Onto Musical Timbral Difference
Tin – Tun	Right	*Mean Frequency (Centroid) of Acoustic Spectrum* Tun has a lower overall spectral centroid due to presence of the fundamental. Tin has a higher centroid because the fundamental is damped by lightly resting one finger on the membrane while striking with another.	*Mean Frequency (Centroid) of Vowel Spectrum* Vowel timbre: /i/ has a higher F2 than /u/, making the centroid of the speech spectrum significantly higher in /i/ than in /u/.
Kat – Ghe	Left	*Rate of Drum Sound Amplitude Decay* Kat is a rapid, nonreverberating sound (closed stroke). Ghe is a longer, reverberating sound (open stroke).	*Rate of Syllable Amplitude Decay* The amplitude envelope of Kat decays significantly faster than Ghe due to the final consonant, which ends the syllable quickly.
Tra – Kra	Right (Tra) or both drums (Kra) (These strokes involve two hits in rapid succession.)	*Timing Between Drum Strokes* In Tra the duration between drum impacts is shorter than in Kra.	*Timing Between Consonant Releases* In Tra the duration between the release of the initial consonant and the release of the /r/ is significantly shorter than in Kra.
Ta – Dha	Right (Ta) or both drums (Dha)	*Presence of Low-Frequency Energy* Ta is a stroke on the right (higher pitched) drum, whereas Dha uses both the right and left (lower pitched drum), giving the composite sound a lower frequency in the case of Dha.	*Voice Fundamental Frequency* F0 of spoken Dha was significantly lower than spoken Ta near the onset of the syllable.

See Table 2.1 for IPA notation of vocables, and for details on how the drums were struck for each sound.

be found in Patel & Iversen, 2003.) The table indicates that tabla drummers are sensitive to a variety of timbral contrasts between drum sounds, and find diverse ways of mapping these onto timbral (or pitch) contrasts in speech.

The study by Patel and Iversen (2003) also provided an example of how a language exploits its special phonetic inventory to capture a musical timbral contrast. This example concerns the vocable /dha/. Spoken /dha/ uses a heavily aspirated form of a /d/ that is unique to Sanskrit-based languages (Ladefoged & Maddieson, 1996). Recall that /dha/ represents a combination stroke on the higher and the lower pitched drum. Why might this sound be particularly apt for representing the combined striking of the two drums? The answer lies in the fine acoustic detail of the drum sound and the corresponding speech sound. On the drums, /dha/ is a combination of two strokes: a /ta/ stroke on the right drum and a /ghe/ stroke on the left. The spectrogram in Figure 2.22a shows that this creates a composite sound with the lowest frequency component contributed by the sound of the left drum (the lower pitched bayan) and higher frequency components contributed by the sound of the right drum (the higher pitched dayan).

Crucially, we found that the frequency of the left drum showed a two-stage structure: a short initial frequency modulation (labeled FM in the figure, lasting about 200 ms), followed by a longer period of stability. When

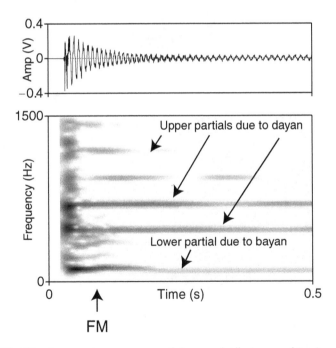

Figure 2.22a Waveform and spectrogram of drummed /dha/, a combination stroke on the dayan and bayan. Note the brief period of frequency modulation (FM) in the bayan sound.

we measured the ratio of energy in the lowest frequency versus the higher frequencies, during versus after the FM, we found that this ratio was significantly larger during the FM portion. Turning to the spoken vocable /dha/, we also noted a clear two-stage pattern in the acoustic structure of this syllable. An initial portion of heavy aspiration (the /h/ sound; lasting about 90 ms) was followed by the vowel /a/ with stable formant structure (Figure 2.22b). The early, aspirated portion is characterized by a particular type of voicing known as aspirated (breathy) voicing, during which the vocal folds are vibrating in an unusual mode. Because of the heavy air stream moving past them they do not fully close on each cycle, which has a dramatic influence on the source spectrum (Ladefoged, 2001). In particular, there is very little energy in higher frequency harmonics of the voice. Thus when we measured the ratio of energy in the fundamental frequency versus in a frequency range spanning the first two formants, we found that this ratio was significantly greater during aspiration. Thus both the drum sound and the speech sound showed a two-stage acoustic structure with the initial stage marked by a dominance of

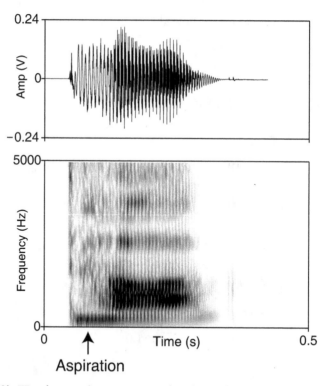

Figure 2.22b Waveform and spectrogram of spoken /dha/. Note the period of heavy aspiration between the onset of the syllable (the release of the /d/) and the onset of stable formant structure in the vowel.

low-frequency energy. This dominance was achieved in completely different ways, but the perceptual end result was similar (Figure 2.22c).

An important question is whether familiarity with the language and music of a particular tradition is needed in order to perceive the similarity between the timbres of the vocables and their associated musical sounds. If not, then this is strong evidence that the mappings are based on real acoustic and perceptual resemblance and not just convention. To investigate this question, we presented vocables and their associated drum sounds in pairs (e.g., spoken and drummed tin and tun) to naïve listeners who knew neither Hindi nor tabla drumming, and asked them to try to guess the correct pairing. We found that listeners performed remarkably well (about 80% correct, on average) for all pairings except /tra/ and /kra/, in which the acoustic difference between the two drum sounds is very hard to discern.

In summary, an empirical study of tabla sounds demonstrates strong connections between the musical and linguistic timbres of a culture, and suggests that similar empirical studies should be conducted in other cultures, particularly in the rich percussive traditions of Africa and the African diaspora.

2.3.4 Consonants and Vowels as Learned Sound Categories in Language

Having described some fundamental aspects of speech acoustics, it is now time to take a cognitive perspective and examine speech sounds as learned sound categories. Evidence abounds that experience with speech produces a mental framework of sound categories that influences the perception of linguistic sound. As with music, such a framework is adaptive because tokens of a given linguistic sound can vary in their acoustic structure. Thus the framework allows a listener to transform acoustically variable tokens into stable mental categories. The following two sections provide evidence for learned sound categories

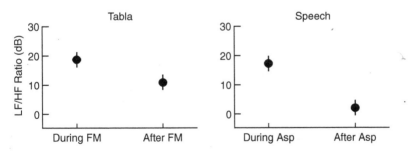

Figure 2.22c Measurements of the ratio of low frequency (LF) to high frequency (HF) energy during the two acoustic stages of the drummed /dha/ and spoken /dha/ (mean and standard error across 30 tokens played/spoken by 6 speakers are shown). In both cases, the early portion of the sound is dominated by low frequency energy, though by completely different mechanisms.

in speech. The first section reviews behavioral evidence from studies of consonant perception, and the second section reviews neural evidence from studies
of vowel perception. I have chosen these particular studies because they invite
parallel studies in music.

Consonants: Perception of Nonnative Contrasts

It has long been known that sounds that function as different categories in one
language can be difficult for speakers of another language to discriminate. A
classic example of this is the perception of English /l/ and /r/ by Japanese speakers (Goto, 1971). In Japanese, these two sounds do not function as different
phonemes, but are broadly consistent with a single /r/-like phoneme.

Iverson et al. (2003) helped illuminate how American English versus Japanese speakers hear this linguistic contrast. They created an "acoustic matrix"
of /ra/ and /la/ syllables that differed systematically in acoustic structure (second
and third formant frequencies, F2 and F3; Figure 2.23a).

They then asked English and Japanese speakers to perform three different
kinds of perceptual tasks with these stimuli. In the first task, listeners simply labeled each stimulus in terms of their own native-language phonemes, and rated
how good an exemplar of that phoneme it was. In the second task, listeners
heard the stimuli in pairs (every possible pairing except self-pairing) and rated
their perceived similarity. In the third task, listeners once again heard stimuli in
pairs, half of which were the same and half of which were different. (When different, they varied in F3 only; F2 was held constant at 1003 Hz.) The task was
simply to say whether the members of a pair were the same or different.

The labeling task showed that English listeners labeled stimuli on the left
half of this acoustic matrix as /ra/ and on the right half as /la/, whereas Japanese
labeled all the stimuli in the matrix as /ra/.[28] The discrimination task revealed
that English listeners showed a peak in discrimination when the two tokens
straddled their two different phoneme categories, whereas Japanese speakers
showed no peak at the corresponding point. Thus English and Japanese listeners were hearing the same physical stimuli in rather different ways. One representation of these perceptual differences came from the similarity-rating task.
The similarity scores were analyzed using multidimensional scaling (MDS), a
technique that maps stimuli in a two-dimensional space such that stimuli that
are perceptually similar lie close together, and vice versa. The resulting maps
for English and Japanese listeners are shown in Figure 2.23b. The order of the
stimuli on each dimension matched the formant frequencies (F2 in the vertical
dimension and F3 in the horizontal dimension), but the two groups of listeners

---

[28] With one minor exception: One stimulus in the matrix was labeled as /wa/ by Japanese
listeners.

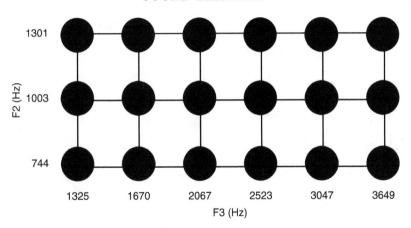

Figure 2.23a Schematic of stimulus grid used by Iverson et al. (2003) to explore the perception of "L" and "R" by American and Japanese listeners. F2 and F3 refer to the second and third speech formant, respectively. The frequencies of F2 and F3 are equally spaced on the mel scale (a psychoacoustic scale for pitch perception).

showed very different perceptual warpings of the acoustic space. Specifically, English speakers were most sensitive to F3 differences, which distinguished /l/ and /r/. In contrast, Japanese speakers were more sensitive to variation in F2. Thus the sound categories of the two languages had warped the perception of a common set of acoustic cues in very different ways.

The existence of such dramatic perceptual differences depending on native language naturally raises the question of how early in development one's native language begins to influence sound perception. In a classic set of studies, Janet Werker and her colleagues investigated the perception of native and non-native consonant contrasts by infant and adult listeners (Werker et al., 1981; Werker & Tees, 1984, 1999). They showed that prior to 6 months of age, Canadian infants could discriminate certain speech contrasts from foreign languages, such as the contrast between two subtly different forms of /t/ in Hindi, even though Canadian adults could not. However, this ability declined rapidly with age and was gone by 1 year of age. (In contrast, infants from Hindi-speaking households maintained this ability as they grew, as would be expected.) This demonstrated that the language-specific framework for sound perception was being formed long before the infants were competent speakers of their native language (cf. Kuhl et al., 1992, for work on vowels).

This work inspired subsequent studies on the perception of other nonnative contrasts. One important finding was that adults can retain the ability to distinguish subtle nonnative contrasts if they involve speech sounds that do not resemble anything in the native language. Specifically, Best et al. (1988) found that both American infants and adults could discriminate between click

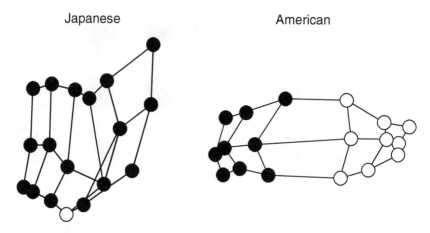

Figure 2.23b Representation of perceived similarity between tokens of the stimulus grid in Figure 2.23a, based on multidimensional scaling. See text for details. Black circles were identified as "R," and white circles were identified as "L" by the American listeners (the white circle in the Japanese data was identified as a "W").

sounds from Zulu, though they had no prior experience with these speech sounds. (Clicks are a rare type of phoneme found in Southern African languages, and are produced by creating suction in the mouth followed by an abrupt release of the tongue.) Findings such as these led to the question of why sensitivity declines from some nonnative contrasts but not others, and helped inspire a number of developmental linguistic models of speech perception (Kuhl, 1993; Best, 1994; Werker & Curtin, 2005). For example, in Best's Perceptual Assimilation Model (PAM), an adult's ability to hear a nonnative contrast depends on the relation of the contrasting phonemes to one's native sound system (cf. Best et al., 2001). If both phonemes assimilate equally well to a native category, discrimination is poor (e.g., Japanese perception of English /l/ vs. /r/). If they assimilate as good versus poor members of a native category, discrimination is better, and if they assimilate two different categories, discrimination is better still. The best discrimination is predicted when the nonnative phonemes fail to assimilate to any native speech sounds: This is the situation Best et al. suggest for the Zulu click study. (As will be discussed in the section on empirical comparative studies, Best and Avery, 1999, later provided intriguing evidence that these click sounds were heard as nonspeech by the English listeners.)

The work of Kuhl, Werker, Best, and their colleagues provides an important background for scientists interested in studying the development of learned sound categories in music. Their research invites parallel studies in the musical domain, as will be discussed further in section 2.4 on sound category learning.

Vowels: Brain Responses to Native Versus
Nonnative Contrasts

A useful tool for studying the structure of sound categories was introduced in section 2.2.3 (subsection "Pitch Intervals and Neuroscience"): the mismatch negativity (MMN). The logic of the MMN paradigm is easily adapted to studies of speech perception. Specifically, a common sound from the native language is presented at the standard, and then another speech sound is presented as the deviant. If the MMN is sensitive only to physical aspects of sounds, then the response to the deviant sound should depend only on its physical distance from the standard. If, however, the MMN shows sensitivity to the linguistic status of the deviant (i.e., a greater response when the deviant becomes a different phoneme in the language), then this is evidence that the brain is responding to sound change in terms of a mental framework of learned sound categories. Such evidence was provided by Näätänen et al. (1997), who studied the MMN to vowels in Finns and Estonians. The standard was a vowel (/e/) that occurred in both languages, and the deviants were four different vowels that ranged between /e/ and /o/ via manipulation of the second formant (F2). Three of these deviants corresponded to vowels used in both languages, but one deviant (/õ/) was a distinctive vowel only in Estonian (in Finnish, this sound simply fell between two other frequently used vowel sounds). Näätänen et al. recorded the MMN in Finns and Estonians to the different deviants, and found that only for the vowel /õ/ did the MMN differ between the two groups. Estonians showed a significantly larger MMN to this sound, suggesting that a learned sound category was modulating the brain response.

As with most MMN studies, the MMN in this study was collected without requiring any task from the participants, who read a book during the brain recordings. Thus the MMN reflects a preattentive response and provides a unique window on mental frameworks for sound perception. The findings of Näätänen et al. have been corroborated in other languages (cf. Näätänen & Winkler, 1999, Phillips et al., 2000, and Kazanina et al., 2006, for MMN research on consonants as sound categories). They have also led to a brain-based approach for studying the development of linguistic sound categories in infants (Cheour et al., 1998). As mentioned in section 2.2.3, the MMN is well suited to studying the development of musical sound categories, and offers a chance to study the development of both kinds of categories in parallel, using a common methodology.

2.4 Sound Category Learning as a Key Link

Our overview of musical and linguistic sound systems has shown that pitch and timbre are organized quite differently in the two domains. For example, ordinary speech does not contain stable pitch intervals, and musical sequences are rarely based on organized timbral contrasts. Thus comparing "like to like" can leave the impression that musical and linguistic sound systems have little in common. From the perspective of cognitive neuroscience, however, the real interest lies in a deeper similarity that lies beneath these surface differences, namely, that both systems depend on a mental framework of learned sound categories (cf. Handel, 1989). Indeed, the fact that the mind has found two entirely different ways of building organized sound category systems suggests that sound category learning is a fundamental aspect of human cognition. Thus a natural focus for comparative research on musical and linguistic sound systems is on the mechanisms that create and maintain learned sound categories. To what extent are these mechanisms shared between domains? One possibility is that these mechanisms have little in common. Indeed, evidence for cognitive and neural dissociations between musical and linguistic sound systems would seem to indicate that this is the case (reviewed in section 2.4.1 below). Another possibility is that music and language share mechanisms for sound category learning to an important degree (McMullen & Saffran, 2004). One might call this "shared sound category learning mechanism hypothesis (SSCLMH)." One implication of this hypothesis is that a clear conceptual distinction must be made between the end *products* of development, which may be domain specific, and developmental *processes,* which may be domain general.

In sections 2.4.2 and 2.4.3, I review studies which support the SSCLMH, focusing on pitch intervals and chords as musical sound categories and vowels and consonants as linguistic sound categories. Because this is a young area of comparative research, in section 2.4.5, I devote some time to pointing the way to future work aimed at exploring shared learning mechanisms. Before embarking on these sections, I first deal with apparent counterevidence in the following section, and show why this evidence is in fact not incompatible with the SSCLMH.

2.4.1 Background for Comparative Studies

There are good reasons to believe that the brain treats spoken and musical sound systems differently. First, focal cortical damage can lead to dramatic dissociations whereby the ability to interpret speech is profoundly impaired, yet the perception of musical sounds is intact, or vice versa (Poeppel, 2001; Peretz & Coltheart, 2003). Second, there is ample evidence from neuropsychology and neuroimaging that the two cerebral hemispheres have different biases in sound processing. Many musical pitch perception tasks show a greater dependence on right hemisphere circuits, whereas many linguistic phonemic tasks show a greater reliance on the left hemisphere (e.g., Zatorre et al., 1996, 2002; Stewart et al., 2006). Third, there are arguments for a "speech mode" of perception that contravenes normal principles of auditory perceptual organization (e.g., Liberman, 1996).

In fact, none of these findings contradicts the idea of shared mechanisms for the *learning* of sound categories in the two domains. I shall treat each finding in turn.

Dissociations

Dissociations for perceiving spoken versus musical sounds after brain damage simply indicate that sound category representations in the two domains, once learned, do not completely overlap in terms of their location in the brain. Whether or not similar mechanisms are used to create these representations is an orthogonal question.

An analogy might be helpful here. Imagine a factory that makes cars and motorcycles, and that keeps the finished vehicles in different rooms. It is possible that damage to the factory (such as a fire) could destroy just the rooms containing cars, or containing motorcycles, but this tells us nothing about the degree of overlap in the tools and processes used to make the two kinds of vehicles.

Given that the auditory system tends to break sounds down into their acoustic components and map these components in orderly ways, it seems likely that long-term representations of spoken and musical sounds will *not* occupy exactly the same regions of cortex. This could simply reflect the fact that the sound categories of speech and music tend to be different in acoustic terms (e.g., relying on timbre vs. pitch, respectively). In fact, studies aimed at localizing brain signals associated with the perception of phonetic versus musical sounds do report some separation (e.g., Tervaniemi et al., 1999, 2000; cf. Scott & Johnsrude, 2003). For example, Tervaniemi et al. (2006) had participants listen to a repeating speech sound (a two-syllable nonsense word) or a musical sound (saxophone tones) that were roughly matched in terms of duration, intensity, and spectral content. Brain scanning with fMRI revealed that both kinds of sounds produced strong activations in bilateral auditory cortex in the superior temporal gyrus (STG). However, as shown in Figure 2.24, speech sounds produced more activation in inferior and lateral areas of the STG than music sounds, which themselves produced more activation in the superior/medial surface of the STG and of Heschl's gyrus (which houses primary auditory cortex). This finding supports the idea that lesions with slightly different locations could selectively impair speech versus music perception.

Hemispheric Asymmetries

The idea that speech and music perception show left versus right hemispheric asymmetry in processing is an old and firmly entrenched idea in neuropsychology. Yet as we shall see, a closer examination of the evidence suggests that both language and music represent their sound categories *bilaterally* in auditory cortex.

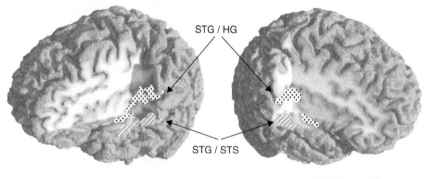

STG / HG

STG / STS

Speech > Music
Music > Speech

Figure 2.24 Brain regions showing significantly more activation during perception of speech versus musical sounds (diagonal lines) or vice versa (stippled dots). STG = superior temporal gyrus, HG = Heschl's gyrus (which contains primary auditory cortex), STS = superior temporal sulcus. From Tervaniemi et al., 2006.

It is well known that tasks that focus participants' attention on phoneme perception are associated with greater left-hemisphere activity in neuroimaging studies, often involving a network that spans left superior temporal auditory temporal cortex and left inferior frontal cortex (Zatorre et al., 1996). In contrast, many tasks involving musical pitch perception show a right hemisphere bias. Zatorre et al. (2002) suggest that this difference between speech and music is due to complementary anatomical and functional specializations of the two auditory cortices for processing the temporal versus spectral structure of sound (cf. Poeppel, 2003). According to this view, perception of the rapid but spectrally coarse timbral contrasts of speech relies more on left hemisphere circuits, whereas analysis of slower but more spectrally refined pitch contrasts of music relies more on right hemisphere circuits.

However, there is intriguing evidence from a variety of studies that hemispheric asymmetries in auditory perception are not just a function of the physical structure of sound. For example, Best and Avery (1999) examined brain lateralization in the perception of Zulu click contrasts by Zulu versus English speakers. Clicks represent a rapid acoustic transition (~ 50 ms), that predict a left hemisphere processing bias according to the theory described above. However, only the Zulu listeners exhibited such a bias. Best and Avery suggest that this was because the English listeners, who were completely unfamiliar with these rare speech sounds, did not process them as speech. In contrast, the Zulu listeners heard the clicks as sound categories from their language. Thus it seems that leftward asymmetries in speech sound processing may be influenced by a sound's status as a learned sound category in the language, and not just by its physical characteristics. Further evidence for this view comes from brain imaging research by Gandour et al. (2000) showing that the perception of tonal contrasts in Thai syllables activates left frontal cortex in Thai listeners (for whom the contrast was linguistically significant) but not in English and Chinese listeners. In other words, when pitch acts as a linguistically significant category, there is evidence for left rather than right hemisphere bias (cf. Wong et al., 2004; Carreiras et al., 2005).

What accounts for this leftward bias for the perception of speech sound categories? Hickok and Poeppel (2004) suggest that it is driven by the interface of two brain systems: a *bilateral* posterior system (in superior temporal auditory regions) involved in mapping phonetic sounds onto speech sound categories, and a *left-lateralized* frontal brain region involved in articulatory representations of speech. According to Hickok and Poeppel, the left hemisphere bias seen in various neural studies of speech perception (including the Zulu and Thai studies) occurs because the tasks given to participants lead them to map between their sound-based and articulatory-based representations of speech, for example, as part of explicitly segmenting words into phonemic components. These authors argue that under more natural perceptual circumstances, speech sounds would be processed bilaterally. In support of this idea, they point out that passive listening to speech is associated with bilateral activation of superior temporal cortex in brain imaging studies. Furthermore, cases of severe and selective difficulty with speech perception following brain damage ("pure word deafness") almost always involve bilateral lesions to the superior temporal lobe (Poeppel, 2001).

What of hemispheric asymmetries for music? When assessing the evidence for musical hemispheric asymmetries, it is crucial to specify exactly which aspect of music is being studied. For example, studies involving the analysis of melodic contour tend to show a right-hemisphere bias, whether the pitch patterns are musical or linguistic (e.g., Patel, Peretz, et al., 1998). However, if one is interested in the cortical representation of sound categories for music, then it is necessary to focus on the perception of categorized aspects of musical sound, such as pitch intervals. In this light, a study of Liégeois-Chauvel et al. (1998) is particularly interesting. They examined music perception in 65 patients who had undergone unilateral temporal lobe cortical excisions for the relief of epilepsy. They found that excisions to *both* hemispheres impaired the use of pitch interval information, whereas only right hemisphere excisions impaired the use of pitch contour information (cf. Boemio et al., 2005). Thus the learned sound categories of musical intervals appear to have a bilateral representation in the brain, analogous to the bilateral representation of speech sound categories argued for by Hickok and Poeppel.

In summary, hemispheric asymmetries for speech and music perception certainly exist, but are more subtle than generally appreciated. Nothing we know about these asymmetries contradicts the idea of shared learning mechanisms for sound categories in the two domains.

A "Speech Mode" of Perception

The idea of special cognitive and neural mechanisms for speech perception has long been a refrain in speech research, ever since the discovery of categorical perception for phoneme contrasts (Liberman et al., 1957, 1967; cf. Eimas et al., 1971). What is at issue is not semantic or syntactic processing, but the basic mapping between sounds and linguistic categories. The demonstration by Kuhl and Miller (1975) of categorical perception for stop consonants in a South American rodent (the chinchilla) was influential evidence against the "specialized mechanisms" view, though it by no means settled the debate (cf. Pastore et al., 1983; Kluender et al., 1987; Hall & Pastore, 1992; Trout, 2003; Diehl et al., 2004). There are still strong proponents of the idea that we listen to speech using different mechanisms than those used for other sounds (Liberman, 1996).

One of the most dramatic forms of evidence for a special mode of speech perception comes from studies of "sine-wave speech" (Remez et al., 1981). Sine-wave speech is created by tracing the center frequencies of speech formants from a spectrogram (such as in Figure 2.21), and then synthesizing a sine wave for each formant that exactly reproduces the formant's pattern of frequency change over time. Sine-wave speech based on the first two or three speech formants (F1, F2, and F3) can sound like meaningless streams of frequency variation to a listener who is unfamiliar with this stimulus. However, once primed to hear the stimulus as speech, listeners experience a dramatic perceptual shift and the seemingly aimless series of frequency glides becomes integrated into a coherent speech percept. (Sound Examples 2.8a–b illustrate this phenomenon. Listen to 2.8a, then 2.8b, and then 2.8a again.)[29] That is, the listener fuses the multiple frequencies into a single stream of consonants and vowels that make up intelligible words (though the "voice" is still inhuman and electronic-sounding). For those who have experienced it, this shift is compelling evidence that there is a special mode of auditory processing associated with hearing sound patterns as speech. Remez et al. (1994) have presented data suggesting that the perception of sine-wave speech violates Gestalt principles of auditory grouping, and argue for the independence of phonetic versus auditory organizational principles.

---

[29] I am grateful to Matt Davis for providing these examples, which are based on three-formant sine-wave speech, in which the amplitude profile of each formant (low-pass filtered at 50 Hz) is used to amplitude-modulate the sine waves (Davis & Johnsrude, 2007).

Although the research of Remez and colleagues provides fascinating evidence for a "speech mode" of perception, there is no logical contradiction between the existence of such a mode and shared processing mechanisms for *developing* learned sound categories in speech and music. That is, the phenomenon of sine-wave speech (turning acoustic patterns into phonemic ones) assumes that sound categories for speech have already developed. What is remarkable about the phenomenon is that the same auditory signal can either activate the representations of these categories or not, depending on the listener's expectations.[30] Thus there is no reason why the same mechanisms that helped form phonemic categories in language could not also serve the formation of pitch interval categories in music. (If this idea is correct, there may be an analog of sine-wave speech for music, i.e., a signal that sounds like one or more aimless streams of gliding pitch variation until one is primed to hear it as music, in which case the sound is interpreted as coherent sequence of musical sound categories; cf. Demany & McAnally, 1994.)

Summary of Background for Comparative Studies

The fact that musical and linguistic sound categories are acoustically distinct and neurally dissociable in the adult brain does not logically demand that their development is based on domain-specific learning processes. In fact, from a cognitive perspective, the notion of shared learning mechanisms makes sense, because a similar problem must be solved in both cases. Recall that the sounds of music and speech are not realized in a precise, Platonic fashion. For example, the "same" pitch interval can vary in size both due to chance variation and to the influence of local melodic context (cf. section 2.2.3). Similarly, different tokens of a given consonant or vowel vary in their acoustic structure depending on phonetic context, even in the speech of a single person. Listeners thus need

---

[30] Those interested in the idea of linguistic versus nonlinguistic modes of perception may find it interesting to consider a phenomenon in certain West African drum ensembles. In such ensembles, the sounds of many drums intertwine, creating a polyrhythmic texture with a unique sound (Locke, 1990). These patterns are nonlinguistic, yet from time to time the lead drummer may use his drum to send a linguistic message by imitating the rhythms and tones of the local language (i.e., a talking drum message; cf. section 2.3.2, subsection "Mapping Linguistic Tone Contrasts Onto Musical Instruments"). Listeners who know the drum language will perceive this as a linguistic message. This raises a number of interesting questions: How does the perception of drum sounds as language interact with their perception as musical sounds? What patterns of activity would be observed in the brain of a person who is listening to nonlinguistic drumming and hears (and understands) an embedded drummed linguistic message, versus in the brain of another listener who hears the same talking drum but does not understand it as language?

to develop a mental framework that allows them to extract a small number of meaningful categories from acoustically variable signals. In the next two subsections, I discuss studies that suggest that the development of sound categories engages processes shared by speech and music.

2.4.2 Relations Between Musical Ability and Linguistic Phonological Abilities

If there are shared mechanisms for learning the sound categories of speech and music, then individual variation in the efficacy of these mechanisms should influence both domains. That is, an individual's ability to learn sound categories in one domain should have some predictive power with regard to sound category learning in the other domain. Recent empirical research on children and adults supports this prediction, because it finds that pitch-related musical abilities predict phonological skills in language.

Anvari et al. (2002) studied the relation between early reading skills and musical development in a large sample of English-speaking 4- and 5-year-olds (50 children per group). Learning to read English requires mapping visual symbols onto phonemic contrasts, and thus taps into linguistic sound categorization skills. The children were given an extensive battery of tasks that included tests of reading, phonemic awareness, vocabulary, auditory memory, and mathematics. (Phonemic awareness refers to the ability to identify the sound components of a word, and a large body of research indicates that children with greater phonemic awareness have advantages in learning to read.) On the musical side, both musical pitch and rhythm discrimination were tested. The pitch tasks included same/different discrimination of short melodies and chords, and the rhythm tasks involved same/different discrimination of short rhythmic patterns and reproduction of rhythms by singing. The most interesting findings concerned the 5-year-olds. For this group, performance on musical pitch (but not rhythm) tasks predicted unique variance in reading abilities, even when phonemic awareness was controlled for. Furthermore, statistical analysis showed that this relation could not be accounted for via the indirect influence of other variables such as auditory memory. Such a finding is consistent with the idea of shared learning processes for linguistic and musical sound categories. Individual variation in the efficacy of these processes could be due to internal factors or to environmental conditions that influence the quality of auditory input (cf. Chang & Merzenich, 2003).

Turning to research on adults, Slevc and Miyake (2006) examined the relationship between proficiency in a second language (L2) and musical ability. In contrast to previous studies on this topic, Slevc and Miyake measured both linguistic and musical skills in a quantitative fashion, and also measured other potentially confounding variables. Working with a group of 50 Japanese adult learners of English living in the United States, they administered language tests that examined receptive and productive phonology, syntax, and lexical knowledge. (The tests of receptive phonology included identifying words that differed by a single phoneme, e.g., "clown" vs. "crown.") The musical tests examined pitch pattern perception, for example, via the detection of an altered note in a chord or in a short melody, as well as accuracy in singing back short melodies. Crucially, they also measured other variables associated with second-language proficiency, such as age of arrival in the foreign country, number of years spent living there, amount of time spent speaking the second language, and phonological short-term memory in the native language. The question of interest was whether musical ability could account for variance in L2 ability beyond that accounted for by these other variables. As in Anvari et al. (2002), the authors used hierarchical regression to tease apart the influence of different variables. The results were clear: Musical ability did in fact predict unique variance in L2 skills. Most relevant for the current discussion, this predictive relationship was confined to L2 receptive and productive phonology, in other words, to that aspect of language most directly related to sound categorization skills in perception.

The studies of Anvari et al. and Slevc and Miyake are notable because they suggest a specific link between sound categorization skills in speech and music, consistent with the idea of shared mechanisms for sound category formation in the two domains. However, their musical tasks were not specifically designed to test sensitivity to musical sound categories and there is thus a need for more refined studies along these lines. One way to do this would be to test sensitivity to pitch intervals, for example, via discrimination of melodies with the same melodic contour but different interval patterns, using transposition to eliminate absolute pitch as a possible cue (cf. Trainor, Tsang, & Cheung, 2002).[31] It would also be desirable to test low-level auditory processing skills (such as temporal resolution and pitch change discrimination), to determine whether sound categorization skills in the two domains are predicted by raw auditory sensitivity (cf. Ramus, 2003, 2006; Rosen, 2003). For example, Wong et al. (2007) have recently found evidence that musical training sharpens the subcortical sensory encoding of linguistic pitch patterns (cf. Overy, 2003; Tallal & Gaab, 2006; Patel & Iversen, 2007).

If there is overlap in the mechanisms that the brain uses to convert sound waves into discrete sound categories in speech and music, then it is conceivable that exercising these mechanisms with sounds from one domain could enhance the ability of these mechanisms to acquire sound categories in the other domain.

---

[31] In performing such tests, it is important to use culturally familiar scales, because one is focusing on learned sound categories in music. Studies using arbitrary, mathematically defined scales are difficult to interpret for this reason (e.g., Foxton et al., 2003).

One way to investigate this question is to ask whether extensive exposure to instrumental music in infants influences language development, especially with regard to the acquisition of phonemic categories (J. Saffran, personal communication). If so, such a finding would have considerable practical significance.

2.4.3 Sound Category–Based Distortions of Auditory Perception

Our perception of the differences between speech sounds (or musical sounds) is not a simple reflection of their raw acoustic differences, but is influenced by their relationship to our learned sound category system (cf. sections 2.2.3 and 2.3.4). Although most early work on the influence of speech categories on auditory perception focused on categorical perception, more recent research has focused on a different phenomenon known as the perceptual magnet effect (PME). The importance of the PME to the current discussion is that it is thought to be driven by a domain-general learning mechanism, in other words, distribution-based learning based on the statistics of the input (Kuhl et al., 1992; Guenther & Gjaja, 1996). Thus if linguistic and musical sound category learning involve shared mechanisms, the PME should be observed in music as well as in speech. This is in fact the case, as described below. First, however, I provide some background on the PME for those unfamiliar with this phenomenon.

The PME is concerned with perception *within* sound categories rather than with perception of contrasts between sound categories, and was first described by Kuhl in the context of vowel perception (1991). Kuhl synthesized a range of vowel stimuli, all intended to be variants of the vowel /i/ (variants differed in the frequency of the first and second formants, F1 and F2). She asked listeners to rate these stimuli as good versus poor exemplars of /i/ using a 7-point scale. The results showed that there was a certain location in (F1,F2) space where vowels received the highest rating. Kuhl chose the highest-rated vowel as the "prototype" (P) vowel. A vowel with a low goodness rating in a different region of (F1,F2) space was designated the "nonprototype" (NP). In a subsequent perception experiment, listeners heard either P or NP repeating as a background stimulus, and had to indicate when this sound changed to another version of /i/. The basic finding was that listeners were *less* sensitive to sound change when the prototype served as the standard, as if the prototype was acting like a perceptual "magnet" that warped the space around it. Kuhl found that infants also showed this effect (though to a lesser extent than adults) but that rhesus monkeys did not, suggesting that this effect might be unique to speech. Subsequent work by other Kuhl and others questioned and refined the concept of the PME, and introduced a number of methodological improvements (Lively & Pisoni, 1997; Iverson & Kuhl, 2000).

The PME has proved somewhat contentious in speech research (e.g., Lotto et al., 1998; Guenther, 2000), but the basic effect seems to be robust when

experimental conditions are appropriate (Hawkins & Barrett-Jones, in preparation). Before turning to musical studies of the PME, several points should be
mentioned. First, the term "prototype" should not be taken to imply a preexisting Platonic category in the mind, but can be thought of as a point of central
tendency in a distribution of exemplars. Second, the distribution of exemplars
is itself subject to contextual effects such as the speaker's gender, age, speaking
rate, and phonetic context, for which listeners may normalize (see section 2.3.3,
subsection "Timbral Contrasts Among Vowels"). Finally, and most importantly
for our current purposes, the PME differs from traditional work on categorical
perception in its emphasis on distribution-based statistical learning.

Acker et al. (1995) first tested the PME in music, using chords instead of
vowels. Chords are collections of simultaneous pitches, and serve a particularly important role in Western tonal music, as will be discussed in Chapter 5.
For the current purposes, one can think of a chord as loosely analogous to a
vowel: a complex of frequencies that acts as a perceptual unit. Acker et al. used
the C major triad of Western music (C-E-G), constructing prototypical and
nonprototypical versions of this chord by varying the tuning of the constituent tones E and G. When asked to perform discrimination tasks in which a
prototypical versus nonprototypical (slightly mistuned) version of the C major
triad served as the reference, listeners performed *better* in the vicinity of the
prototype, precisely the opposite of what was found in language. Acker et al.
therefore suggested that in music, category prototypes acted as anchors rather
than magnets.

Based on this work, it appeared that the PME might not apply to music.
However, subsequent research has shown that the results of Acker et al. may
not be representative of most listeners. This is because these researchers had
only studied musically trained subjects. More recently, Barrett (1997, 2000)
performed a similar study, but included both musicians and nonmusicians. She
replicated the earlier results for musicians, but found that nonmusicians showed
worse discrimination in the vicinity of the category prototype, in other words,
the classic perceptual magnet effect. How could this be explained?

Barrett proposed an interesting solution to this puzzle. She argued that musicians are trained to pay good deal of attention to sounds in the vicinity of
prototypes in order to tune their instruments. Nonmusicians, in contrast, are
well served if they can simply distinguish one chord from another, and likely
pay little attention to the precise tuning of chords. Barrett hypothesized that in
general, listeners expend no more energy than necessary in focusing their attention on acoustic details within a category.[32] Barrett proposed that differences

---

[32] Interestingly, this idea was inspired by a theory from speech production research,
namely that speakers expend no more energy than necessary in making acoustic contrasts, given the needs of their listener (Lindblom, 1990).

in attention to prototypes result in prototypical chords acting as "perceptual repellors" for musicians and "perceptual attractors" for nonmusicians. She thus refined the notion of a "perceptual magnet" and proposed that aspects of the *listener* determine whether a magnet acts as an attractor or a repellor.

In this light, recent research on the PME in nonlinguistic sounds has proved particularly interesting. Guenther et al. (1999) conducted a study in which listeners heard narrow-band filtered white noise with different center frequencies. One group received categorization training, in which they learned to identify stimuli in a certain frequency region as members of a single category. The other group received discrimination training, and practiced telling stimuli in this region apart (with feedback). When the two groups were tested on a subsequent discrimination task, the categorization group showed a reduction in their ability to discriminate stimuli in the training region versus in a control region, in other words, a PME. In contrast, the discrimination group showed the reverse effect. In subsequent research, Guenther and colleagues have combined neural network models of auditory cortex with fMRI studies in order to probe the neural mechanisms of the PME. Based on this work, they have suggested that a clumped distribution of exemplars, combined with a drive to sort stimuli into perceptually relevant categories, result in changes to auditory cortical maps such that prototypes to have smaller representations than nonprototypes (Guenther et al., 2004). According to this model, prototypes are more difficult to discriminate from neighboring tokens simply because they are represented by fewer cortical cells. Importantly, the researchers see this as a domain general mechanism for learning sound categories, an idea supported by their work with nonspeech stimuli.

In summary, comparative PME research supports the notion of domain-general developmental mechanisms for sound category perception, and illustrates how our understanding of sound categorization processes can benefit from research that flows seamlessly across linguistic and musical auditory processing.

2.4.4 Decay in Sensitivity to Nonnative Sound Categories

A well-established idea in research on speech is that the perceptual sensitivities of an infant become tuned to the native sound system. Recall from section 2.3.4 (subsection on consonants) that infants are initially sensitive to many subtle phonetic contrasts, including those that do not occur in their native language. Early in life they lose sensitivity to nonnative contrasts as they learn the sounds of their native language. In other words, the infant goes from being a "citizen of the world" to being a member of a specific culture.

Is a similar pattern observed in musical development? If so, this could suggest common mechanisms for sound category learning in the two domains. In fact, there is one study that seems to indicate a similar developmental process in music. However, there are problems with this study. I review the study here because it is often cited as support for the notion that musical development involves a decay in sensitivities to nonnative pitch intervals, when in fact this has yet to be clearly demonstrated.

Lynch et al. (1990) studied the ability of American infants and adults to detect mistunings in melodies based on culturally familiar versus unfamiliar musical scales/intervals. The familiar scales were the Western major and minor scales, and the unfamiliar scale was the Javanese pelog scale, which contains different intervals. A 7-note melody based on a given scale was played repeatedly, and on some repetitions the 5th note (the highest note in the melody) was mistuned by raising its frequency. Infants and adults were compared on their ability to detect these changes. In a finding reminiscent of classic work on speech perception (Werker & Tees, 1984), infants showed equally good discrimination with the familiar and unfamiliar scale, whereas adult nonmusicians showed better performance on the familiar scales.

However, subsequent research by Lynch and others changed the picture. Using a different version of their testing paradigm in which the mistuning was randomly located rather than always on the same note, Lynch and Eilers (1992) found that 6-month-old Western babies did in fact show a processing advantage for the culturally familiar scale, a finding that was replicated a few years later (Lynch et al., 1995). They speculated that this increase in task demands may have uncovered an innate processing advantage for the simpler frequency ratios found in the Western versus Javanese scales.

It should be noted that the findings of Lynch and colleagues are tempered by a particular methodological choice that may have influenced their results. In the studies described above, the repeating background melody always occurred at the same absolute pitch level. This choice has been criticized by other researchers (Trainor & Trehub, 1992), who point out that only when the background melody is continuously transposed can one be sure that discrimination is really based on sensitivity to intervals, and not on absolute frequencies.

Thus although the Lynch et al. studies were pioneering in aiming to do comparable research on the development of pitch categories in music and phonological categories in speech, well-controlled studies of this issue have yet to be done. The following section suggests a specific direction that such studies might take.

2.4.5 Exploring a Common Mechanism for Sound Category Learning

Sections 2.4.2 and 2.4.3 above reviewed evidence consistent with the hypothesis that music and language share mechanisms for the formation of learned sound categories (the "shared sound category learning mechanism hypothesis," or SSCLMH; cf. section 2.4.1). One such mechanism was already alluded to in section 2.4.3 when discussing the perceptual magnet effect. This is statistical learning, which involves tracking patterns in the environment and acquiring implicit knowledge of their statistical properties, without any direct feedback. That is, statistical learning is driven by distributional information in the input rather than by explicit tutoring.

Statistical learning is a good candidate for a sound category learning mechanism shared by speech and music. Statistical learning has already been demonstrated for other aspects of language learning, such as segmentation of word boundaries from sequences of syllables (Saffran et al., 1996). Furthermore, empirical work suggests that statistical learning plays a role in various aspects of music perception, ranging from the creation of tonal hierarchies (cf. Chapter 5) to the shaping of melodic expectations (e.g., Krumhansl, 1990, 2000; Oram & Cuddy, 1995; Cohen, 2000; Huron, 2006). The question, then, is how one would go about exploring whether music and speech both rely on statistical learning in the development of sound categories.

One idea for comparative research is to build on existing findings regarding the role of statistical learning of speech sound categories. It is well established that experience with a native language influences phonetic discrimination (cf. section 2.3.4). For example, over time infants lose sensitivity to certain phonetic contrasts that do not occur in their language, and gain sensitivity for other, difficult phonetic contrasts in their native tongue (Polka et al., 2001; cf. Kuhl et al., in press). Recently there has been growing interest in the mechanisms that account for these perceptual changes. Maye et al. (2002, 2003, in press) have addressed this issue via speech perception studies with infants and adults. In these studies, two sets of participants are exposed to different distributions of the same set of speech tokens, and then tested for their ability to discriminate between specific tokens from this set. Two such distributions are illustrated in Figure 2.25.

The x-axis of the figure shows the acoustic continuum along which speech stimuli are organized, namely, voice onset time (VOT, the time between the release of a consonant and the onset of vibration of the vocal folds). In this case, the stimuli form a continuum between a prevoiced /da/ on the left edge and a short-lag /ta/ on the right end. One group of participants heard tokens that followed a bimodal distribution (dotted line), whereas the other heard a unimodal distribution (solid line).

The key aspect of this design is that there are tokens that occur with equal frequency in the two distributions (e.g., the tokens with VOT = −50 and 7 ms, in other words, tokens 3 and 6 counting from the left edge of the x-axis). The question of interest is whether the ability to discriminate these tokens depends on the distribution in which they are embedded. Maye and Weiss (2003) addressed this question with 8-month-old infants. The researchers found that only infants exposed to the bimodal distribution showed evidence of discriminating tokens 3 and 6, whereas infants exposed to the unimodal distribution (and

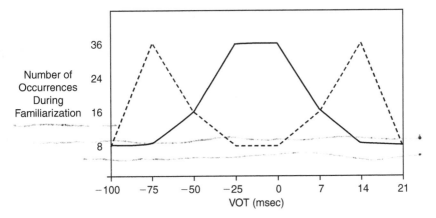

Figure 2.25 Distribution of stimuli along an acoustic continuum from /da/ to /ta/. One group of infants heard stimuli from a bimodal distribution (dashed line), whereas another group heard stimuli from a unimodal distribution (solid line). Importantly, both groups heard tokens 3 and 6 (–50 ms and 7 ms VOT, respectively) equally often.

a control group with no exposure) did not discriminate these tokens. Importantly, the amount of exposure prior to test was small, less than 3 minutes. This converges with other research showing that statistical learning is a remarkably rapid, powerful learning mechanism (e.g., Saffran et al., 1996).

It would be a straightforward matter to construct an experiment similar to this using musical materials, such as an interval that varied between a major third and a minor third in terms of pitch steps. (Alternatively, one could use two intervals that do not occur in Western music, if one wanted to avoid culturally familiar materials.) As a practical issue, it will be of interest to see whether neural measures (such as the mismatch negativity; cf. sections 2.2.3 and 2.3.4, subsections on brain responses) can complement behavioral techniques as assays of discrimination, because the former may ultimately prove easier to collect from infants (cf. Trainor et al., 2003; McMullen & Saffran, 2004; Kuhl et al., in press).

Taking a step back, comparative studies of sound category formation in speech and music are worth pursuing because they can identify general principles by which the brain creates and maintains sound categories. Furthermore, comparative work can help address the emerging idea that the mental framework for sound perception is not a frozen thing in the mind, but is adaptive and is constantly tuning itself (Kraljic & Samuel, 2005; Luce & McLennan, 2005; McQueen et al., 2006). This perspective is in line with the observation of substantial individual variation in perception of nonnative speech contrasts (Best et al., 2001), and a large degree of individual variation in musical sound categories, even among trained musicians (e.g., Perlman & Krumhansl, 1996, and references therein).

2.5 Conclusion

Linguistic and musical sound systems illustrate a common theme in the study of music-language relations. On the surface, the two domains are dramatically different. Music uses pitch in ways that speech does not, and speech organizes timbre to a degree seldom seen in music. Yet beneath these differences lie deep connections in terms of cognitive and neural processing. Most notably, in both domains the mind interacts with one particular aspect of sound (pitch in music, and timbre in speech) to create a perceptually discretized system. Importantly, this perceptual discretization is not an automatic byproduct of human auditory perception. For example, linguistic and musical sequences present the ear with continuous variations in amplitude, yet loudness is not perceived in terms of discrete categories. Instead, the perceptual discretization of musical pitch and linguistic timbre reflects the activity of a powerful cognitive system, built to separate within-category sonic variation from differences that indicate a change in sound category. Although music and speech differ in the primary acoustic feature used for sound category formation, it appears that the mechanisms that create and maintain learned sound categories in the two domains may have a substantial degree of overlap. Such overlap has implications for both practical and theoretical issues surrounding human communicative development.

In the 20th century, relations between spoken and musical sound systems were largely explored by artists. For example, the boundary between the domains played an important role in innovative works such as Schoenberg's *Pierrot Lunaire* and Reich's *Different Trains* (cf. Risset, 1991). In the 21st century, science is finally beginning to catch up, as relations between spoken and musical sound systems prove themselves to be a fruitful domain for research in cognitive neuroscience. Such work has already begun to yield new insights into our species' uniquely powerful communicative abilities.

Appendix 1: Some Notes on Pitch

This is an appendix for section 2.2.2.

Pitch is one of the most salient perceptual aspects of a sound, defined as "that property of a sound that enables it to be ordered on a scale going from low to high" (Acoustical Society of America Standard Acoustical Terminology; cf. Randel, 1978). The physical correlate of pitch is frequency (in cycles per second, or Hertz), and in a constant-frequency pure tone, the pitch is essentially equal to the frequency of the tone. (A pure tone contains a single frequency, as in a sinusoidal sound wave. Apart from frequency, duration and amplitude play a small role in the pitch of pure tones.)

In the case of periodic sounds made from a fundamental frequency and a series of upper harmonics that are integer multiples of this fundamental (such as the sound of a clarinet or of the human voice uttering a vowel), the pitch corresponds to the fundamental frequency. In sounds with a more complex spectral structure, pitch is not always a simple reflection of the physical frequency structure of the sound. This is illustrated by the phenomenon of the "missing fundamental," in which the perceived pitch is lower than any of the frequency components of the sound.

The complex nature of pitch perception was driven home to me when a colleague and I were conducting neural experiments on the perception of tones with three frequency components: 650, 950, and 1250 Hz. We asked participants in our study to identify the perceived pitch of this composite tone by adjusting a pure tone until it matched the pitch of the composite. To our surprise, some of the subjects place the pure tone at exactly 650 Hz, whereas others placed it much lower near 325 Hz (a "missing fundamental"). Both groups of subjects were utterly confident of their judgment, and measurements of their brain activity showed differences between those who heard the missing fundamental and those who did not. This illustrates how perceived pitch is not determined by the physical makeup of a sound, but is a perceptual construct (Patel & Balaban, 2001).

Pitch perception has become a subfield of research in its own right, and is an active area in which psychologists, neuroscientists, and engineers regularly interact (Shamma & Klein, 2000; Moore, 2001; Plack et al., 2005).

Appendix 2: Semitone Equations

This is an appendix for section 2.2.2, subsection "Introduction to Musical Scales."

The exact size of a semitone (st) can be computed as:

$$1 \text{ st} = 2^{(1/12)} \approx 1.0595$$

In this equation, the 2 represents the doubling of frequency in one octave, and the 1/12 represents a division of this frequency range into 12 equal-sized steps on the basis of pitch ratios.

Because the semitone is a ratio-based measure, the ratio between any two frequencies $F1$ and $F2$ (in Hz) can be expressed in semitones as:

$$st = 12 \times \log_2(F1/F2).$$

To compute this same interval in cents (c):

$$c = 1{,}200 \times \log_2(F1/F2)$$

To convert a distance of X semitones between two frequencies $F1$ and $F2$ into a frequency ratio R:

$$R = 2^{(X/12)}$$

Appendix 3: Theories for the Special Perceptual Qualities of Different Pitch Intervals

This is an appendix for section 2.2.2, subsection "Introduction to Musical Scales."

In order to get a flavor for theories that posit a special perceptual status for certain pitch intervals, we will focus largely on one interval: the musical fifth. After the octave, the fifth is the most important interval in Western music, and also serves as an important interval in a wide range of other musical traditions, ranging from large musical cultures in India and China to the music of small tribes in the islands of Oceania (Jairazbhoy, 1995; Koon, 1979, Zemp, 1981). Some of the explanations for the special status of the fifth are given below.

A.3.1 Sensory Consonance and Dissonance as the Basis for Musical Intervals

One idea for the special status of certain intervals (such as the fifth) dates back to Hermann von Helmholtz (1885), and is related to the interaction of different frequency components of a sound. It has long been known that when two pure tones close in frequency are sounded simultaneously (for example, A3 and A#3, or 220 Hz and 233.08 Hz), the result is a composite tone with amplitude fluctuation (or "beating") due to the physical interference of the two sound waves. As the frequencies are moved apart, this physical interference begins to subside, but there is still a sensation of roughness due to the fact that the two tones are not fully resolved by the auditory system. That is, within the auditory system the two tones lie within a "critical band," exciting similar portions of the basilar membrane (the membrane that helps resolve sounds into their frequency components as part of sending auditory signals to the brain). Once the tones are no longer within the same critical band (approximately 3 semitones), the sensation of roughness disappears.

Generalizing this idea, if one plays two complex tones simultaneously, each of which consists of a fundamental and its harmonics, the harmonics of Tone 1 that lie close to the harmonics of Tone 2 will interact with them to create roughness. The sensory consonance/dissonance theory of musical intervals predicts that the overall dissonance of two simultaneous complex tones is equal to the sum of the roughness produced by each pair of interacting harmonics. According to this theory, the octave is maximally consonant because the fundamental and all the harmonics of the upper tone line up exactly with harmonics of the lower (Figure A.1), and the fifth is the next most consonant interval because the frequency components of the upper tone either line up

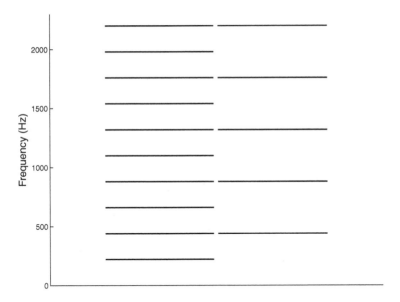

Figure A.1 Alignment of frequency partials of two harmonic tones whose fundamentals are one octave apart: A3 (left column, fundamental frequency of 220 Hz) and A4 (right column, fundamental frequency of 440 Hz).

with the harmonics of the lower or fall far enough between them to avoid interaction (Figure A.2).

In contrast, the minor second (an interval of 1 semitone) is highly dissonant because several of the harmonics of the two tones lie close enough to each other in frequency to create roughness (Figure A.3).

One appealing aspect of this theory is that it can provide a quantitative ranking of perceived consonance of different musical intervals between complex harmonic tones, and this prediction can be tested against perceptual data in which listeners rate consonance or dissonance of these same intervals (Plomp & Levelt, 1965; Kameoka & Kuriyagawa, 1969a,b). For example, the theory predicts high consonance for the fifth and fourth and low consonance/high dissonance for the minor second (a one semitone interval) and major seventh (an 11 semitone interval), predictions that accord well with intuition and experiment.

It should be noted that research on sensory consonance and dissonance has had its shortcomings. One such shortcoming is that the task given to listeners in judging tone pairs often confounds aesthetic and sensory qualities of a stimulus. Participants are often asked to judge "how pleasing" or "agreeable"

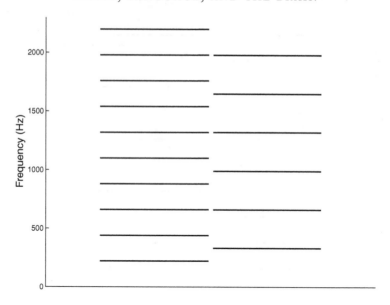

Figure A.2 Alignment of frequency partials of two harmonic tones whose fundamentals are a fifth (seven semitones) apart: A3 (left column, fundamental frequency of 220 Hz) and E4 (right column, fundamental frequency of ~ 330 Hz).

a given interval is, with the assumption that intervals that are more consonant are more pleasing. In fact, there may be individual differences in the degree to which people prefer consonant or dissonant intervals. It is known, for example, that there are cultures in which rough-sounding intervals such as the second are considered highly pleasing, as in certain types of polyphonic vocal music in Bulgaria. Presumably Bulgarian listeners hear these small intervals as rough, but they find this attractive rather than unattractive (cf. Vassilakis, 2005). Thus in their instructions to listeners, researchers need to clearly distinguish sensory attributes of roughness or smoothness from aesthetic judgment about these qualities, or else risk confounding two different sources of variability in individual responses. (An analogy can be made to the perception of flavor in food. Some cultures find spicy food distasteful, whereas others find it attractive. Thus in a taste test with spicy foods, one needs to be clear about whether one is asking the taster to rate how "pleasant" they find the food versus how "spicy" they find it. Both cultures will likely agree on which foods are spicy, but may disagree on whether this is appealing or not.) Another weakness of this research is that the predictions of the model, which should be culture-independent, have been tested only against data collected in contexts in which Western European music is widely heard (Germany, Japan, and the United States). Thus newer

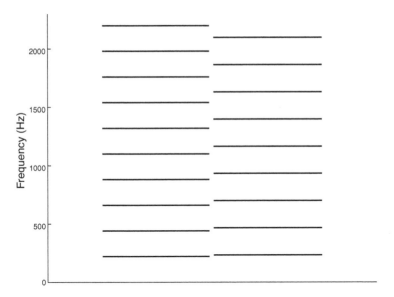

Figure A.3 Alignment of frequency partials of two harmonic tones whose fundamentals are a minor second (one semitone) apart: A3 (left column, fundamental frequency of 220 Hz) and A♯3 (right column, fundamental frequency of ~ 233 Hz).

data, collected in a standardized way in variety of cultural contexts, is needed to test the model adequately.

A.3.2 Pitch Relationships as the Basis for Musical Intervals

In the sensory consonance/dissonance theory of intervals described above, the special status of the fifth is its perceptual smoothness, which is second only to the octave. But what is smoothness? A lack of roughness. Thus the theory is ultimately framed in negative terms. An alternative idea for the prevalence of the fifth is based on the idea that this interval has a positive quality that makes it attractive. One recent theory along these lines focuses on patterns of neural activity in the auditory nerve, and in particular the temporal structure of neural impulses that result from different combinations of tones. Tramo et al. (2003) have presented data suggesting that the fifth generates a neural pattern that invokes not only the pitches of the lower and upper notes of the interval, but also a pitch one octave below the lower note, and other harmonically related notes. In contrast, the neural pattern to dissonant intervals such as the minor second does not suggest any clear pitches (cf. Cariani, 2004).

One might call this the "pitch-relationship theory" of musical intervals (cf. Parncutt, 1989). According to this theory, the fifth is special because it projects a clear sense of multiple, related pitches, including the "missing fundamental" that lies an octave below the lower note.[33] Of course, to distinguish it from the sensory consonance/dissonance theory, it is necessary to examine other intervals in which the two theories make different predictions. To date, no such direct comparison has been made. A direct comparison might be possible using the perception of three simultaneous tones (triadic chords) that have perceptually distinct qualities. For example, the major triad (e.g., C-E-G, three tones separated by intervals of 4 and 3 st) is considered far more consonant and stable than the augmented triad (e.g., C-E-G♯, three tones separated by intervals of 4 and 4 st). This difference is not predicted on the basis of interacting frequency partials (Parncutt, 1989; Cook, 2002), and may be better accounted for by the pitch-relationship theory (cf. Cook & Fujisawa, 2006).

A.3.3 The Overtone Series as the Basis for Musical Intervals

Many complex periodic sounds, including the sounds made by vibrating strings and by the human vocal folds, have a harmonic structure, consisting of a discrete set of frequencies ("partials") with one lowest frequency (the fundamental) accompanied by a set of upper partials that are integer multiples of this fundamental frequency (harmonics of the fundamental). Consider a harmonic sound with a fundamental frequency of 100 Hz. The harmonics will be 200 Hz, 300 Hz, 400 Hz, and so on. Taking the frequency ratios between successive frequencies gives 1:2, 2:3, 3:4, and so on. Thus the intervals of the octave, fifth, fourth, and so on are in every harmonic sound encountered by the auditory system.

This observation has often been used to claim a natural basis for the intervals that constitute the Western major scale, with the implicit assumption that the order in which the intervals occurs in the harmonic series is related to the perceived consonance of tone combinations with those frequency ratios. The exact form that this argument has taken has varied over time, with different people emphasizing different sources of harmonic sounds. Some have focused on vibrating strings (Bernstein, 1976), with the implication that musical intervals are a fact of nature, whereas others have focused on the voice (Terhardt, 1984), with the implication that appreciation of these intervals arises through exposure to the harmonic structure of speech. In one recent variant of the "argument from speech" (Schwartz et al., 2003), researchers have studied the frequency structure of running speech and found that the frequency partial with the most energy in the voice is often not the fundamental (frequency partial #1), but partial #2 or #4.

---

[33] Because the ratio of the upper to lower note in a musical fifth is 3:2, the missing fundamental is half the frequency of the lower note, giving a ratio of 3:2:1.

Like all even-numbered partials, these two partials have an upper partial that is 3/2 their frequency (for example, partial #6 is always 3/2 the frequency of partial #4). Thus the researchers were able to show empirically that the frequency with the strongest energy peak in the speech spectrum is often accompanied by another concentration of energy at an interval of a fifth above this peak. The authors then argue that the fifth has a special status in music precisely because it is "speech-like" in a statistical sense, and hence highly familiar. They then apply similar arguments to other intervals of the Western musical scale.

A.3.4 Future Directions in Research on the Basis of Musical Intervals

The three preceding sections have outlined different approaches to explaining why one particular interval (the fifth) is important in musical scales. All three approaches have a universalist flavor, which is reasonable because this interval appears in the musical scales of many diverse cultures, suggesting that something about the human auditory system biases people toward choosing this interval in building pitch relations in their musical sound systems. Which theory best explains the prevalence of the fifth is an open question. Indeed, the theories are not mutually exclusive, and all the forces described above may play a role.

Although there is good reason to believe that the fifth has a basis in auditory perception, can the other intervals of the Western major scale be explained in this universalist framework? Those who study music in non-Western cultures are justifiably skeptical of strong universalist forces due to the variability in scale systems. Furthermore, limitations of the above approaches in explaining even the Western scale have been noted (see, for example, Lerdahl & Jackendoff, 1983:290, for a critique of the overtone theory). To determine which of these theories has the most merit in a cross-cultural framework will require cross-cultural data on interval perception, collected using consistent methods. Also, the theories will need to make sufficiently different quantitative predictions about interval perception, or else no amount of empirical research will be able to distinguish between them.

What directions can future research on musical intervals take? For those interested in the idea of universal auditory predispositions for certain musical intervals, one direction involves testing individuals unfamiliar with certain intervals to see whether they nevertheless show some special perceptual response to them. This has been the motivation behind research on musical interval perception in infants. For example, Schellenberg and Trehub (1996) tested the ability of 6-month-old Canadian infants to detect a change in the size of a repeating melodic interval (i.e., an interval formed between two sequentially presented sounds). They found that detection was better when the standard interval was a fifth or fourth and the deviant interval was a tritone than vice versa, and suggested that this demonstrated an innate bias for the former intervals, which are based on small whole-number ratios. Unfortunately, one cannot rule out the influence of prior musical exposure on this result, because before 6 months of age infants are exposed to a good deal of music, especially lullabies (Unyk et al., 1992). In Western melodies, intervals of a fifth or fourth are more common than of a tritone (Vos & Troost, 1989), meaning that the processing advantage of the former intervals could simply reflect greater prior exposure to these intervals. Thus the result would be much stronger if infants came from households in which there was no ambient music.[34] Alternatively, Hauser and McDermott (2003) have suggested that one way to address innate biases in interval perception is to test nonhuman primates whose exposure to music and speech has been tightly controlled. If such primates showed a processing advantage for the musical fifth, despite lack of any exposure to music or speech, this would be strong evidence that certain intervals are innately favored by the primate auditory nervous system.[35]

Appendix 4: Lexical Pitch Scaling as a Proportion of the Current Range

This is an appendix for section 2.3.2, subsection "A Closer Look at Pitch Contrasts Between Level Tones in Tone Languages."

In mathematical terms:

$$T = 100 \times (F - L)/R$$

Where T = the tone's range-normalized scaling in percent, F = the tone frequency, L = the bottom of the individuals' speaking range, and R = the speaking range. F, L, and R are expressed in Hz.

---

[34] One possible source of such households would be cultural groups in which music is frowned upon for cultural or religious reasons (e.g., certain pious Muslims). Care must be taken, however, that there are no other sources of musical intervals in the environment: for example, from the chanting of holy texts. Another way to seek such households would be to advertise for individuals who do not listen to music at home and whose infants have had minimal exposure to songs, musical toys, and television or radio shows with music. One hopes there are not many such households, but given human diversity, some are likely to exist.

[35] In conducting such research it will be important to know if the vocalizations of the primates are harmonic. If so, then any bias for the fifth could reflect exposure to harmonic intervals in the spectra of their own communication systems, rather than innate auditory biases (à la Terhardt, 1984, and Schwartz et al., 2003). Furthermore, if nonhuman primates do *not* show a bias for the fifth, it is not clear what conclusions can be drawn. Given that virtually all non-human primate auditory research is done with monkeys (rather than with apes, which are genetically much closer to humans), it is possible that differences in the auditory systems of monkeys and humans would be responsible for the negative finding. Thus the only easily interpretable outcome of this research would be if the primates did show a processing advantage for the fifth.

Chapter 3
_____
Rhythm

3

Rhythm

3.1 Introduction

The comparative study of spoken and musical rhythm is surprisingly underdeveloped. Although hundreds of studies have explored rhythm within each domain, empirical comparisons of linguistic and musical rhythm are rare. This does not reflect a lack of interest, because researchers have long noted connections between theories of rhythm in the two domains (e.g., Selkirk, 1984; Handel, 1989). The paucity of comparative research probably reflects the fact that specialists in one domain seldom have the time to delve into the intricacies of the other. This is regrettable, because cross-domain work can provide a broader perspective on rhythm in human cognition. One goal of this chapter is to equip researchers with conceptual and empirical tools to explore the borderland between linguistic and musical rhythm. As we shall see, this is a fertile area for new discoveries.

Before embarking, it is worth addressing two overarching issues. The first is the definition of rhythm. The term "rhythm" occurs in many contexts besides speech and music, such as circadian rhythms, oscillations in the brain, and the rhythmic calls of certain animals. In most of these contexts, "rhythm" denotes periodicity, in other words, a pattern repeating regularly in time. Although periodicity is an important aspect of rhythm, it is crucial to distinguish between the two concepts. The crux of the matter is simply this: Although all periodic patterns are rhythmic, not all rhythmic patterns are periodic. That is, periodicity is but one type of rhythmic organization. This point is especially important for understanding speech rhythm, which has had a long (and as we shall see, largely unfruitful) association with the notion of periodicity. Thus any definition of rhythm should leave open the issue of periodicity. Unfortunately, there is no universally accepted definition of rhythm. Thus I will define rhythm as the systematic patterning of sound in terms of timing, accent, and grouping. Both speech and music are characterized by systematic temporal, accentual, and phrasal patterning. How do these patterns compare? What is their relationship in the mind?

The second issue is the very notion of rhythm in speech, which may be unfamiliar to some readers. One way to informally introduce this concept is to consider the process of learning a foreign language. Speaking a language with native fluency requires more than mastering its phonemes, vocabulary, and grammar. One must also master the patterns of timing and accentuation that characterize the flow of syllables in sentences. That is, each language has a rhythm that is part of its sonic structure, and an implicit knowledge of this rhythm is part of a speaker's competence in their language. A failure to acquire native rhythm is an important factor in creating a foreign accent in speech (Taylor, 1981; Faber, 1986; Chela-Flores, 1994).

The following two sections (3.2 and 3.3) give overviews of rhythm in music and speech, respectively, focusing on issues pertinent to cross-domain comparisons. (Such comparisons are made within each section where appropriate.) These overviews motivate a particular way of looking at rhythmic relations between speech and music. This new perspective is introduced in the final section of the chapter, together with empirical evidence spanning acoustic, perceptual, and neural studies.

3.2 Rhythm in Music

The following discussion of rhythm in music focuses on music that has a regularly timed beat, a perceptually isochronous pulse to which one can synchronize with periodic movements such as taps or footfalls. Furthermore, the focus is on music of the Western European tradition, in which beats are organized in hierarchies of beat strength, with alternation between stronger and weaker beats. This form of rhythmic organization has been the most widely studied from a theoretical and empirical standpoint, and is also the type of rhythm most often compared with speech, either implicitly or explicitly (Pike, 1945; Liberman, 1975; Selkirk, 1984).

It is important to realize, however, that this is just one way in which humans organize musical rhythm. It would be convenient if the rhythmic structure of Western music indicated general principles of rhythmic patterning. Reality is more complex, however, and only a comparison of different cultural traditions can help sift what is universal from what is particular. To illustrate this point, one can note musical traditions in which rhythm is organized in rather different ways than in most Western European music.

One such tradition involves the Ch'in, a seven string fretless zither that has been played in China for over 2,000 years (van Gulik, 1940). The musical notation for this instrument contains no time markings for individual notes, indicating only the string and type of gesture used to produce the note (though sometimes phrase boundaries are marked). The resulting music has no sense of a beat. Instead, it has a flowing quality in which the timing of notes emerges from the gestural dynamics of the hands rather than from an explicitly regulated temporal scheme. The Ch'in is just one of many examples of unpulsed music from around the globe, all of which show that the mind is capable of organizing temporal patterns without reference to a beat.

Another tradition whose rhythms are quite different from Western European music is Balkan folk music from Eastern Europe (Singer, 1974; London, 1995). This music has salient beats, but the beats are not spaced at regular temporal intervals. Instead, intervals between beats are either long or short, with the long interval being 3/2 the length of the shorter one. Rhythmic cycles are built from repeating patterns of long and short intervals, such as S-S-S-L, S-S-L-S-S (note that the long element is not constrained to occur at the end of the cycle). One might think that such an asymmetric structure would make the music difficult to follow or synchronize with. In fact, listeners who grew up with this music are adept at following these complex meters (Hannon & Trehub, 2005), and much of this music is actually dance music, in which footfalls are synchronized to the asymmetric beats.

As a final example of a rhythmic tradition with a different orientation from Western European music, Ghanian drumming in West Africa shows a number of interesting features. First, the basic rhythmic reference is a repeating, non-isochronous time pattern played on a set of hand bells (Locke 1982; Pantaleoni, 1985). Members of a drum ensemble keep their rhythmic orientation by hearing their parts in relation to the bell, rather than by focusing on an isochronous beat. Furthermore, the first beat of a rhythmic cycle is not heard as a "downbeat," in other words, a specially strong beat (as in Western music); if anything, the most salient beat comes at the *end* of the cycle (Temperley, 2000). Finally, this music emphasizes diversity in terms of the way it can be heard. As different drums enter, each with its own characteristic repeating temporal pattern, a polyrhythmic texture is created that provides a rich source of alternative perceptual possibilities depending on the rhythmic layers and relationships one chooses to attend to (Locke 1982; Pressing, 2002). This is quite different from the rhythmic framework of most Western European music, in which the emphasis is on relatively simple and perceptually consensual rhythmic structures. One possible reason for this difference is that Western music has major preoccupations in other musical dimensions (such as harmony), and a relatively simple rhythmic framework facilitates complex explorations in these other areas. Another reason may be that tempo in Western European music is often flexible, with salient decelerations and accelerations of the beat used for expressive purposes. A fairly simple beat structure may help a listener stay oriented in the face of these temporal fluctuations (cf. Temperley, 2004).

Thus it would be an error to assume that the rhythmic structure of Western European music reflects basic constraints on how the mind structures rhythmic patterns in terms of production or perception. As with every musical tradition, the rhythmic patterns of Western European music reflect the historical and musical concerns of a given culture. On the other hand, a comparative perspective reveals that certain aspects of rhythm in Western European music (such as a regular beat and grouping of events into phrases) are also found in numerous other cultures, which suggests that these aspects reflect widespread cognitive proclivities of the human mind.

The discussion below relies at times on one particular melody to illustrate various aspects of rhythmic structure in Western music. This is the melody of a children's song, indexed as melody K0016 in a database of Bohemian folk melodies (Schaffrath, 1995; Selfridge-Feld, 1995). Figure 3.1 shows the melody in Western music notation and in "piano roll" notation with each tone's pitch plotted as a function of time (the melody can be heard in Sound Example 3.1).

The melody was chosen because it is historically recent and follows familiar Western conventions, yet is unlikely to be familiar to most readers and is thus free of specific memory associations. It also illustrates basic aspects of rhythm in a simple form. Beyond this, there is nothing special about this melody, and any number of other melodies would have served the same purpose.

3.2.1 The Beat: A Stable Mental Periodicity

The phenomenon of a musical beat seems simple because it is so familiar. Almost everyone has tapped or danced along to music with a beat. A regular beat is widespread in musical cultures, and it is worth considering why this might be so. One obvious function of a beat is to coordinate synchronized movement, such as dance. (The relationship between dance and music is widespread

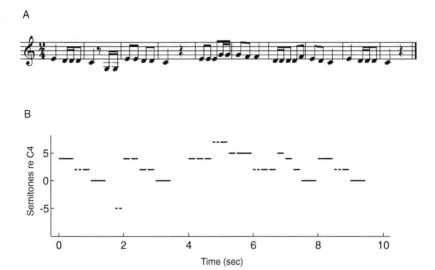

Figure 3.1 A simple melody (K0016) in (A) music notation and (B) piano roll format. In (B), the y-axis shows the semitone distance of each pitch from C4 (261.63 Hz).

in human societies; indeed, some cultures do not even have separate terms for music and dance.) A second obvious function of a beat is to provide a common temporal reference for ensemble performance. Indeed, a cross-cultural perspective reveals that ensemble music without a periodic temporal framework is a rare exception. Perlman (1997) points to one such exception in Javanese music known as *pathetan,* noting that "Except for certain isolated phrases, *pathetan* has no unifying metric framework. . . . Rhythmic unison is not desired, and the musicians need not match their attacks with the precision made possible by a definite meter" (p. 105). A detailed discussion of pathetan by Brinner (1995:245–267) suggests that it is an exception that proves the rule: without a metric frame, players substitute close attention to a lead melodic instrument (typically a *rebab* or bowed lute) in order to coordinate and orient their performance. Thus when periodicity in ensemble music is withdrawn, its functional role is filled in other ways.

From a listener's perspective, perception of a beat is often linked to movement in the form of synchronization to the beat. For many people, this synchronization is a natural part of musical experience requiring no special effort. It may come as a surprise, then, that humans are the only species to spontaneously synchronize to the beat of music. Although synchrony is known from other parts of the animal kingdom, such as the chorusing of frogs or the synchronized calls of insects (Gerhardt & Huber 2002, Ch. 8; Strogatz, 2003), human synchronization with a beat is singular in a number of respects (see Chapter 7, section 7.5.3, for further discussion of this point). Of course, beat perception does not automatically cause movement (one can always sit still), but the human uniqueness of beat synchronization suggests that beat perception merits psychological investigation. Research in music cognition has revealed several interesting facts about beat perception.

First, there is a preferred tempo range for beat perception. People have difficulty following a beat that is faster than every 200 ms and slower than every 1.2 seconds. Within this range, there is a preference for beats that occur roughly every 500–700 ms (Parncutt, 1994; van Noorden & Moelants, 1999). It is interesting to note that this is the same range in which people are the most accurate at making duration judgments, in other words, they neither overestimate nor underestimate the duration of temporal intervals (Eisler, 1976; cf. Fraisse, 1982). Furthermore, this is the range in which listeners are the most accurate in judging slight differences in tempo (Drake & Botte, 1993). It is also interesting to note that in languages with stressed and unstressed syllables, the average duration between stressed syllables has been reported to be close to or within this range (Dauer, 1983; Lea, 1974, described in Lehiste, 1977).

Second, although people usually gravitate toward one particular beat tempo, they can tap at other tempi that are simple divisors or multiples of their preferred tapping rate (e.g., at double or half their preferred rate; Drake, Jones, & Baruch, 2000). For example, consider Sound Example 3.2, which presents K0016 along with two different indications of the beat. Both are perfectly possible, and it is likely that most people could easily tap at either level depending on whether they focus on lower or higher level aspects of rhythmic structure. Drake, Jones, and Baruch (2000) have shown that people vary in the level they synchronize with in music, and that their preferred level correlates with their spontaneous tapping rate. Furthermore, although individuals naturally gravitate to one particular level, they can move to higher or lower levels if they wish (e.g., by doubling or halving their tapping rate) and still feel synchronized with the music. Thus when speaking of "the beat" of a piece, it is important to keep in mind that what a listener selects as the beat is just one level (their *tactus*) in a hierarchy of beats.

Third, beat perception is robust to moderate tempo fluctuations. In many forms of music, the overall timing of events slows down or speeds up within phrases or passages as part of expressive performance (Palmer, 1997). People are still able to perceive a beat in such music (Large & Palmer, 2002) and synchronize to it (Drake, Penel, & Bigand, 2000), indicating that beat perception is based on flexible timekeeping mechanisms.

Fourth, there is cultural variability in beat perception. Drake and Ben El Heni (2003) studied how French versus Tunisian listeners tapped to the beat of French versus Tunisian music. The French tapped at a slower rate to French music than to Tunisian music, whereas the Tunisians showed the opposite pattern. Drake and Ben Heni argue that this reflects the fact that listeners can extract larger-scale structural properties in music with which they are familiar. These findings indicate that beat perception is not simply a passive response of the auditory system to physical periodicity in sound: It also involves cultural influences that may relate to knowledge of musical structure (e.g., sensitivity to how notes are grouped into motives; cf. Toiviainen & Eerola, 2003).

Fifth, and of substantial interest from a cognitive science standpoint, a perceived beat can tolerate a good deal of counterevidence in the form of accented events at nonbeat locations and absent or weak events at beat locations, in other words, syncopation (Snyder & Krumhansl, 2001). For example, consider Sound Examples 3.3 and 3.4, two complex temporal patterns studied by Patel, Iversen, et al. (2005) with regard to beat perception and synchronization. The patterns begin with an isochronous sequence of 9 tones that serves to indicate the beat, which has a period is 800 ms. After this "induction sequence," the patterns change into a more complex rhythm but with the same beat period. Participants were asked to synchronize their taps to the isochronous tones and then continue tapping at the same tempo during the complex sequence. Their success at this task was taken as a measure of how well they were able to extract a beat from these sequences. In the "strongly metrical" (SM) sequences (Sound Example 3.3), a tone occurred at every beat position. In the "weakly metrical" (WM) sequences, however, about 1/3 of the beat positions were silent (Sound Example 3.4). (NB: The SM and WM sequences had exactly the same set of interonset intervals, just arranged differently in time; cf. Povel & Essens, 1985.) Thus successful beat perception and synchronization in WM sequences required frequent taps at points with no sound.

All participants were able to synchronize with the beat of the SM sequence: Their taps were very close in time to the idealized beat locations. (In fact, taps typically preceded the beat by a small amount, a finding typical of beat synchronization studies, indicating that beat perception is anticipatory rather than reactive.) Of greater interest was performance on the WM sequences. Although synchronization was not as accurate as with the SM sequences as measured by tapping variability, most participants (even the musically untrained ones) were able to tap to the beat of these sequences, *though from a physical standpoint there was little periodicity at the beat period.* That is, most people tapped to the silent beats as if they were physically there, illustrating that beat perception can tolerate a good deal of counterevidence.

The above facts indicate that beat perception is a complex phenomenon that likely has sophisticated cognitive and neural underpinnings. Specifically, it involves a mental model of time in which periodic temporal expectancies play a key role (Jones, 1976). This may be one reason why it is unique to humans.

Beat perception is an active area of research in music cognition, in which there has long been an interest in the cues listeners use to extract a beat. Temperley and Bartlette (2002) list six factors that most researchers agree are important in beat finding (i.e., in inferring the beat from a piece of music). These can be expressed as preferences:

1. For beats to coincide with note onsets
2. For beats to coincide with longer notes
3. For regularity of beats
4. For beats to align with the beginning of musical phrases
5. For beats to align with points of harmonic change
6. For beats to align with the onsets of repeating melodic patterns

Because beat perception is fundamental to music and is amenable to empirical study, it has attracted computational, behavioral, and neural approaches (e.g., Desain, 1992; Desain & Honing, 1999; Todd et al., 1999; Large, 2000; Toiviainen & Snyder, 2003; Hannon et al., 2004; Snyder & Large, 2005; Zanto et al., 2006) and has the potential to mature into a sophisticated branch of music cognition in which different models compete to explain a common set of behavioral and neural data. Its study is also attractive because it touches on larger issues in cognitive neuroscience. For example, synchronization to a beat provides an opportunity to study how different brain systems are coordinated in perception and behavior (in this case, the auditory and motor systems). A better understanding of the mechanisms involved in beat perception and synchronization could have applications for physical therapy, in which synchronization with a beat is being used to help patients with neuromotor disorders (such as Parkinson's disease) to initiate and coordinate movement (Thaut et al., 1999; cf. Sacks, 1984, 2007).

3.2.2 Meter: Multiple Periodicities

In Western European music, beats are not all created equal. Instead, some beats are stronger than others, and this serves to create a higher level of periodicity in terms of the grouping and/or accentuation of beats. For example, the beats of a waltz are grouped in threes, with an accent on the first beat of each group, whereas in a march beats are grouped into twos or fours, with primary accent on the first beat (in a four-beat march, there is secondary accent on the third beat).

Waltzes and marches are but two types of meter in a broad diversity of meters used in Western European music, but they serve to illustrate some general features of meter in this tradition. First, the meters of Western music are dominated by organization in terms of multiples of two and three in terms of how many beats constitute a basic unit (the measure), and how many subdivisions of each beat there are. For example, a waltz has three beats per measure, each of which can be subdivided into two shorter beats, whereas a march has two (or four) beats per measure, each of which can also be subdivided into two beats. Many other possibilities exist, for example two beats per measure, each of which is subdivided into three beats.[1] The key point is that meter typically has at least one level of subdivision below the beat (London, 2002, 2004:34), in addition to periodicity above the beat created by the temporal patterning of strong beats. One way to represent this is via a metrical grid, which indicates layers of periodicity using rows of isochronous dots. One of these rows represents the tactus, with the row above this showing the periodic pattern of accentuation above the tactus. Other rows above or below the tactus show other psychologically accessible levels of periodicity (Figure 3.2 shows a metrical grid for K0016).

Thus one should be able to tap to any of these levels and still feel synchronized with the music. (The use of dots in metrical grids indicates that meter concerns the perceptual organization of points in time, which in physical terms would correspond to the perceptual attacks of tones; Lerdahl & Jackendoff, 1983.) In grid notation, the relative strength of each beat is indicated by the number of dots above it, in other words, the number of layers of periodicity it participates in. Dots at the highest and lowest level must fall within the "temporal envelope" for meter: Periodicities faster than 200 ms and slower than ~4–6 s

---

[1] This corresponds to a time signature of 6/8, in contrast to a waltz, which has a time signature of 3/4. As one can see, although 6/8 = 3/4 in mathematical terms, these ratios refer to rather different forms of organization in a musical context.

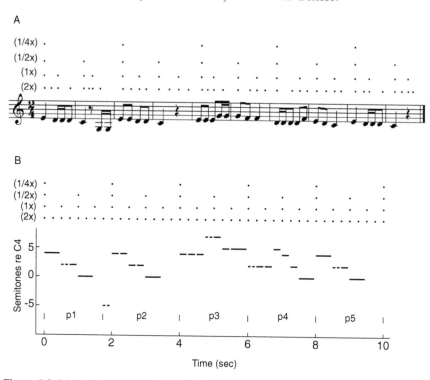

Figure 3.2 Metrical structure of K0016. A typical tactus is shown by the metrical level labeled 1x. Phrase boundaries are indicated below the piano roll notation (p1 = phrase 1, etc.).

are unlikely to be spontaneously perceived as part of a metric framework. (Note that the upper end of this envelope is substantially longer than the ~1.2 second limit for following a beat mentioned in section 3.2.1. That shorter limit refers to beat-to-beat intervals, whereas 4–6 s refers to the highest metrical levels, and is likely to be related to our sense of the psychological present (cf. London, 2002, 2004:30).[2]

Before moving on, the relationship between accent and meter should be discussed. This is an important relationship, because strong beats are perceptually accented points in the music. This kind of accent does not always rely on

---

[2] An apparent exception occurs in long rhythmic cycles of Indian classical music (e.g., cycles of 16 beats or more), in which the strong accent on the first beat of each cycle can be separated by 10 seconds or more, yet plays an important perceptual role in the music. However, this may be an exception that proves the rule, as explicit counting of the beats by the audience is part of the listening tradition in this music. That is, conscious effort is expended in order to keep track of where the music is in its long metrical cycle.

physical cues such as intensity or duration (note, for example, that all tones in K0016 are of equal intensity), and emerges from the detection of periodicity at multiple time-scales. There are of course many physical (or "phenomenal") accents in music due to a variety of factors, including duration, intensity, and changes in melodic contour. There are also "structural accents" due to salient structural points in the music, for example, a sudden harmonic shift or the start of a musical phrase (Lerdahl & Jackendoff, 1983). The interplay of different accent types is one of the sources of complexity in music (Jones, 1993), particularly the interplay of metrical accents with off-beat phenomenal or structural accents. For example, syncopation in music illustrates the successful use of phenomenal accents "against the grain" of the prevailing meter. This raises a key point about the musical metrical grid, namely that it is a *mental* pattern of multiple periodicities in the mind of a listener, and not simply a map of the accentual structure of a sequence. This point will become relevant in the discussion of metrical grids in language.

The influence of musical meter on behavior, perception, and brain signals has been demonstrated in a number of ways. Sloboda (1983) had pianists perform the same sequence of notes set to different time signatures (in music, the time signature indicates the grouping and accentuation pattern of beats, i.e., the meter). The durational patterning of the performances differed substantially depending on the meter, and in many cases a given pianist did not even realize they were playing the same note sequence in two different meters. A demonstration of meter's effect on synchronization comes from Patel, Iversen, et al. (2005), who showed that tapping to a metrical pattern differs from tapping to a simple metronome at the same beat period. Specifically, taps to the first beat of each metric cycle (i.e., the "downbeats" in the strongly metrical sequences of Sound Example 3.3) were closer to the physical beat than taps on other beats. Importantly, these downbeats (which occurred every four beats) were identical to other tones in terms intensity and duration, so that the influence of downbeats on tapping was not due to any physical accent but to their role in creating a four-beat periodic structure in the minds of listeners.

In terms of meter's influence on perception, Palmer and Krumhansl (1990) had participants listen to a sequence of isochronous tones and imagine that each event formed the first beat of groups of two, three, four or six beats. After a few repetitions, a probe tone was sounded and participants had to indicate how well it fit with the imagined meter. The ratings reflected a hierarchy of beat strength (cf. Jongsma et al., 2004). Turning to neural studies, Iversen, Repp, and Patel (2009) had musically trained participants listen to a metrically ambiguous repeating two-note pattern and mentally impose a downbeat in a particular place. Specifically, in half of the sequences they imagined that the first tone was the downbeat, and in the other half they imagined that the second tone was the downbeat. Participants were instructed not to move or to engage in motor imagery. Measurement of brain signals from auditory regions using magnetoencephalography (MEG) revealed that when a note was interpreted as the downbeat, it evoked an increased amount of neural activity in a particular frequency band (beta, 20–30 Hz) compared to when it was not a downbeat (even though the tones were physically identical in the two conditions).[3] A control experiment showed that the pattern of increased activity closely resembled the pattern observed when the note in question was in fact physically accented (Figure 3.3). These results suggest that the perception of meter involves the active shaping of incoming signals by a mental periodic temporal-accentual scheme.

3.2.3 Grouping: The Perceptual Segmentation of Events

Grouping refers to the perception of boundaries, with elements between boundaries clustering together to form a temporal unit. This can be illustrated with K0016. In listening to this melody, there is a clear sense that it is divided into phrases, schematically marked in Figure 3.4.

The perceptual boundaries of the first two phrases are marked by silences (musical rests). Of greater interest are the boundaries at the end of the third and the fourth phrases, which are not marked by any physical discontinuity in the tone sequence, but are nevertheless salient perceptual break points.

As emphasized by Lerdahl and Jackendoff (1983), grouping is distinct from meter, and the interaction of these two rhythmic dimensions plays an important role in shaping the rhythmic feel of music. For example, anacrusis, or upbeat, is a rhythmically salient phenomenon involving a slight misalignment between grouping and meter, in other words, a phrase starting on a weak beat (such as phrase 2 of K0016).

Psychological evidence for perceptual grouping in music comes from a number of sources. Memory experiments show that if a listener is asked to indicate whether a brief tone sequence was embedded in a previously heard longer tone sequence, performance is better when the excerpt ends at a group boundary in the original sequence than when it straddles a group boundary (Dowling, 1973; Peretz, 1989). This suggests that grouping influences the mental chunking of sounds in memory. Further evidence for grouping comes from studies that show how grouping warps the perception of time. For example, clicks placed near phrase boundaries in musical sequences perceptually migrate to those boundaries and are heard as coinciding with them (Sloboda & Gregory, 1980; Stoffer,

---

[3] Neural activity in the beta frequency band has been associated with the motor system, raising the possibility that meter perception in the brain involves some sort of coupling between the auditory and motor system, even in the absence of overt movement.

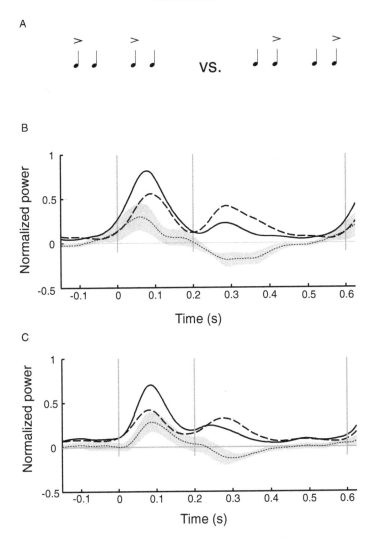

Figure 3.3 (A) Repeating two-note rhythmic pattern, in which the listener imagines the downbeat on either the first tone (left) or second tone (right). (B) Evoked neural responses (measured over auditory brain regions) to the two-tone pattern subjectively interpreted in two different ways, in other words, with the downbeat on tone 1 versus tone 2. (The onset times of tones 1 and 2 are indicated by thin, vertical, gray lines at 0 and 0.2 s). The solid and dashed black lines show across-subject means for the two imagined beat conditions (solid = beat imagined on tone 1, dashed = beat imagined on tone 2). Data are from the beta frequency range (20–30 Hz). The difference is shown by the dotted line, with shading indicating 1 standard error. (C) Evoked neural responses in the beta frequency range to a two-tone pattern physically accented in two different ways, with the accent on tone 1 (solid line) versus tone 2 (dashed line).

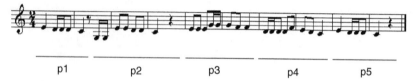

Figure 3.4 K0016 segmented into melodic phrases (p1 = phrase 1, etc.).

1985). More evidence for perceptual warping based on grouping comes from a study by Repp (1992a), in which participants repeatedly listened to a computer-generated isochronous version of the opening of a Beethoven minuet. The task was to detect a lengthening in 1 of 47 possible positions in the music. Detection performance was particularly *poor* at phrase boundaries, probably reflecting an expectation for lengthening at these points (Repp further showed that these were the points at which human performers typically slowed down to mark the phrase structure). Finally, in a gating study of recognition for familiar melodies in which successively longer fragments of tunes were heard until they were correctly identified, Schulkind et al. (2003) found that identification performance was highest at phrase boundaries.[4] Thus there is abundant evidence that grouping plays a role in musical perception.

What cues do listeners use in inferring grouping structure in music? Returning again to K0016, the ends of phrases 3 and 4 are marked by local durational lengthening and lowering of pitch. It is notable that these cues have been found to be important in the prosodic marking of clause endings in speech (Cooper & Sorensen, 1977). Even infants show sensitivity to these boundary cues in both speech and music (Hirsh-Pasek et al., 1987; Krumhansl & Jusczyk, 1990; Jusczyk & Krumhansl, 1993). For example, infants prefer to listen to musical sequences in which pauses are inserted after longer and lower sounds rather than at other locations, presumably because in the former case the pauses coincide with perceptual boundaries. Of course, there is much more to grouping than just these two cues. Deliège (1987) found that salient changes in intensity, duration, pitch, and timbre can all play a role in demarcating the edges of groups. Another factor that is likely to be important is motivic repetition, for example, a repeating pattern of

[4] Schulkind et al. (2003) conducted an interesting analysis of melodic structure that helps suggest why phrase boundaries might be important landmarks in melody recognition. They examined the temporal distribution of pitch and temporal accents in melodies, in which pitch accents were defined as notes that were members of the tonic triad or points of contour change, and temporal accents were defined as relatively long notes and metrically accented notes. They found that accent density was higher at phrase boundaries than within phrases. (For those unfamiliar with the concept of a tonic triad, it is explained in Chapter 5). Thus the edges of phrases are structural slots that attract accents of various kinds.

the same overall duration and internal durational patterning. When these different cues are in conflict, people can disagree about where they hear grouping boundaries (Peretz, 1989). The interaction of different factors in grouping perception is a topic that draws continuing interest, because data on the perceived segmentation of pieces is relatively easy to collect (Clarke & Krumhansl, 1990; Deliège et al., 1996; Frankland & Cohen, 2004; Schaefer et al., 2004).

Grouping plays a prominent role in modern cognitive theories of music, in which it is conceived of as hierarchical, with lower level groups nested within higher level ones. For example, a theoretical analysis of grouping in K0016 would add layers above and below the phrase layer. Below the phrase layer, each phrase would be parsed into smaller groups (motives); above the phrase layer, phrases would be linked into higher level structures. For example, one might unite Phrases 1 and 2 into a group, followed by a group consisting of Phrases 3 and 4, and a final group coincident with Phrase 5. One of the most developed theoretical treatments of hierarchical grouping in music is that of Lerdahl and Jackendoff (1983), who propose certain basic constraints on grouping structure such as the constraint that a piece must be fully parsed into groups at each hierarchical level, and that boundaries at higher levels must coincide with those at lower levels. Evidence for multiple layers of grouping structure in music comes from research by Todd (1985), who showed that the amount of lengthening at a given phrase boundary in music is predicted by the position of that boundary in a hierarchical phrase structure of a piece.

The hierarchical view of grouping structure in music shows strong parallels to theories of prosodic structure in modern linguistic theory, notably the concept of the "prosodic hierarchy" (Selkirk, 1981, Nespor & Vogel, 1983). The prosodic hierarchy refers to the organization of sonic groupings at multiple levels in speech, ranging from the syllable up to the utterance. A key conceptual point made by all such theories is that these groupings are not simple reflections of syntactic organization. To take a well-known example, consider the difference between the syntactic bracketing of a sentence in 3.1a versus its prosodic phrasal bracketing 3.1b (Chomsky & Halle, 1968):

(3.1a) This is [the cat [that caught [the rat [that stole [the cheese]]]]]

(3.1b) [This is the cat] [that caught the rat] [that stole the cheese]

Prosodic grouping reflects a separate phonological level of organization that is not directly determined by syntactic structure. Instead, other linguistic factors play an important role, such as the semantic relations between words and the desire to place focus on certain elements (Marcus & Hindle, 1990; Ferreira, 1991). Furthermore, there are thought to be purely rhythmic factors such as a tendency to avoid groups that are very short or very long, and a tendency to balance the lengths of groups (Gee & Grosjean, 1983; Zellner Keller, 2002). The prosodic grouping structure of a sentence is by no means set in stone: There are differences among individuals in terms of how they group the words of the same sentence, and the grouping structure of a sentence can vary with speech rate (Fougeron & Jun, 1998). Nevertheless, grouping is not totally idiosyncratic, and psycholinguists have made good progress in predicting where speakers place prosodic boundaries in a sentence based on syntactic analyses of sentences (Watson & Gibson, 2004).

Although Example 3.1 above only shows one level of prosodic phrasing, modern theories of the prosodic hierarchy posit multiple levels nested inside one another. Theories vary in the number of levels they propose (Shattuck-Hufnagel & Turk, 1996),[5] so for illustrative purposes only one such theory is discussed here. Hayes (1989) posits a five-level hierarchy comprised of words, clitic groups, phonological phrases, intonational phrases, and utterances. Figure 3.5 shows a prosodic hierarchy for a sentence according to this theory, with the syntactic structure also shown for comparison. (Note that a clitic group combines a lexical word that has a stressed syllable with an adjacent function word—an unstressed syllable—into a single prosodic unit. See Hayes, 1989, for definitions of other units.)

One form of evidence offered for the existence of a given level in the prosodic hierarchy is a systematic variation in the realization of a phonemic segment that depends on prosodic structure at that level. For example, Hayes (1989) discusses /v/ deletion in English speech as an example of a rule that operates within the clitic group. Thus it is acceptable to delete the /v/ in American English when saying, "Will you [save me] a seat?" because "save me" is a clitic group. (That is, if you listen carefully to an American English speaker say this phrase rapidly, "save" is often acoustically realized as "say," though it is intended as—and heard as—"save".) In contrast, the /v/ is not deleted when saying "[save] [mom]" because [save] and [mom] are two separate clitic groups. Other evidence that has been adduced for prosodic constituents includes preferences for interruption points between, rather than within, constituents (Pilon, 1981), and speeded word spotting at the boundaries of constituents (Kim, 2003).

Evidence that the prosodic hierarchy has multiple levels comes from phonetic modifications of speech that vary in a parametric fashion with the height of the prosodic boundary at the phoneme's location (this corresponds to the number of coincident prosodic boundaries at that point, as higher level boundaries are always coincident with lower level ones). For example, Cho and Keating (2001) showed that in Korean, the voice-onset time of stop consonants is larger at higher prosodic boundaries, and Dilley, Shattuck-Hufnagel, and Ostendorf (1996) have shown that the amount of glottalization of word-onset vowels is greater at higher level boundaries.

---

[5] In a survey of 21 typologically different languages, Jun (2005) found that all languages had at least one grouping level above the word, and most had two.

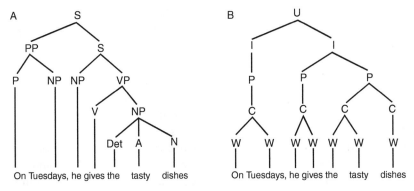

Figure 3.5 (A) Syntactic and (B) prosodic hierarchy for a sentence of English. Abbreviations for (A): S = sentence, PP = prepositional phrase, NP = noun phrase, VP = verb phrase, Det = Determiner, A = adjective, N = Noun, V = Verb. Abbreviations for (B): U = utterance, I = Intonation phrase, P = phonological phrase, C = clitic group, W = word. Adapted from Hayes, 1989.

Another phenomenon that supports the notion of hierarchical grouping in speech is variation in perceived juncture between words (Jun, 2003). In connected speech, words are acoustically run together and the silent intervals that do occur (e.g., due to stop consonants) are not necessarily located at word boundaries (cf. Chapter 2, section 2.3.3, subsection "A Brief Introduction to the Spectrogram"). Nevertheless, words are perceived as separated from one another. Unlike with written language, however, the perceived degree of spacing is not identical between each pair of words: Rather, some word boundaries seem stronger than others. For example, the sentence in 3.1c below contains juncture markings from a system devised by Price et al. (1991). In this system, a researcher listens repeatedly to a given sentence and places numerals from 0 to 6 between each pair of words to indicate the degree of perceived separation between them. A "break index" of 0 indicates the weakest perceived juncture, in other words, between the words of a clitic group. At the opposite extreme, a break index of 6 indicates the end of a sentence.

(3.1c) Only 1 one 4 remembered 3 the 0 lady 1 in 1 red 6.

Wightman et al. (1992) studied the relationship between these break indices and speech duration patterns in a large speech corpus, and found a correlation between perceived boundary strength and amount of lengthening of the syllable preceding the boundary (cf. Gussenhoven & Rietveld, 1992).[6] This finding is

---

[6] More specifically, the lengthening was confined to the syllabic rime (the vowel and following consonants). Interestingly, this asymmetric expansion of the syllable due to prosodic boundaries differs from temporal changes in a syllable due to stress (Beckman et al., 1992).

strikingly reminiscent of the research on music by Todd (1985) described above. Another parallel to music is that durational lengthening interacts with pitch and amplitude cues in determining the perceived strength of prosodic boundaries (Streeter, 1978; de Pijper & Sanderman, 1994).

In conclusion, grouping is a fundamental rhythmic phenomenon that applies to both musical and linguistic sequences. In both domains, the mind parses complex acoustic patterns into multiple levels of phrasal structure, and music and language share a number of acoustic cues for marking phrase boundaries. These similarities point to shared cognitive process for grouping across the two domains, and indicate that grouping may prove a fruitful area for comparative research. As discussed in section 3.5, empirical work is proving these intuitions correct.

3.2.4 Durational Patterning in Music

Up to this point, the discussion of musical rhythm has been concerned with points and edges in time: beats and grouping boundaries. A different set of issues in rhythm research concerns how time gets filled, in other words, the durational patterning of events.

Duration Categories in Music

In music, the durational patterning of events is typically measured by the time intervals between event onsets within a particular event stream: This defines a sequence of interonset intervals (IOIs). For example, the sequence of IOIs between the tones of a melody defines the durational patterning of that melody. Typically, durations tend to be clustered around certain values reflecting the organization of time in music into discrete categories. Fraisse (1982) pointed out that two categories that figure prominently in Western musical sequences are short times of 200–300 ms and long times of 450–900 ms (cf. Ross, 1989). He argued that these two duration categories were not only quantitatively different but also different in terms of their perceptual properties: Long intervals are perceived as individual units with distinct durations, whereas short intervals are perceived collectively in terms of their grouping patterns rather than in terms of individual durations.

There is empirical evidence that durations in musical rhythms are perceived in terms of categories (Clarke, 1987; Schulze, 1989). For example, Clarke (1987) had music students perform a categorical perception experiment on rhythm. Participants heard short sequences of tones in which the last two tones had a ratio that varied between 1:1 and 1:2. Listeners had to identify the final duration ratio as one or the other of these, and also had to complete a task that required them to discriminate between different ratios. The results showed a steep transition in the identification function, and increased discrimination when stimuli were near the boundary versus within a given region. (Clarke also found that the location of the boundary depended on the metrical context in which the sequence was perceived, providing another example of the influence of meter on perception; cf. section 3.2.2.)

In speech, the duration of basic linguistic elements (such as phonemes and syllables) is influenced by a number of factors. For example, there are articulatory constraints on how fast different sounds can be produced, which creates different minimum durations for different sounds (Klatt, 1979). There are also systematic phonological factors that make some sounds longer than others. For example, in English, the same vowel tends to be longer if it occurs before a final stop consonant that is voiced rather than unvoiced (e.g., the /i/ in "bead" vs. "beet"), and this difference influences the perception of the final stop as voiced or voiceless (Klatt, 1976). A simple phonological factor that influences syllable duration is the number of phonemes in the syllable: Syllables with more phonemes tend to be longer than those with fewer phonemes (e.g., "splash" vs. "sash"; Williams & Hiller, 1994). Atop these sources of variation are other sources including variations in speaking style (casual vs. clear), and variations in speech rate related to discourse factors, such as speeding up near the end of a sentence to "hold the floor" in a conversation (Schegloff, 1982; Smiljanic & Bradlow, 2005). Given all these factors, it is not surprising that the durations of speech elements do not tend to cluster around discrete values. Instead, measurements of syllable or phoneme duration typically reveal a continuous distribution with one main peak. For example, Figure 3.6a shows a histogram of syllable durations for a sample of spoken English.

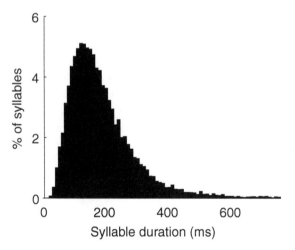

Figure 3.6a Histogram of syllable durations in a corpus of spontaneous speech in American English. Data are from approximately 16,000 syllables. Mean syllable duration = 191 ms, sd = 125 ms. Syllables with duration >750 ms are not shown (<1% of total). Histogram bin size = 10 ms. Analysis based on data from Greenberg, 1996.

Having said this, it is important to note that durational categories do occur in some languages. For example, there are languages with phonemic length contrasts in which the same word can mean entirely different things when a short versus long version of the same vowel or consonant is used. In some languages, such as Estonian, there can even be three-way length contrasts. For example, "sata" can mean three entirely different things ("hundred," "send," and "get") depending on the length of the first /a/. It would be interesting to study length contrasts in a given vowel phoneme and examine the amount of temporal variability within each duration category in connected speech. This could be compared to temporal variability of a given duration category in music, to see whether the perceptual system has a similar tolerance for within-category variability in the two domains.[7]

Expressive Timing in Music

If the perceptual system cared only about musical durations as a sequence of discrete categories, then computer renditions of musical pieces based on exact renderings of music notation would be perfectly acceptable to listeners. Although such mechanical performances do occur in some settings (e.g., rhythm tracks in some modern popular music), in other contexts, such as the classical piano repertoire, such performances are rejected as unmusical. Not surprisingly then, physical measurements of human performances reveal considerable deviations from notated durations. For example, Figure 3.6b shows a histogram of IOIs, all of which represent realizations of notes with the *same notated duration* (an eighth note or quaver) from a famous pianist's rendition of Schumann's Träumerei (Repp, 1992b).[8] Had the piece been performed by a machine, all of these IOIs would be a single value. Instead, considerable variation is seen. The crucial fact about this variation is that it is not "noise": It largely represents structured variation related to the performer's interpretation of the piece (Palmer, 1997; Ashley, 2002). For example, Repp (1992b) studied several famous pianists' renderings of Träumerei and found that all showed slowing of tempo at structural boundaries, with the amount of slowing proportional to the importance of the boundary (cf. Todd, 1985). At a finer timescale, Repp found that within individual melodic phrases there was a tendency to accelerate at the beginning and slow near the end, with the pattern of IOIs following a smooth parabolic function. Repp speculated that this pattern may reflect principles of

---

[7] In doing this research, it would be important to be aware of durational lengthening in the vicinity of phrase boundaries in both speech and music: If there are different degrees of preboundary lengthening in the two domains, then events near boundaries should be excluded from the analysis as this would be confounded with variability measures.

[8] I am grateful to Bruno Repp for providing me with this data.

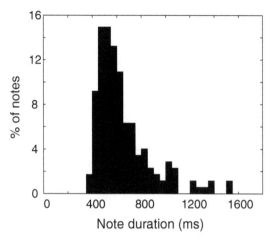

Figure 3.6b Histogram of durations of eighth notes from a performance of Schumann's Träumerei by Claudio Arrau. The large values in the right tail of the histogram are due to phrase-final ritards. Data are from approximately 170 eighth notes. Mean note duration = 652 ms, sd = 227 ms. Notes with duration > 1,600 ms are not shown (<1% of total). Histogram bin size = 50 ms.

human locomotion, in other words, a musical allusion to physical movement (cf. Kronman & Sundberg, 1987).

The above paragraph focuses on the role of IOIs in expressive timing. IOIs are the basis of "expressive timing profiles," time series that show the actual pattern of event timing versus the idealized pattern based on notated duration. Although studies of these profiles have dominated research on expressive timing, it is important not to overlook another aspect of expressive timing, namely, articulation. Although IOI refers to the time interval between the onsets of successive tones, articulation refers to the time between the *offset* of one tone and the onset of the next. If there is little time between these events (or if the tones overlap so that the offset of the prior tone occurs after the onset of the following tone, which is possible in piano music), this is considered "legato" articulation. In this type of articulation, one tone is heard as flowing smoothly into the next. In contrast, staccato articulation involves a salient gap between offset and onset, giving the tones a rhythmically punctuated feel. In addition to IOI and articulation patterns, another important cue to musical expression is the patterning of tone intensity.

Due to the fact that timing, articulation and intensity in music can be measured with great precision using modern technology (e.g., using pianos with digital interfaces, such as the Yamaha Disklavier), expression has been a fruitful area of research in studies of music production. There has also been some research on expressive features in perception. For example, listeners can reliably identify performances of the same music as expressive, deadpan (mechanical), or exaggerated (Kendall & Carterette, 1990), and can identify the performer's intended emotion on the basis of expressive features (Gabrielsson & Juslin, 1996).

Palmer (1996) has shown that musically trained listeners can identify a performer's intended metrical and phrase structure on the basis of expressive cues. One clever demonstration of the perceptual importance of expressive timing was provided by Clarke (1993), who used naturally performed short melodies. For each melody, Clarke extracted its expressive timing profile, manipulated it, and then reimposed it on a mechanical performance of the melody, thus creating a Frankensteinian melody with structure and expression mismatched. For example, in one condition the original note-by-note expressive timing profile was shifted several notes to the right. Musicians judged the originals versus the mismatched melodies in terms of the quality of performance, and favored the originals. Thus listeners are sensitive to the way expressive timing aligns with the structure of musical passages.

Expressive timing in music has an interesting relationship to prosodic structure in speech. Just as a musical passage played by different performers will have different expressive timing patterns, the same sentence spoken by different speakers will have a different temporal patterning of syllables and phonemes. In the past, researchers have suggested that these individualistic aspects of performance are "normalized away" in memory for musical and spoken sequences, arguing that the abstract memory representation favors a less detailed, more categorical structure (Large et al., 1995; Pisoni, 1997). More recent research, however, suggests that listeners retain some temporal information in memory for speech and music (Bradlow et al., 1999; Palmer et al., 2001). For example, Palmer et al. (2001) familiarized listeners with particular performances of short melodic sequences, and then later tested the ability to recognize these performances against other performances of the same sequences. The different performances were generated by a pianist who produced the same short melodic sequences as part of longer melodies that differed in their metrical structure (3/4 vs. 4/4 time). As a result of the differing metrical structure, the same melodic sequence was produced with different patterns of articulation and intensity. For each such melodic sequence, both musicians and nonmusicians were able to recognize the original version they had heard when presented with it versus another version. Furthermore, even 10-month-old infants discriminated between familiar and unfamiliar performances, orienting longer toward the former. Palmer et al. relate these findings to research in speech perception showing that listeners retain stimulus-specific acoustic properties of words along with abstract linguistic properties (Luce & Lyons, 1998).

Another line of research relating timing in music to speech prosody concerns "tempo persistence." Jungers et al. (2002) had pianists alternate between listening to short melodies and sight-reading different short melodies. The participants were told to attend to both the heard and performed melodies for a later memory test. In fact, the real question of interest was the relationship between the tempo of the heard and performed melodies. The heard melodies occurred in blocks of slow and fast tempi, and Jungers et al. found that the tempo of performed melodies was influenced by the tempo of heard melodies: The pianists played more slowly after slow melodies and faster after fast melodies. A similar experiment using spoken sentences rather than melodies showed a similar tempo persistence effect in speech. These findings are reminiscent of research on "accommodation" in sociolinguistics, which has shown that when people of different social backgrounds meet, their speech becomes more alike (cf. Giles et al., 1991).

In an interesting follow-up study, Dalla Bella et al. (2003) studied tempo persistence across modalities. Listeners (both musicians and nonmusicians) alternated between hearing melodies and reading sentences aloud. The musicians showed a tempo persistence effect: They spoke faster after hearing faster melodies. However, the nonmusicians showed no such effect. Furthermore, when the musicians did the reverse experiment (in which they alternated between hearing sentences and sight-reading melodies), there was no evidence of tempo persistence. Dalla Bella et al. suggest that musicians may be better than nonmusicians at beat extraction in music, and that this may drive the effect of tempo persistence seen in their first study. Following this logic, I would suggest that the lack of an effect in their second study indicates that speech perception does not involve extraction of a beat.

3.2.5 The Psychological Dimensions of Musical Rhythm

The interactions of beat, meter, accent, grouping, and expressive timing make musical rhythm a psychologically rich phenomenon (and this is just within the confines of Western European music!). Some idea of this richness is suggested by the work of Gabrielsson, who has conducted studies in which a variety of rhythms are compared and classified by listeners using similarity judgments and adjective ratings (reviewed in Gabrielsson, 1993). Statistical techniques such as multidimensional scaling and factor analysis are used to uncover the perceptual dimensions involved in the experience of musical rhythms. This research has revealed an astonishingly large number of dimensions (15), which group broadly into those concerned with structure (e.g., meter, simplicity vs. complexity), motion (e.g., swinging, graceful), and emotion (e.g., solemnity vs. playfulness). Although much of the cognitive science of musical rhythm focuses on structural issues, it is important to keep the links to motion and emotion in mind, for these connections are part of what distinguishes musical rhythm from speech rhythm, a point to which I will return at the end of the discussion of rhythm in speech.

3.3 Rhythm in Speech

Although the study of rhythm in poetry has a long history, dating back to ancient Greek and Indian texts, the study of rhythm in ordinary language is a relatively recent endeavor in linguistics. Researchers have taken at least three approaches to this topic. The first approach is typological, and seeks to understand the rhythmic similarities and differences among human languages. The driving force behind this work has been idea that linguistic rhythms fall into distinct categories. For example, in one widespread typological scheme (discussed in the next section), English, Arabic, and Thai are all members of a single rhythmic class ("stress-timed languages"), whereas French, Hindi, and Yoruba are members of a different class ("syllable-timed languages"). As is evident from this example, membership in a rhythmic class is not determined by the historical relationship of languages; rhythm can unite languages that are otherwise quite distant both historically and geographically.

The second approach to speech rhythm is theoretical, and seeks to uncover the principles that govern the rhythmic shape of words and utterances in a given language or languages. This research, which includes an area called "metrical phonology," seeks to bring the study of the linguistic rhythm in line with the rest of modern linguistics by using formalized rules and representations to derive the observed rhythmic patterning of utterances.

The third approach is perceptual, and examines the role that rhythm plays in the perception of ordinary speech. One prominent line of research in this area concerns the perceptual segmentation of words from connected speech. Another, smaller line of research examines the effects of rhythmic predictability in speech perception.

The goal of this part of the chapter is to introduce each of these areas and make comparisons to musical rhythm when appropriate. Before commencing, it is worth introducing a concept that occurs in each section: the notion of prominence in speech. In many languages, it is normal to produce the syllables of an utterance with differing degrees of prominence. This is true even when a sentence is said with no special emphasis on any particular word. For example, when speaking the following sentence, note how the syllables marked by an x are more prominent than their neighbors:

       x   x   x   x   x   x

(3.2) She wrote all her novels with a blue pen that she inherited from her aunt.

The most important physical correlates of prominence are duration, pitch movement, vowel quality, and loudness.[9] Prominence in speech raises many

---

[9] Perceived loudness incorporates both physical intensity and the distribution of energy across different frequency bands, in other words, "spectral balance." The latter may be

interesting questions. How many different degrees of prominence can listeners reliably distinguish (Shattuck-Hufnagel & Turk, 1996)? Do languages differ in the extent to which they rely on particular acoustic cues to prominence in production and perception (Berinstein, 1979; Lehiste & Fox, 1992)? Empirical data on these issues is still relatively sparse, and we will not delve into them here. Instead, most sections below treat prominence as a binary quantity referred to as "stress," following the tradition of much work on speech rhythm. An exception occurs in section 3.3.2, where degrees of prominence are discussed in the context of modern linguistic theories of speech rhythm.

Before embarking on the following sections, a word should be said about the concept of stress in linguistics. Stress is recognized as one aspect of word prosody in human languages; tone and lexical pitch accent are two other aspects. Just as not all languages have lexical tone (cf. Chapter 2 for a discussion of tone languages) or lexical pitch accent,[10] not all languages have lexical stress, in other words, a systematic marking of certain syllables within a word as more prominent than others. Importantly, these three aspects of word prosody are not mutually exclusive. For example, there are tone languages with stress (e.g., Mandarin) and without it (e.g., Cantonese), and pitch-accent languages with or without stress (e.g., Swedish and Japanese, respectively; Jun, 2005). Thus in the discussion below, it should be kept in mind that stress is a widespread but not universal feature of human language.

3.3.1 Rhythmic Typology

Four approaches to rhythmic typology are described below. Behind all of these approaches is a common desire to understand the relationships of the world's linguistic rhythms.

Periodicity and Typology

The most influential typology of language rhythm to date is based on the notion of periodicity in speech. This typology has its roots in the work of Kenneth Pike (1945), who proposed a theory of speech rhythm based on a dichotomy between languages in terms of syllable and stress patterns. He dubbed certain languages (such as Spanish) "syllable-timed," based on the idea that syllables

---

a more salient and reliable cue than the former (Sluijter & van Heuven, 1996, Sluijter et al., 1997).

[10] In a pitch-accent language, a word can have entirely different meaning depending on its pitch pattern. The difference between a tone language and a pitch-accent language is that in the former there is a prescribed pitch for each syllable, whereas in pitch-accent languages a certain syllable of a word may have lexical specification for pitch (Jun, 2005).

mark off roughly equal temporal intervals. These stood in contrast to "stress-timed" languages such as English, which were characterized by roughly equal temporal intervals between stresses. To illustrate stress-timed rhythm, Pike invited the reader to "notice the more or less equal lapses of time between the stresses in the sentence":

     x   x   x   x

(3.3) The teacher is interested in buying some books.

Pike then asked the reader to compare the timing of stresses in the above sentence with the following one, and notice the similarity "despite the different number of syllables" (p. 34):

    x x   x   x

(3.4) Big battles are fought daily.

Pike argued that in stress-timed languages the intervals between stressed syllables (referred to as "feet") were approximately equal despite changing numbers of syllables per foot. To achieve evenly timed feet, speakers would stretch or compress syllables to fit into the typical foot duration. Pike believed that learning the rhythm of a language was essential to correct pronunciation. He noted, for example, that Spanish speakers learning English "must abandon their sharp-cut syllable-by-syllable pronunciation and jam together—or lengthen where necessary—English vowels and consonants so as to obtain rhythm units of the stress-timing type" (p. 35).

Abercrombie (1967:34–36, 96–98) went further than Pike and proposed a physiological basis for stress versus syllable timing. This bold step was based on a specific hypothesis for how syllables are produced. Abercrombie believed that each syllable was associated with a contraction of muscles associated with exhalation (the intercostal muscles of the rib cage), and that some contractions were especially strong: These latter contractions produced stressed syllables. He referred to these two types of contractions as "chest pulses" and "stress pulses" (thus only some chest pulses were stress pulses; cf. Stetson 1951). Abercrombie proposed that in any given language, one or the other kind of pulse occurred rhythmically. He then equated rhythm with periodicity: "Rhythm, in speech as in other human activities, arises out of the periodic recurrence of some sort of movement. . . " (p. 96). Furthermore, he claimed that "as far as is known, every language in the world is spoken with one kind of rhythm or with the other" (p. 97), naming English, Russian, and Arabic as examples of stress-timed languages, and French, Telugu, and Yoruba as examples of syllable-timed languages. Just as Pike had done, he noted that a language could not be both stress-timed and syllable-timed. Because there are variable numbers of syllables between stresses, equalizing the duration of interstress intervals meant that "the rate of syllable succession has to be continually adjusted, in order to fit varying numbers of syllables into the same time interval."

It is hard to overestimate the impact of Pike and Abercrombie on the study of rhythm in speech. The terms "stress-timed" and "syllable-timed" have become part of the standard vocabulary of linguistics. A third category, "mora-timing," is also in standard use, and is used to describe the rhythm of Japanese speech. The mora is a unit that is smaller than the syllable, usually consisting of a consonant and vowel, but sometimes containing only a single consonant or vowel. Ladefoged (1975:224) stated that "each mora takes about the same length of time to say," thus arguing for the rough isochrony of morae.[11] Since the publication of Abercrombie's book, many languages have been classified into one of these two categories (Dauer, 1983; Grabe & Low, 2002), and many research studies have examined the issue of isochrony in speech. In this sense, the stress versus syllable-timed theory of speech rhythm has been very fruitful. It provided a clear, empirically testable hypothesis together with a physiological justification.

In another sense, however, the theory has been an utter failure. Empirical measurements of speech have failed to provide any support for the isochrony of syllables or stresses (see references in Bertinetto, 1989).[12] To take just a few examples from the many papers that have tested the isochrony hypothesis, Dauer (1983) showed that English stress feet grow in duration with increasing number of syllables, rather than maintaining the even duration necessary for isochrony (cf. Levelt, 1989:393). Roach (1982) compared English, Russian, and Arabic to French, Telugu, and Yoruba and demonstrated that the former stress-timed languages could not be discriminated from the latter syllable-timed ones on the basis of the timing of interstress intervals. Finally, Beckman (1982) and Hoequist (1983) showed that morae are not of equal duration in Japanese.

Given that the notion of periodicity in ordinary speech was empirically falsified over 20 years ago, why do the labels of stress-timing, syllable-timing, and mora-timing persist? One reason may be that it matches subjective intuitions about rhythm. For example, Abercrombie himself (1967:171) noted that the idea of isochronous stress in English dates back to the 18th century. Another reason is suggested by Beckman (1992), who argues that this tripartite scheme persists because it correctly groups together languages that are perceived as rhythmically similar, even if the physical basis for this grouping is not clearly understood (and is not isochrony of any kind).

---

[11] As an example, Ladefoged points out that the word *kakemono* (scroll) takes about the same amount of time to say as "nippon" (Japan), and attributes this to the fact that both words contain four morae: [ka ke mo no] and [ni p po n].

[12] Abercrombie's theory of syllables as rooted in chest pulses has also been falsified. It should be noted that Abercrombie was a pioneering scientist who established one of the first laboratories devoted to basic research in phonetics (in Edinburgh). His ideas about speech rhythm are but a tiny slice of his work, and though wrong, stimulated a great deal of research.

The key point of the current section, then, is that periodicity, which plays such an important role in much musical rhythm, is not part of the rhythm of ordinary speech. The next section explores a different approach to speech rhythm, one that sets aside notions of isochrony.

Phonology and Typology

The fact that speech is not isochronous should not lead us to discard the idea of speech rhythm. That is, research can move forward if one thinks of rhythm as systematic timing, accentuation, and grouping patterns in a language *that may have nothing to do with isochrony*. One productive approach in this framework is the phonological approach to rhythmic typology. The fundamental idea of this approach is that the rhythm of a language is the *product* of its linguistic structure, not an organizational *principle* such as stress or syllable isochrony (Dauer, 1983; cf. Dasher & Bolinger, 1982). In this view, languages are rhythmically different because they differ in phonological properties that influence how they are organized as patterns in time. One clear exposition of this idea is that of Dauer (1983, 1987), who posited several factors that influence speech rhythm.

The first factor is the diversity of syllable structures in a language.[13] Languages vary substantially in their inventory of syllable types. For example, English has syllables ranging from a single phoneme (e.g., the word "a") up to seven phonemes (as in "strengths"), and allows up to three consonants in onset and coda. In sharp contrast, languages such as Japanese (and many Polynesian languages) allow few syllable types and are dominated by simple CV syllables. Romance languages such as Spanish and French have more syllable types than Japanese or Hawaiian but avoid the complex syllables found in languages such as English and Dutch, and in fact show active processes that break up or prevent the creation of syllables with many segments (Dauer, 1987).

The diversity of syllables available to a language influences the diversity of syllable types in spoken sentences. For example, Dauer (1983) found that in a sample of colloquial French, over half the syllable tokens had a simple CV structure, whereas in a similar English sample, CV syllables accounted for only about one-third of the syllable tokens. These differences are relevant to rhythm because syllable duration is correlated with the number of phonemes per syllable, suggesting that sentences of English should have more variable syllable durations (on average) than French sentences.

---

[13] Syllables are generally recognized as having three structural slots: the onset consonant(s), the nucleus (usually occupied by a vowel), and the following consonants (referred to as the coda). A syllable with one consonant in the onset and none in the coda is represented by CV, whereas CCVC means two consonants in the onset and one in the coda, and so on.

The second factor affecting speech rhythm is vowel reduction. In some languages, such as English, unstressed syllables often have vowels that are acoustically centralized and short in duration (linguists commonly refer to this sound as "schwa," a neutral vowel sounding like "uh"). In contrast, in other languages (such as Spanish) the vowels of unstressed syllables are rarely if ever reduced, contributing to a less variable pattern of vowel duration between stressed and unstressed syllables.

The third rhythmic factor proposed by Dauer is the influence of stress on vowel duration. In some languages, stress has a strong effect on the duration of a vowel in a syllable. For example, one recent measurement of spoken English finds that vowels in stressed syllables are about 60% longer than the same vowels in unstressed syllables (Greenberg, 2006). In contrast, studies of Spanish suggest that stress does not condition vowel duration to the same degree (Delattre, 1966).

Dauer suggested that languages traditionally classified as stress-timed versus syllable-timed differ in the above phonological features, with stress-timed languages using a broader range of syllable types, having a system of reduced vowels, and exhibiting a strong influence of stress on vowel duration. This nicely illustrates the perspective of speech rhythm as a product of phonology, rather than a causal principle (e.g., involving periodicity).[14]

Dauer's proposal leads to testable predictions. Specifically, the three factors she outlines (diversity in syllable structure, vowel reduction, and the influence of stress on vowel duration) should all contribute to a greater degree of durational variability among the syllables of stress-timed versus syllable-timed utterances. Surprisingly, there is little published data on durational variability of syllables in sentences of stress versus syllable-timed languages. One reason for this may be that the demarcation of syllable boundaries in speech is not always straightforward. Although people generally agree on how many syllables a word or utterance has, there can be disagreement about where the boundaries between syllables are, even among linguists. For example does the first "l" in the word "syllable" belong to the end of the first syllable or to the beginning of the second syllable, or is it "ambisyllabic," belonging to both syllables? Although it is true that syllable measurements are subject to decisions that may vary from one researcher to the next, this should not impede empirical research: It simply means that measurements should be accompanied by an indication of where each syllable boundary was placed. I return to this point below.

---

[14] Dauer also suggested that stress- and syllable-timed languages had a different relationship between stress and intonation: In the former, stressed syllables serve as turning points in the intonation contour, whereas in the latter, intonation and stress are more independent. As intonation is not discussed in this chapter, this idea will not be pursued here.

Before turning to another phonological approach to speech rhythm, it is worth noting that the phonological properties listed by Dauer do not always co-occur. Thus Dauer argued against the idea of discrete rhythmic classes and for the notion of a rhythmic continuum. In support of this idea, Nespor (1990) has noted that Polish has complex syllable structure but no vowel reduction (at normal speech rates), and Catalan has simple syllable structure but does have vowel reduction. Thus there is currently a debate in the field of speech rhythm as to whether languages really do fall into discrete rhythm classes or whether there is a continuum based on the pattern of co-occurrence of rhythmically relevant phonological factors (cf. Arvaniti, 1994; Grabe & Low, 2002). Only further research can resolve this issue, particularly perceptual research (as discussed below in section 3.3.1, subsection "Perception and Typology").

I now turn briefly to a different phonological theory of speech rhythm, proposed by Dwight Bolinger (1981). Although Bolinger focused on English, his ideas are quite relevant to typological issues. The foundation of Bolinger's theory is the notion that there are two distinct sets of vowels in English: full vowels and reduced vowels. By "reduced" vowels Bolinger does not simply mean vowels in unstressed syllables that are short and acoustically centralized (i.e., a phonetic definition). He argues for a phonological class of reduced vowels in English, which behave differently from other vowels. Bolinger places three vowels in this class, an "ih"-like vowel, and "uh"-like vowel, and a "oh"-like vowel (more similar to "uh" than to the full vowel "o"). Phonetically all of these vowels occur in the central region of vowel space, near the schwa vowel /ə/ of English (see Figure 2.19: Bolinger's "ih" and "oh" vowel are not shown in that figure, but the former would occur just to the left and up from /ə/, and the latter would occur just to the right and up from /ə/). Bolinger (1981:3–9) presents arguments to support the notion that these vowels are a phonologically distinct subclass, in other words, that they behave in certain ways that full vowels do not. Space limitations prevent a detailed discussion of these arguments. Here I will focus on two claims Bolinger makes about full and reduced vowels that are relevant for speech rhythm.

First, he claims that syllables containing full and reduced vowels tend to alternate in English sentences. Second, he claims that there is a "lengthening rule" such that "when a long syllable is followed by a short one, the short one borrows time from it and makes it relatively short" (p. 18). (By a "long" syllable, he means a syllable with a full vowel, and by a "short" syllable, he means a syllable with a reduced vowel; there is no claim for a particular duration ratio between the two types of syllables.) To illustrate this rule, Bolinger offers the following example (note that the first sentence is from an ad for a special type of soap):

(3.5) Gets out dirt plain soap can't reach.

        L   L L   L   L   L   L

(3.6) Takes a-way the dirt that com-mon soaps can nev-er reach
       Lˉ S Lˉ S Lˉ   S Lˉ   S Lˉ   S Lˉ S L

In the example above, I have indicated the shortened L's of the second sentence by Lˉ (after Faber, 1986). The point of this example is that each Lˉ of
sentence 3.6 is shorter than the L's of sentence 3.5, and this occurs (according to Bolinger) because each S "borrows time" from the preceding L. Note
that sentence 3.6 has strict alternation between L and S. This is a special case:
Bolinger makes no claims for strict alternation, only a claim for a tendency
(thus sequences such as L L S S S L S L L . . . are perfectly possible). I suspect
Bolinger chose the sentences in 3.5 and 3.6 as examples because he felt that
each (Lˉ S) pair in sentence 3.6 is not terribly different in duration from each
L in sentence 3.5: This is suggested by his graphical placement of the L's in the
two sentences above one another, in his original text. However, the durational
equivalence of L and (Lˉ S) is not part of Bolinger's claim. This is an important
point. Bolinger's theory may be relevant to the subjective impression of isochrony (because of the rough alternation of L and S and the lengthening rule), but
it has no isochrony principle.

Faber (1986) argues that Bolinger's theory is superior to stress-timing theory
when it comes to teaching the rhythm of English to foreign students (cf. Chela-
Flores, 1994). He also points out that Bolinger's theory can be used to explain
characteristic timing patterns that stress-timing theory cannot account for, such
as why "cart" is shorter in:

(3.7) Ask Mr. Carter
           L - S

than in:

(3.8) Ask Mr. Cartwright.
           L   L

Or why "man" is shorter in:

(3.10) Have you seen the manor?
             L- S

than in:

(3.10) Have you seen the manhole?
             L   L

Bolinger's theory of speech rhythm is distinct from the theory outlined by
Dauer in that it deals not just with the variability syllable duration but with the
patterning of duration. Specifically, Bolinger argues that the characteristic rhythm
of English is due to the rough *alternation* of syllables with full and reduced
vowels, and to the way full vowels *change* duration when intervening reduced

syllables are added. This is already enough to suggest a basis for typological distinctions between languages. For example, one might test the idea that stress-timed languages have more contrast in adjacent vowel durations than do syllable timed languages, and that stress-timed languages have lengthening rules of the type suggested by Bolinger for English (Bolinger himself does not suggest these ideas, but they are an obvious corollary of his work). If Bolinger had stopped here, he would already have made a valuable contribution to speech rhythm research. Bolinger's theory has one further component, however, that represents a fundamental divergence from the theory outlined by Dauer.

Once again focusing on English, Bolinger suggested that just as there are two kinds of vowels (full and reduced), there are also two kinds of rhythm. The first is the rhythmic patterning already described, in other words, the rough alternation of long and short syllables and the lengthening rule. Above this level, however, is a second level of rhythmic patterning concerned with temporal relations between accents cued by pitch. Note that this idea entails the notion that syllabic rhythm is fundamentally about duration and does not rely on pitch as a cue. In other words, "there is a basic level of temporal patterning that is independent of tonal patterning" (Bolinger 1981:24, citing Bruce, 1981). Bolinger argues that this temporal patterning would be observable even in speech spoken on a monotone. Speech is not spoken on a monotone, however, and Bolinger argues that syllables accented by pitch form a second level of rhythmic patterning in which the fundamental rule is *a tendency to separate pitch accents so that they do not occur too closely together in time*. The mechanism for avoiding "accent clash" is to move adjacent accents away from each other, a phenomenon sometimes called "stress-shift" in English. (One oft-cited example of stress shift is when "thirtéen" becomes "thírteen mén"; Liberman & Prince, 1977.) The term "stress-shift" is somewhat unfortunate, because there is evidence that what is shifting is pitch accent, not syllable duration or amplitude (Shattuck-Hufnagel et al., 1994).

The idea that speech rhythm involves temporal patterning at two distinct linguistic levels merits far more empirical research than it has garnered to date. I will return to this idea in section 3.3.4.

Duration and Typology

Until very recently, the measurement of duration has had a largely negative role in the study of speech rhythm, namely in falsifying claims for the periodicity of stresses or syllables. The insights of the phonological approach, however, have created a new positive role for durational measurements. A key feature of this work has been the abandonment of any search for isochrony, and a focus on durational correlates of phonological phenomena involved in speech rhythm. Ramus and colleagues (1999), inspired by the insights of Dauer, examined the durational pattering of vowels and consonants in speech, based on ideas about how syllable structure should influence this patterning. For example, languages that use a greater variety of syllable types (i.e., stress-timed languages) are likely to have relatively less time devoted to vowels in sentences than languages dominated by simple syllables, due to the frequent consonant clusters in the former languages. By similar reasoning, the durational variability of consonantal intervals in sentences (defined as sequences of consonants between vowels, irrespective of syllable or word boundaries) should be greater for languages with more diverse syllable structures. This latter point is schematically illustrated in 3.11, in which boundaries between syllables are marked with a dot and consonantal intervals are underlined:

(3.11a) CV.CCCVC.CV.CV.CVCC   "stress-timed" language

(3.11b) CV.CV.CVC.CV.CV.CVC.CV   "syllable-timed" language

Note how the greater diversity of syllable types in 3.11a leads to greater variation in the number of consonants between vowels (likely to translate into greater durational variability of consonantal intervals) as well as a lower vowel to consonant ratio (likely to translate into a lower fraction of utterance duration spent on vowels).

These ideas were borne out by empirical measurements. Figure 3.7 (from Ramus et al., 1999) shows a graph with percent of duration occupied by vowels

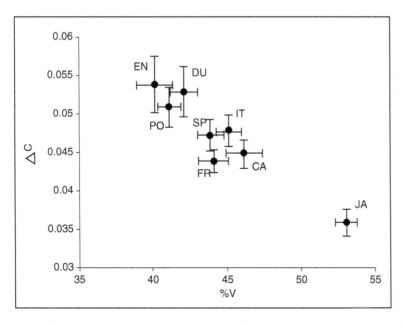

Figure 3.7 Percentage of sentence duration occupied by vowels versus the standard deviation of consonantal intervals within sentences for 8 languages. (CA = Catalan, DU = Dutch, EN = English, FR = French, IT = Italian, JA = Japanese, PO = Polish, SP = Spanish.) Error bars show +/- 1 standard error. From Ramus, Nespor, & Mehler, 1999.

(%V) versus consonantal interval variability (ΔC) within sentences in eight languages. (The data for each language came from 20 sentences read by four speakers, i.e., five sentences per speaker.)

What is interesting about this graph is that languages traditionally classified as stress-timed (English and Dutch) have low %V and high ΔC values, and occupy a different region of the graph than languages traditionally classified as syllable timed (French, Italian, and Spanish). Furthermore, Japanese, which linguists place in a different rhythmic category (mora-timed) is isolated from the other languages. (The location of Polish and Catalan in this graph is discussed in the next section, on perception.) This demonstrated an empirical correlate of traditional linguistic rhythmic classes, and has inspired other researchers to examine more languages in this framework. One interesting study is that of Frota and Vigário (2001), who examined the rhythm of Brazilian Portuguese versus European Portuguese (henceforth BP and EP). Linguists had often claimed that these two varieties were rhythmically different, with EP being stress-timed, and BP being syllable-timed or having mixed rhythmic characteristics. This makes Portuguese a fascinating topic for speech rhythm research, because one can study sentences with exactly the same words but spoken with different rhythms. (British English and Singapore English provide another such opportunity, because the former is stress-timed and the latter has been described as syllable-timed; see Low et al., 2000.) Frota and Vigário compared sentences spoken by European and Brazilian speakers of Portuguese, and found that EP had significantly a higher ΔC and lower %V than BP, as predicted by Ramus et al.'s findings.[15]

One important question about this line of research concerns the perceptual relevance of ΔC and %V. Ramus et al. focused on these measures because of their interest in the role of rhythm in infant speech perception. There is evidence that newborns and young infants can discriminate languages that belong to different rhythmic classes (Mehler et al., 1988, 1996; see also the next section). Mehler and colleagues (1996) have argued that this ability helps bootstrap language acquisition: Once a given rhythmic class is detected, class-specific acquisition mechanisms can be triggered that direct attention to the units that are relevant for segmenting words from connected speech (e.g., stresses in the case of English, syllables in the case of French, as discussed in section 3.3.3, subsection "The Role of Rhythm in Segmenting Connected Speech"). For this theory to work, infants must have some basis for discrimi-

---

[15] Although Ramus et al. (1999) related differences in ΔC and %V to syllable structure, Frota and Vigário (2001) point out that in the BP/EP case, differences in these variables are driven by vowel reduction, because syllable structures are similar in the two varieties. See Frota and Vigário (2001) for details. Frota and Vigário also provide a very useful discussion of the ΔC parameter and the need to normalize this variable for overall sentence duration/speech rate (see also Ramus, 2002a).

nating rhythmic class. Thus Ramus et al. (1999) sought an acoustic correlate of rhythmic class that would require minimal knowledge about linguistic units. ΔC and %V are two such parameters, because one only need assume that the infant can distinguish between vowels and consonants (see Galves et al., 2002, for an acoustic correlate of ΔC that does not even require segmentation into vowels and consonants).

One may ask, however, if ΔC and %V are directly relevant to the perception of speech rhythm, or if they are simply correlated with another feature that is more relevant to rhythm perception. That is, one could argue that these measures are global statistics reflecting variability in syllable structure, and are not themselves the basis of rhythm perception in speech (cf. Barry et al., 2003). A more promising candidate for perceptual relevance may be variability in syllable duration, which is likely to be correlated with variability in syllable structure and with vowel reduction. Because the syllable is widely regarded as a fundamental unit in speech rhythm, and because both adults and infants are sensitive to syllable patterning (e.g., van Ooyen et al., 1997), it would be worth examining the corpus of sentences used by Ramus et al. for syllable duration variability to see if this parameter differentiates traditional rhythmic classes. This would also be a straightforward test of Dauer's ideas, as the phonological factors she outlines imply that syllable duration variability should be higher in sentences of stress-timed than of syllable-timed languages.

Surprisingly, there has been little empirical work comparing sentence-level variability in syllable duration among different languages. As noted in the previous section, this may reflect the difficulties of assigning syllable boundaries in connected speech. From a purely practical standpoint, it is easier to define phoneme boundaries, using criteria agreed upon by most phoneticians (e.g., Peterson & Lehiste, 1960). However, this should not stop research into syllabic duration patterns, because these patterns are likely to be perceptually relevant. To illustrate both the feasibility and the challenges of a syllable-based approach, examples 3.11c and d below show a sentence of English and French segmented at syllable boundaries (the segmentations were done by myself and Franck Ramus, respectively). Periods indicate syllable boundaries that we felt were clear, whereas square brackets indicate phonemes that seemed ambiguous in terms of their syllabic affiliation. In the latter case, one must decide where to place the syllable boundary. For example, if the phoneme sounds ambisyllabic then the boundary can be placed in the middle of the phoneme, or if it sounds like it has been resyllabified with the following vowel, the boundary can be placed before the phoneme.

(3.11c) The .last .con.cert .gi.ven .at .the .o[p]era .was .a .tre.men.dous .suc.cess

(3.11d) Il. fau.dra .beau.coup .plus .d'ar.gent .pour .me.ne[r] à .bien .ce .pro.jet

It is likely that different researchers will vary in how they make these judgment calls. Nevertheless, this is not an insurmountable problem for rhythm research.

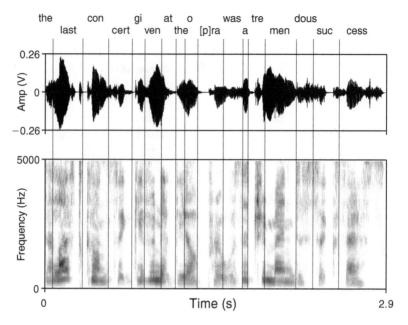

Figure 3.8a A sentence of British English segmented into syllables. (Note that "opera" is pronounced "opra" by this speaker.)

In fact, if different researchers define syllable boundaries in slightly different ways but nevertheless converge on the rhythmic differences they find between languages, this is strong evidence that the observed differences are robust.[16] Figure 3.8a and 3.8b show my markings of syllable boundaries in the waveform and spectrograms of these two sentences (the sentences can be heard in Sound Examples 3.5a and b; note that in sentence 3.5a, "opera" is pronounced "opra").

For these sentences, the variability of syllable durations as measured by the coefficient of variation (the standard deviation divided by the mean) is .53 for the English sentence and .42 for the French sentence. Making similar measurements on all the English and French sentences in the Ramus database yields the data in Figure 3.8c. As can be seen, on average English sentences have more variable syllable durations than do French sentences (the difference is statistically significant, $p < 0.01$, Mann-Whitney U test). It would be interesting to

---

[16] Individual researchers who are comparing syllable duration patterns across two languages can also handle the problem of syllable boundary identification by making all such decisions in a manner that is conservative with regard to the hypothesis at hand. For example, if comparing languages A and B with the hypothesis that syllables are more variable in duration in the sentences of language A, then any judgment calls about syllable boundaries should be made in such a way as to work against this hypothesis.

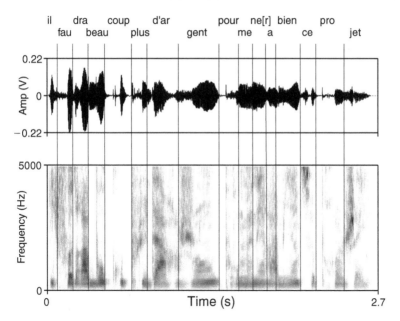

Figure 3.8b A sentence of French segmented into syllables.

have similar variability measurements for numerous languages that have been classified as stress- versus syllable-timed: Would these measurements divide the languages into their traditional rhythmic classes? (See Wagner & Dellwo, 2004, for a promising start.)

Turning now to the ideas of Dwight Bolinger, recall Bolinger's claim that syllables containing full and reduced vowels tend to alternate in English. This leads to an empirical prediction, namely that the durational contrast between adjacent vowel durations in English sentences should be greater than in languages of a different rhythmic class, such as French or Spanish. In fact, there is research supporting this prediction, though it was not inspired by Bolinger's work but by an interest in the role that vowel reduction plays in the rhythm of stress- versus syllable-timed languages. Low, Grabe, and Nolan (2000) set out to explore the idea that vowel reduction contributes to the impression of stress-timing via its impact on vowel duration variability in sentences. They tested this idea by examining vowel duration patterning in a stress-timed versus a syllable-timed variety of English (British vs. Singapore English). Crucially, they developed an index of variability that was sensitive to the patterning of duration. Their "normalized pairwise variability index" (nPVI) measures the degree of contrast between successive durations in an utterance. An intuition for the nPVI can be gained by examining Figure 3.9, which schematically depicts two sequences of events of varying duration (the length of each bar corresponds to the duration of the event).

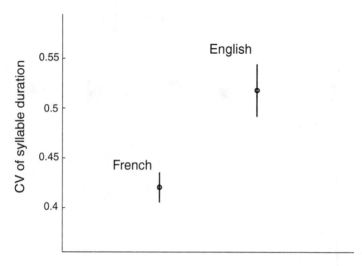

Figure 3.8c The coefficient of variation (CV) of syllable duration in 20 English and 20 French sentences. Error bars show +/- 1 standard error.

In sequence A, neighboring events (e.g., events 1 and 2, 2 and 3) tend to have a large contrast in duration, and hence the sequence would have a large nPVI. Now consider sequence B, which has the same set of durations as sequence A, arranged in a different temporal order. Now neighboring events tend to have low contrast in duration, giving the sequence a low nPVI value. Hence the two sequences have a sharp difference in durational contrastiveness, even though they have exactly the same overall amount of durational variability, for

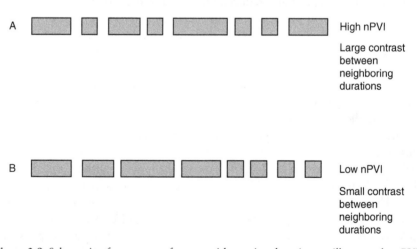

Figure 3.9 Schematic of sequences of events with varying duration, to illustrate the nPVI (longer bars = longer durations). See text for details.

example, as measured by the standard deviation of durations. (See this chapter's appendix 1 for the nPVI equation.)

Because the nPVI is fundamentally a measure of contrast, the use of the term "variability" in its name is somewhat unfortunate, as variability and contrast are not necessarily correlated, as shown in Figure 3.9. In fact, it is quite possible to have two sequences A and B in which the variability of durations in A is greater than B, but the nPVI of durations is greater in B than of A (an example is given in section 3.5.1). Thus a better term for this measure might have been the "normalized pairwise contrastiveness index."

I have delved into the details of the nPVI because it has proven quite fruitful in the study of speech rhythm and in the comparative study of linguistic and musical rhythm (discussed in 3.5.1). Grabe and Low (2002) have used the nPVI to examine the patterning of vowel durations in sentences of a number of languages, and have shown that several languages traditionally classified as stress-timed (such as German, Dutch, British English, and Thai) have a larger vocalic nPVI than a number of other languages traditionally classified as syllable timed (such as French, Italian, and Spanish). This supports Bolinger's idea that durational alternation of vowels is important to stress-timed rhythm.[17] Inspired by this work, Ramus (2002b) measured the vowel nPVI for all eight languages in his database and found the results shown in Figure 3.10.

Figure 3.10 plots the nPVI for vocalic intervals against the rPVI for intervocalic intervals (i.e., consonantal intervals). (The rPVI, or "raw pairwise variability index," is computed in the same way as the nPVI but without the normalization term in the denominator; cf. this chapter's appendix 1. Grabe and Low [2002] argue that normalization is not desirable for consonantal intervals because it would normalize for cross-language differences in syllable structure.) Focusing on the nPVI dimension, the stress-timed languages (English and Dutch) are separated from the syllable-timed languages (Spanish, Italian, and French), which provides additional support for Bolinger's ideas.[18] Furthermore,

---

[17] The correlation between nPVI and rhythm class is not perfect, however. Grabe and Low (2002) found a high vowel nPVI value for Tamil, a language which has been classified as syllable-timed (cf. Keane, 2006). It should be noted that Grabe and Low's (2002) results should be considered preliminary because only one speaker per language was studied. Subsequent work has applied the nPVI to cross-linguistic corpora with fewer languages but more speakers per language (e.g., Ramus, 2002b; Lee & Todd, 2004; Dellwo, 2004).

[18] It should be noted that both Grabe and Low (2002) and Ramus (2002b) measured the nPVI of vocalic intervals, defined as vowels and sequences of consecutive vowels irrespective of syllable and word boundaries, whereas Bolinger's arguments are focused on individual vowels. This is not a serious problem because most vocalic intervals are individual vowels due to the strong tendency for vowels to be separated by consonants in speech. For example, in the database used by Ramus (eight languages, 160 sentences),

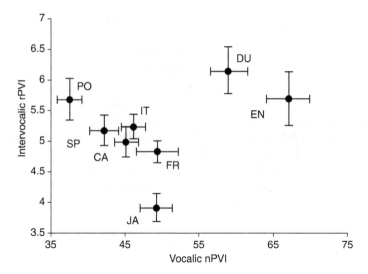

Figure 3.10 Vocalic nPVI versus Consonantal (intervocalic) rPVI for sentences in eight languages. (CA = Catalan, DU = Dutch, EN = English, FR = French, IT = Italian, JA = Japanese, PO = Polish, SP = Spanish.) Error bars show +/- 1 standard error. From Ramus, 2002a.

Polish is now far from the stress-timed languages, which is interesting because there is perceptual evidence that Polish is rhythmically different from these languages due to its lack of vowel reduction (see section 3.3.1, subsection "Perception and Typology"). Japanese is similar to French in terms of nPVI, however, suggesting that nPVI alone is not enough to sort languages into traditional rhythmic classes. Adding a second dimension of rPVI for consonantal intervals, however, does segregate out Japanese, which has very low durational contrast between successive consonantal intervals. This suggests that at least two phonetic dimensions may be needed to capture differences between rhythmic classes (see also Ramus et al., 1999).

One interesting linguistic application of the nPVI has been to the ontogeny of speech rhythm. It has been claimed that the rhythm of English-speaking children is syllable-timed in contrast to the stress-timed rhythm of adult speech (Allen & Hawkins, 1978). Grabe et al. (1999) conducted an nPVI study that

there are 2,725 vowels, out of which 2,475 (91%) are singletons, in other words, a single vowel flanked by a consonant on either side (or if the vowel is the first or last phoneme of the sentence, a single vowel flanked by a following or preceding consonant, respectively). Thus it is likely that nPVI measurements based on individual vowels would produce qualitatively similar results as those based on vocalic intervals (cf. Patel et al., 2006).

supported this claim. They measured the nPVI of vowels in the speech of English versus French speaking 4-year-olds and their mothers. They found that English children had significantly lower nPVI values than their mothers, whereas French children resembled their mothers in having a low nPVIs. That is, both English and French children spoke with a syllable-timed rhythm (though the nPVI of the English children was already larger than that of their French counterparts). It would be interesting to track nPVI as a function of age in English and French children, to study the developmental time course of speech rhythm in the two languages.

All nPVI studies to date have focused on a single rhythmic layer in language: the temporal patterning of vowels or consonants. In the spirit of Bolinger's idea that rhythm may involve multiple levels of temporal organization, it would be worth using the nPVI to explore the relationship of durational patterns at various rhythmically relevant levels in speech (cf. Asu & Nolan, 2006). For example, within English sentences, one could compute the nPVI of interstress intervals (ISIs) relative to the nPVI of syllable durations by measuring both of these quantities in each sentence and then taking the ratio of the former to the latter. It may be that the subjective impression of isochrony in English arises in part from a lower durational contrast between ISIs than between syllables, which would make this ratio significantly less than 1. I return to this idea in section 3.3.4.

This section has reviewed a few different acoustic correlates of speech rhythm. Due to the success of this work, it seems certain that more such correlates will be proposed and explored in the future (e.g., Gut, 2005). Ultimately, the usefulness of such measures will depend on whether they group together languages that are perceived as rhythmically similar and divide languages perceived as rhythmically different. Perceptual studies are thus fundamental to research on rhythmic typology, and it is to such studies that we turn next.

Perception and Typology

All typological theories of language rhythm are ultimately rooted in perception. In the past, linguists have defined rhythm categories (such as stress vs. syllable timing) based on their auditory impressions of languages, and then researchers have sought to identify phonological and acoustic correlates of these classes. The recent success in finding durational correlates of traditional rhythm classes is a testament to the intuition of linguists in their aural rhythmic judgments. However, it is also apparent that the old categorization system has its shortcomings. For example, some languages straddle different categories (e.g., Polish and Catalan, see above), and many languages do not fit neatly into any of the existing categories (Grabe & Low, 2002). Thus the old system is cracking at the seams, and a new science of rhythm classification is called for. Such a science must have as its foundation a body of perceptual data that provides a measure of the rhythmic similarities and differences between languages. These data will allow researchers to construct a perceptual map of language rhythms and determine to what extent the rhythms of human languages fall into distinct clusters (vs. forming a continuum). It will also help suggest new avenues for empirical research into the acoustic foundations of speech rhythm.

Fortunately, perceptual work on the rhythmic differences between languages has already begun. An innovative study by Ramus and Mehler (1999) devised a method for studying the perception of speech rhythm posited on the idea that if a listener can tell two languages apart when the only cues are rhythmic, then the languages belong to distinct rhythmic classes. Speech resynthesis techniques were used to selectively remove various phonetic differences between languages and focus attention on rhythm. Sound Examples 3.6 and 3.7 illustrate Ramus and Mehler's technique on a sentence of English and Japanese. Each sentence is presented in four versions, which convert the original sentence to an increasingly abstract temporal pattern of vowels and consonants. In the first transformation, each phoneme is replaced by a particular member of its class: all fricatives replaced by /s/, vowels by /a/, liquids (l & r) by /l/, plosives by /t/, nasals by /n/, and glides by /ai/ (a condition they called "saltanaj," pronounced "sal-tan-ai"). The original intonation of each sentence is preserved. In the second transformation, all consonants are replaced by /s/ and all vowels by /a/ (a condition they call "sasasa"). In the final transformation, the voice pitch is flattened to a monotone, leaving the temporal pattern of vowels and consonants as the only difference between the languages (a condition the authors refer to as "flat sasasa"). Ramus and Mehler found that French adults could discriminate between English and Japanese in all three conditions, supporting the hypothesis that the rhythms of English and Japanese are indeed perceptually distinct.

Focusing on the flat sasasa transformation, Ramus et al. (2003) also tested French adults' ability to discriminate the rhythms of English, Polish, Spanish, and Catalan. The results indicated that Polish could be discriminated from the other languages, whereas Catalan could not be discriminated from Spanish, though it was distinct from English and Polish. (Recall that on phonological grounds, Polish and Catalan seemed intermediate between stress-timed and syllable-timed languages; cf. section 3.3.1, subsection "Phonology and Typology.") These perceptual data suggest that Polish does belong in a separate rhythmic category than English, whereas Catalan belongs in the same category as Spanish. This finding has implications for maps of the acoustic correlates of speech rhythm, such as Figure 3.7. In that map, Polish clustered with stress-timed languages, indicating that a different acoustic dimension is needed to separate perceived rhythmic classes. Indeed, Ramus et al. (1999, 2003) have noted that Polish can be separated out from all other languages in their original study on a dimension that measures the variability of vowel duration in a sentence, ΔV, because Polish has a very low vowel duration variability compared to all other languages in their sample.[19] Thus perceptual work on speech has already suggested that if one wishes to preserve the notion of rhythm classes in language, at least four classes are needed: stress-timed, syllable-timed, mora-timed (represented by Japanese), and one other yet-to-be-named category represented by Polish.[20]

Another line of perceptual research concerned with rhythmic typology has focused on newborns and infants. This choice of subjects may seem surprising, but these studies are motivated by the idea that very young humans are sensitive to speech rhythm and use it to guide learning of fine-grained sound patterns of language (Mehler et al., 1996). Nazzi et al. (1998) studied newborn rhythm perception using low-pass filtered speech. This removes most of the phonetic information but preserves syllable, stress, and pitch patterns. They showed that French newborns are able to discriminate English from Japanese, but not English from Dutch, suggesting that the latter are members of the same rhythmic class. They also showed that the newborns could discriminate English and Dutch from Spanish and Italian, but not English and Spanish from Dutch and Italian, suggesting that the former pairings more accurately capture perceptual rhythmic classes (cf. Nazzi et al., 2000, for converging findings with 5-month-old infants). These findings support the authors' hypothesis that babies can discriminate languages *only* when they belong to different rhythmic classes, a notion that they dub the "rhythm hypothesis" for language acquisition. If this is true, then the ears of infants may be particularly important instruments in mapping human speech rhythms in future research.[21]

The studies of Ramus, Nazzi, and colleagues raise a number of points for future research on the perception of speech rhythm. First, it is important to design stimuli and tasks that focus attention on those aspects of speech rhythm that play a role in normal speech perception. For example, a danger of the flat sasasa condition it that when a language with a highly variable syllable structure (such as English) is compared to a language dominated by simple syllables (such as Japanese), a salient perceptual difference between the resulting flat

---

[19] Polish also has the lowest vocalic nPVI of all languages in the Ramus et al. (1999) database (Ramus, 2002a; cf. Figure 3.10).

[20] It would be desirable for future research on rhythmic classes to suggest new names for rhythmic classes, as the current names (stress-timed, syllable-timed, and mora-timed) are implicitly bound up with the (failed) notion of isochrony.

[21] One possible confound in the elegant study of Nazzi et al. (1998) is the presence of intonation, which may have played a role in the infants' discrimination. Indeed, Ramus et al. (2000) found that French newborns could distinguish Dutch from Japanese using resynthesized saltanaj speech, but that their discrimination ability was much weaker when the original F0 contours of the sentences were replaced by the same artificial contours (Ramus, 2002b). He also notes that intonation can be removed entirely using flat sasasa resynthesis, but that the resulting sound patterns are problematic for use with newborns and infants, who may find them boring or distressing.

sasasa stimuli is the more frequent occurrence of long-duration /s/ sounds in the former stimulus (which result from transforming consonant clusters into single, long /s/ sounds). Thus discrimination could simply be based on listening for frequent long /s/ sounds rather than on attending to temporal structure.

Second, research on the perceptual taxonomy of language rhythms should not only be based on discrimination tasks, but should also incorporate similarity judgments. Musical studies of rhythmic similarity provide a good model for such research (Gabrielsson, 1973, 1993). In this research, rhythms are presented in a pairwise fashion and listeners rate their perceived similarity using a numerical scale. The resulting ratings are studied using multidimensional scaling to uncover perceptual dimensions used by listeners in classifying rhythms. This paradigm could easily be adapted to study speech rhythm, using low-pass filtered speech with minimal pitch variation as stimuli. Such studies should be sensitive to the idea that the important perceptual dimensions for rhythm may be relational, for example, a high contrastiveness between successive syllable durations while simultaneously having a lower durational contrastiveness between interstress intervals (cf. the end of section 3.3.1, subsection "Duration and Typology").

Finally, a fundamental issue for all future studies of rhythmic typology is the extent to which perceived rhythmic similarities and differences between languages depend on the native language of the listener. The theory of stress, syllable, and mora timing was proposed by native English speakers, and it is an open question whether speakers of other languages perceive rhythmic cues in the same way that English speakers do. For example, it has recently been demonstrated that French listeners have some difficulty distinguishing nonsense words that differ only in the location of stress, whereas Spanish listeners have no such difficulty (Dupoux et al., 2001). This likely reflects the fact that Spanish has contrastive stress: Two words can have the same phonemes but a different stress pattern, and this can change the meaning of the word entirely (e.g., *sábana* vs. *sabána,* which mean "sheet" and "savannah" respectively; cf. Soto-Faraco et al., 2001). French does not have this property, and Dupoux et al. suggest that this difference is responsible for the "stress deafness" they found in their French listeners. Results such as this raise a fundamental question: Is there a single map of perceived rhythmic similarities and differences among languages, or does the geography of the map differ according to the native language of the listener? Only empirical work can resolve this issue, but it seems a real possibility that native language influences the perception of rhythmic relations between languages.

3.3.2 Principles Governing the Rhythmic Shape of Words and Utterances

For those interested in comparing rhythm in language and music, it is important to be familiar with a branch of theoretical linguistics known as "metrical phonology." Metrical phonology deals with speech rhythm, but it does so in a manner quite different from the approaches described so far. First and foremost, rhythmic prominence is treated as hierarchical. That is, prominence is incrementally assigned *at each level* of the prosodic hierarchy according to systematic principles. For example, in a given theory it may be the case that all syllables begin with a basic amount of prominence, then the lexically stressed syllable of each word (or clitic group) is assigned an additional degree of prominence, then a phrase-level prominence is added to a particular word of a phrase (e.g., the "nuclear stress rule" in English), and so on. In this view, prominence is not simply a binary phonetic feature called "stress" that syllables either have or do not. Rather, prominence is an acoustic projection of the hierarchical prosodic structure of an utterance, and as such, has several degrees that serve to indicate a syllable's position in an utterance's rhythmic hierarchy (Halle & Vergnaud, 1987; Halle & Idsardi, 1996; Shattuck-Hufnagel & Turk, 1996).[22]

One of the clearest expositions of metrical phonology is in Selkirk's 1984 book, *Phonology and Syntax: The Relation Between Sound and Structure.* One goal of this book is to show how one can go from a string of words to a representation of the syllabic prominence pattern of the spoken utterance in a rule-governed fashion. The relative prominence of syllables is represented using a "metrical grid" that treats each syllable as a point in abstract time (Figure 3.11), meaning that prominence patterns are considered without regard to their exact timing.

Two aspects of the linguistic metrical grid, introduced by Liberman (1975), embody "the claim that the rhythmic organization of speech is quite analogous to that of music" (Selkirk, 1984:9). First, as noted above, prominence is treated hierarchically, analogously to hierarchical theories of musical meter (Cooper & Meyer, 1960; Lerdahl & Jackendoff, 1983). Above the basic level of the syllable are several other levels. The second level marks stressed syllables, and is the level of the basic "beat," in analogy to the tactus in music (Selkirk, 1984:10, 40). The third level marks the primary lexical stress of each word, and the fourth level marks the main accent of each phrase. This "text-to-grid" assignment of

---

[22] An early conceptual link between hierarchical theories of linguistic rhythm and theories of musical structure was made by Jackendoff (1989), who noted a structural equivalence between one type of prosodic tree structure used to depict hierarchical prominence relations in language and a type of tree used by Lerdahl and Jackendoff (1983) to indicate the relative structural importance of events in a span of musical notes. Jackendoff speculated that the coincidence of these two formalisms might reflect the fact that language and music use different specializations of general-purpose mental principles for assigning structure to temporal patterns, in other words, principles that parse sound sequences into recursive hierarchies of binary oppositions of structural importance. As noted by Jackendoff, however, prosodic trees have been largely abandoned in theories of speech rhythm.

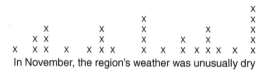

Figure 3.11 A metrical grid for a sentence of English. From Selkirk, 1984.

beats provides the input on which rhythmic principles operate. These principles, which represent the second link to musical meter, amount to a tendency to alternate between stronger and weaker elements at *each level* of the hierarchy. The principles are enforced by rules that can add, delete, and move beats to make the pattern at each level more congruous with an alternating pattern. For example, a rule of "beat addition" might add a beat at the second level to avoid a long series of unstressed syllables. At the third level, a rule of "beat movement" might shift the primary stress/accent of word to avoid the adjacency of primary lexical stress/accent (as when "thirteen" becomes "thírteen mén"; Liberman and Prince, 1977, Shattuck-Hufnagel et al.,1994; Grabe & Warren, 1995). The ideal goal is that strong beats at any given level are separated by no more than two weak beats at that level (the "principle of rhythmic alternation"). Thus metrical phonology derives the prominence pattern of a sentence using ideas directly inspired by theories of musical meter.

The notion that speech has multiple rhythmically relevant levels is an interesting abstract similarity between rhythm in language and music, because a fundamental property of musical meter is the existence of perceptually salient temporal pattering on multiple timescales (cf. section 3.2.2). Furthermore, just as musical meter involves at least one psychologically accessible rhythmic level below the beat and one or two levels above it, metrical phonology proposes rhythmic levels below and above the "beat" of stressed syllables. That is, both theories concern the patterning of time intervals at several timescales.

Although the picture painted by metrical phonology is an elegant one, it should be noted that its claims are by no means universally accepted by speech scientists (Cooper & Eady, 1986), and that the patterns of prominence it proposes are typically constructed from the intuitions of linguists rather than from acoustic and perceptual data collected in laboratory settings. However, there is hope that the field can be put on an empirical footing. For example, there is phonetic evidence for four degrees of prominence in speech (at least in stress-timed languages), corresponding to reduced vowels, full vowels, stressed syllables, and accented syllables (Terken & Hermes, 2000). For the current purposes, metrical phonology is interesting because it draws attention to a number of issues in which comparisons of linguistic and musical rhythm are instructive. One of these issues (multiple layering in rhythmic structure) leads to ideas for empirical comparative studies of rhythm in speech and music, and is discussed further in section 3.3.4. Two other issues are discussed below.

Differences Between Linguistic and Musical Metrical Grids

Although the hierarchies posited by metrical phonology were inspired by Western music, some very important differences between the meters of music and language are readily apparent. Most notably, temporal periodicity in musical meter is much stricter than anything found in speech, and this difference has dramatic cognitive consequences. The regular periodicities of music allow meter to serve as a mental framework for sound perception, such that an event can be perceived as metrically prominent even if is physically quite weak, as in syncopated rhythms. By comparison, the prominences of language are not regular enough to allow for anything as abstract as syncopation. As a result, linguistic metrical grids are not abstract periodic mental patterns (like musical metrical grids) but are simply maps of heard prominences, full of temporal irregularities. For example, Dauer (1983) reports that the average interstress interval in speech was around 450 ms, with a standard deviation of approximately 150 ms. Dividing the standard deviation by the mean yields a coefficient of variation of about 33%. This variability is markedly different from music, in which perceived beats occur in a much more evenly spaced fashion. For example, when tapping to music, adults show a coefficient of variation of about 5%. Thus "metrical grids" in language should perhaps be called "prominence grids," to avoid the implication of an abstract mental periodicity.

Questioning the Principle of Rhythmic Alternation in Speech

Setting aside questions of temporal periodicity, one can ask if speech and music share a more abstract similarity in terms of a tendency to arrange prominences in alternating patterns of strong and weak elements. If so, this might suggest a basic cognitive relationship between rhythm in language and music. Evidence in favor of a principle of alternation in language comes from studies showing that English speakers adjust prominence patterns to make them more regular. For example, Kelly and Bock (1988) had speakers pronounce nonsense words embedded in sentences, such as:

(3.12a) The full teplez decreased.
(3.12b) Throw the teplez badly.

The focus of interest was whether speakers stressed the first or second syllable of the nonsense word. Overall, speakers tended to stress the first syllable, in accordance with a general trend in English for disyllabic nouns to have initial stress. However, this tendency was significantly weaker when the nonsense word was preceded by a stressed syllable (as in sentence 3.12a), as if speakers wanted to spread out the occurrence of stresses. Further evidence for alternation of stress patterns in speech production comes from Cutler (1980), who examined sentences in which speakers inadvertently omitted a syllable, such as:

```
     x      x       x     x
```
(3.13a) Next we have this bicential rug

versus the intended sentence:

```
     x      x       x     x
```
(3.13b) Next we have this bicentennial rug

Much more often than chance, the errors served to shorten a long run of unstressed syllables, thus tending to promote the alternation of stressed and unstressed syllables.

Although these findings seem to support a positive principle of alternation, it is also possible that they reflect the action of a negative principle that seeks to break up clusters of prominent syllables or clusters of nonprominent syllables (i.e., "stress clashes" and "stress lapses," Nespor & Vogel, 1989). Some support for the latter view comes from the observation that the regularizing tendencies reported by Kelly and Bock (1988) and Cutler (1980) are actually rather weak. In the former study, subjects placed initial stress on the target nonsense word in the majority of cases, whether or not the immediately preceding syllable was stressed. The presence of a prior stressed syllable simply lowered the proportion of initial stress from 80% to 70%, suggesting only a mild tendency to maintain an alternating stress pattern in speech. Similarly, Cutler's study is based on collecting relatively rare syllable omission errors, meaning that speakers usually manage quite well with irregular prominence patterns.

Thus at the current time it is impossible to rule out the hypothesis that the tendency to alternate stronger and weaker syllables in speech is the result of nonrhythmic forces that seek to keep prominences at a comfortable distance from each other. In fact, research on Greek suggests that the *alternation* of prominence may not even be a universal pattern for human languages, because Greek tolerates long sequences of unstressed syllables (Arvaniti, 1994). Thus it may be that the only universal principle regarding prominence patterns in language is that prominences that are too close together are subject to linguistic mechanisms for clash avoidance (see Arvaniti, 1994, for evidence from Greek; and Nespor, 1990, for references to studies of clash avoidance mechanisms in numerous languages). The reason such mechanisms exist may ultimately be rooted in the mechanics of articulation. Stressed syllables tend to be made with larger jaw movements than unstressed syllables (de Jong, 1995), and it may be biomechanically advantageous to avoid crowding larger jaw movements together when speaking at the fast rates typical of normal conversation.

3.3.3 The Perception of Speech Rhythm

The role of rhythm in speech perception has been the focus of at least four different lines of research. Two of these have obvious conceptual connections to musical rhythm: the study of perceived isochrony in speech and the investigation of the role of rhythmic predictability in perception. The third line has investigated the role of speech rhythm in the perceptual segmentation of words from connected speech. Although not obvious at first, this research is in fact quite pertinent to comparative perceptual studies of rhythm in language and music. The final (and most recent) line of work concerns the role that rhythm plays in perception of nonnative accents. Although no conceptual link has yet been made between this work and music research, it is briefly described because it is a promising new area for empirical work on speech rhythm.

The Perception of Isochrony in Speech

As noted in section 3.3.1 (subsection "Periodicity and Typology"), the idea that linguistic rhythm involves regular temporal intervals (e.g., between stresses or syllables) has received no empirical support from measurements of speech. However, all such measurements have been based on data from speech production, in other words, on waveforms or spectrograms of spoken utterances. In an influential paper, Lehiste (1977) made the interesting suggestion that periodicity may be stronger in perception than in production. That is, the ear may ignore or compensate for surface irregularities in judging periodicity in speech. She based this idea on empirical work in which she examined the ability of listeners to identify the longest or shortest interstress interval (ISI) in short sentences of four ISIs, and to do the same task on nonspeech analogs of the sentences in which the stresses were replaced by clicks and the speech by noise. She found that listeners performed better in the nonlinguistic condition, and suggested that if listeners had difficulty judging ISI duration differences in speech, this would lead to a sense that ISIs were similar in duration, in other words, an impression of isochrony. (Of course, it may not be speech per se that makes small duration differences difficult to detect; it could be that the presence of semantic meaning in language preoccupies the listener's attention so that fine duration judgments are difficult. Thus an important control condition for future studies of this sort is to use a language with which the listener is unfamiliar.)

Lehiste went on to study the just noticeable difference (JND) in duration for sequences of four noise-filled intervals, reasoning that this would establish a conservative estimate of the JNDs for ISIs in speech. She used three basic reference durations in her noise sequences (300, 400, and 500 ms). In each sequence, three of the four intervals had the same duration, and the fourth was increased or decreased in nine 10-ms steps. She found that reliable judgments identifying one interval as longer or shorter than the others required changes of between

30 and 100 ms. She argued that JNDs for ISIs in speech are no better than this and are likely to be worse, and thus that physical measurements of isochrony need to take this "perceptual tolerance" into account (cf. Kristofferson, 1980).

Lehiste's work is interesting because it raises the possibility that listeners hear more isochrony than is really there in speech. Some evidence offered in favor of this argument comes from Donovan and Darwin (1979), who had individuals listen to English sentences and then imitate the timing of each sentence's stress pattern by tapping. The subjects also performed this task with sequences of noises whose timing mimicked the stress pattern of sentences. The critical finding was that when imitating speech, subjects tapped with less temporal variability than the actual timing of stressed syllables, whereas when imitating noise they did not show this pattern.

Although these findings are intriguing, further work has suggested that this paradigm may be flawed. Scott et al. (1985) replicated the findings of Donovan and Darwin for English, but also found that subjects showed regularization of tapping to French (which is not considered to have periodic stress), as well as to garbled speech. This suggests that the observed regularization may be a side consequence of the greater difficulty of remembering acoustically complex stimuli versus noise patterns.

Thus Lehiste's ideas merit further investigation, because they raise the important issue of how perceived timing patterns relate to the physical intervals measured in speech. Nevertheless, there is nothing in Lehiste's work that supports the idea that speech is perceived as isochronous under ordinary circumstances. As noted in section 3.3.2 (subsection "Differences Between Linguistic and Musical Metrical Grids"), the variability of ISI durations in speech is on the order of 33%. For a 500-ms average ISI, this is 150 ms, which is above the threshold for subjective isochrony suggested by Lehiste.

Lehiste's ideas do point in one interesting direction in terms of comparative studies of speech and music, namely a direct comparison of the threshold for detecting temporal irregularities in perceptually isochronous sequences (e.g., a repeating syllable "ta ta ta ta") versus a repeating musical sound of equivalent acoustic complexity.[23] If speech can tolerate more durational variability than music and still sound isochronous, this raises interesting questions about different mechanisms for time perception in the two domains.

One could also examine the threshold for detecting tempo change in isochronous sequences in speech and music. Current data suggest that for nonmusician listeners, the threshold for tempo change detection in sequences of musical sounds is 5%–8% (Drake & Botte, 1993; cf. Rivenez et al., 2003). Would the threshold be higher if speech sounds were used?

[23] Such a study will have to be careful to try and match acoustic properties of the onset of the spoken and musical sound. For example, if a musical sound with a sharp attack is used, such as a piano tone, then a speech sound with a plosive onset (such as /ta/) should be used rather than one with a gradual onset (such as /la/).

The Role of Rhythmic Predictability in
Speech Perception

A number of researchers have argued that the ability to predict the location
of stressed syllables in English is perceptually beneficial (e.g., Martin, 1972;
Shields et al., 1974; Cutler & Foss, 1977). The reasoning behind this idea
is based on certain assumptions: Stressed syllables carry important semantic
information, and a listener's attention is limited, so that it is useful to expend
attentional resources on those points in time where stresses occur. Thus the
ability to anticipate stress location can help guide attention in an efficient manner. This idea suggests a point of contact between rhythm perception in speech
and music, because there are theories linking rhythm and attention in music
psychology (Jones, 1976; Large & Jones, 1999; Barnes & Jones, 2000). In order to determine if this is really a meaningful parallel, however, two questions
must be answered. First, is there evidence that rhythmic predictability plays an
important role in speech perception? Second, are the mechanisms for rhythmic
prediction similar in speech and music?

The best evidence for a role of rhythmic predictability in speech perception
comes from studies using phoneme-monitoring tasks. In these experiments, listeners are told to listen to one sentence at a time and press a button when they
hear a target phoneme (such as /d/). Cutler and Darwin (1981) conducted a
study in which sentences were recorded that had high, low, or neutral emphasis
on a given target word. For example, sentences 3.14a and b below were used
to record high versus low emphasis on the word "dirt" (in the sentences below,
the word bearing the main emphasis of the sentence is italicized):

(3.14a) She managed to remove the *dirt* from the rug, but not the grass stains.

(3.14b) She managed to remove the dirt from the *rug*, but not from their clothes.

Cutler and Darwin then spliced the neutral version of the target word into
high and low emphasis sentences, so that the target phoneme /d/ (and the rest of
the word that began with this phoneme) were acoustically identical in the two
cases. A faster reaction time to the target phoneme in high-emphasis sentences
would indicate that the *prediction* of stress was influencing speech processing.
This is precisely what was found: Listeners were reliably faster in detecting the
target phoneme in high-stress sentences. Of particular interest is that this difference persisted even when fundamental frequency variation was removed from
the two sentence types, suggesting that patterns of duration and amplitude were
sufficient to predict the upcoming stress.

Cutler and Darwin's study focused on target words that either did or did not
bear the main contrastive stress of the entire sentence. That is, they were not
studying the perception of just any stressed syllable, but of a particularly salient
stressed syllable in a sentence. Pitt and Samuel (1990) conducted a study in
which the context manipulation was not so extreme: They used sentences that

predicted stress or nonstress at a target point due to rhythmic and syntactic factors, for example, the first syllable of the word "permit" in:

(3.15a) The guard asked the visitor if she had a permit to enter the building.

(3.15b) The waiter decided he could not permit anyone else in the restaurant.

In sentence 3.15a, the context leads one to expect stressed syllable at the target location, both because the syntax of the sentence predicts a noun (a word category that tends to start with a stressed syllable in English) and for the rhythmic reason that the prior stress in the sentence is quite far away (the first syllable of "visitor"). In sentence 3.15b, the context leads one *not* to predict a stressed syllable, both because the syntax predicts a verb (a word category that tends to start with a weak syllable in English), and because the prior stress is quite nearby (on "could" or "not").

Like Cutler and Darwin, Pitt and Samuel used a splicing technique to ensure that the physical target word was the same in the two contexts, and asked listeners to respond when they heard a target phoneme (e.g., /p/ in the above example). Unlike Cutler and Darwin, however, they found no significant difference in reaction time to the target phoneme as function of the preceding context. Thus it appears that although rhythm may help listeners predict sentence level emphasis, it does not play a strong role in predicting lexical stress, even when reinforced by syntax. This casts some doubt on the idea that rhythm plays an important role in guiding attention to the majority of stressed syllables in spoken sentences. Clearly, more work is needed to determine to what extent stress is predictable under normal circumstances.

Even if a significant role for rhythmic prediction in speech is demonstrated, however, it is quite possible that the mechanisms that underlie rhythmic prediction in speech and music are quite different. In music, rhythmic predictability reflects the periodic structure of temporal intervals. In speech, the basis for rhythmic predictability (e.g., predicting when a stress will occur) is unlikely to involve periodic time intervals, because there is no evidence that such intervals exist in normal speech. A first step in studying the basis of rhythmic prediction in speech would be to study the stimuli used by Cutler and Darwin (1981), especially those stimuli in which fundamental frequency variation was removed. What temporal and/or amplitude patterns helped guide listeners' expectations in that study?

Thus at the current time, the hypothesis that rhythmic predictability in speech confers an advantage by guiding attention to semantically important parts of utterances is not well supported by empirical evidence. In music, it is clear that rhythmic predictability has an adaptive value: it allows the formation of a temporal expectancy scheme that plays an important role in musical perception (e.g., beat perception), and it guides the coordination of ensemble performance and the synchronization of movements in dance. Because speech does not have a regular beat, what functional role would rhythmic predictability play? One idea suggested by Lehiste (1977) is that it plays a role in signaling phrase boundaries in speech. Specifically, she suggested that one method speakers have for disambiguating syntactically ambiguous sentences is by signaling a structural boundary via lengthening of an interstress interval (ISI). For example, she studied speakers' productions of sentences such as "The old men and women stayed at home," which is syntactically ambiguous (either just the men were old or both the men and women were old). She found that when speakers said this sentence in such a way to make one or the other interpretation clear, the sequence "men and women" was very different in duration, being substantially longer when a syntactic boundary was intended between "men" and "women." Furthermore, she conducted a follow-up study in which the same sentences were resynthesized using a monotone, and the duration of the critical ISI was manipulated by uniformly expanding the duration of the phonemes within it, so that the relative durations of segments remained the same. She found that listeners were able to perceive the intended meaning solely on the basis of the length of the critical ISI, suggesting that ISI duration can signal a phrase boundary.

A subsequent study by Scott (1982) set out to test Lehiste's hypothesis against the more conventional notion that phrase boundaries are signaled by phrase-final lengthening. She found evidence for a weak version of Lehiste's hypothesis, in that there appeared to be some cases in which listeners used ISI patterns, but others in which they relied on traditional phrase-final lengthening. Nevertheless, the evidence was suggestive enough for this line of research to merit further study. A key conceptual point, however, is that evidence that ISI duration plays a role in creating perceived boundaries in speech is not equivalent to evidence for isochrony. The expectation for how long an ISI should be need not be based on an expectation for isochrony, but could be based on expectations for how long a given ISI should be given the number (and type) of syllables within it and the current speech rate (cf. Campbell, 1993). According to this view, a prosodic break is more likely to be heard when an ISI is significantly longer than expected, and rhythmic predictability is simply implicit knowledge of the statistical relation between ISI duration and the number and type of syllables in an ISI. This would allow a functional role for rhythmic predictability without any recourse to notions of isochrony.

The Role of Rhythm in Segmenting Connected Speech

To a native listener, spoken sentences consist of a succession of discrete words, yet this perception is an illusion. As pointed out in Chapter 2, word boundaries in language do not map in any simple way onto acoustic breaks in the speech signal, and as anyone who has listened to sentences in a foreign language can attest, it is far from obvious where the word boundaries in connected speech are. This problem is particularly relevant for infants, who are constantly faced with multiword utterances (van de Weijer, 1999) and who do not have the benefit of an existing vocabulary to help them identify where one word ends and the next begins.

A substantial body of research in psycholinguistics indicates that the rhythmic properties of a language assist a listener in segmenting speech. Work on English, for example, has pointed to a segmentation strategy based on stress: Listeners expect strong syllables to be word-initial. This likely reflects the predominance of words with initial stress in the English lexicon (Cutler & Carter, 1987), and manifests itself in a number of different ways in perception. For example, Cutler and Butterfield (1992) showed that when listeners missegment speech, they tend to place word boundaries before stressed syllables, as when "by loose analogy" is misheard as "by Luce and Allergy." Furthermore, when English speakers are asked to spot real monosyllabic words embedded in larger polysyllabic nonsense words, they find it easier when the real word does not straddle two stressed syllables. "Mint," for example, is easier to spot in "mintef" than in "mintayf," presumably because in the latter word the strong second syllable "tayf" triggers segmentation, thus splitting "mint" into two parts (Cutler & Norris, 1988). Cutler (1990) has dubbed the strategy of positing a word onset at each strong syllable the "metrical segmentation strategy."

Research on segmentation in other languages has revealed that stress-based segmentation is by no means universal. French and Spanish speakers, for example, favor syllabically based segmentation (Mehler et al., 1981; Pallier et al., 1993), whereas Japanese speakers favor moraic segmentation (Otake et al., 1993). Thus segmentation relies on units that are phonologically important in the native language. One striking finding of this cross-linguistic research is that the native language's segmentation strategies are applied *even when listening to a foreign language,* showing that segmentation tendencies are not simply a reaction to a particular speech rhythm, but a perceptual habit of a listener (see Cutler, 2000, for a review). One possibility suggested by Cutler is that this habit is a residue of early language learning, when rhythmic segmentation played an important role in bootstrapping lexical acquisition.

The relevance of this research to comparative studies of language and music is that it shows that experience with a language's rhythm leaves a permanent influence on a listener in terms of segmenting speech patterns, whether or not these patterns come from the native language. From this observation it is but one step to ask if experience with the native language influences how one segments nonlinguistic rhythmic patterns. This question is taken up in section 3.5.2 below.

The Role of Rhythm in the Perception of Nonnative Accents

When a person listens to their native language, s/he usually has a keen sense of whether or not it is being spoken with a native accent. Recent research on speech rhythm has taken advantage of this fact by having listeners judge the degree of perceived "foreign accentedness" in utterances spoken by nonnative speakers.

Empirical rhythmic measurements are then taken of speech of the different non-native speakers. By examining the correlation between perceived degree of foreign accent and the quantitative rhythmic measures, researchers hope to identify the perceptual cues listeners use in gauging speech rhythm patterns.

Using this approach, White and Mattys (2007) examined Spanish speakers of English and found that the greater their vowel duration variability within sentences, the more native-sounding they were rated by English speakers. This probably reflects vowel reduction: Spanish speakers who learn to reduce vowels in unstressed syllables (a characteristic of English, but not of Spanish; cf. section 3.3.1, subsection "Phonology and Typology") are likely to sound more like native speakers. A consequence of vowel reduction within sentences is that vowel duration variability increases, because some vowels become very short.

As noted in section 3.3.1 (subsection "Duration and Typology"), another empirical measure of rhythm influenced by vowel reduction is the nPVI, which measures the degree of durational contrast between adjacent vowels in a sentence rather than overall durational variability. White and Mattys found that the vowel nPVI of Spanish speakers of English was positively correlated with how native they sounded. Crucially, however, vowel duration variability was a better predictor of accent judgment than was nPVI. This suggests that vowel duration variability may be more perceptually relevant for speech rhythm than durational contrastiveness.

This is a very promising approach, because different rhythmic measures can be pitted against each other to see which best predicts perceptual data. However, the findings to date must be considered tentative because of an uncontrolled variable. This is variability in the degree to which nonnative speakers accurately produce the phonemes of the second language (i.e., the individual vowels and consonants). When judging a speaker's degree of foreign accent, listeners almost certainly base their judgments on some combination of segmental and suprasegmental cues. This is a problem because some nonnative speakers may produce native-sounding prosody but nonnative sounding segmental material, or vice versa. To compound the problem, different listeners may vary in the extent to which they weight segmental versus suprasegmental cues in judging how "foreign" a given nonnative speaker sounds. Thus to truly focus listeners' attention on rhythm, segmental cues must be made uniform. Resynthesis techniques, such as those used by Ramus and colleagues (cf. section 3.3.1, subsection "Perception and Typology") might provide one way to make sentences spoken by different nonnative speakers uniform in terms of phonemic material while preserving prosodic differences.

3.3.4 Final Comments on Speech Rhythm: Moving Beyond Isochrony

Although the history of speech rhythm research is tightly bound up with notions of periodicity (e.g., the isochrony of stresses or syllables), the evidence reviewed above suggests that the case for periodicity in speech is extremely weak. Thus progress in the study of speech rhythm requires conceptually decoupling "rhythm" and "periodicity," a point made in the introduction of this chapter. It is quite clear that speech has rhythm in the sense of systematic temporal, accentual, and grouping patterns of sound, and languages can be similar or different in terms of these patterns. However, the rhythms of language are not based on the periodic occurrence of any linguistic unit. Instead, the patterning is largely the *by-product* of phonological phenomena, such as the structure of syllables, vowel reduction, the location of lexical prominence, stress clash avoidance, and the prosodic phrasing of sentences. These phenomena lead to differences in the way utterances are organized in time.

The notion that rhythm in language is primarily *consequence* rather than *construct* stands in sharp contrast to rhythm in music, in which patterns of timing and accent are a focus of conscious design. Another salient difference between rhythm in speech and music, related to the lack of a periodic framework for speech rhythm, is the fact that speech rhythm conveys no sense of motion to a listener (cf. section 3.2.5). Do these differences mean that rhythm in language and music cannot be meaningfully compared? Absolutely not. As demonstrated in section 3.5 below, empirical comparisons are not only possible, they can be quite fruitful. They have had nothing to do with periodicity, however.

For those interested in cross-domain studies of rhythm, it is heartening to note that there is renewed interest in empirical studies of rhythm in speech production and speech perception (Ramus et al., 1999; Ramus & Mehler, 1999; Low et al., 2000; Grabe & Low, 2002; Lee & Todd, 2004, White & Mattys, 2007), and that there is much room for further work. For example, there is a need for more empirical data on listeners' judgments of how native-sounding a foreign speakers' utterances are, from the standpoint of rhythm. Such studies will need to employ creative ways of isolating the rhythm of speech from other phonetic dimensions of language, for example, using resynthesized speech in which phonetic content and pitch contours can be completely controlled (cf. Ramus & Mehler, 1999). There is also a need for studies that measure temporal patterning at multiple linguistic levels and that quantify relations between levels. It may be that important perceptual dimensions of speech rhythm are relational, such as having a high degree of contrast between adjacent syllable durations while simultaneously having a low degree of contrast between the duration of interstress intervals (some data pertinent to this idea are given at the end of this section). This is an area in which collaborations between linguists and music researchers would be especially useful.

In the remainder of this section, I would like to consider why periodicity has been (and continues to be) such an enduring concept in speech rhythm research. Below I offer several reasons for this historical phenomenon.

The simplest reason, of course, is the mistaken notion that rhythm *is* periodicity, or that rhythm *is* a regular alternation between strong and weak beats, rather than the broader notion of rhythm as systematic temporal, accentual, and phrasal patterning of sound, *whether or not this patterning is periodic*. Indeed, one need not look beyond music to see that a definition of rhythm *as* periodicity or *as* strong-weak beat alternation is overly simplistic: Many widespread musical forms lack one and/or the other of these features yet are rhythmically organized (cf. section 3.2).

The second reason that the notion of periodicity has endured may be the idea that it has a useful function in speech perception, such as making salient information predictable in time. There are psychological theories of auditory perception that propose that attention can be allocated more efficiently when events are temporally predictable, based on the idea that auditory attention employs internal oscillatory processes that synchronize with external rhythmic patterns (e.g., Jones, 1976; Large & Jones, 1999). Such theories provide a rationale for those interested in the idea that periodicity in speech is perceptually adaptive. Alternatively, those interested in periodicity might claim that it is useful because it creates a framework within which deviations are meaningful. This is the basis of Lehiste's idea that lengthening of interstress intervals in English can be used to mark phrase boundaries (cf. section 3.3.3, subsection "The Role of Rhythmic Predictability in Speech Perception"). The principal drawback of these perception-based arguments for periodicity is that the evidence for them is very weak. Although further research is needed, the current evidence suggests that periodicity does not have an important role to play in normal speech perception. This should not be surprising: The comprehension of speech *should be* robust to variation in the timing of salient events, because such variations can occur for a number of reasons. For example, a speaker may suddenly speed up or slow down for rhetorical reasons within a conversation. Under such conditions, relying on periodicity for comprehension seems a maladaptive strategy.

The third reason for periodicity's allure may be the belief that because various temporal patterns in human physiology (e.g., heartbeat, walking, chewing) exhibit periodic structure, speech is also likely to be periodic, perhaps even governed by rhythmic pattern generators. However, the use of rhythmic neural circuits for speech is not particularly plausible. The constant use of novel utterances in language means that articulators must be coordinated in different ways each time a new sentence is produced. Furthermore, the maneuvers that produce particular speech sounds depend on the local context in which they occur. Thus the motor patterns of speech cannot be predicted in advance with a high degree of precision. Without stereotyped movement patterns, evolution has no grounds for placing the control of speech in a rhythmic neural circuit. An analogy here is to multifingered touch-typing, a behavior involving the sequencing of overlapping movements of multiple articulators (the fingers). Although touch-typing is highly temporally organized, the resulting sequences are not based on periodic movements.

So far I have focused on negative reasons for the persistence of the concept of periodicity in speech. I will now briefly speculate on the positive reasons for the persistence of this concept, in other words, why periodicity in speech has been such an intuitively appealing notion to speech researchers, particularly those whose native language is English. (It is notable that the idea of periodicity in speech was promulgated by linguists who were English speakers, and that arguments for stress isochrony in English have been present since at least the 18th century; cf. Abercrombie, 1967:171; Kassler, 2005). First, it seems that English speakers find the interstress interval (ISI) to be a salient temporal unit in speech. For example, in a preliminary study, Cummins (2002) asked English listeners to repeat nonsense phrases such as "manning the middle" in time with an external pacing cue, so that the two stressed syllables were perceptually aligned with a periodically repeating two-tone pattern (for example, "man" would align with a high tone, and "mid" with a low tone; cf. Cummins & Port, 1998). This is equivalent to aligning the start and end of the ISI with two tones. Cummins also tested speakers of Italian and Spanish because these languages have lexical stress, permitting phrases to be constructed in a manner analogous to the English phrases (such as "BUSca al MOto" in Spanish, stress indicated by capitalization). Cummins observed that although English speakers learned the task quickly and performed accurately, Spanish and Italian speakers took much longer, were uncomfortable with the task, and produced a great deal of variability in their results. Cummins suggests that this difference is due to the fact that the ISI is not a salient perceptual unit for speakers of Italian and Spanish, despite the fact that there is lexical stress in these languages.

This intriguing finding raises the question of why ISI is salient to English listeners. Does it play some functional linguistic role? As discussed in section 3.3.3 (subsection "The Role of Rhythmic Predictability in Speech Perception"), ISI duration may play a role in signaling linguistic boundaries to English listeners, even if ISIs are not isochronous. Currently there is not enough evidence to say confidently what role the ISI plays, but let us assume for a moment that English speakers and listeners are sensitive to it as an entity. Given the empirical observations about the large variability in ISI duration in English (e.g., coefficients of variation around 33%; Dauer, 1983), why would listeners ever feel that ISIs were isochronous? One answer may concern the relative degree of variability in ISI durations compared to syllable durations. As suggested above, the impression of isochrony may be due in part to a lower degree of contrast between successive ISI durations relative to successive syllable durations. For example, consider Figure 3.12, which shows the same sentence as Figure 3.8a and Sound Example 3.5a ("the **last concert given** at the **opera** was a **tremendous success**").

Syllable boundaries are marked with vertical lines (as in Figure 3.8), but now stressed syllables (indicated in by boldface above) have been marked with

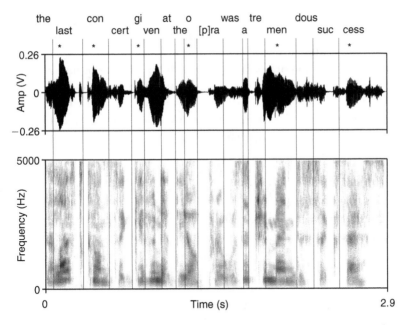

Figure 3.12 The English sentence of Figure 3.8a, with stresses marked by asterisks (*).

an asterisk. The asterisk was placed at the vowel onset of the stressed syllable, in other words, near its perceptual attack (its "P-center"; Morton et al., 1976; Patel et al., 1999). In this sentence, the nPVI of syllable durations is 59.3, and the nPVI of ISIs is 28.4, making the ratio $nPVI_{ISI}/nPVI_{syll}$ equal to 0.48. Thus in this particular case, the amount of durational contrast between adjacent ISIs is only about half of that between adjacent syllables.

I have computed similar ratios for each of the 20 sentences of British English from Ramus's database.[24] For 15 out of 20 sentences, this ratio was less than 1. The overall mean ratio across the 20 sentences was .83 (std = .45), and was significantly less than 1 ($p < .0001$ by a one-tailed t-test). An even stronger effect was observed when one computes the ratio of ISI duration variability to syllable duration variability (using the coefficient of variation, i.e., CV_{ISI}/CV_{syll}) Here 17 out of 20 sentences had a value less than 1, and the mean was .69 (std = .25), again significantly less than 1. Thus if the ear is sensitive to temporal patterning at the levels of both syllables and stresses, the low durational variability of ISIs *relative to the variability of syllable durations* might contribute to a sense that stresses are temporally regular. Of course, for this explanation to have any merit it must be shown that the ratio of ISI to syllable variability differentiates stress-timed from syllable-timed

[24] I am grateful to Laura Dilley for marking stressed syllables in these sentences.

languages. Languages such as Italian and Spanish would be good candidates for testing this hypothesis, because they are syllable-timed languages in which stress can be reliably marked.

Although the notion of isochrony in speech continues to beguile researchers, I suspect that it will have little or no role in the most fruitful research on speech rhythm in the coming years. Isochrony was important to the birth of speech rhythm studies, but it is a concept whose usefulness is exhausted. It is time to move on to a richer view of speech rhythm.

3.4 Interlude: Rhythm in Poetry and Song

As in the rest of this book, the focus of this chapter is on comparing ordinary speech to instrumental music. However, no comparison of rhythm in language and music is complete without a discussion of poetry and song. In these art forms, words are carefully chosen and consciously patterned for rhythmic effect. Of course, poetry and song are but two of numerous vocal genres with organized rhythms. In the United States certain styles of preaching in African American churches are notable for their rhythmic patterning, a taste of which can be heard in Martin Luther King Jr.'s famous "I Have a Dream" speech. In other cultures, it is possible to identify numerous genres of speech in which rhythmic design plays a role (see Agawu, 1995, for a fascinating case study of the range of rhythmically regulated forms of speech in an African society). The focus here is on poetry and song, however, because these have received the greatest amount of empirical research in terms of rhythm.

3.4.1 Rhythm in Poetry

The study of poetic rhythm has been the focus of a good deal of research by literary scholars (for introductions, see Gross, 1979; Fussell, 1979; Hollander, 2001). In this tradition, poetic "meter" refers to the abstract patterning scheme which governs the temporal structure of a poem, whereas "rhythm" refers to the actual patterning of durations and accents. For example, a great deal of English verse is written in iambic pentameter, a verse form consisting of 5 iambic feet, in which an iamb is a (weak + strong) syllable pattern. Naturally there are many exceptions to this pattern within iambic pentameter poetry: A particularly common one is the substitution of a trochaic foot, or (strong + weak) syllable pattern at the onset of a line. Thus the rhythm of a particular line may violate the overall meter of the poem.

Literary prosodists argue that listeners internalize the regularities of meter and perceive departures from this scheme as variation from a stable background (Richards, 1979:69; Adams, 1997:12). That is, meter is seen as having an intimate relationship with expectancy. This idea is related to the notion of musical meter as an abstract mental scheme, but differs from musical meter in an important way. Musical meter refers to *temporal* periodicity, whereas poetic meter involves *configurational* periodicity, in other words, the focus is on the repetition of some basic prosodic unit rather than on temporal periodicity per se. For example, in iambic pentameter it is the weak + strong configuration of the iambic foot that is the design focus, not the isochrony of stressed syllables. In various forms of French and Chinese verse, the number of syllables per line is strictly regulated, but there is no focus on making syllables periodic (equal in duration).

It is interesting to note that different languages tend to favor different kinds of poetic meters. For example, English verse has often tended toward purely stress-based forms in which regulation of the number of stresses per line is the focus, independent of the number of syllables (e.g., the meter of *Beowulf*, with four stresses per line). In contrast, English verse based on regulating the number of syllables per line without regard to stress is rare (Fussell, 1979:62–75). This likely reflects the powerful role of stress in ordinary English speech rhythm. Indeed, Fussell has argued that "a meter customary in a given language is customary just because it 'measures' the most characteristic quality of the language" (Fussell, 1974:498). Thus stress plays a dominant role in English poetry, but little role in French, in which the number of syllables per line is a more common concern. Japanese, in turn, often regulates the number of morae per line, as in the 5–7–5 mora structure of the haiku.

Lerdahl and Halle (1991) and Lerdahl (2003) have sought to unify the theoretical treatment of rhythm in poetry and music, using shared concepts such as hierarchical grouping structure and metrical grids. Our focus here, however, is on empirical research. Over the past few decades, poetic rhythm has attracted the interest of a number of speech scientists, who have made quantitative measurements of the temporal patterns of poetry. For example, the phonetician Gunnar Fant and colleagues have studied the acoustics of iambic versus trochaic lines of verse in Swedish (1991b). The researchers found that in iambic feet, the weak syllable is about 50% as long as the following strong syllable, whereas in trochaic feet, the weak syllable is about 80% of the duration of the preceding strong syllable (cf. Nord et al., 1990). This difference is likely due to preboundary lengthening, which acts to increase the duration of the final syllable in each foot (i.e., the strong syllable in an iamb and the weak syllable in a trochee). Thus iambic and trochaic feet are not simply mirror images of each other in terms of their temporal profiles: Iambic feet are much more temporally asymmetric.

These observations may be relevant to the study of the aesthetic effect of the two kinds of feet in poetic lines. For example, Adams (1997:55–57) notes that trochaic meters are often associated with awe and the suspension of reality, as in Blake's poem, "The Tyger," in which trochaic patterns dominate the first three lines of the first stanza:

(3.16)
Tyger! Tyger! burning bright
In the forests of the night
What immortal hand or eye
Could frame thy fearful symmetry?

This aesthetic property of trochaic meter may be partly due to its more uniform profile of syllabic durations, which goes against the grain of normal English speech rhythm and thus gives the resulting speech an incantatory feel.

Another prominent phonetician who has long conducted research on poetic rhythm is Ilse Lehiste (1991). In one set of studies, Lehiste examined the relationship between the timing of feet and of the lines in which feet are embedded. She found that the temporal variability of lines is lower than one would predict based on the variability of feet duration, suggesting that speakers make temporal compensations between feet in order to keep lines within a certain duration. That is, lines act as a unit of temporal programming in the recitation of poetry (Lehiste, 1990). Ross and Lehiste (1998, 2001) have also examined the interplay of linguistic and poetic rhythm in framing the temporal patterns of Estonian verse and folksongs.

3.4.2 Rhythm in Song

For languages with clearly defined stress, such as English, each phrase or sentence comes with a distinct pattern of stronger and weaker syllables. When words in these languages are set to metrical music, a relationship is established between the syllabic accent patterns and musical metrical accent patterns. Sensitivity to these relationships is part of the skill of writing music with words, and empirical research suggests that composers exploit this relationship for artistic ends.

Palmer and Kelly (1992) studied vocal lines in themes from Gilbert and Sullivan's 14 operettas, focusing on compound nouns (like the single word "blackbird") and adjective-noun pairs (like the two word phrase "black bird"). In English, compound nouns receive stress on the first syllable, whereas adjective-noun pairs receive stress on the second syllable. They studied how such words were aligned with the metrical structure of the music, and found that the stressed syllable tended to align with a metrically strong beat in the music. Given the complex texts of Gilbert and Sullivan's songs, this strategy of alignment may contribute a sense of precision and balance to the lyrics of these operettas.

Temperley (1999) looked at a different genre of vocal music, namely rock songs. In contrast to Palmer and Kelly, he found that verbal stress frequently *anticipated* metrical accent in rock songs by a fraction of a beat, as in the

Beatles' "Here Comes the Sun" (Figure 3.13). This systematic anticipation contributes a sense of syncopation and rhythmic energy to the song, and provides an example of how the systematic *misalignment* of verbal and musical stress adds dynamic energy to music.

The relationship between rhythm in speech and song is a fertile area that merits much more empirical investigation than it has received to date. In the remainder of this section, I outline three directions that this research could take. The first pertains to cultural differences in the prevalence of certain types of musical rhythms. For example, Yamomoto (1996) notes that children's songs based on triple rhythms (e.g., 6/8 time signature) are rare in Japan but common in Britain, and suggests that this might be due to differences in English versus Japanese speech rhythm. If Yamomoto is correct, one would predict that Japanese- versus English-speaking children would differ in how easily they can learn songs in these meters. Another language with which one could test a similar idea is Greek. Recall from section 3.3.2 (subsection "Questioning the Principle of Rhythmic Alternation in Speech") that Arvaniti (1994) showed that Greek, a language of the Balkan region, tolerates a more irregular alternation between stressed and unstressed syllables than does English. Also recall from section 3.2 that the Balkan region features music with irregularly spaced beats. Would Greek-speaking children find it easier to learn the irregular meters of Balkan songs than English-speaking children (cf. Hannon & Trehub, 2005)? In the studies outlined above, it would of course be essential that the two groups of children be matched for prior musical exposure to different musical meters. It may thus be best to work with immigrants who speak the native language at home but whose children are exposed to Western music. In such a case, if learning experiments reveal the predicted cultural differences, this would support the interesting hypothesis that a culture's speech rhythm predisposes it toward or away from certain musical rhythms.

A second direction for research in this area is to examine verbally improvised music that is accompanied by a rhythmic musical context, such as contemporary rap music. If the vocal and musical lines can be recorded on different audio tracks, and points of verbal and musical stress can be independently identified,

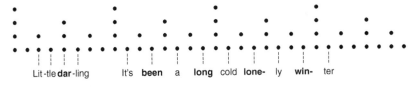

Figure 3.13 A musical metrical grid for a portion of the Beatles' "Here Comes the Sun." The lyrics are aligned below the grid, and linguistically stressed syllables are indicated in boldface: Note how most such syllables slightly precede strong metrical positions in the music. From Temperley, 1999.

then one could study temporal relations between verbal and musical accent points as a piece unfolds in time. It would be particularly interesting to study these relations in novice versus expert rap musicians, to see if part of being an expert in this genre is greater flexibility and/or precision in the manner in which the alignment of the two types of accents is handled. In a study such as this, identifying precise points in time for verbal and musical accent will be essential, and the issue of the perceptual attack time of syllables and of musical tones ("P-centers") comes to the fore (Morton et al., 1976; Gordon, 1987; Patel et al., 1999).

A final possible line of research is suggested by a correspondence between Richard Strauss and Romain Rolland in 1905 about musical text setting (Myers, 1968).[25] Strauss emphasizes the clear-cut relationship between syllabic accent in speech and metrical accent in music: "In German 'she' on the strong beat of a bar is absolutely impossible. For example, in a bar of 4/4, the first and third beat always have a necessary stress which can only be made on the radical [stressed] syllable of each word." He also expresses his frustration over variability in the alignment of word stress and musical stress in French opera: "Yesterday, I again read some of Debussy's Pélleas et Mélisande, and I am once more very uncertain about the principle of the declamation of French when sung. Thus on page 113, I found: 'Cheveúx, chéveux, dé cheveux.' For heaven's sake, I ask you, of these three ways there can all the same only be *one* which is right."

Rolland replies by emphasizing the mutability and subtlety of French word accent:

> The natural value of "cheveux" is chevéux. But a man in love will, when saying this word, put quite a special stress on it: "tes chéveux." . . . You see, the great difficulty with our language is that for a very large number of words, accentuation is variable,—never arbitrary, but in accordance with logical or psychological reasons. When you say to me: . . ." Of these 3 (cheveux) *only one can be right,* what you say is doubtless true of German, but not for French.

What this correspondence suggests is that German text setting is more rigid in its alignment of verbal and musical accent, whereas French is more permissive in terms of accent alignment between text and music. Indeed, Dell and Halle (in press; cf. Dell, 1989) report that French text-setting is quite tolerant of mismatches between verbal and musical accent, except at the ends of lines, where alignment tends to be enforced. They contrast this high degree of "mismatch tolerance" in French songs to a much lower degree found in English songs. The correspondence between Strauss and Rolland, and the work of Dell and Halle, suggest that languages have salient differences in the way they align music and text in terms of rhythmic properties, though quantitative work is

---

[25] I am grateful to Graeme Boone for bringing this correspondence to my attention.

needed to confirm this. These writings also lead to ideas for cross-cultural perceptual studies testing sensitivity to accent mismatches in songs. Specifically, listeners could be presented with different versions of a song that have text and tune aligned in different ways, with one version having many more accent mismatches. Listeners could then be asked to judge in which version the words and music go best together. One might predict that German listeners judging German songs (or English listeners judging English songs) would be more selective in terms of the pairings that sound acceptable than French listeners judging French songs.

3.5 Nonperiodic Aspects of Rhythm as a Key Link

One major theme of this chapter is that languages have rhythm (systematic temporal, accentual, and grouping patterns), but that this rhythm does not involve the periodic recurrence of stresses, syllables, or any other linguistic unit. Initially it may seem that "giving up on periodicity in speech" would mean that there is little basis for comparing rhythm in music and language. In fact, the opposite is true. By abandoning a fixation on periodicity one is freed to think more broadly about speech rhythm and its relationship to musical rhythm. As we shall see below, a focus on nonperiodic aspects of linguistic rhythm is proving fruitful in terms of comparing language and music at structural and neural levels.

3.5.1 Relations Between Musical Structure and Linguistic Rhythm

The notion that a nation's instrumental music reflects the prosody of its language has long intrigued music scholars, especially those interested in "national character" in music. Gerald Abraham explored this idea at length (1974, Ch. 4), noting as one example an observation of Ralph Kirkpatrick on French keyboard-music: "Both Couperin and Rameau, like Fauré and Debussy, are thoroughly conditioned by the nuances and inflections of spoken French. On no Western music has the influence of language been stronger" (p. 83). In a more succinct expression of a similar sentiment, Glinka (in *Theater Arts,* June 1958) wrote: "A nation creates music, the composer only arranges it" (cited in Giddings, 1984:91).

Until very recently, evidence for this idea has been largely anecdotal. For example, Garfias (1987) has noted that in Hungarian each word starts with a stressed syllable, and that Hungarian musical melodies typically start on strong beats (i.e., anacrusis, or upbeat, is rare). Although this is an interesting observation, it is possible that this is due to the fact that many such melodies come from folk songs. In this case, the linguistic influence on musical rhythm would be mediated by text. A more interesting issue, implied by Kirkpatrick, is whether linguistic rhythm influences the rhythm of instrumental music, in other words, music that is not vocally conceived.

One approach to this question was suggested by Wenk (1987). He proposed that cultures with rhythmically distinct languages should be examined to see if differences in musical rhythm reflect differences in speech rhythm. Wenk focused on English and French, prototypical examples of a stress-timed versus a syllable-timed language. Wenk and Wioland (1982) had previously argued that a salient rhythmic difference between the two languages was that English grouped syllables into units *beginning* with a stressed syllable, whereas French grouped syllables into units *ending* with a stressed syllable, as in:

x   x   x

(3.17a) / Phillip is / studying at the uni/versity

x   x   x

(3.17b) / Philippe / étudie / à l'université

Wenk and Wioland further argued that the stress at the ends of rhythmic groups in French was marked primarily by durational lengthening. Based on this idea, Wenk (1987) predicted that phrase-final lengthening would be more common in French versus English instrumental music. He tested this idea by having a professional musician mark phrase boundaries in English versus French classical music. The number of phrases in which the final note was the longest note in the phrase was then tallied for both cultures. Wenk found that it was indeed the case that more such phrases occurred in French than in English music.

Wenk's study was pioneering in its empirical orientation, but it also had limitations that make it difficult to accept these findings as a firm answer to the question of interest. Only one composer from each culture was examined (Francis Poulenc and Benjamin Britten), and from the oeuvre of each composer, only one movement from one piece was selected. Furthermore, no comparable empirical data for language rhythm were collected (e.g., the degree of phrase-final lengthening in English vs. French speech).

Despite its limitations, Wenk's study outlined a useful approach, namely to identify empirical rhythmic differences between two languages and then determine if these differences are reflected in the music of the two cultures. Pursuing this idea in a rigorous fashion entails three requirements. First, an empirical measure of speech rhythm is needed to quantify rhythmic differences between languages. Second, this same measure should be applicable to music so that language and music could be compared in a common framework. Third, both the linguistic and musical samples needed to be broad enough to insure that the findings are not idiosyncratic to a few speakers or composers.

Joseph Daniele and I conducted a study that set out to meet these crite-ria (Patel & Daniele, 2003a). Like Wenk, we focused on British English and French due to their distinct speech rhythms and because they have been the locus of strong intuitions about links between prosody and instrumental music (e.g., Hall, 1953; Abraham, 1974; Wenk 1987). Our work was inspired by recent phonetic research on empirical correlates of stress-timed versus syllable-timed speech rhythm (cf. section 3.3.1, subsection "Duration and Typology"). In particular, the work of Low, Grabe, and Nolan (2000) attracted our attention because it focused on something that could be measured in both speech and mu-sic, namely the durational contrast between successive elements in a sequence. Their measure, called the normalized pairwise variability index, or nPVI, had been applied to vowels in sentences from stress-timed and syllable-timed lan-guages, and had been shown to be higher in stress-timed languages, likely due to the greater degree of vowel reduction in these languages (Grabe & Low, 2002; Ramus, 2002a; Lee & Todd, 2004; see the above-mentioned subsection of 3.3.1 for background on the nPVI).

Two aspects of this measure made it appealing for use with music. First, the nPVI a is purely relative measure of contrast. That is, the durational difference between each pair of intervals is measured *relative to* the average duration of the pair. This normalization, which was originally introduced to control for fluctuations in speech rate, makes the nPVI a dimensionless quantity that can be applied to both language and music. (For example, nPVI can be computed from speech durations measured in seconds and from musical durations measured in fractions of a beat.) Second, the nPVI has been applied to vowels. Vowels form the core of syllables, which can in turn be compared to musical tones (i.e., in setting words to music it is quite common for each note to be assigned to one syllable).[26] Our strategy, then, was to apply the nPVI to tone sequences from British and French instrumental music, to determine if differences emerged that reflected the rhythmic differences between British English and French speech.

Figure 3.14 shows the nPVI to British English versus continental French speech, based on measurements of vowel durations in sentences uttered by na-tive speakers of each language. (The sentences are short, news-like utterances from the corpus of Nazzi et al., 1998.)[27]

---

[26] Although this is true for English and French, it should be noted that in Japanese it is the mora and not the syllable that gets mapped onto a musical note (Hayes, 1995a).

[27] The nPVI values for English and French speech shown in Figure 3.14 are taken from Patel et al. (2006), rather than from Patel and Daniele (2003a). Both studies show a significant difference between the two languages (English nPVI > French nPVI), but the 2006 study is based on more accurate measurements. See Patel et al. (2006) for measure-ment details, and for a list of all sentences analyzed.

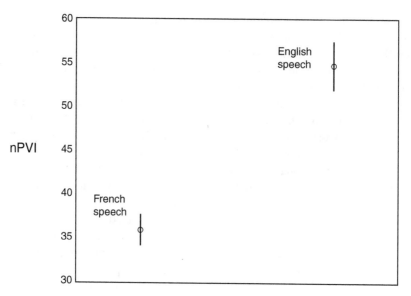

Figure 3.14 The nPVI of British English and French sentences. Error bars show +/- 1 standard error. Data from Patel, Iversen, & Rosenberg, 2006.

The nPVI is significantly higher for English than for French speech. Figure 3.15 gives an intuition for why this is the case by illustrating the pattern of vowel duration for one English and French sentence in this corpus (cf. Sound Examples 3.8a, b).

For example, in the top panel, the first two values (about 120 ms and 40 ms) are the durations of the first two vowels in the sentence (i.e., the vowels in "Finding"), and so on. Note how successive vowels tend to differ more in duration for the English sentence than for the French sentence. In the English sentence, some vowels are very short (often due to vowel reduction), whereas other vowels are quite long (often due to stress). This leads to a greater tendency for durational contrast between neighboring vowels, which is reflected in the nPVI score.

As mentioned above, an appealing aspect of the nPVI is that it can be applied to music in order to measure the durational contrast between successive notes. Western music notation indicates the relative duration of notes in an unambiguous fashion, as shown in Figure 3.16.

In the figure, the first note of each theme is arbitrarily assigned a duration of 1, and the durations of the remaining notes are expressed as a multiple or fraction of this value. (Any numerical coding scheme that preserves relative duration of notes would yield the same nPVI, because it is a normalized measure.) In this example, the nPVI of the Debussy theme is lower than that of the Elgar theme, even though the raw variability of note duration in the Debussy theme is

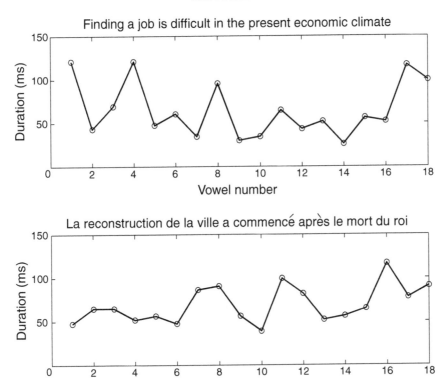

Figure 3.15 Vowel durations in an English and a French sentence. Note the greater degree of short-long contrast in the English sentence between adjacent vowel durations. The nPVI for the English sentence is 54.9, and for the French sentence is 30.0.

greater than that in the Elgar theme (as measured by the coefficient of variation, in other words, the standard deviation divided by the mean). This emphasizes the fact that the nPVI indexes the degree of contrast between successive elements in a sequence, not the overall variability of those elements.

Our source of musical material was a standard reference work in musicology, *A Dictionary of Musical Themes,* Second Edition (Barlow & Morgenstern, 1983), which focuses on the instrumental music of Western European composers. In choosing composers to include in our study we were guided by two factors. First, the composers had to be from a relatively recent musical era because measurements of speech prosody are based on contemporary speech, and languages are known to change over time in terms of sound structure. Second, the composers had to be native speakers of British English or French who lived and worked in England or France. Using these guidelines, we examined all English and French composers from Barlow and Morgenstern who were born in the 1800s and died in the 1900s, and who had at least five musical

D122: Debussy - Quartet in G minor for Strings, 1st movement, 2nd theme

E72:   Elgar - Symphony No. 1 in A flat, Opus 55, 4th movement, 2nd theme

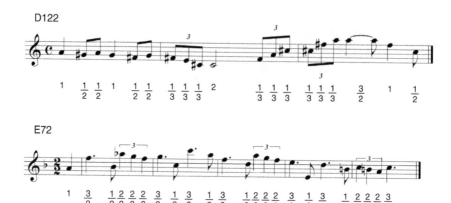

Figure 3.16 Two musical themes with the relative durations of each note marked. nPVI of D122 = 42.2, of E72 = 57.1. Themes are from Barlow & Morgenstern, 1983. From Patel & Daniele, 2003a.

themes in the dictionary that were eligible for inclusion in the study (see Patel & Daniele, 2003a, for inclusion criteria, and for the rationale of using music notation rather than recorded music for nPVI analysis). We chose composers who spanned the turn of the century because this era is noted by musicologists as a time of "musical nationalism" in Europe.

Based on our criteria, 16 composers were included in the study, including English composers such as Elgar, Delius, and Vaughan Williams, and French composers such as Debussy, Poulenc, and Saint-Saëns. About 300 musical themes were represented, and one musical nPVI value was computed for each theme. The results of our analysis of musical nPVI are shown in Figure 3.17, along with the speech nPVI values. Remarkably, the two cultures have significantly different musical nPVI values, with the difference being in the same direction as the linguistic nPVI difference (see Patel & Daniele, 2003a, and Patel et al., 2006, for further details).

Thus there is empirical evidence that speech rhythm is reflected in musical rhythm, at least in turn-of-the century classical music from England and France. How is this connection between language and music mediated? Some musicologists have proposed that national character arises from composers adapting folk melodies into their compositions. Because such melodies are typically from songs, it may be that the rhythm of words influences the rhythm of these melodies, thus giving the melodies a language-like rhythmic pattern. However, we believe that this may not be the best explanation for our finding, because our

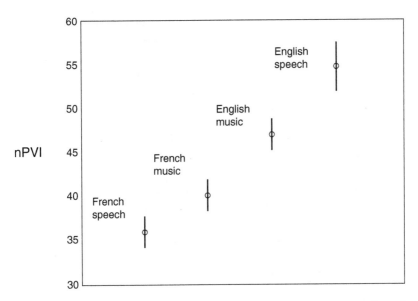

Figure 3.17 The nPVI of British English and French musical themes. Error bars show +/- 1 standard error. Data from Patel & Daniele, 2003a, and Patel, Iversen, & Rosenberg, 2006.

study included numerous composers who are not thought to be strongly influenced by folk music, such as Elgar and Debussy (Grout & Palisca, 2000). Instead, we feel there may be a more direct route from language to music. It is known from studies of language acquisition that the perceptual system is sensitive to the rhythmic patterns of language from a very early age (Nazzi et al., 1998; Ramus, 2002b). Composers, like other members of their culture, internalize these patterns as part of learning to speak their native language. (One mechanism for this internalization is a process called statistical learning, which is discussed in more detail in the next chapter.) We suggest that when composers write music, linguistic rhythms are "in their ears," and they can consciously or unconsciously draw on these patterns in weaving the sonic fabric of their music. This does not imply that the connection between linguistic and musical rhythm is obligatory. Rather, this link is likely to be greater in historical epochs where composers seek a national character for their music.

Our findings for English and French speech and music immediately raised two questions. Would the musical nPVI difference be observed if a broader sample of English and French themes and composers were studied? Perhaps more importantly, would our result generalize to other cultures in which stress- versus syllable-timed languages are spoken? Fortunately, Huron and Ollen (2003) provided answers to these questions. Using an electronic version of *A Dictionary of Musical Themes* created by Huron, they computed the nPVI of a much larger sample of English and French musical themes (about 2000 themes, composed between the mid-1500s and mid-1900s). They confirmed that the nPVI of English music was significantly higher than that of French music, though the difference was smaller than that found by Patel and Daniele (likely due to less stringent sampling criteria). They also computed the musical nPVI for a range of other nations, analyzing almost 8,000 themes from 12 nationalities over more than 3 centuries. Of the nationalities they examined, five can be assigned to stress-timed languages and three to syllable timed languages (Fant et al., 1991a; Grabe & Low, 2002; Ramus, 2002b). These are listed in Table 3.1 along with their musical nPVI values. (The data in table 3.1 represent corrected values of the original table in Huron & Ollen, 2003, kindly provided by David Huron. See this chapter's appendix 2 for data from more cultures.)

Four out of the five nations with stress-timed languages (American, Austrian, English, and Swedish) do indeed have higher musical nPVI values than the three nations with syllable-timed languages, providing support for the idea that stress-timed and syllable-timed languages are associated with distinctive musical rhythms. However, German music is a notable exception: It has a low musical nPVI value despite the fact that German is a stress-timed language with a high nPVI value for speech (Grabe & Low, 2002; Dellwo, 2004).

However, there may be a historical reason why German music has a low nPVI, namely the well-known influence of Italian music on German music (Kmetz et al., 2001). Because Italian music has a low nPVI, stylistic imitation of this music might outweigh any linguistic influence of the German language on the nPVI of German music. One way to test this idea is to examine the nPVI

Table 3.1 Musical nPVI Values for Eight Different Nationalities

	Musical nPVI	
	Mean	S.E.
Nationalities With Stress-Timed Languages		
American	46.7	1.0
Austrian	45.1	0.6
English	45.6	0.9
German	43.2	0.6
Swedish	50.0	2.4
Nationalities With Syllable-Timed Languages		
French	43.4	0.7
Italian	41.4	1.0
Spanish	42.5	1.9

in historical perspective, for example, as a function of each composer's birth year. When themes from 14 German composers were examined in this fashion a striking trend emerged, as shown in Figure 3.18 (Patel & Daniele, 2003b; Daniele & Patel, 2004).

Over the course of 250 years, nPVI almost doubled, a trend that is highly statistically significant. (Interestingly, this trend is also evident for the six Austrian composers we included in our study.) Given what is known about the history of the German language, this is unlikely to reflect a change in the rhythm of German from syllable-timed to stress-timed during this period (C. Heeschen, personal communication). Instead, it most likely reflects historical changes in musical style, perhaps including a waning influence of Italian music on German music over this period. In fact, the finding would be consistent with the idea that Italian music had a strong influence on German music during the Baroque era (1600–1750), less influence during the Classical era (1750–1825), and the least influence during the Romantic era (1825–1900). More generally, it suggests

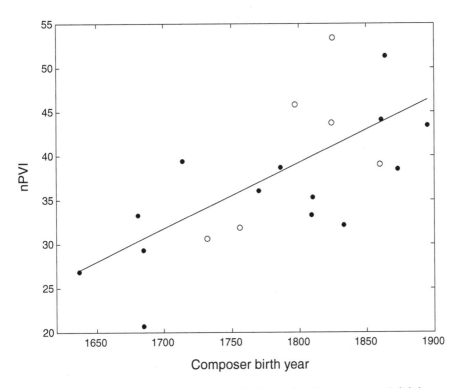

Figure 3.18 nPVI as a function of composer birth year for 20 composers. (Solid dots = German composers; open dots = Austrian composers.) The best-fitting linear regression line is shown. From Patel & Daniele, 2003b.

that in studying linguistic influences on speech rhythm, it is important to keep in mind historical influences that can run counter to linguistic influences.[28]

Taking a step back, musical nPVI research demonstrates that the rhythmic structure of speech and music can be fruitfully compared without any resort to notions of periodicity. It is worth noting that the research done so far hardly exhausts what can be done using this measure. For example, one could apply the nPVI to recordings of performed music rather than to music notation. One could also examine the nPVI of performances of the same piece of instrumental music by musicians who speak stress-timed versus syllable-timed languages, to see if the native language influences temporal patterns in music performance (cf. Ohgushi, 2002). Finally, one could study improvised music, for example, by studying jazz musicians who speak different dialects with different rhythmic qualities (e.g., in the United States, perhaps a northeast dialect versus a southern dialect). In this case, the nPVI could be used to investigate whether the temporal pattern of speech is reflected in the rhythm of improvised music.

3.5.2 Relations Between Nonlinguistic Rhythm Perception and Speech Rhythm

The idea that nonlinguistic rhythm perception can be influenced by one's native language has been articulated by both linguists and music researchers. Over 50 years ago, Jakobson, Fant, and Halle (1952:10–11) made the following claim:

> Interference by the language pattern affects even our responses to nonspeech sounds. Knocks produced at even intervals, with every third louder, are perceived as groups of three separated by a pause. The pause is usually claimed by a Czech to fall before the louder knock, by a Frenchman to fall after the louder; while a Pole hears the pause one knock after the louder. The different perceptions correspond exactly to the position of word stress in the languages involved: in Czech the stress is on the initial syllable, in French, on the final and in Polish, on the penult.

The groupings suggested by Jakobson et al. can be schematically represented as follows, in which each x represent a knock and the upper case X's are louder:

(3.18) X x x X x x X . . . = (X x x) Czech

= (x x X) French

= (x X x) Polish

---

[28] Unlike German music, English and French music do not show a significant increase in nPVI over the equivalent time period, based on themes in Barlow and Morgenstern's dictionary (Greig, 2003). This raises an interesting musicological puzzle: Why do German and Austrian music show such a strong historical change in this measure of rhythm, whereas English and French music do not?

The claim of Jakobson et al. is certainly provocative, but there has been no empirical evidence to support it. Nevertheless, the idea of a link between native language and nonlinguistic rhythm perception persists. For example, Stobart and Cross (2000) have documented a form of music from the Viacha people of the Bolivian highlands in which the local manner of marking the beat is different from what most English-speaking listeners perceive. Sound Example 3.9 illustrates this music with an Easter song played on a small guitar (*charango*). The position at which the Viacha clap or tap their foot to the beat can be heard at the end of the excerpt. This tendency to mark the shorter event in each group of two notes as the beat is contrary to the tendency of English speakers to hear the pattern iambically, that is, with the beat on the second event of each pair. Stobart and Cross speculate that the tendency to mark the beat trochaically (on the first member of each group) is related to stress patterns in words of the local language, Quechua.

The two examples above differ in that the former concerns segmentation (rhythmic grouping), whereas the latter concerns beat perception. Note, however, that neither refers to notions of periodicity in speech. Instead, they both refer to patterns of lexical stress and how this influences nonlinguistic auditory perception. Thus once again we see that interesting claims about rhythmic relations between music and language can be made without any reference to periodicity in speech.

How can one assess whether the native language influences the perception of nonlinguistic rhythm? As a first step, it is necessary to demonstrate that there are cultural differences in nonlinguistic rhythm perception. Rhythmic segmentation or grouping is of particular interest in this regard, as intimated by Jakobson et al. (1952). This is because psycholinguistic research indicates that that the rhythm of one's native language leads to segmentation strategies that are applied even when listening to a foreign language. The idea that the native language can influence nonlinguistic rhythmic segmentation is thus just one step away from this idea (cf. section 3.3.3, subsection "The Role of Rhythm in Segmenting Connected Speech").

Yet at the current time, it is widely believed that elementary grouping operations reflect general auditory biases not influenced by culture. This belief stems from a century-old line of research in which researchers have investigated rhythmic grouping using simple tone sequences (Bolton, 1894; Woodrow, 1909). For example, listeners are presented with tones that alternate in loudness (. . . loud-soft-loud-soft . . .) or duration (. . . long-short-long-short . . .) and are asked to indicate their perceived grouping. Two principles established a century ago, and confirmed in numerous studies since, are widely accepted:

1. A louder sound tends to mark the beginning of a group.
2. A lengthened sound tends to mark the end of a group.

These principles have come to be viewed as universal laws of perception, underlying the rhythms of both speech and music (Hayes, 1995b; Hay & Diehl, 2007). However, the cross-cultural data have come from a limited range of cultures (American, Dutch, and French). Are the principles truly universal? A study by Kusumoto and Moreton (1997) suggested otherwise, finding that American versus Japanese listeners differed with regard to Principle 2 above. This study motivated a replication and extension of this work by Iversen, Patel, and Ohgushi (2008), described below.

Iversen et al. had native speakers of Japanese and native speakers of American English listen to sequences of tones. The tones alternated in loudness ("amplitude" sequences, Sound Example 3.10a) or in duration ("duration" sequences, Sound Example 3.10b), as shown schematically in Figure 3.19.

Listeners told the experimenters how they perceived the grouping. The results revealed that Japanese and English speakers agreed with principle 1): both reported that they heard repeating loud-soft groups. However, the listeners showed a sharp difference when it came to principle 2.) Although English speakers perceived the "universal" short-long grouping, many Japanese listeners strongly perceived the opposite pattern, in other words, repeating long-short groups. (cf. Figure 3.19). Because this finding was surprising and contradicted a "law" of perception, Iversen et al. replicated it with listeners from different parts of Japan. The finding is robust and calls for an explanation. Why would native English and Japanese speakers differ in this way?

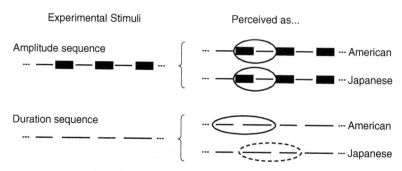

Figure 3.19 *Left side:* Schematic of sound sequences used in the perception experiment. These sequences consist of tones alternating in loudness ("amplitude sequence," top), or duration ("duration sequence," bottom). In the amplitude sequence, thin bars correspond to softer sounds and thick bars correspond to louder sounds. In the duration sequence, short bars correspond to briefer sounds and long bars correspond to longer sounds. The dots before and after the sequences indicate that only an excerpt of a longer sequence of alternating tones is shown. *Right side:* Perceived rhythmic grouping by American and Japanese listeners, indicated by ovals. Solid black ovals indicate preferences that follow "universal" principles of perception, while the dashed black oval indicates a preference that violates the purported universals.

Assuming that that these different perceptual biases are not innate, they key question is what aspect of auditory experience might be responsible for this difference. Two obvious candidates are music and speech, because these sound patterns surround humans throughout their life. Both patterns present the ear with sequences of sound that must be broken into smaller coherent chunks, such as phrases in music, or phrases and words in speech. Might the temporal rhythm of these chunks differ for music or speech in the two cultures? That is, might short-long patterns be more common in American music or speech, and long-short be more common in Japanese music or speech? If so, then learning these patterns might influence auditory segmentation generally, and explain the differences we observe.

Focusing first on music, one relevant issue concerns the rhythm of how musical phrases begin in the two cultures. For example, if most phrases in American music start with a short-long pattern (e.g., a "pick-up note"), and most phrases in Japanese music start with a long-short pattern, then listeners might learn to use these patterns as segmentation cues. To test this idea, we examined phrases in American and Japanese children's songs (because we believe these perceptual biases are probably laid down early in life). We examined 50 songs per culture, and for each phrase we computed the duration ratio of the first to the second note and then counted how often phrases started with a short-long pattern versus other possible patterns (e.g., long-short, or equal duration). We found that American songs show no bias to start phrases with a short-long pattern. Interestingly, Japanese songs show a bias to start phrases with a long-short pattern, consistent with our perceptual findings. However, the musical data alone cannot explain the cultural differences we observe, because this data cannot explain the short-long grouping bias of American listeners.

Turning to language, one basic difference between English and Japanese concerns word order (Baker, 2001). For example, in English, short grammatical (or "function") words such as "the," "a," "to," and so forth, come at the beginning of phrases and combine with longer meaningful (or "content") words (such as a noun or verb). Function words are typically "reduced," having short duration and low stress. This creates frequent linguistic chunks that start with a short element and end with a long one, such as "the dog," "to eat," "a big desk," and so forth. This fact about English has long been exploited by poets in creating the English language's most common verse form, iambic pentameter.

Japanese, in contrast, places function words at the ends of phrases. Common function words in Japanese include "case markers," short sounds that can indicate whether a noun is a subject, direct object, indirect object, and so forth. For example, in the sentence "John-san-ga Mari-san-ni hon-wo age-mashita," ("John gave a book to Mari") the suffixes "ga," "ni," and "wo" are case markers indicating that John is the subject, Mari is the indirect object and "hon" (book) is the direct object. Placing function words at the ends of phrases creates frequent chunks that start with a long element and end with a short one, which is just the opposite of the rhythm of short phrases in English (cf. Morgan et al., 1987).

Apart from short phrases, the other short meaningful chunks in language are words. Because our perception experiment focused on two-element groups, we examined the temporal shape of common disyllabic words in English and Japanese. English disyllabic words tend to be stressed on the first syllable (e.g., MO-ney, MAY-be; Cutler & Carter, 1987), which might lead one to think that they would have a long-short rhythmic pattern of syllable duration. To test this, we examined syllable duration patterns for the 50 most common disyllabic words in the language (from a corpus of spontaneous speech), and measured the relative duration of the two syllables. Surprisingly, common words with stress on the first syllable did not have a strong bias toward a long-short duration pattern. In contrast, common words with stress on the second syllable, such as "a-BOUT," "be-CAUSE," and "be-FORE," had a very strong short-long duration pattern. Thus the average duration pattern for common two-syllable words in English was short-long (Figure 3.20).

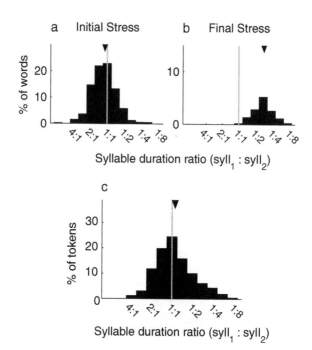

Figure 3.20 Distribution of syllable duration ratios for common two-syllable words in spontaneous speech in American English. Separate histograms are shown for initial-stress versus final-stress words in (a) and (b), and combined data are shown in (c), weighted by word frequency. Averages indicated by arrowheads. The overall distribution in (c) has a significant short-long bias (average ratio = 1 : 1.11).

This means that a short-long rhythm pattern is reflected at both the level of small phrases and common disyllabic words in English. We also examined syllable duration patterns in the 50 most common disyllabic words in Japanese. In contrast to English, the average duration pattern for such words was long-short. Thus once again, linguistic rhythm mirrored the results of the perception experiment.

Taking a step back, our results show that the perception of rhythmic grouping, long thought to follow universal principles, actually varies by culture. Our explanation for this difference is based on the rhythms of speech. Specifically, we suspect that learning the typical rhythmic shape of phrases and words in the native language has a deep effect on rhythm perception in general. If our idea is correct, then rhythmic grouping preferences should be predictable from the temporal structure of small linguistic chunks (phrases and words) in a language.

These findings highlight the need for cross-cultural work when it comes to testing general principles of auditory perception. Much of the original work on rhythmic grouping of tones was done with speakers of Western European languages (e.g., English, Dutch, and French). Although these languages do indeed have important differences, they all follow the pattern of putting short function words at the onset of small linguistic phrases, which may account for the similarity of perceptual grouping in these cultures. A more global perspective reveals that languages with phrase-final short function words are widespread, but exist largely outside of Europe, for example, in India and East Asia (Haspelmath et al., 2005). We predict that native speakers of these languages will group tones of alternating duration like Japanese listeners do (long-short).

An important future direction for this work concerns the development of rhythmic grouping preferences in childhood. Do infants have an innate bias for a particular grouping pattern (e.g., short-long), which is then modified by experience (cf. Trainor & Adams, 2000)? Or are they rhythmic "blank slates"? Regarding the perception of rhythm by adults, if speakers of different languages perceive nonlinguistic rhythm differently, this could help explain reports of differences between Westerners and Japanese in the performance of simple musical rhythms (Ohgushi, 2002; Sadakata et al., 2004). That is, simple rhythms may be performed differently in different cultures because they are perceived differently during learning. This would indicate that experience with speech shapes nonlinguistic rhythm cognition at a very basic level.

3.5.3 Neural Relationships Between Rhythm in Speech and Music

In this chapter, I have claimed that certain aspects of speech rhythm and musical rhythm show a striking similarity, such as the grouping of events into phrases, whereas other aspects are fundamentally different, such as the role of temporal periodicity. To what extent do neural data support this claim? Is there evidence that some aspects of rhythm in speech and music are handled by similar brain systems, whereas other aspects show little neural overlap?

Focusing first on grouping, there is evidence for overlap in brain processing of phrase boundaries in both domains. This evidence comes from electrical brain responses (event-related potentials, ERPs) in normal individuals. Steinhauer et al. (1999) demonstrated that the perception of phrase boundaries in language is associated with a particular ERP component termed the "closure positive shift" (CPS), a centro-parietal positivity of a few hundred milliseconds that starts soon after the end of an intonational phrase. Further studies using filtered or hummed speech (to remove lexical cues and leave prosodic cues) showed that the CPS is sensitive to prosodic rather than syntactic cues to phrase boundaries (Steinhauer & Friederici, 2001; Pannekamp et al., 2005). Inspired by this work, Knösche et al. (2005) examined the ERPs in musicians to the ends of musical phrases, and found a component similar to the CPS reported by Steinhauer et al. Using MEG, they also identified brain areas that were likely to be involved in the generation of the CPS in music. These areas included the anterior and posterior cingulate cortex and the posterior hippocampus. Based on the roles these areas play in attention and memory, the researchers argue that the musical CPS does not reflect the detection of a phrase boundary per se, but memory and attention processes associated with shifting focus from one phrase to the next.

The studies of Steinhauer et al. and Knösche et al. point the way to comparative neural studies of grouping in language and music. There is much room for further work, however. For example, in the Knösche et al. study the sequences with phrase boundaries have internal pauses, whereas the sequences without phrase boundaries do not. It would be preferable to compare sequences with and without phrase boundaries but with identical temporal structure, for example, using harmonic structure to indicate phrasing (cf. Tan et al., 1981). This way, ERPs associated with phrase boundaries cannot be attributed to simple temporal differences in the stimuli. It would also be desirable to conduct a within-subjects study of brain responses to phrases in language and music. Such comparative work should attend to the absolute duration of musical versus linguistic phrases, as the neural processes involved in grouping may be influenced by the size of the temporal unit over which information is integrated (Elbert et al., 1991; von Steinbüchel, 1998).

Turning to the question of periodicity, if speech rhythms and periodic musical rhythms are served by different neural mechanisms, then one would predict neural dissociations between linguistic rhythmic ability and the ability to keep or follow a beat in music. The neuropsychological literature contains descriptions of individuals with musical rhythmic disturbance after brain damage, or "acquired arrhythmia" (e.g., Mavlov, 1980; Fries & Swihart, 1990; Peretz, 1990; Liégeois-Chauvel et al., 1998; Schuppert et al., 2000; Wilson et al., 2002; Di Pietro et al., 2003). Two notable findings from this literature are that rhythmic abilities can be selectively disrupted, leaving pitch processing skills relatively intact, and that there are dissociations between rhythmic tasks requiring simple discrimination of temporal patterns and those requiring the evaluation or pro-duction of periodic patterns (e.g., Peretz, 1990). For example, Liégeois-Chauvel et al. (1998) found that patients with lesions in the anterior part of the left or right superior temporal gyrus were much more impaired on a metrical task than on a temporal discrimination task. The metrical task involved identifying a pas-sage as a waltz or a march, whereas the temporal discrimination task involved a same different judgment on short melodic sequences that differed only in terms of their duration pattern. In the metrical task, patients were encouraged to tap along with the perceived beat of the music to help them in their decision. Wilson et al. (2002) describe a case study of a musician with a right temporo-parietal stroke who could discriminate nonmetrical rhythms but who could not discriminate metrical patterns or produce a steady pulse.

Unfortunately, none of these studies explicitly set out to compare rhythmic abilities in speech and music. Thus the field is wide open for comparative stud-ies that employ quantitative measures of both speech and musical rhythm after brain damage. It would be particularly interesting to study individuals who were known to have good musical rhythmic abilities and normal speech be-fore brain damage, and to examine whether disruptions of speech rhythm are associated with impaired temporal pattern discrimination, impaired metrical abilities, or both.

Another population of individuals who would be interesting to study with regard to speech and musical rhythm are individuals with "foreign accent syn-drome" (Takayama et al., 1993). In this rare disorder, brain damage results in changes in speech prosody that give the impression that the speaker has ac-quired a foreign accent. It remains to be determined if this disorder is associated with systematic changes in speech rhythm, but if so, one could examine if such individuals have any abnormalities in their musical rhythmic skills.

Of course, a difficulty in studying acquired arrhythmia and foreign accent syndrome is that such cases are quite rare. Thus it would be preferable to find larger populations in which either speech rhythm or musical rhythmic abili-ties were impaired, in order to conduct comparative research. One popula-tion that holds promise for comparative studies are tone-deaf or "congenital amusic" individuals who have severe difficulties with music perception and production which cannot be attributed to hearing loss, lack of exposure to music, or any obvious nonmusical social/cognitive impairments (Ayotte et al., 2002). One advantage of working with such individuals is that they can easily be found in any large community through a process of advertising and careful screening (Ayotte et al., 2002; Foxton et al., 2004). Such individuals appear to have problems with basic aspects of pitch processing, such as discriminating small pitch changes or determining the direction of small pitch changes (i.e., whether pitch goes up or down) (Peretz & Hyde, 2003; Foxton et al., 2004). Interestingly, they do not seem to be impaired in discriminating simple temporal patterns and can synchronize successfully to a simple metronome. However, they do have difficulty synchronizing to the beat of music (Dalla Bella & Peretz, 2003). Of course, it could be that the difficulty in synchronizing with music is simply due to the distraction caused by a stimulus with pitch variation, due to deficits in pitch processing (cf. Foxton et al., 2006). Thus future studies of beat perception in congenital amusia should use complex rhythmic sequences with no pitch variation, such as those used in the study of Patel, Iversen, et al. (2005) described in section 3.2.1 above (cf. Sound Examples 3.3. and 3.4). If musically tone-deaf individuals cannot synchronize to the beat of such sequences, this would suggest that the mechanisms involved in keeping a beat in music have nothing to do with speech rhythm (because the speech of musically tone-deaf individuals sounds perfectly normal).[29]

I suspect that future research will reveal little relationship between speech rhythm abilities in either production or perception and musical rhythm abilities involving periodicity (such as metrical discrimination or beat perception and synchronization). This would support the point that periodicity does not play a role in speech rhythm.

3.6 Conclusion

Speech and music involve the systematic temporal, accentual, and phrasal patterning of sound. That is, both are rhythmic, and their rhythms show both important similarities and differences. One similarity is grouping structure: In both domains, elements (such as tones and words) are grouped into higher

---

[29] Of course, before any firm conclusions can be drawn, the speech rhythm of tone-deaf individuals would need to be quantitatively measured to show that it did not differ from normal controls (for example, using the nPVI). Also, it is possible that tone-deaf individuals cannot keep a beat because their pitch perception problem has caused an aversion to music, so that they have not had enough exposure to music to learn how to keep a beat. Thus it would be preferable to work with individuals who have normal pitch perception and who enjoy music, but who cannot keep a beat. The existence of such "rhythm-deaf" individuals is intuitively plausible, as there are certainly people who like music but claim to have "two left feet" when it comes to dancing, and/or who cannot clap along with a beat. It should be possible to find a population of such people through a process of advertising and screening, akin to the procedures used to find congenital amusics.

level units such as phrases. A key difference is temporal periodicity, which is widespread in musical rhythm but lacking in speech rhythm. Ironically, the idea that speech has periodic temporal structure drove much of the early research on speech rhythm, and was the basis for a rhythmic typology of languages which persists today (stress-timed vs. syllable-timed languages). It is quite evident, however, that the notion of isochrony in speech is not empirically supported. Fortunately, much recent empirical research on speech rhythm has abandoned the notion of isochrony, and is moving toward a richer notion of speech rhythm based on how languages differ in the temporal patterning of vowels, consonants, and syllables. A key idea that motivates this research is that linguistic rhythm is the product of a variety of interacting phonological phenomena, and not an organizing principle, unlike the case of music.

It may seem that breaking the "periodicity link" between speech and music would diminish the chance of finding interesting rhythmic relations between the domains. In fact, the converse is true. Changing the focus of comparative work from periodic to nonperiodic aspects of rhythm reveals numerous interesting connections between the domains, such as the reflection of speech timing patterns in music, and the influence of speech rhythms on nonlinguistic rhythmic grouping preferences. Although many more connections await exploration, it seems clear that some of the key processes that extract rhythmic structure from complex acoustic signals are shared by music and language.

Appendix 1: The nPVI Equation

This is an appendix for section 3.3.1, subsection "Duration and Typology."
The nPVI equation is:

$$\text{nPVI} = 100 / (m-1) \times \sum_{k=1}^{m-1} \left| (d_k - d_{k+1}) / ((d_k + d_{k+1}) / 2) \right|$$

In this equation, m is the number of durations in the sequence (e.g., vowel durations in a sentence) and d_k is the duration of the kth element. The nPVI computes the absolute value of the difference between each successive pair of durations in a sequence, normalized by the mean of these two durations (this normalization was originally introduced to control for fluctuations in speech rate). This converts a sequence of m durations to a sequence of $m - 1$ contrastiveness scores. Each of these scores ranges between 0 (when the two durations are identical) and 2 (for maximum durational contrast, i.e., when one of the durations approaches zero). The mean of these scores, multiplied by 100, yields the nPVI of the sequence. The nPVI value for a sequence is thus bounded by lower and upper limits of 0 and 200, with higher numbers indicating a greater degree of durational contrast between neighboring elements.

Appendix 2: Musical nPVI Values
of Different Nations

This is an appendix for Chapter 3, section 3.5.1, Table 3.1. Data kindly provided by David Huron.

In the tables below, ♯ C = number of composers, *sd* = standard deviation.

Nationality	Mean	♯ Themes	♯ C	*sd*
American	46.7	478	32	22.4
Armenian	43.1	33	1	22.2
Austrian	45.1	1,636	22	23.7
Austro-Hung	45.9	14	1	18.7
Belgian	48.7	41	6	19.4
Bohemian	44.4	30	1	22.9
Brazilian	41.5	5	1	18.3
Catalan	48.9	12	1	16.8
Cuban	36.0	17	2	17.9
Czech	46.9	266	6	24.3
Danish	51.0	7	1	24.6
English	45.6	741	27	24.4
Finnish	44.9	169	2	25.3
Flemish	25.2	3	1	3.8
French	43.4	1,343	52	25.2
German	43.2	2,379	39	26.8
Hungarian	45.4	244	8	25.4
Irish	44.1	16	3	25.7
Italian	41.4	572	46	23.9
Mexican	28.4	13	2	19.3
Norwegian	45.2	122	2	20.3
Polish	50.2	60	8	18.7
Romanian	42.4	26	2	21.3
Russian	41.3	853	25	23.4
Spanish	42.5	108	8	19.3
Swedish	50.0	12	3	29.3

Data from the above table regrouped by language: English = American, English, Irish; French = French, Belgian; German = German, Austrian, Austro-Hungarian; Slavic = Russian, Czech, Polish, Bohemian; Spanish = Spanish, Catalan, Cuban, Mexican; Scandinavian = Danish, Norwegian, Swedish (not Finnish)

Language	Mean	# Themes	# C	sd
English	46.0	1,235	62	23.6
French	43.6	1,384	58	25.0
German	44.0	4,029	62	25.6
Slavic	43.1	1,209	40	23.5
Spanish	41.0	150	13	19.4
Scandinavian	45.9	141	6	21.3

Melody

4

Melody

4.1 Introduction

Melody is an intuitive concept that is hard to define. Standard dictionary definitions often prove unsatisfactory. For example, "pitched sounds arranged in musical time in accordance with given cultural conventions and constraints" (Ringer, 2001:363) invokes "musical time." Yet the notion of melody is not confined to music, because linguists have long used the term to refer to organized pitch patterns in speech (Steele, 1779; 't Hart et al., 1990). It may seem that dropping "musical" from the above definition would solve this problem, but the resulting description would allow very simple tone sequences, such as the alternating two-tone pattern of European ambulance sirens. Such patterns hardly qualify as "melodic."

Can a single definition of melody be found that encompasses both music and speech? One possibility is "an organized sequence of pitches that conveys a rich variety of information to a listener." This definition emphasizes two points. First, melodies are tone sequences that pack a large informational punch. For example, speech melody can convey affective, syntactic, pragmatic, and emphatic information. Musical melody can also convey a broad variety of information, as detailed in section 4.2 below. The second point is that a tone sequence qualifies as a melody by virtue of the rich mental patterns it engenders in a listener. That is, melody perception is a constructive process by which the mind converts a sequence of tones into a network of meaningful relationships.

How do melody in speech and music compare in terms of structure and cognitive processing? A first step in addressing this question is to define the scope of the problem. This chapter focuses on that aspect of speech melody known as intonation, in other words, organized pitch patterns at the *postlexical* level (Jun, 2003, 2005). Such patterns do not influence the semantic meaning of individual words. This is in contrast to lexical pitch contrasts, which occur in tone languages such as Mandarin and Yoruba and in pitch-accent languages such as Swedish and Japanese. (Although section 4.4 of this chapter touches on lexical pitch contrasts, a more detailed treatment of the relation between lexical tones and music is given in Chapter 2.) Furthermore, this chapter examines music's relation to *linguistic* intonation, that aspect of speech melody that conveys structural (vs. affective) information (cf. section 4.1.2). Music's relation to affective intonation is explored in Chapter 6 (on meaning in music and language). Linguistic and affective intonation are treated in different chapters because they are conceptually distinct and are associated with different bodies of research. Thus henceforth in this chapter, "intonation," "linguistic melody," and "speech melody" refer to linguistic intonation unless otherwise specified.

4.1.1 Important Differences Between Musical and Linguistic Melody

Any systematic comparison of musical and linguistic melody must acknowledge at the outset that there are important differences between them. First and foremost, most musical melodies are built around a stable set of pitch intervals, whereas linguistic melodies are not (cf. Chapter 2). Although the precise set of intervals in musical melodies varies by culture, the organization of pitch in terms of intervals and scales is a salient difference between music and ordinary speech. The consequences of this difference are profound. For example, a stable system of intervals allows musical melodies to make use of a tonal center, a focal pitch that serves as a perceptual center of gravity for the melody. An interval system also allows the creation of a hierarchy of pitch stability in melodies, as discussed in section 4.2.6. In contrast, the "tones" of intonation have no such organization: Each tone is used where it is linguistically appropriate and there is no sense in which some are more stable or central than others.[1] Another consequence of an interval system is that when combined with a temporal grid provided by beat and meter, a scaffolding is created for an elaborate set of structural relations between tones, as discussed in section 4.2.2. This is likely part of what makes musical melodies so aesthetically potent. In contrast, the network of pitch relations in intonation contours is not nearly as rich. As a result, intonation contours are aesthetically inert, as evidenced by the fact that people rarely hum intonation contours or find themselves captivated by the pitch patterns of speech.[2] This is quite sensible, as a musical melody is an

---

[1] It has been noted that the low pitch at the end of declarative utterances is often quite stable for a given speaker, likely reflecting physiological factors (Lieberman, 1967; Liberman & Pierrehumbert, 1984). This form of pitch stability, however, has nothing to do with structural relations between intonational tones.

[2] The Czech composer Leoš Janáček (1854–1928) is an interesting exception. Janáček was fascinated by speech melodies and filled many notebooks with musical transcriptions of intonation contours (Wingfield, 1999; Pearl, 2006; Patel, 2006a).

aesthetic object, a sound sequence that is an end in itself, whereas a linguistic intonation contour is simply a means to an end, in other words, pitch in the service of quotidian linguistic functions. If a musical melody is "a group of tones in love with each other" (Shaheen, quoted in Hast et al., 1999), then a linguistic melody is a group of tones that work together to get a job done.

A second difference between musical and linguistic melody is that the perception of the latter appears to be influenced by a particular kind of expectation that is unique to speech. This expectation concerns a phenomenon known as "declination," a gradual lowering of the baseline pitch and narrowing of pitch range over the course of an utterance. This phenomenon may have a physiological basis in the decline of air pressure driving vocal fold vibration (Collier, 1975).[3] Listeners appear to take this phenomenon into account when making judgments about the equivalence of pitch movements in earlier versus later portions of an utterance (Pierrehumbert, 1979; Terken, 1991). For example, Terken constructed synthetic intonation contours for the 7-syllable nonsense syllable utterance/mamámamamamáma/, with pitch accents on the second and sixth syllable, as shown schematically in Figure 4.1.

In one condition, there was no baseline declination and the participants' task was to adjust the height of the second pitch movement so that it had the same prominence as the first movement. Terken found listeners made the second peak significantly lower than the first, as if they were influenced by an expectation for F0 declination over the course of the utterance. (That is, a physically smaller movement later in a sentence seemed just as prominent as a larger movement earlier in the sentence, because of an implicit expectation that pitch range is narrower later in an utterance.) Interestingly, Terken also included a condition in which listeners were instructed to equalize the peak *pitch* of the two movements, rather than to equate their prominence. In this case, the listeners behaved differently: They made the two peaks much closer in pitch, even though the height of the second peak was still adjusted to be below the first peak. This demonstrated that listeners use different strategies when judging pitch versus prominence, which in turn implies differences in the perceptual mechanisms mediating spoken and musical melodies.

A third difference concerns neuropsychological dissociations between melody in speech and music. For example, musical tone-deafness, which is discussed in detail later in this chapter, is associated with severe problems with

---

[3] Indeed, such a tendency has even been noted in the calls of nonhuman primates (Hauser & Fowler, 1992). However, it is important to note that declination is not always present: It is less frequent in spontaneous speech than prepared speech (Umeda, 1982) and is often suppressed in questions (Thorsen, 1980). Nevertheless, it is frequent enough to create expectations that influence pitch perception in a sentence context, as described in the text.

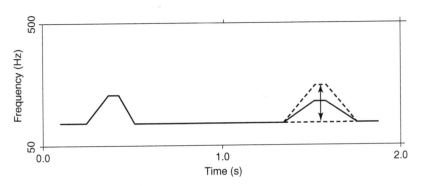

Figure 4.1 Schematic diagram of intonation contours used by Terken, 1991. See text for details.

melodic production and perception. In terms of production, musically tone-deaf individuals often make contour errors when singing (e.g., going up in pitch when the original melody goes down), a kind of error that is rarely made by ordinary individuals, even those with no musical training (Giguère et al., 2005; Dalla Bella et al., 2007). In terms of perception, they are typically unaware when music is off-key (including their own singing), and have difficulty discriminating and recognizing melodies. Despite these severe problems with musical melody, these individuals do not suffer from any obvious problems with speech intonation production or perception (Ayotte et al., 2002).

   Given the differences outlined in this section, it may seem the prospects for finding structural or cognitive relations between melody in speech and music are dim. In fact, such a judgment is premature. Section 4.2 below explores musical melody and identifies several meaningful parallels to speech. Section 4.3 then examines two modern lines of research on linguistic intonation that suggest significant links to musical melody. After a brief interlude in section 4.4 (on linguistic and musical melody in song), the final section of the chapter discusses two areas in which empirical research is demonstrating interesting connections between the structure and processing of spoken and musical melody.

4.1.2 A Brief Introduction to Linguistic Intonation

As background for the discussions that follow, it is worth providing some basic information on linguistic intonation (further detail is given in section 4.3) The primary determinant of speech melody is the fundamental frequency (F0) of the voice, which is the basic rate of vibration of the vocal folds. Speakers influence F0 via the tension of their vocal folds and via air pressure beneath the folds (subglottal pressure): Greater tension or air pressure leads to faster vibration and higher pitch, and vice versa.[4] The average range of F0 variation over the course of an utterance is about one octave (Hudson & Holbrook, 1982; Eady, 1982), and the average F0 of women is about one octave above that of adult men.[5]

Through its structured use in speech, linguistic intonation can convey syntactic, pragmatic, and emphatic information, as well as signaling prosodic grouping patterns (Cutler et al., 1997). The English language provides examples of the first three of these functions, and French provides a good example of the fourth. Syntactically, pitch can help to disambiguate the structure of spoken utterances. For example, in a sentence such as "The investigator found the uncle of the businessman who was wanted by the police," there is ambiguity regarding the relative clause "who was wanted by the police": it may modify one of two nouns: "uncle" or "businessman." Listeners' syntactic interpretation of the sentence is influenced by pitch: They tend to interpret the relative clause as modifying the noun that bears a salient pitch accent (Schafer et al., 1996, cf. Speer et al., 2003). An example of pitch's role in pragmatics is the use of a pitch rise at the end of certain English utterances to mark them as questions (e.g., "You're going" vs. "You're going?"). The role of pitch in emphasis is well known: Combined with other cues (such as duration), pitch in English can be used to place focus on a particular word in a sentence, as in "I wanted to go TONIGHT, not tomorrow." Finally, the role of pitch in signaling prosodic grouping structure is illustrated by French, which uses pitch rises to mark the boundaries of short phrases within sentences (as discussed further in section 4.2.1).

Scientific research on intonation typically relies on the F0 contours of sentences. One such contour is shown in Figure 4.2, for the sentence "Having a big car is not something I would recommend in this city," as spoken by a female speaker of British English (cf. Sound Example 4.1).

A salient aspect of F0 evident in this figure, and in speech generally, was articulated by Joshua Steele over two centuries ago: "the melody of speech moves rapidly up or down by slides, wherein no graduated distinction of

---

[4] Although this chapter will focus on F0 as the physical correlate of speech melody, it is important to note that from a psychoacoustic standpoint the sensation of pitch in speech is derived not directly from F0 but is inferred from the frequency spacing of the harmonics of F0. That is, the pitch of the voice is an example of the perception of the "missing fundamental," as is evident from the fact that the pitch of the male voice (~100 Hz) is easily heard over telephones, even though telephones filter out frequencies below 300 Hz. Harmonics 3–5 are thought to be especially important in voice pitch perception (see Moore, 1997, for more details).

[5] For a discussion of the possible evolutionary basis of this sex difference, see Ohala (1983, 1994).

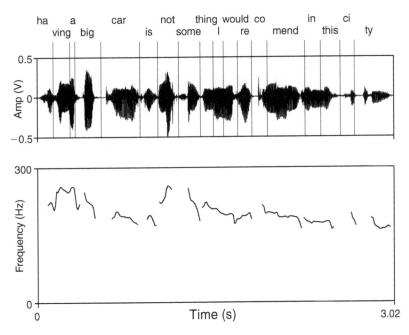

Figure 4.2 A sentence of British English spoken by a female speaker. Top: Acoustic waveform, with syllable boundaries marked by thin vertical lines. Bottom: F0 contour.

tones or semitones can be measured by the ear; nor does the voice . . . ever dwell distinctly, for any perceptible space of time, on any certain level or uniform tone, except the last tone of which the speaker ends or makes a pause" (Steele, 1779:4).[6] The sinuous trajectory of F0 in speech stands in contrast to the sequence of discrete pitches produced by many musical instruments, and raises a fundamental question: How can spoken melodies can be compared to musical ones?

Fortunately for speech-music research, modern linguistics has a number of systems of intonation analysis in which F0 contours are mapped onto sequences of discrete tones. Two such systems are briefly introduced here. They are discussed in more detail in section 4.3, because of their particular relevance to speech-music comparisons.

The first such system, based on a phonological analysis of intonation, is illustrated in Figure 4.3.

[6] Steele's observations about speech intonation, particularly its rapid rate of change, were remarkably prescient. Empirical work suggests that the movements of voice pitch in speech may in fact be near their physiological speed limit (Xu & Sun, 2002).

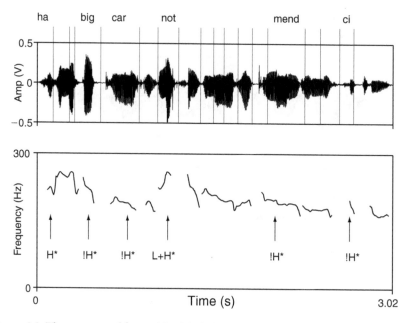

Figure 4.3 The sentence of figure 4.2 with the F0 contour marked for intonational tones according to the ToBI system. Upward arrows indicate the time points in the F0 contour that correspond to these tones. In the waveform, only those syllables that bear a tone are transcribed. Notation for tones: H = High, L = low, * = tone associated with a stressed syllable, L+H = bitonal low-high accent, ! = downstepped tone. (Downstep is discussed in section 4.3. For simplicity, edge tones have been omitted in this figure.)

This figure shows the F0 contour in Figure 4.2 annotated with phonological "tones" that mark the pitch accents in the sentence according to a prominent theory of speech intonation, the "autosegmental metrical" (AM) theory. The tone labels are taken from the "tones and break indices," or ToBI, system of conventions, which has its origins in AM theory (Beckman et al., 2005). As detailed later in this chapter, this theory posits that intonation contours can be decomposed into sequences of discrete linguistic tones, which are associated with specific points in the F0 contour. The remainder of the intonation contour, which lies between these points, is considered a mere interpolation, so that most of the F0 trajectory is not linguistically significant. AM theory typically uses just two pitch levels: high (H) and low (L), though these do not correspond to fixed frequency values. Instead, they represent phonological categories whose precise realization in terms of pitch values depends strongly on context.

A different system of intonation analysis is illustrated in Figure 4.4.

In contrast to the AM model, the "prosogram" model (Mertens, 2004a, 2004b) has its roots in psychoacoustic research on pitch perception in speech (as detailed in section 4.3.2). It aims to depict the pitch pattern of a sentence as

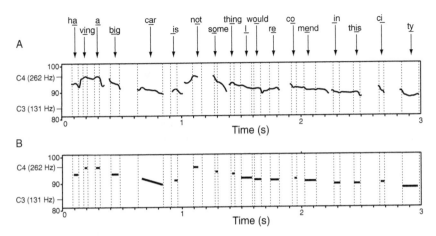

Figure 4.4 Illustration of the prosogram, using the sentence of Figure 4.2. (A) shows the original F0 contour, and (B) shows the prosogram. In both graphs the vertical axis shows semitones relative to 1 Hz (thus 90 st corresponds to 181 Hz; cf. this chapter's appendix), and musical C3 and C4 are marked for reference. In (B), syllable tones were computed based on the F0 of each vowel. (The choice of the unit of analysis for computing syllable tones is discussed in section 4.3.2.) The temporal onset and offset of each vowel is indicated by vertical dashed lines in (A) and (B). In the syllable transcription above the sentence, vowels have been underlined, and an arrow connects each vowel to its corresponding region in the F0 contour.

it is perceived by human listeners. The most notable feature of the prosogram is that it parses the continuous F0 contour into a sequence of syllable tones, many of which have a fixed pitch. In Figure 4.4, for example, all but one syllable ("car") have been assigned level tones. Although this makes the prosogram look a bit like the "piano roll notation" of a musical melody (cf. Figure 3.1), it is important to note that the level tones of a prosogram (and the pitch intervals between them) do not adhere to any musical scale. (See Figure 4.4 caption for an explanation of the y-axis units on the prosogram, and this chapter's appendix for formulae relating these units to values in Hz.)

Unlike the AM approach to intonation, the prosogram model assigns a tone to each syllable, and thus may seem at odds with the AM approach. However, the models are not contradictory. Recall that tone labeling in AM theory reflects the idea that the listener's language interpretation system cares only about a few points in the intonation contour, because these define the relevant linguistic contrasts. That is, AM theory is focused on phonology. The prosogram model, in contrast, is concerned with specifying *all* the pitches that a listener hears when perceiving intonation. Thus the prosogram model is focused on phonetics. The models are not contradictory because even if a listener's cognitive system *cares* only about a few pitches in a sentence, it is clear that the listener *hears* more than just these pitches, because most of the duration of a spoken utterance is accompanied by an F0 contour.

Although further work is needed to integrate the AM and prosogram approaches (cf. Hermes, 2006), this issue will not occupy us in this chapter. For the current purposes, the relevant point is that there are well-motivated systems of intonation analysis that employ discrete tones rather than continuous F0 contours. This allows a number of theoretical and empirical comparisons to be drawn between speech and music (cf. sections 4.3.1 and 4.5.1). For those who are skeptical of both of these approaches to intonation, however, it is worth noting that a good deal of the chapter does not depend on a commitment to either AM or prosogram theory.

4.2 Melody in Music: Comparisons to Speech

As pointed out in the introduction, a musical melody is more than a mere succession of pitches: It is a network of interconnected patterns in the mind *derived* from a sequence of pitch variation. That is, the human perceptual system converts a two-dimensional sequence (pitch vs. time) into a rich set of perceived relationships. One way to appreciate this richness is to list these relationships. This section provides one such list with nine items, and considers each item in terms of comparisons to speech intonation perception. The list is not exhaustive, but it covers many of the fundamental relations in musical melodies. The focus is on the perception of a simple melody by a listener familiar with Western European tonal music, because such melodies have received the greatest amount of empirical research to date. For illustrative purposes, I rely from time to time on a particular musical melody from this tradition, a generic melody chosen because it represents certain general features of melodic structure (the melody K0016, introduced in Chapter 3; cf. Figure 3.1 and Sound Example 3.1).

4.2.1 Grouping Structure

Grouping refers to the perceptual clustering of tones into chunks larger than single tones but smaller than the entire melody, as discussed in Chapter 3. For example, in listening to the 33 tones of K0016, there is a clear sense that the tones are grouped into five phrases (cf. Figure 3.4). The first two phrase boundaries are demarcated by silences (musical rests), but the boundaries of Phrases 3 and 4 are not marked by any physical discontinuity in the sequence. Instead, these boundaries are preceded by tones that are long and /or low compared to other tones in the same phrase. Although the five phrases marked in Figure 3.4 constitute the most perceptually obvious grouping level in K0016, theories of grouping structure posit that these phrases are but one layer in a hierarchical grouping structure, with lower level groups embedded in higher level ones (e.g., Lerdahl & Jackendoff, 1983; cf. Chapter 3, section 3.2.3).

As discussed in Chapter 3, grouping plays a prominent role in the study of prosody. What is the relationship between grouping and intonation in speech? Research on the perception of prosodic boundaries reveals that salient pitch events can serve as grouping cues in speech (de Pijper & Sanderman, 1994), just as they can in musical melodies (Lerdahl & Jackendoff, 1983). Furthermore, several modern theories of intonation posit that grouping structure has a close relationship with pitch patterning in an utterance. For example, autosegmental-metrical (AM) theory posits that English sentences can have two levels of intonational grouping: the "intermediate phrase" (abbreviated "ip") and the "intonational phrase" (abbreviated "IP"; Beckman & Pierrehumbert, 1986), both of which are marked by pitch events in the intonation contour called "edge tones." (In the case of the ip, the edge tone is called a "phrase tone" or "phrase accent," and in the case of the IP, it is called a "boundary tone.") This is illustrated in Figure 4.5 (cf. Sound Example 4.2).

Figure 4.5 shows the waveform and F0 contour of a sentence of British English: "In this famous coffee shop you will eat the best donuts in town."

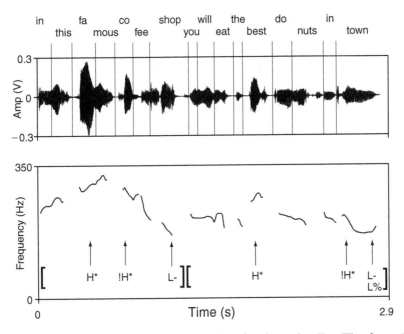

Figure 4.5 A sentence of British English spoken by a female speaker. Top: Waveform with syllable boundaries marked by thin vertical lines. Bottom: F0 contour with ToBI tones, as in Figure 4.3. Brackets indicate intermediate phrases according to an AM analysis of the sentence. L- indicates a low edge tone (phrase accent) at the end of each intermediate phrase, and L% indicates a boundary tone at the end of the full intonational phrase.

According to AM analysis of the sentence, this sentence has two intermediate phrases. The first ip ends with "shop," and its right boundary is marked by a lowering in pitch, thought to reflect the presence of a low phrase accent, indicated by L- (cf. section 4.3.1). The next intermediate phrase terminates at the end of the sentence. This point is also marked by a pitch fall, thought to reflect the combined effect of the low phrase accent marking the end of the second ip and the low boundary tone at the end of the full IP (L- and L%, respectively).

Pitch lowering is known to be a salient cue to phase boundaries in speech and music (e.g., Jusczyk & Krumhansl, 1993). It is important to note, however, that phrase boundaries in speech can also be marked by pitch *rises*. To take an example from French, several theories of French intonation posit that words in French sentences are grouped into short prosodic phrases (e.g., the "accentual phrases" of Jun & Fougeron, 2000, 2002). Notably, it is quite common for such phrases to end with a rising pitch movement if they are not the final phrase in the sentence (cf. Delattre, 1963; Di Cristo, 1998). This is illustrated in Figure 4.6, which shows a sentence of French together with its F0 contour ("La femme du pharmacien va bientôt sortir fair son marché"; cf. Sound Example 4.3). As shown in the figure, the sentence is divided into four accentual phrases: (La femme) (du pharmacien) (va bientôt sortir) (fair son marché).

The right boundaries of all but the final accentual phrase are marked by a rising pitch movement. This association of pitch rises with prosodic grouping boundaries is part of the characteristic melody of spoken French. This stands in contrast to English, in which intermediate phrases do not have a bias to "end high" and often end on a low pitch (Grover et al., 1987).

This example illustrates an important point about intonation. Part of what makes one language's intonation different from another is the way in which salient pitch movements align with the grouping structure of a sentence. An informal but compelling demonstration of the perceptual importance of this difference comes from the work of Gunnar Fant and colleagues. These scientists are using speech synthesis to explore intonation patterns in different languages. This approach permits them to graft the intonational patterns of one language onto the words of another. This is illustrated in Sound Examples 4.4a,b, which present two versions of an English sentence ("Along three of the walls there was a stage of rough wooden boards covered with straw"). The first version has English words and English intonation, whereas the second version has English words but French intonation, resulting in the perceptual impression of English spoken with a decidedly French accent. In particular, note how the phrases that end with "walls" and "boards" in the French accent version end on an upward pitch movement, but on a downward pitch movement in the original English version.

Thus it would appear that the relationship between melody and grouping structure is a promising area for comparative speech-music research. For

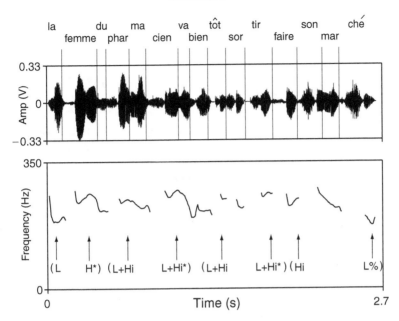

Figure 4.6 A sentence of French spoken by a female speaker. Top: Waveform with syllable boundaries marked by thin vertical lines. Bottom: F0 contour with phonological tones, according to an AM-style model of French intonation (Jun & Fougeron, 2002). Tone alignment points are marked as in Figure 4.3. Parentheses indicate accentual phrases (APs). The initial tone or tones of each AP (L or L+Hi) are phrase tones, whereas the final tones (H* or L+H*) are pitch accent tones. L% indicates the boundary tone at the end of the intonational phrase.

example, one could study the relationship between grouping boundaries and salient pitch peaks in French versus English musical melodies. Are pitch peaks likely to occur closer to the end of phrases in French music than in English music? Does the answer depend on whether songs (in which melodies are written to go with words) or instrumental music is analyzed? In conducting such a study, one must of course decide how to identify phrase boundaries in musical melodies; ideally this would involve perceptual data collected from groups of listeners in segmentation experiments (cf. Deliège, 1987; Frankland & Cohen, 2004)

One can also ask the inverse question: Do the pitch patterns of spoken phrases in one's native language influence grouping predispositions in music? For example, if French and English speakers were asked to indicate phrase boundaries in musical melodies, would French speakers show a greater tendency to hear boundaries after pitch rises than English speakers? If so, this would suggest that experience with linguistic pitch patterns influences the parsing of musical melodies.

4.2.2 Beat and Meter

A salient perceptual feature of many musical melodies is a steady beat to which one can synchronize by tapping (see Chapter 3, section 3.2.1 for an extended discussion and for examples using K0016). Most research on beat perception in melodies has focused on the temporal structure of tone sequences, under the assumption that the pitch pattern of a melody contributes little to the sense of a beat. However, empirical research indicates that pitch patterns can make a modest contribution to beat perception, for example, via accents created by melodic contour peaks or valleys (Hannon et al., 2004).

As discussed in Chapter 3, there is no evidence that speech has a regular beat, or has meter in the sense of multiple periodicities. If one abstracts away from regular timing, however, it is interesting to note that pitch variation contributes to rhythm in both domains via the role it plays in making certain events more prominent or accented. For example, contour peaks are perceptually accented points in musical melodies (Thomassen, 1983; Huron & Royal, 1996), which can participate in rhythm by either reinforcing or contradicting the underlying beat (for example, in K0016 the contour peak in the fourth phrase is in a nonbeat position, providing a sense of syncopation in this phrase; cf. Sound Example 3.1). In the intonation of English, salient pitch accents occur on a subset of the stressed syllables in an utterance, thus marking out a second layer of temporal structure over and above the patterning of stressed syllables (Jun, 2005; Ladd, 1996: Ch. 2). The linguist Bolinger has argued that the temporal patterning of these accents is part of the rhythm of an utterance (cf. Ch. 3, section 3.3.1, subsection "Phonology and Typology").

4.2.3 Melodic Contour

The sequential patterns of ups and downs in a melody, regardless of precise interval size, define its pitch contour. (A pitch contour can therefore be specified by a sequence of symbols that simply stand for "up," "down," or "same," rather than a sequence of numbers specifying the direction and size of intervals between pitches.) A pitch contour and its temporal pattern define a melodic contour. Dowling and others (Dowling, 1978; Dowling et al., 1995) have shown over a long series of experiments that melodic contour plays an important role in immediate memory for unfamiliar melodies. This has been demonstrated by showing that when listeners are asked to say if a melody is an exact transposition of a previously heard novel melody, they often give false positive responses to melodic "lures" that share the same contour as the original but not its precise intervals. As more time is given between the two melodies, the tendency for false positives declines and discrimination of exact transpositions from same contour lures improves, suggesting that the mental representation of a novel melody is gradually consolidated in terms of pitch interval categories (cf. Chapter 2, section 2.2.3, subsection "Pitch Intervals and Melody Perception"). This finding is consistent with the view that adults represent familiar melodies in terms of precise interval sizes, a view supported by adults' equal accuracy at detecting contour-violating versus contour-preserving changes to such melodies (Trehub et al., 1985).

This view of melodic contour implies that contour-based representations of melodies are "coarse-grained" schema that lack the detail of representations based on musical intervals. Thus it makes sense that melodic contour is one of the first aspects of music to be discriminated by infants, who have not yet developed the interval-based tonal schema of their culture (Trehub et al., 1984, 1987; Ferland & Mendelson, 1989; Trainor & Trehub, 1992; Trehub, Schellenberg, & Hill, 1997). Five-year-old children also seem to rely heavily on contour in melody perception, as they are worse than adults at detecting contour-preserving changes to unfamiliar tone sequences (Schellenberg & Trehub, 1999). Overall, developmental studies such as these suggest that contour-based processing is a kind of default processing of tone sequences, which gradually yields in importance to more detailed processing based on the learned sound categories of musical intervals (cf. Chapter 2). Of course, this is not to say that contour ceases to play a significant role in music perception for experienced listeners. For example, researchers have shown that melodies with fewer changes in melodic contour direction are perceived as simpler than melodies with more such changes (Boltz & Jones, 1986; Cuddy et al., 1981), and that familiar melodies can be recognized even if the interval pattern is somewhat distorted, as long as contour is preserved (Dowling & Harwood, 1986). Furthermore, neuroimaging research suggests that melody perception involves the dynamic integration of contour and interval processing (Patel & Balaban, 2000; Patel, 2003a).

Contour-based processing almost certainly has its origins in intonation perception. Starting early in life, prelinguistic infants in many cultures are exposed to a special speech register known as infant-directed speech, or "motherese" (Fernald, 1985; Fernald et al., 1989). One characteristic of infant-directed speech is the use of exaggerated and distinctive intonation contours to arouse or soothe infants and convey approval, disapproval, and so forth (Fernald & Kuhl, 1987). It is thus adaptive for infants to be sensitive to pitch contour cues from an early age, as these contours play a functional role in emotional communication. Even if infants are not exposed to motherese, as is claimed for some cultures (Ochs & Schieffelin, 1984), normal language acquisition inevitably involves learning the structural equivalence of intonation patterns that are similar in contour but not identical in terms of exact pitch movements. For example, if two different speakers utter "Go in front of the BANK, I said," using a pitch rise to mark the work BANK as contrastive, they might use different size pitch movements. Nevertheless, the sentence has the same pragmatic meaning, and a listener must learn to grasp this equivalence, which lies in the similarity in pitch contour despite differences in absolute pitch patterns. Thus one can expect all normal language listeners to arrive at competence with pitch contour perception.

The considerations outlined above suggest that the perception of melodic contour could be a fruitful area for comparative speech-music research. In fact, this is proving to be the case. Section 4.5.2 explores the cognitive and neural relations between contour processing in the two domains.

4.2.4 Intervallic Implications

When a musical melody is stopped at a point at which it sounds incomplete, listeners typically have expectations for what the next note will be, even when the melody is unfamiliar. This can be demonstrated by having listeners rate how well different tones continue a melody (Krumhansl et al., 2000), or by having them continue the melody by singing (Carlsen, 1981). In both cases, responses are far from random, and are thought to reflect a combination of culture-specific knowledge and universal Gestalt principles of auditory processing (Krumhansl et al., 1999, 2000). It is the latter principles that are of interest with regard to comparisons with speech intonation.

The most prominent theory of the Gestalt principles governing note-to-note musical expectancies is the "implication-realization" theory of Narmour (1990), which has inspired a good deal of empirical research pioneered by Krumhansl (1991, 1995a, 1995b; cf. Cuddy & Lunney, 1995). This model proposes five innate principles governing the expectancy for a following note given an existing musical interval (hence the term "intervallic implication") (Schellenberg, 1996). Schellenberg (1997) identified various redundancies between these principles and proposed a simplified two-factor model that is discussed here (cf. Schellenberg et al., 2002; Krumhansl et al., 2000). The first factor is referred to as "pitch proximity": Listeners expect a subsequent tone to be close in pitch to the last pitch they heard. The second factor is referred to as "pitch reversal," and actually describes two tendencies. The first is an expectation that after a large interval, the following tone will reverse the direction of the melody. The second is an expectation that reversals of any kind will create a symmetric pattern so that the upcoming tone will be close in frequency (within 2 semitones) to the penultimate tone of the sequence (for example, A-C-A, or A-E-B). Thus pitch reversal requires consideration of the two previous tones heard by a listener. (The discussion of pitch reversal below focuses on reversal per se rather than symmetry.)

Schellenberg et al. (2002) tested the proximity and reversal principles in experiments in which children and adults rated different possible continuations of melodies. The authors found that pitch proximity was an equally good predictor of expectancy across age groups, but that pitch reversal was a good predictor only in the adult group. This developmental difference shows that pitch reversal is not a hardwired principle of auditory processing, raising the question of where the principle comes from. Might it come from implicit learning of patterns in musical melodies? The tendency for reversals to follow pitch jumps is in fact widespread in musical melody, likely reflecting the simple fact that pitch jumps tend to approach the edge of a melody's range, forcing a subsequent move in the opposite direction (von Hippel & Huron, 2000). However, if this is a widespread feature of music, why doesn't it play a role in children's musical expectancies?

Schellenberg et al. suggest that children's lack of expectancy for pitch reversal may result from the exposure of children to infant-directed speech (or child-directed speech with similar prosodic properties). Specifically, they suggest that in infant directed speech large pitch movements are often followed by further movement in the same direction, rather than reversals. Thus the effect of speech might wash out the effect of music on the development of expectancies for pitch reversals. Although speculative, this proposal is notable for advancing the idea that expectations for pitch patterns in musical melodies are shaped not only by experience with music, but also by experience with the pitch patterns of speech. Direct evidence for the idea would require quantifying the statistical regularities of spoken and musical melodies in a common framework, which could be done using methods that will be discussed in section 4.5.1 of this chapter.

4.2.5 Motivic Similarity

A fundamental aspect of melody perception in music is the recognition of motivic similarity between different parts of a melody. For example, the first and last phrase of K0016 are identical (cf. Sound Example 3.1), which helps to provide this melody with a sense of closure. Motivic similarity need not be so literal: People can recognize similarity without identity. Because similarity is a graded feature influenced by many factors, ranging from surface acoustic features (such as timbre and articulation) to midlevel structural features (such as melodic contour) to abstract features (such as implied harmony), its empirical study presents a challenging problem (Schmuckler, 1999; McAdams & Matzkin, 2001), and progress in this area has been slow.

To what extent do the principles that govern the perception of motivic similarity in music draw on mechanisms of similarity perception in intonation? To answer this question one first needs a clear understanding of the basis for intonational similarity judgments in speech. There is some research on this topic, based on the idea that a language has only a limited number of linguistically distinctive intonation contours. For example, commenting on the intonation of British English, Halliday (1970:6) remarked:

> There is no limit to the number of different pitch contours that it is theoretically possible to produce. . . . But not all the variations in pitch that the speaker uses . . . are significant. The very large set of possible pitch contours can be thought of as being grouped into a small number of distinct pitch contours . . . rather in the same way that we group the [many] colours that we can tell apart into a small set

which we can recognize as different colours, and which we label "yellow," "red,"
"green," and so on.

Perceptual research on intonation supports Halliday's idea. One set of studies based on similarity judgments of affectively neutral intonation contours
suggests that Dutch listeners recognize six basic intonation patterns underlying the diversity of observed pitch sequences in their language, based on
specific types of rises and falls that occur within pitch contours ('t Hart et al.,
1990:82–88). This research provides an excellent starting point for those interested in cross-domain research on motivic similarity in speech and music (see
also Gussenhoven & Rietveld, 1991; Croonen, 1994: Ch. 7).

4.2.6 Tonality Relations: Pitch Hierarchies

"Tonality relations" in music refer to psychological relations between tones
resulting from the systematic ways in which tones are employed in relation to
each other. For example, Western tonal melodies typically adhere to a musical scale based on 7 out of 12 possible pitches per octave (cf. Chapter 2 for a
discussion of musical scales), and departures from this structure are perceptually quite salient to listeners enculturated in this tradition ("sour notes," discussed later in this section). Furthermore, tones within melodies are organized
such that some pitches are more structurally central or stable than others. This
can be illustrated with K0016. Consider Figure 4.7a, in which each note of
K0016 has been marked with a number representing each tone's position or
scale degree in the scale from which the melody is built (e.g., scale position 1 is
do, 2 is *re*, 3 is *mi*, etc., and –5 is *so* in the octave below).

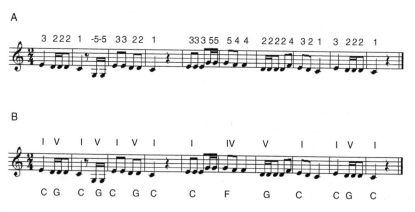

Figure 4.7 (A) K0016 with scale degree of each tone marked. Note that –5 corresponds
to scale degree 5 in the lower octave. (B) Harmonization of K0016. The letters below
the staff give the chords in the key of C major, whereas the Roman numerals above the
staff indicate chord functions (I = tonic, IV = subdominant, V = dominant). For readers
unfamiliar with these harmonic terms, they are defined in Chapter 5.

Note that scale degree 1 (the "tonic") plays a central role in this melody. It is the final tone of phrases 1, 2, 4, and 5, and thus serves as a resting point within the melody and at the melody's end. Furthermore, it always occurs on a beat and is of long duration (cf. Chapter 3, Figure 3.2). Scale degree 1 thus acts a perceptual "center of gravity" for the entire melody, a role that can be contrasted with the role of scale degree 2. Degree 2 is far more common than degree 1 in this melody (13 vs. 4 occurrences), yet degree 2 never serves as a resting point: Instead, it almost always leads back to degree 1. Furthermore, it is never long in duration, and frequently occurs off the beat. Thus scale degrees 1 and 2, though neighbors in frequency, vary dramatically in their perceptual stability. This contrast between physical and psychological similarity of tones 1 and 2 is characteristic of tonal music. That is, stable tones within a musical scale are often flanked by unstable tones. This is shown in Figure 4.8, which shows empirical data from a set of classic experiments by Krumhansl and Kessler (1982; cf. Steinke et al., 1997).

In these experiments, listeners heard a brief musical context such as a short chord sequence within a given key[7] followed by a brief pause and then one of the 12 possible pitches within the octave (the "probe tone"). Listeners were asked to rate how well the tone fit into or went with the preceding musical material, on a scale of 1–7 (in which 7 indicated the best fit). The rating given to each tone can be thought of as a measure of its tonal stability in the given musical context. As can be seen, large asymmetries in stability exist among the 12 tones of the chromatic scale in a major-key or minor-key context. (The figure is oriented to the key of C but represents data from tests of different keys: All data have been transposed to the key of C.)

Focusing on the probe-tone profile for the major-key context, note that the most stable tone (C, or scale degree 1) is flanked by scale tones of low stability (D and B, or scale degrees 2 and 7). Also note that the highly stable tones C, E, and G (degrees 1, 3, and 5) are not neighbors in frequency, but are separated by at least 3 semitones. Thus the pitch hierarchy (or "tonal hierarchy") shown in Figure 4.8 makes adjacent scale degrees distinctly different in terms of their structural roles, providing a psychological pull that works directly against Gestalt auditory principles that make frequency neighbors psychologically similar (e.g., as members of a single auditory stream). The tension between these two types of relations may be one of the forces that animate musical melodies.[8]

---

[7] For those unfamiliar with the concepts of chords or keys, they are explained in Chapter 5.

[8] Although this chapter focuses on Western European tonal music, it is important to note that pitch hierarchies are not unique to this tradition. Some form of a tonal center or tonic is widespread in musical melodies of different cultures, in both in art music and folk music (e.g., Herzog, 1926; Castellano et al., 1984; Kessler et al., 1984).

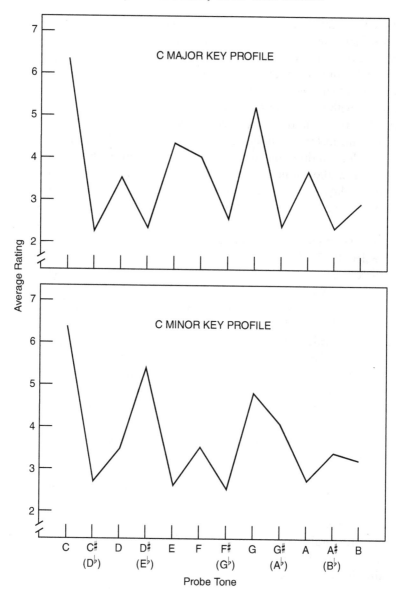

Figure 4.8 Probe tone profiles, indicating listeners' judgments of how well a given tone fits with a preceding musical context. From Krumhansl & Kessler, 1982.

The influence of tonal relations on melody perception has been demonstrated in a number of ways. Bigand (1997) had participants listen to increasingly long fragments of a melody and judge the stability of each fragment's end, in other words, the feeling that the melody could naturally stop versus the feeling that it must continue. Stability judgments varied widely over the course of a single melody, demonstrating the dynamic nature of melody perception (cf. Boltz, 1989). Two main contributing factors to this variance were the final tone's position in the pitch hierarchy and its duration (cf. Sound Examples 4.5a,b).

Another demonstration of the power of tonality relations is the well-known phenomenon of the "sour note," demonstrated in Sound Example 4.6. Sour notes are notes that are perceptually salient because they violate the norms of tonality relations. Unlike what the name implies, there is nothing inherently wrong with a sour note: It is perfectly well-tuned note that would sound normal in another context (and which presumably would not sound sour to someone unfamiliar with tonal music). Its sourness has to do with its lack of membership in the prevailing scale. Furthermore, its degree of sourness is a function of its position in the tonal hierarchy (Janata et al., 2003). Listeners with no explicit musical training can detect such notes, indicating that a basic level of musical syntactic knowledge can be acquired without any formal training. Indeed, the inability to detect such notes is indicative of musical tone deafness or "congenital amusia" (Kalmus & Fry, 1980; Drayna et al., 2001; Ayotte et al., 2002), a disorder discussed later in this chapter.

In summary, pitches in musical melodies are organized into scales that feature salient hierarchies of stability. These hierarchies are reflected in the systematic use of different scale degrees for different structural purposes (e.g., scale degree 1 as a stable resting point). As a result, different scale degrees take on distinct psychological qualia in the fabric of the music. As noted by Huron (2006:173), "In a given context, a tone will sound stable, complete, and pleasant. In another context, that exact same tone will feel unstable, incomplete, and irritating." It is a remarkable fact of tonality that individual pitches can come to life in this way.

At present, there is no evidence of anything resembling scales or pitch hierarchies in speech melody. As noted in section 4.1.1, there is no sense in which some intonational tones are more stable or central than others. This is a very salient difference between musical and spoken melody, but it should not overshadow the many other points of contact between melody in the two domains.

4.2.7 Tonality Relations: Event Hierarchies

The hierarchical stability relations between pitches described in the previous section were atemporal schema derived from experience with musical melodic patterns. Musical melodies also have pitch hierarchies of a different sort concerning temporal relations between pitches in individual sequences, in other words, "event hierarchies" (Bharucha, 1984a). The basic idea of an event hierarchy is that some pitches in a melody act as its structural skeleton, whereas others serve to elaborate or ornament this skeleton. This notion is central to Western European music theory (e.g., the theories of Schenker (1969), Meyer (1973), and Lerdahl and Jackendoff (1983; cf. Cook, 1987a), and is also found in the music theory of many non-Western cultures, including China and India. For example, in one Chinese folk tradition, musicians speak of ornamentation as "adding flowers" to a basic melodic structure (Jones, 1995). The ability to distinguish structural from ornamental pitches is thought to play an important role in melody perception, such as in a listener's ability to recognize one melody as an elaborated version of another (cf. Lerdahl & Jackendoff, 1983).

Empirical research has shown that pitch hierarchies, in combination with rhythmic factors, play an important role in shaping event hierarchies in tonal music. Evidence for musical event hierarchies is discussed in Chapter 5, section 5.2.2. Here the pertinent question is whether speech intonation exhibits event hierarchies. Surprisingly, at least one modern approach to intonation (AM theory) suggests that the answer may be "yes," though the event hierarchies of intonation have nothing to do with pitch hierarchies based on differing degrees of perceived stability. This issue is taken up in section 4.3.1.

4.2.8 Tonality Relations: Implied Harmony

Melodies in Western tonal music typically have implied harmony, a background chord progression from which important tones of the melody are drawn (for those unfamiliar with the concept of a musical chord, chords and chord syntax are discussed in Chapter 5). Thus there is a hierarchical level of pitch organization beneath the tones of the melody, with its own principles of combination and patterning. To illustrate this point, Figure 4.7b shows a harmonic analysis in terms of underlying chords for K0016, and Sound Example 4.7 presents K0016 with a chordal accompaniment to make this harmony explicit. The structure of the chord sequence underlying a melody plays a role in melody perception for both musicians and nonmusicians, influencing judgments of the musical coherence of melodies as well as memory for melodies (Cuddy et al., 1981; Povel & Jansen, 2001). There is also evidence from studies of song learning that listeners abstract the underlying harmonic structure of a melody. Sloboda and Parker (1985) had listeners sing back unfamiliar melodies presented to them on a piano. An analysis of their errors of recall (e.g., interval errors) showed that they preserved the overall contour of the melody and the background harmonic progression (cf. Davidson et al., 1981).

Although there is nothing resembling chord structure or harmony in speech intonation, there is intriguing evidence from speech synthesis that local pitch events may combine into larger structures that have their own principles of patterning. In one approach to intonation synthesis (the IPO model, described in section 4.3.2), intonation contours are constructed from standardized pitch movements arranged in sequences ('t Hart & Collier, 1975; 't Hart et al., 1990). Researchers have found that synthesis of acceptable intonation patterns involves arranging small pitch movements nonrandomly into local "configurations" (linking certain kinds of rises and falls), which in turn are sequenced to form contours spanning a single clause. Not all possible sequences of configurations form acceptable contours, in other words, constraints on contour formation also exist. This multilevel organization is reminiscent of the organization of successive pitches into chords and chords into sequences, and both may reflect a general propensity to organize pitch sequences into patterns at multiple hierarchical levels (cf. Ladd, 1986).

4.2.9 Meta-Relations

The preceding eight sections have discussed different kinds of perceptual relations engendered by musical melody. There are also relations between these relations, in other words, meta-relations. For example, a slight misalignment of grouping and beat can add rhythmic energy to a melody in the form of anacrusis or upbeat, as in the onset of phrase 2 of K0016. Another meta-relation concerns the relation between the tonal hierarchy and rhythm. Boltz (1991) has found that melodies in which tonally stable pitches occur at regular temporal intervals (e.g., at the ends of phrases) are remembered more accurately than melodies without this feature.

Are there any meta-relations in musical melodies that one can compare to speech intonation? One relevant line of research in this regard concerns the perceptual interactions of accents due to pitch and rhythm, in other words, the "joint accent structure" of melodic sequences (Jones, 1987, 1993). Joint accent structure refers to the temporal relation between salient points in the pitch pattern of a melody, such as contour peaks (Huron & Royal, 1996), and salient points in the temporal pattern of a melody, such as lengthened tones. Evidence suggests that listeners are sensitive to the relative timing of these points in music: Their alignment and periodicity relations can influence memory for melodies (Jones & Ralston, 1991) and how well people can synchronize their taps with accents in melodies (Jones & Pfordresher, 1997). For the purposes of comparing melody in music and speech, the issue of temporal alignment between pitch peaks and long events is of interest, because contour peaks and lengthened events can be identified in both musical melodies and in intonation contours. To illustrate this idea, consider Figure 4.9, which shows the pitch and duration of each vowel for a sentence of French: "Les mères sortent de plus en plus rapidement de la maternité" as uttered by a female speaker (cf. Sound Example 4.8).

The pitch values in the figure were computed from a prosogram analysis of the sentence (cf. Figure 4.4, and section 4.3.2), and are shown in terms of semitones from the lowest pitch in the sentence. Note the salient peaks in both the pitch and duration time series. It would be interesting to determine if the alignment of pitch and duration peaks in French sentences shows any statistical regularities, and if these regularities differ from the patterns found in other

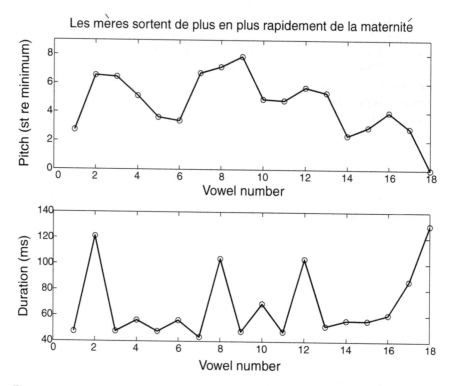

Figure 4.9 The pitch and duration of each vowel in a sentence of French: "Les mères sortent de plus en plus rapidement de la maternité" as spoken by a female speaker. Top: Pitch values as computed from a prosogram, shown as semitones from the vowel with the lowest pitch. Bottom: Duration of each vowel in ms.

languages (e.g., British English). If so, one could then examine melodies from the music of two cultures, and ask if linguistic alignment differences are reflected in the alignment of melodic contour peaks and long tones in music.

4.2.10 Musical Versus Linguistic Melody: Interim Summary

Section 4.2 has reviewed a number of key aspects of melody perception, and found that in many cases one can draw a parallel with some aspect of speech intonation perception. This raises an obvious question. If there are interesting parallels between musical and linguistic melody perception, then why do melodies in the two domains "feel" so different in terms of subjective experience? For example, musical melodies can get "caught in one's head" for days, whereas spoken melodies rarely capture our interest as sound patterns.

One reason for this may be that musical melodies engender a much richer set of perceptual relations. For example, section 4.2 lists eight basic relations invoked by a simple musical melody, and this is by no means an exhaustive list (cf. Meyer, 1973; Narmour, 1990; Patel, 2003a). Furthermore, there are many possible meta-relations between these relations. (In fact, given just eight relations, the number of possible pairwise meta-relations is 28!) This may be why musical melody perception is psychologically so distinct from intonation perception. It is not only that musical melodies have perceptual relations that spoken melodies do not (such as beat, interval structure, and the tonality relations built on interval structure); it is the fact that these additional relations lead to many more meta-relations. Thus the possible perceptual relations in musical melodies are far more numerous and intricate than those in speech melodies.

The greater intricacy of musical melodies should not deter the search for links between melody in the two domains. On the contrary, a solid understanding of the components of musical melody perception can help guide the search for meaningful connections with language. Based on the review in section 4.2, one link that stands out as particularly promising is melodic contour perception. For this reason, the topic is taken up in greater detail in section 4.5.2, which draws on data from cognitive neuroscience to further explore this connection between music and language.

4.3 Speech Melody: Links to Music

Although section 4.2 focused on musical melody and its connections to speech, in this section the perspective is reversed. That is, speech intonation is given priority and the focus is on what modern research on intonation suggests about connections with music. One challenge for this perspective is selecting among the many available theories of intonation available today (Hirst & Di Cristo, 1998). Here I focus on two theories, chosen because of their relevance to comparative speech-music research.

Before delving into these theories, it worth returning to a point made earlier in this chapter about an important difference between melody in speech and music (cf. section 4.1.1). Unlike musical melody, speech intonation is not built around a stable set of pitch intervals. Why is this the case? Given the enormous range of linguistic diversity, why is there not a single known language that uses stable pitch intervals for intonation? Such a system is theoretically possible, because interval-based pitch contrasts are found in the vocal music of virtually every culture.

The likely reason is that spoken language mixes affective and linguistic intonation in a single acoustic channel. Affective intonation is an example of a gradient signaling system: Emotional states and the pitch cues signaling them both vary in a continuous fashion.[9] For example, high average pitch and wide-ranging, smooth pitch contours convey a happy rather than a sad affective state to a listener (Juslin & Laukka, 2003). Furthermore, there are other nonlinguistic factors that influence pitch height and pitch range in a continuous way, such as the loudness with which one speaks (Shriberg et al., 2002). This means that intonation cannot utilize a frequency grid with fixed spacing between pitches. Instead, the pitch contrasts of linguistic intonation must be realized in a flexible and relative way (Ladd, 1996; cf. Chapter 2, section 2.3.2, subsection "A Closer Look at Pitch Contrasts Between Level Tones in Tone Languages"). The lack of a stable interval structure is the single most salient difference between musical and spoken melodies, and is likely why theories of musical melody and theories of speech melody have had so little conceptual contact.[10] Despite this fact, it is possible to identify interesting connections between linguistic and musical melody, as we shall see.

One other point worth mentioning is that that the linguistic use of intonation is more diverse than has generally been appreciated. For example, to a speaker of English it might seem that using pitch to put focus on certain words in sentences is a universal property of intonation, but a comparative perspective reveals that this is not the case. Somali uses linguistic morphemes to mark focus on words, rather than intonation (Antinucci, 1980; Lecarme, 1991). Another example of intonational diversity concerns the relationship between rising pitch at the end of yes–no questions versus falling pitch at the end of statements. Although this pattern is common in Western European languages, it is by no means universal. For example, questions in Standard Hungarian have high pitch on the penultimate syllable of a sentence, followed by a sharp pitch fall on the final syllable, so that "it is not overstating the case to say that many Hungarian questions sound like emphatic statements to native speakers of English . . ." (Ladd, 1996:115). Furthermore, in Belfast English, statements are produced with a final pitch rise as often as questions (Grabe, 2002). These are but two examples, but they serve to indicate that generalizations about linguistic intonation must be made with care (Ladd, 2001).

4.3.1 Intonation and Phonology

One of the most influential frameworks for intonation research today is "autosegmental-metrical" (AM) theory, which has its origins in the work of

---

[9] Of course, intonation is not the only cue to affect in speech (for example, voice quality also plays an important role; cf. Chapter 6 and Ladd et al., 1985). Also, there are cases in which affect influences intonation patterns in a more categorical (vs. continuous) fashion (Ladd, 1996: Ch. 1).

[10] One of the few points of contact has been articulated by Fred Lerdahl (2003), who has applied the theoretical machinery of musical pitch analysis to derive intonation contours for lines of spoken poetry.

Bruce (1977) and Pierrehumbert (1980). This approach tends to be practiced by researchers whose primary focus is linguistic structure rather than auditory perception. Because a detailed discussion of AM theory is beyond the scope of this book (see Ladd, 1996, and forthcoming), here I give only a brief introduction oriented toward comparative language-music research. I also focus on English, in which most research in the AM framework has taken place, though AM-style descriptions exist for an increasingly diverse range of languages (Jun, 2005).

A basic tenet of AM theory is that the linguistic aspects of intonation are based on *categorical* distinctions involving sequences of discrete pitch events. Specifically, the continuous F0 contours of speech are viewed as reflecting a sequence of distinct "pitch accents" and "edge tones" associated with certain points in the physical F0 contour. The rest of the intonation contour is considered a mere interpolation between these events, so that most of the F0 trajectory is not linguistically significant. That is, F0 contours in speech are seen as the result of moving between certain well-defined targets in pitch and time, a view quite analogous to the conception of melody in music (especially vocal music, in which voice pitch often moves in a sinuous manner, e.g., Seashore, 1938; Sundberg, 1987; cf. Bretos & Sundberg, 2003).

Pitch accents in the AM model are built from a basic inventory of tones. For example, in one current theory that informs the ToBI system of analysis (Beckman et al., 2005), there are two tones, associated with two contrastive pitch levels: high and low (H and L). Different types of pitch accents can built from these tones, for example, H*, L*, L*+H, and L+H* (see Table 4.1).The star means that the given tone is associated with a stressed syllable). The first two of these involve single tones, whereas the latter two are "bitonal" and involve a rising pitch movement from low to high. It has been argued that in English these different pitch accents signal the pragmatic status particular words (e.g., Pierrehumbert & Hirschberg, 1990; cf. Wennerstrom, 2001). This builds on a long-held idea among linguists that the units of intonation have discourse meaning (e.g., Pike, 1945; Bolinger, 1958; cf. Ladd, 1987).

In addition to pitch accents, the AM approach posits that intonation contours have tones that mark the edges of phrases. Words in English sentences are claimed to be grouped into prosodic phrases at two levels: smaller intermediate

Table 4.1 The Discourse Meanings of Different Pitch Accents in AM Theory

H*	Indicates new information
L+H*	Indicates contrasting information
L*	Indicates currently accessible (not new) information
L*+H	Indicates information whose relevance is uncertain

phrases, or "ip's" whose edges are marked by a high or low phrase tone (H-, L-) and larger intonational phrases, or "IP's" whose edges are marked by a high or low boundary tone (H%, L%). As with pitch accents, a pragmatic meaning has been suggested for phrase tones and boundary tones: They serve to indicate whether an ip or an IP is related to the preceding or following ip/IP. In contrast to pitch accents, edge tones do not convey perceptual prominence.

An important aspect of AM theory with regard to comparison with music concerns the sequential relations between the basic elements (pitch accents and edge tones). How constrained are these relations? Pierrehumbert and Hirschberg (1990) argued that the meaning of intonation contours is "compositional," in other words, each element contributes a particular pragmatic meaning and the contour as a whole (i.e., the intonational "tune" or sequence of elements) conveys no additional meaning above and beyond the simple sum of the parts. This suggests that tunes are subject to minimal constraints in terms of the sequencing of elements, and that for the most part tones are chosen independently of the tones that immediately precede them. This stands in sharp contrast to musical melody, in which tones are patterned at both local and global scales. There is evidence, however, that intonational sequences do have sequential constraints (cf. Ladd, 1996: Ch. 6). For example, Grabe et al. (1997) showed that the meaning of an initial H or L boundary tone depended on whether it was followed by a H or L pitch accent. More recently, Dainora (2002) examined a large corpus of speech that had been labeled with AM notation and searched for statistical constraints on sequences of pitch accents and edge tones. She found strong evidence that tones are not chosen independently of the tones that precede them. For example, the identity of an edge tone (as L or H) is influenced by the particular types of pitch accents that precede it. Thus intonational tunes do have some statistical regularities, though the constraints appear to be quite weak compared to musical melodies. Dainora found that these regularities could be captured by a second-order Markov model (a statistical model in which an element's identity depends upon only the identity of the two preceding elements).

A word needs to be said about the two distinct tonal levels in the AM system. Because these are abstract levels they do not correspond directly to specific pitch values or a specific pitch interval between H and L, but simply indicate the relative pitch height of a tone with regard to neighboring tones. In fact, the mapping between these abstract levels and actual frequency values (referred to as "scaling") is a complex issue that is the focus of ongoing research. Such research suggests that multiple factors are involved in scaling, including the degree of prominence of a word, declination (the general tendency for F0 values to decrease over the course of an utterance; cf. Section 4.1.1), and the local context in which tones occur. For example, a high tone may be "downstepped" (lowered in frequency) when it occurs in certain tonal contexts, or the pitch target of a tone may not be realized because of undershoot due to tonal crowding. As a consequence of these complexities, H and L tones do not correspond to fixed frequency values, but are simply relative positions within a pitch range that is itself subject to change (Pierrehumbert, 2000). Consequently, analysis of intonation contours in terms of H and L tones is not something that can be done automatically on the basis of pitch contours, but requires training in AM theory and is done by individuals who listen to sentences while examining a visual display of the F0 contours.

One interesting area of empirical research motivated by the AM model is the precise timing of tones with respect to phonetic boundaries (referred to as "tonal alignment"). Research on alignment has given rise to the idea that the abstract tones of AM are implemented as phonetic "tonal targets": particular points in the intonation contour (often peaks or valleys in the F0 trajectory) that have stable relationships to certain phonetic landmarks, such as the edges of stressed syllables (Arvaniti et al., 1998; Ladd et al., 1999). For example, it has been proposed that certain types of tonal targets in Greek occur at a certain short distance in time *after* the end of a stressed syllable. One interesting line of evidence for the perceptual significance of tonal alignment concerns the speech of impersonators. Zetterholm (2002) studied a professional Swedish impersonator who was good at imitating the voice of a famous Swedish personality. Focusing on the production of one particular word that occurred several times in recordings of the impersonator's natural voice and of his voice while impersonating, Zetterholm showed that the impersonator systematically changed the alignment of the tonal peak of this word from a value characteristic of the impersonator's native dialect to a value characteristic of the dialect of the imitated person. Turning to linguistic differences in alignment, Atterer and Ladd (2004) found that pitch rises in German showed later alignment than comparable pitch rises in English, and that native speakers of German carried over their alignment patterns when speaking English as a second language.

Some readers may find the AM approach overly abstract in positing a categorical structure beneath the continuous acoustic variation of F0. A comparison to vowel perception is helpful here. No one disputes that every language has an inventory of linguistically distinct vowels, each of which forms a distinct perceptual category for listeners of that language. Yet in the acoustics of speech, a given vowel does not correspond to a fixed acoustic pattern. Not only does a vowel's acoustics vary across speakers due to vocal tract differences and the resulting differences in formant values (Peterson & Barney, 1952), within the speech of a single speaker a vowel's acoustic realization varies due to coarticulation and other factors, such as undershoot due to rapid speech (Lindblom, 1990). Nevertheless, listeners are able to abstract away from this diversity and hear the distinct linguistic categories beneath them; indeed, this ability is present even in infants (Kuhl, 1983). Vowel perception shows that the mind is quite adept at parsing graded variation in a continuous acoustic space (in this case, of formant values) into discrete linguistic categories.

The AM approach treats intonation in much in the same way that phonology treats vowels, positing discrete mental categories underneath a continuous and variable phonetic surface. Of course, it is easier to demonstrate perceptual discreteness with vowels than with intonation. Changing a vowel alters the semantic meaning of a word in a categorical fashion (e.g., *bet* vs. *beet*), so that listeners can readily agree that different vowels correspond to distinct linguistic categories. It is more difficult to demonstrate that pitch contrasts signal distinct pragmatic categories to listeners. Simply asking listeners what a given pitch accent "means" is not an optimal strategy, as listeners are not used to making explicit judgments about pragmatic (as opposed to semantic) meanings. Thus indirect tests of discreteness in intonation perception are needed. One interesting approach, pioneered by Pierrehumbert and Steele (1989), is to use an imitation paradigm in which a participant is asked to mimic as closely as possible the intonation of a short utterance with a particular F0 pattern. Using computer editing of sound, the F0 pattern of the model utterance is varied in small increments between two extremes representing two different hypothesized pitch accent types. Examination of the F0 patterns produced by participants suggests a bimodal distribution, as if listeners are parsing the continuum of F0 variation into two distinct categories (cf. Redi, 2003; Dilley, 2005).

What sorts of links between language and music does the AM approach suggest? At a very general level, the AM approach draws attention to the idea that speech melody has two facets: an abstract phonological structure of underlying pitch contrasts and a physical realization of pitch versus time (cf. Cutler et al., 1997). This view of melody is quite analogous to the way musical melody is conceptualized: The same musical melody sung by different people will differ in fine-grained acoustic details of the pitch trajectory, but will nevertheless articulate the same set of underlying pitch contrasts.

Although this is a general conceptual similarity between melody in the two domains, the AM approach also suggests a much more specific point of contact between melody in speech and music. Recall that an important aspect of AM theory is that only certain points in the F0 contour are considered to be linguistically significant. For example, consider the AM analysis of the sentence in Figure 4.5. As can be seen, this sentence has four pitch accents (two high tones and two downstepped high tones, labeled as H* and !H*, respectively) and three edge tones (L- tones at the end of each ip, plus a L% tone at the end of the entire utterance, which combines forces with the L- tone in the final ip in terms of influencing the F0 contour). Recall that the asterisk notation indicates that the given tone is associated with a stressed syllable. (Note that not all stressed syllables receive a pitch accent in this sentence. For example, "eat" and the first syllable of "donuts" are stressed but are not associated with a phonological tone. This is not unusual: AM analyses of English sentences often identify pitch accents on just a subset of the stressed syllables of the utterance.) Yet although

AM theory identifies just a few points in a pitch contour as linguistically significant, listeners almost certainly *hear* pitch on each syllable of a sentence (cf. the prosogram, discussed in section 4.3.2). Hence built into AM theory is the notion of an event hierarchy, with some pitch events in a sequence being more structurally important than others.

As we saw in section 4.2.7, the notion of an event hierarchy is central to modern theories of melody perception in music, in which it is common to think of melodies as having some tones that are more structurally important than others. This suggests that the mental processing of a tone sequence in terms of an event hierarchy of relative importance may have its origins in the perception of speech intonation. This is a question that is open for research. A first step in addressing the issue would be to seek empirical evidence for event hierarchies in speech melody. For example, one might try discrimination experiments in which the same sentence is presented twice with a slight difference in its F0 contour. The question of interest is whether a difference of a given size is more salient if it occurs at a point that AM theory indicates is structurally important than if it occurs in an "interpolation" region. If this was demonstrated, and if it could not be explained on a simple psychoacoustic basis, it would open the way to exploring event hierarchies in speech melodies and their relationship to musical melodic structure.

4.3.2 Intonation and Perception

I now turn to a different line of research on intonation, one that has roots in the study of auditory perception. This approach originated at the Institute for Perception Research in The Netherlands, or the IPO, which represents the initials of the Dutch name of that institute ('t Hart et al., 1990). Research at the IPO was motivated by the desire to synthesize sentences with natural-sounding intonation in different languages, and was enabled by speech technology that allowed full control over F0 contours in synthetic speech.

Prior to the IPO approach, most intonation research used impressionistic transcriptions of pitch based on the ears of the individual doing the transcribing. Indeed, this approach dates back to Joshua Steele's 1779 book, *An Essay Toward Establishing the Melody and Measure of Speech to Be Expressed and Perpetuated by Peculiar Symbols.* Steele worked by ear, using sliding fingerings on a bass viol to mimic intonation in order to transcribe it. (Steele borrowed the convention of the musical staff for transcription, but instead of using fixed pitches, he used short curved lines to indicate the pitch movement occurring on each syllable; cf. Kassler, 2005.) Several other notation systems were developed by later British and American researchers, using a variety of symbols to indicate how voice pitched moved up and down over the course of an utterance. Because of technological limitations, these pioneering researchers worked without the benefit of actual measurements of F0 over time. Naturally this meant that the notations were impressionistic and subject to a good deal of individual variation.

A major technical advance that led to the IPO approach was the ability to measure the fundamental frequency contour of a sentence, and then to resynthesize the sentence with the original contour or with an altered contour imposed by the researcher. Researchers could then test the perceptual significance of systematic alterations in the contour. This powerful "analysis-by-synthesis" approach transformed intonation research from an impressionistic endeavor to a quantitative, perception-based science. For example, the researchers quickly made a remarkable discovery: It was possible to replace the original contour with a simpler version that was perceptually equivalent to the original. This process of "close-copy stylization" of F0 is shown in Figure 4.10.

The dotted line shows the original F0 contour of an English sentence, whereas the solid line is the close-copy stylization. The close-copy contains the minimum number of straight line segments that produces a sentence that is perceptually equal to the original. The success of this stylization procedure led to the idea that listeners extract a few structurally significant pitch movements from the details of the actual F0 curve of a sentence. One reason that the details are not relevant to perception may be that they are inevitable byproducts of the machinery of speech. For example, the vowels /i/ and /u/ tend to have

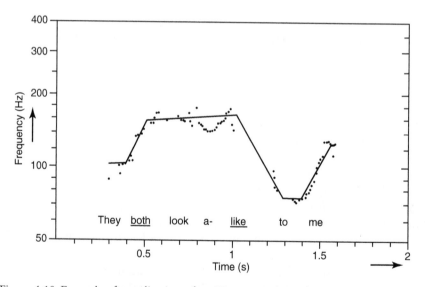

Figure 4.10 Example of a stylization of an F0 contour for a sentence of English (accented syllables are underlined). The original F0 contour is shown with dots, and the close-copy stylization is shown with solid lines. Note that frequency is plotted on a logarithmic scale, in other words, a fixed distance along this axis represents a fixed ratio between F0 values, rather than a fixed numerical difference. From 't Hart et al., 1990.

higher pitch than the vowels /a/ and /ae/ (Whalen & Levitt, 1995), perhaps because raising the tongue for a high vowel causes upward tension on the hyoid bone and an involuntary tensing of the vocal folds (Ladefoged, 1964:41). Also, vowels following a voiceless consonants (such as /p/ and /f/) tend to start on a higher pitch than vowels following voiced consonants (such as /b/ and /v/), due to vocal fold biomechanics (Löfqvist et al., 1989). Effects such as these produce "microintonation": small pitch deflections that are not intended by the speaker. The perceptual equivalence of original and close-copy intonation contours suggests that these fluctuations are not relevant to listeners.

For the current purposes, the significance of the IPO approach is that it showed that the raw F0 contour of a sentence, although an accurate physical description of the speech signal, is not the most accurate representation of intonation as it perceived by human listeners. This helped open the way to studies of "F0 stylization," in other words, transformations of the F0 contour into simpler representations meant to capture how spoken pitch patterns are perceived by human listeners (cf. Rossi, 1971, 1978a, 1978b; Harris & Umeda, 1987; Hermes, 2006). F0 stylization is important for speech-music comparisons, as we shall see. Before expanding on this point, however, it should be noted that the IPO approach went beyond stylization to seek an inventory of standardized pitch movements from which natural-sounding speech melodies could be constructed. Speech melodies in the IPO approach consist of standardized pitch movements arranged in sequences (cf. de Pijper, 1983; Collier, 1991). The movements were differentiated by their direction, size, and duration, yielding an inventory of basic pitch rises and falls.[11] Pitch movements were used to mark important words and structural boundaries, and took place between pitch levels of an abstract frequency grid that declined over the course of an utterance, as shown in Figure 4.11 (cf. section 4.1.1 for a discussion of declination).

In terms of comparisons to music, an interesting feature of the IPO approach is the organization of spoken melodic patterns at multiple hierarchical levels. At the most local level, pitch movements are combined nonrandomly into "configurations" (i.e., the linking of certain kinds of rises and falls). At the next level, configurations are linked together to form "contours" spanning a single clause

---

[11] One difference between the IPO approach and the AM approach is that the former treats pitch movements as the primitives of intonation, whereas the latter treats pitch levels as the primitives. Evidence for the latter view includes the observation that the beginning and endpoints of pitch movements are more stable than the duration or slope of these movements (Arvaniti et al., 1998; Ladd et al., 1999). This difference in perspective is not irreconcilable, however: It is relatively easy to recast the IPO approach into a target-based framework, because movements always take place between well-defined start and endpoints. Furthermore, it may be that listeners hear some pitch events in intonation as level pitches and others as movements (cf. the prosogram, described later in this section).

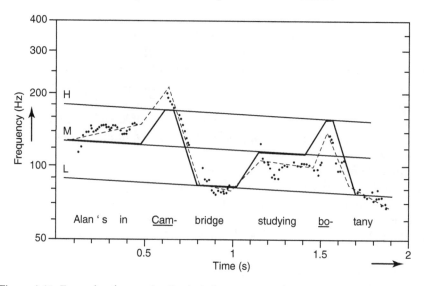

Figure 4.11 Example of a standardized pitch movements for a sentence of British English (accented syllables are underlined). The original F0 contour is shown with dots, the close-copy stylization is shown with dashed lines, and the stylized movements are shown with a solid line. The stylized movements move between abstract reference lines that decline in frequency over time (H = high, M = mid, L = low). From 't Hart et al., 1990.

('t Hart et al., 1990:81). Not all possible sequences of configurations form acceptable contours; instead, constraints on contour formation exist and can be indicated in the form of a branching flow chart or transition network of pitch movements. This approach to the grammar of melody has interesting parallels to the principles governing variation of musical melodies within "tune families" (McLucas, 2001). As is evident from this description, the IPO approach eventually became a quasi-phonological model of intonation, which specified linguistically significant intonational contrasts and their patterning in utterances.

From the current perspective, however, the important legacy of the IPO approach is the notion of pitch stylization (cf. Hermes, 2006). This approach has been further developed by other researchers. One of the most notable achievements in this regard is the prosogram model, which was introduced in section 4.1.2 (Mertens 2004a, 2004b). The prosogram is based on empirical research that suggests that pitch perception in speech is subject to three perceptual transformations. The first is the segregation of the F0 contour into syllable-sized units due to the rapid spectral and amplitude fluctuations in the speech signal (House, 1990). The second is a threshold for the detection of pitch movement within a syllable (the "glissando threshold"; 't Hart 1976). If the rate of pitch change within a syllable (in semitones/second) does not exceed this threshold, then the syllable is perceived as having a level pitch corresponding to a temporal integration of F0 within the syllable (d'Alessandro & Castellengo, 1994; d'Alessandro & Mertens, 1995).[12] This is a crucial feature in terms of comparing speech and music, as discussed below. The third transformation, which is less relevant for the current purposes, applies when the glissando threshold is exceeded. This is a threshold for detection of a change in the direction of a pitch glide within a syllable (the "differential glissando threshold"). If the differential glissando threshold is exceeded, then a single syllable is perceived as having more than one pitch movement. Thus for example, a single syllable can be perceived as having a pitch rise followed by a pitch fall, if the syllable is long enough and there is enough pitch change within it.

A key question about the prosogram concerns the units to which it assigns tones. Although perceptual research suggests that listeners segregate F0 contours into syllable-sized units (House, 1990), it also appears that pitch changes during syllable onsets do not play a significant role in perception. This may be because such regions are often the locus of microintonation effects (cf. Hermes, 2006). Hence it appears that the syllable rime (the syllable stripped of its onset consonants, i.e., the vowel plus following consonants) is the primary domain that conveys pitch information to a listener. Figure 4.12 shows a rime-based prosogram analysis of the same sentence depicted in Figure 4.4.

Recall that Figure 4.4 was computed using vowels rather than rimes as the unit of prosogram analysis. As can be seen from comparing these two figures, the patterning of tones in terms of pitch is very similar in the two prosograms. (The rime-based tones are often longer, of course, because they include more of the F0 contour.) The similarity of these representations suggests that vowels provide a reasonable unit of analysis for the prosogram, especially if one is interested in the pitch (vs. durational) patterning of tones. This is fortunate, because identification of vowels is phonetically simpler than identification of rimes (which require linguistic decisions about syllable boundaries). Thus in practice, prosogram computation requires only that the user supply the timing of vowel onsets and offsets in an utterance. The prosogram then computes perceived tones according to the second and third transformations mentioned in the preceding paragraph.[13]

Stepping back from the details of prosogram computation, Figures 4.4b and 4.12 reveal why the prosogram is so useful for speech-music comparisons. The

---

[12] The glissando threshold used in computing the prosograms in Figures 4.4 and 4.12 is $0.32/T^2$ semitones/second, in which T is the duration (in seconds) of the vowel (in Figure 4.4) or rime (in Figure 4.12). If the rate of pitch change was greater than this threshold, the vowel (or rime) was assigned a frequency glide. The choice of this threshold is based on perceptual research on the threshold for detecting pitch movements in speech, combined with experiments in which prosogram output is compared to human transcriptions of intonation ('t Hart, 1976; Mertens, 2004b).

[13] A recent version of the prosogram can perform automatic segmentation of a sentence into syllabic nuclei, removing the need for the user to supply vowel or rime boundaries.

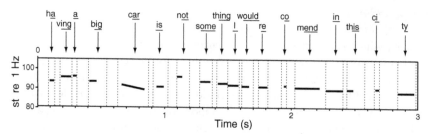

Figure 4.12 Illustration of a rime-based prosogram of the same sentence depicted in Figure 4.4. (Axis conventions as in Figure 4.4.) Note the similarity between the pitches of this prosogram and the prosogram in Figure 4.4B, which was computed using a vowel-based analysis. The temporal onset and offset of each rime is indicated by vertical dashed lines. In the syllable transcription above the sentence, rimes have been underlined, and an arrow connects each rime to the corresponding region of the prosogram. When a prosogram tone occupies only a portion of a rime (e.g., in the 6th syllable, "is"), this is typically due either to lack of voicing or low signal amplitude in some part of the rime.

representation of intonation in terms of syllable tones is quite music-like, because most tones are level pitches. From a cognitive perspective, this is interesting because it implies that the auditory image of speech intonation in a listener's brain has more in common with music than has generally been believed. From a practical perspective, the dominance of level pitches means that spoken and musical melodies can be compared using quantitative measurements of pitch patterns. This approach informs the empirical comparative work on spoken and musical melody described below in section 4.5.1.[14]

4.4 Interlude: Musical and Linguistic Melody in Song

In keeping with the rest of this book, the focus of this chapter is on the relationship between spoken language and instrumental music. Nevertheless, it is worth touching briefly on song, because the artful combination of words and music creates a natural area for the study of melodic relations between speech and music. An interesting question about song is how its musical melody relates to the pitch pattern of the spoken lyrics. This is particularly relevant

[14] The prosogram is freely available from http://bach.arts.kuleuven.be/pmertens/prosogram/, and runs under Praat, which is freely available from http://www.fon.hum.uva.nl/praat/.

for tone languages, in which pitch makes lexical distinctions between word meanings. In such languages, distorting the spoken pitch pattern can affect intelligibility, raising the question of to what extent song melodies are constrained by the melody of speech. As far back as 1934, the ethnomusicologist George Herzog asked, "Does music slavishly follow speech-melody in [tone] languages, or does it merely accept raw material with which to work? Is there a clash between melodic patterns based on speech, and purely musical melodic patterns or tendencies? And how far can musical elaboration distort the speech-melody pattern of the song-text without making it incomprehensible to the listener?" (p. 454). Since Herzog's time, many studies have been published on the relation of speech melody and song melody in tone languages (Feld & Fox, 1994, p. 31, cite 10 such studies; for an exemplary quantitative study, see Richard, 1972).

A case of strong correspondence between speech and song melody occurs in Cantonese opera (Yung, 1991). Southern coastal Cantonese has nine linguistic tones, consisting of five level tones and four contour tones (cf. Chapter 2 for a definition of these types of linguistic tones). Yung notes that close correspondence between the contour of a spoken text and its associated musical melody is characteristic of the genre. However, he also notes that in other parts of China such close matching between text and music is not observed, suggesting that the key factor is not intelligibility. Instead, he argues that the close correspondence springs from practical concerns. Singers of Cantonese opera often must memorize operas very quickly, and often have to sing different operas each day for several days. Typically, they are given a script a few days before a performance, and must perform without music notation or rehearsal. In this situation, Yung suggests that singers compose as they perform, using "the relatively less defined pitches of linguistic tones as a guide . . . in creating a series of well-defined pitches to form the melodic line of the music" (pp. 416–417). Thus the case of Cantonese opera is likely to be unusual in terms of the strong influence of speech melody on song.

A more representative case is reported by Herzog (1934), who studied songs in Jabo, a tone language from Liberia with four discrete levels. He found a definite relationship between the shape of song melodies and the pattern of linguistic tones on the underlying words, but he also found that the relationship was not a slavish one. A given linguistic tone did not have a one-to-one correspondence with a given musical tone, and musical considerations such as motivic similarity and balancing of phrase structure often led the music to contradict the shape suggested by the speech melody. Presumably, these factors left enough of the speech melody intact so that the meanings of words were clear from context. Thus it may be that the only strong predictive power of speech melody in tone languages is in suggesting what a song melody will *not* be: namely, it will rarely have a contour completely contrary to that of the spoken melody (cf. Blacking, 1967; Wong & Diehl, 2002).

Research on the relation of spoken and musical melodies in non-tone languages is much less developed than in tone languages. In one study, Arnold and Jusczyk (2002) examined spoken and sung versions of three nursery rhymes. The spoken versions were made by individuals who were unfamiliar with the musical melodies that normally accompanied them, and who read them as texts of connected prose (rather than as verse organized into couplets). To conduct cross-domain comparison, musical pitch contours were analyzed simply in terms of high and low pitch targets, in other words, maxima and minima in the song's F0 track that were aligned with stressed syllables. Speech contours were analyzed in terms of the ToBI system of analysis to identify high and low tones (cf. section 4.3.1). The authors found that pitch targets in the sung version did tend to correspond in type (high or low) to those realized on the same words in the text, though the amount of correspondence varied widely across the three nursery rhymes. Clearly, this is an area that is open for research. One idea for quantifying the degree of correspondence between linguistic intonation and musical melody in songs is to use the prosogram to identify the melodic contour of the lyrics when they are spoken, and then to compare this contour to the musical melodic contour to which the text is set in a song. It would be interesting to know if songs with melodies congruent with the spoken pitch contour have an advantage in terms of how easily they are learned or remembered (cf. Patel, 2006a).

4.5 Melodic Statistics and Melodic Contour as Key Links

The purpose of this section is to delve into two areas in which direct comparisons of musical and linguistic melody are proving fruitful. Section 4.5.1 addresses structure, and shows that a specific aspect of the statistics of speech intonation is reflected in instrumental music. Section 4.5.2 concerns processing, and provides evidence that perception of melodic contour in speech and music engages overlapping cognitive and neural machinery. This latter section also outlines a hypothesis (the "melodic contour deafness" hypothesis) that aims to account for the apparent dissociation of musical and linguistic melody perception in musically tone-deaf individuals. As we shall see, one implication of this hypothesis is that a behavioral dissociation is not the same as a neural dissociation.

4.5.1 Melodic Statistics

Analysis of intonation in terms of the syllable tones of the prosogram (section 4.3.2) opens the way to quantitative comparisons of melody in speech and music. For example, musical melodies are characterized by a number of statistical regularities that appear cross-culturally (summarized in Huron, 2006). To what extent are these regularities unique to music versus shared with speech? If some regularities are shared, what is the cognitive significance of this fact?

One well-known regularity of musical melodies is the predominance of small ("conjunct") intervals between successive pitches. Figure 4.13 shows the relative frequency of intervals of different sizes in a sample of Western music (Vos & Troost, 1989). The general pattern is similar to that seen when melodies from a range of cultures are sampled (Huron, 2006:74).

As is clear from the figure, musical melodies are dominated by small intervals. Another way of putting this is that most melodic motion is by small steps (of 2 semitones or less). The predominance of small intervals is reflected in listeners' expectations for how novel melodies will continue when stopped midstream (cf. section 4.2.4), showing that this is a perceptually relevant feature of melodies.

Why do small intervals dominate melodies? The two most commonly proffered reasons are motor and perceptual. The motor explanation suggests that small intervals are easier to produce in succession than large ones, with the voice and with most instruments (cf. Zipf, 1949:336–337). The perceptual explanation suggests that too many large pitch movements risk splitting a melody into separate perceptual streams, destroying the perceptual cohesion between successive tones (Bregman, 1990; cf. Narmour, 1990). Of course, the motor and perceptual explanations are not mutually exclusive: Indeed, they may reinforce each other. One can thus group them into a single category of "constraint-based explanations" based on the notion of intrinsic constraints on production and perception.

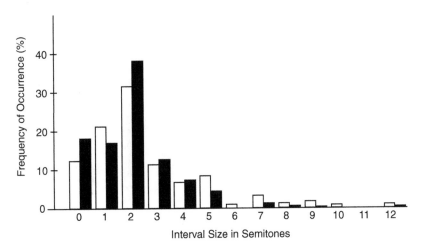

Figure 4.13 Histograms showing the relative proportion of pitch intervals of different sizes in Western melodies (classical and rock: white bars; folk, dark bars). From Vos & Troost, 1989.

An alternative to constraint-based theories is the idea is that the preference for small intervals in music arises out of experience with speech. That is, if speech melodies are dominated by small pitch movements, and if listeners absorb the statistics of spoken pitch patterns in their environment, then this might influence their proclivities in terms of shaping musical melodies. This hypothesis invokes a perceptual mechanism known as "statistical learning," which has been discussed in Chapters 2 and 3. Statistical learning refers to tracking patterns in the environment and acquiring implicit knowledge of their statistical properties, without any direct feedback. Statistical learning is discussed in more detail later in this chapter. For now, the relevant point is that statistical learning may provide one mechanism for a cross-domain influence of speech on music.

How can one test this idea? The first step is to determine if speech melodies are in fact dominated by small pitch movements. Consider once again the prosogram in Figure 4.4b. The intervals between adjacent level tones are listed in Table 4.2. (Note that that there are 18 tones in the prosogram of Figure 4.4b, but only 15 intervals appear in Table 4.2. This is because one of the prosogram tones is a glide, and intervals are computed only between immediately adjacent level tones.) One fact that is immediately apparent from this table is that most intervals are quite small, reminiscent of the pattern found in music. How representative is this pattern? Figure 4.14 shows a histogram of intervals between level tones in a corpus of 40 English and French sentences that have been analyzed using prosograms like that in Figure 4.4b.

As can be seen, intonational pitch patterns are dominated by small pitch movements. In Figure 4.14, 56% of all intervals between level tone pitches are

Table 4.2 The Size of Pitch Intervals in Semitones Between Adjacent Level Tones in a Prosogram of an English Sentence (cf. Figure 4.4b)

Interval Number	Size in Semitones
1	2.56
2	−0.01
3	−2.51
4	4.96
5	−1.72
6	−0.83
7	−1.64
8	−0.56
9	−0.21
10	0.54
11	−0.90
12	−1.02
13	0.01
14	0.47
15	−1.89

less than or equal to 2 semitones. One notable difference between the distribution of intervals in speech and music is that in musical melodies intervals of 2 semitones are more common than intervals of 1 or 0 semitones (see Figure 4.13). No such tendency is seen in speech. (In Figure 4.14, the percentage of intervals between 0-1, 1-2, and 2-3 semitones, respectively, are 35%, 21%, and 19%). This predominance of 2-semitone intervals in musical melodies likely reflects the fact that intervals of 2 semitones are more common than intervals of 1 semitone in musical scales (cf. Chapter 2). Despite this difference between music and speech, the larger point is that speech melodies, like musical melodies, are dominated by small pitch intervals. This is probably not a peculiarity of English and French; it is likely to hold for languages generally.

Finding that small intervals predominate in speech melodies is consistent with the idea that music reflects speech. However, it is also consistent with the idea that pitch patterns in speech and music are subject to the same set of motor and perceptual constraints. This illustrates a basic problem in interpreting commonalities between statistical regularities in music and speech: Such commonalities could be due to the operation of some physiological or perceptual factor that influences both speech and music, rather than to any cross-domain influence.

Hence if one is interested in the possibility of speech influencing music, some strategy is needed to eliminate the problem of common external influences. One such strategy is to look for quantifiable *differences* between the statistics of speech intonation in different cultures, and to see if these differences are reflected in instrumental music of these cultures. Because there is no way that

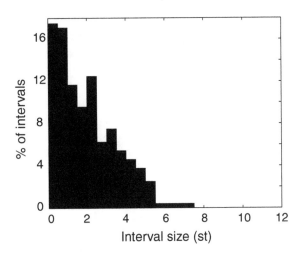

Figure 4.14 Histogram showing the relative proportion of pitch intervals of different sizes (n = 543 total) between level tones in prosograms of British English and French sentences. Histogram bin size = 0.5 st.

general motor or perceptual factors can explain differences in speech melody between languages, a reflection of linguistic differences in music makes a stronger case for cross-domain influence.

This "difference-based" approach to comparing language and music has been applied by Patel, Iversen, and Rosenberg (2006) to the speech and instrumental classical music of England and France. This study complemented an earlier study with a similar approach, which focused on rhythm (Patel & Daniele, 2003a; cf. Chapter 3, section 3.5.1). Once again, the topic of investigation was the provocative claim (made by a number of musicologists and linguists over the past 50 years) that a culture's instrumental music reflects the prosody of its native language. For example, the linguist Hall (1953) suggested a resemblance between Elgar's music and the intonation of British English.

In addressing this idea, we used the same corpus of speech and music as in our earlier work on rhythm. That is, the speech corpus consisted of short, newslike utterances read by native speakers of each language, whereas the musical corpus consisted of themes from instrumental classical music by 16 composers whose lives spanned the turn of the 20th century (such as Elgar and Debussy). Although we focused on just two cultures, a principal goal of this research was to establish methods of broad applicability in comparative speech-music studies.

We computed prosograms for all sentences in our speech corpus, resulting in representations like that in Figure 4.4b. Then, focusing on just the level pitches (which represented about 97% of pitches assigned by the prosogram algorithm, the rest being glides), we computed two measures of melodic statistics for each sentence. The first was variability in pitch height, which simply measured how widely spread the level pitches were around their mean pitch. The second was variability in pitch interval size within a sentence, in which an interval was defined as the jump in pitch between immediately successive level pitches. This measure serves to indicate whether steps between successive level pitches tend to be more uniform or more variable in size.

Initially it may seem odd to focus on pitch intervals in speech. Although the human perceptual system is quite sensitive to interval patterns in music (in which, for example, a melody can be recognized in any transposition as long as its interval pattern is preserved), music features well-defined interval categories such as minor second and perfect fifth, whereas speech does not (cf. section 4.1.1). Might the perceptual system attend to interval patterns in speech despite the lack of stable interval structure? Recent theoretical and empirical work in intonational phonology suggests that spoken pitch intervals may in fact be important in the perception of intonation, even if they do not adhere to fixed frequency ratios (Dilley, 2005; cf. Hermes, 2006). If this is the case, then one can understand why composers might have implicit knowledge of the "spoken interval statistics" of their language, which might in turn be reflected in the music that they write.

We used semitones in our measurements of pitch height and pitch intervals in speech, reflecting the perceptual scaling of intonation (Nolan, 2003).[15] We also used semitones in measuring pitch height and pitch intervals in music, working directly from music notation. The height measurements revealed no significant difference in variability between English and French speech, nor between English and French music. The results of interval measurements were more revealing. Spoken French had significantly lower pitch interval variability than spoken English, and music mirrored this pattern. That is, French musical themes had significantly lower interval variability than English themes, Put another way, as the voice moves from one syllable to the next in speech, the size of each pitch movement is more uniform in French than in English speech. Similarly, as a melody moves from one note to the next, the size of the pitch movement is more uniform in French than in English music. Figure 4.15 shows the results of the pitch interval variability measures combined with our previous findings on rhythm. Note that the measure of variability on the vertical axis is "melodic interval variability" (MIV), defined as 100 times the coefficient of variation (CV) of interval size (CV = standard deviation/mean). Scaling the CV by 100 serves to put MIV in the same general range of absolute values as nPVI.

We call Figure 4.15 an "RM space" (rhythm-melody space) plot, because it shows the position of a given language or music in a two-dimensional space with rhythm on one axis and melody on the other. One appealing thing about RM space is that the "prosodic distance" between two languages can be quantified via the length of a line connecting the points representing the mean (nPVI, MIV) of the two languages (see Patel et al., 2006 for details). In Figure 4.15, the prosodic distance between English and French speech is 27.7 RM units. In contrast, the line connecting the English and French music is only about 1/3 as long (8.5 RM units). Thus the musical difference is smaller than the linguistic one. This is not surprising, given that music is an artistic endeavor with substantial intracultural variation and (unlike speech) no a priori reason to follow rhythmic or melodic norms. What is remarkable is that despite this variation, quantitative differences emerge between the music of the two nations that reflect linguistic differences.

By what route do speech patterns find their way into music? One oft-heard proposal is that composers borrow tunes from folk music, and these tunes bear the stamp of linguistic prosody because they were written with words. This might be termed the "indirect route" from speech to music. If this is the case,

---

[15] Earlier work by Hermes and Van Gestel (1991) had suggested ERBs should be used in measuring pitch distances in speech. The precise choice of units for speech is unlikely to influence the results reported here. Our measure of pitch variability, the coefficient of variation (CV), is a dimensionless quantity that would allow one to measure pitch distances in speech and music in different units (ERBs vs. semitones), and still compare variability across domains with the CV as a common metric.

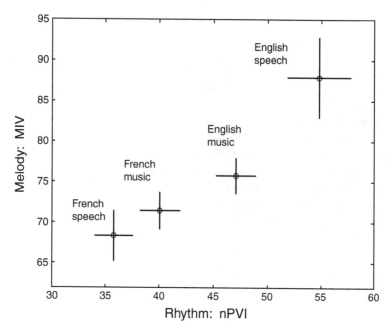

Figure 4.15 Rhythm-melody (RM) space for speech and music. Error bars show +/− 1 standard error. See text for details.

then there are no strong cognitive implications for speech-music relations, because the speech-music resemblance is simply the result of borrowing of music that has been consciously shaped to fit linguistic phrases.

We favor a different hypothesis, however. This is the idea that implicit learning of prosodic patterns in one domain (ordinary speech) influences the creation of rhythmic and tonal patterns in another domain (instrumental art music). This might be termed the "direct route" between speech and music, because contact between speech and music need not be mediated by an intermediate speech-music blend (such as songs). One advantage of the direct-route hypothesis is that it can account for the reflection of speech in music not thought to be particularly influenced by folk music (e.g., much of Debussy's and Elgar's work; Grout & Palisca, 2000).

The direct-route hypothesis centers on the notion of statistical learning of prosodic patterns in the native language. Recall that statistical learning refers to tracking patterns in the environment and acquiring implicit knowledge of their statistical properties, without any direct feedback. Statistical learning of prosodic patterns in one's native language likely begins early in life. Research on auditory development has shown that infants are adept at statistical learning of phonetic/syllabic patterns in speech and of pitch patterns in nonlinguistic tone sequences (Saffran et al., 1996, 1999) Thus it seems plausible that statistical learning of rhythmic and tonal patterns in speech would also begin in infancy, especially because infants are known to be quite sensitive to the prosodic patterns of language (Nazzi et al., 1998; Ramus, 2002b). Of course, statistical learning of tone patterns need not be confined to infancy. Adult listeners show sensitivity to the distribution of different pitches and to interval patterns in music (Oram & Cuddy, 1995; Saffran et al., 1999; Krumhansl, 2000; Krumhansl et al., 1999, 2000). Importantly, statistical learning in music can occur with atonal or culturally unfamiliar materials, meaning that it is not confined to tone patterns that follow familiar musical conventions.

It is worth emphasizing that the direct-route hypothesis does not imply that speech prosody influences musical structure in a deterministic fashion. It simply implies that composers can be influenced by their implicit knowledge of their native language's rhythm and melody. Music is an artistic medium, after all, and composers are free to do what they like. In particular, the influence of music of other cultures may override native linguistic influences on musical structure (see Patel & Daniele, 2003b; Daniele & Patel, 2004).

Two final points deserve mention. First, it remains to be explained why English speech should have a greater degree of pitch interval variability than French. One idea is that British English may use three phonologically distinct pitch levels in its intonation system, whereas French may only use two (cf. Willems, 1982; Ladd & Morton, 1997; cf. Figure 4.11 for one model of English intonation based on three distinct pitch levels). A compelling explanation, however, awaits future research. Second, our study focused on a very simple aspect of melodic statistics (pitch variability). More sophisticated analyses of melodic statistics are clearly called for. One idea is to study the alignment of pitch and duration patterns, to see if differences in the "joint accent structure" of speech melody between languages are reflected in music (cf. section 4.2.9, and Patel et al., 2006).

4.5.2 Melodic Contour Perception

Melodic contour refers to a melody's pattern of ups and downs of pitch over time, without regard to exact interval size. As discussed in section 4.2.3, melodic contour perception is important in both music and speech. Yet it is not obvious on a priori grounds whether the processing of melodic contour in the two domains is mediated by common cognitive and neural machinery. One might imagine that the lack of stable pitch interval structure in speech, combined with a speech-specific tendency for pitch declination (cf. section 4.1.1) would lead linguistic melodic contours to be processed differently from musical melodic contours. Indeed, Peretz and Coltheart (2003) have proposed a modular model of music processing in which melodic contour analysis is a domain-specific aspect of music perception, not shared with speech. Thus cross-domain studies of melodic contour perception are relevant to debates on the overlap of musical and linguistic processing in the brain.

In terms of evidence from cognitive neuroscience, reports of selective impairments of music, or "selective amusia," are of particular relevance for the cross-domain study of melodic contour processing. The two sections below discuss melodic contour processing in two populations: individuals with "acquired amusia" and those with "congenital amusia," or musical tone-deafness.

Melodic Contour Perception in Acquired Amusia

Acquired amusia refers to deficits in musical perception and/or production abilities following brain damage that are not simply due to hearing loss or some other peripheral auditory disorder (Marin & Perry, 1999; Peretz, 2006). The condition is reported relatively rarely, probably due to social factors. That is, individuals who experience dramatic changes in music perception after brain damage may not seek medical attention for this problem, or may not be directed by their physicians toward a neuropsychologist who studies music. From the standpoint of brain localization, amusia has been associated with damage to diverse regions of the brain (not just the auditory cortices), though there are a preponderance of cases with right-hemisphere damage in the published literature (Griffiths, 2002; Stewart et al., 2006).

Patel, Peretz, et al. (1998) examined intonation perception in two amusic individuals with different kinds of music perception deficits. The first participant, CN, was an "associative amusic" who was able to discriminate musical pitch and rhythm patterns but was unable to identify culturally familiar tunes, suggesting a selective difficulty in accessing stored representations for familiar tunes (Peretz, 1996). The second participant, IR, was an "apperceptive amusic" who could not discriminate musical pitch and rhythm patterns. Thus her deficit was at a lower level than that of CN.

To test the intonation perception of these individuals, Patel, Peretz, et al. (1998) used sentence pairs in which the members of the pair were lexically identical but had different intonation. Furthermore, computer editing of each sentence pair was used to ensure that the timing of syllables in the two sentences was identical and that intensity differences were minimized, so that the only salient cue for discrimination was pitch. These sentence pairs could take one of two forms: "statement-question pairs" in which one version of a sentence was a statement and the other a question (such as "He wants to buy a house next to the beach" spoken as a statement vs. a question), and "focus-shift pairs" in which the two sentences had contrastive focus on a different word (such as "Go in FRONT of the bank, I said" vs. "Go in front of the BANK, I said").

In addition to these linguistic stimuli, pairs of nonlinguistic tone sequences were also presented for discrimination. These tone sequences were created from the intonation contours of the sentence pairs, replacing each syllable of a sentence with a tone whose pitch was fixed at the Hz value midway between the maximum and minimum F0 values for that syllable (Figure 4.16). The linguistic and nonlinguistic stimuli were thus matched for overall length and pitch range.

Tone onsets occurred at the vowel onset times of corresponding syllables, and tone offsets were determined by the offset of F0 within each syllable. Thus each tone sequence had the same temporal rhythm as the syllables in the parent sentence. All tones had a complex frequency structure consisting of a fundamental and a few harmonics of decreasing amplitude. An example of a sentence pair and its melodic analogs are given in Sound Examples 4.9a–d. (Note that the sentences are in French, as the study was conducted with French-speaking amusics. Similar sound examples in English are provided later.) The rationale behind the study was that if the amusics' perceptual deficits were confined to

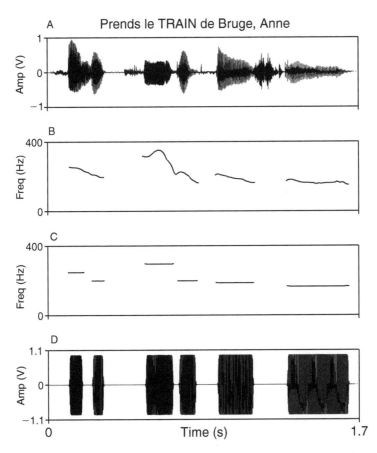

Figure 4.16 Illustration of the process of converting the intonation contour of a sentence into a discrete tone analog. The waveform of a French sentence is shown in (A) and its F0 contour in (B). In (C), the F0 of each syllable has been set to a fixed value. (D) shows the waveform of the tone analog. Adapted from Patel, Peretz, et al., 1998.

music, they should perform well on discriminating the sentences but have difficulty with the tone sequences, in other words, a dissociation between speech and nonlinguistic tone sequence processing should be observed. On the other hand, if intonation and tone-sequence processing overlap in the brain, then similar performance on the two types of sequences should be found.[16]

The results of the study supported the second conclusion. CN did well on both the linguistic and nonlinguistic sequences, whereas IR had difficulty discriminating both types of sequences. Furthermore, IR's problems could not be attributed to simple low level perceptual problems in perceiving pitch patterns, because further experiments showed that she could accurately label individual statements and questions as either "statement" or "question," and could identify which word in a given focus-shift sentence carried the main emphasis. Thus it appeared that IR's intonation *perception* was only mildly compromised, but her memory for melodic contours suffered (cf. Belleville et al., 2003). This interpretation was supported by a comparison of the lesion profiles of CN and IR. Compared to CN, IR had additional damage in left primary auditory cortex and right frontal cortex (Figure 4.17).

The latter lesion is likely to be associated with a memory-based deficit, because right frontal and temporal cortex has been implicated in pitch memory tasks in both speech and music (Zatorre et al., 1994). This suggested that both intonation and nonlinguistic tone sequences rely on common brain regions when melodic contours must be retained in working memory (cf. Semal et al., 1996).[17]

Melodic Contour Perception in Musical Tone Deafness

For those interested in comparing melody perception in music and speech, the phenomenon of musical tone-deafness (henceforth mTD) is of particular interest. Also referred to as "congenital amusia" (Peretz & Hyde, 2003), mTD

---

[16] Note that this study was conducted before the authors were aware of the prosogram, and thus the construction of tonal analog of intonation was based on intuitive criteria rather than on an explicit algorithm for F0 stylization. Nevertheless, the resulting pitch sequences do bear some resemblance to sequences that would be generated by a prosogram, although they lack any glides (cf. section 4.3.2).

[17] Another amusic who has been studied with a similar paradigm has also demonstrated equivalent difficulties with intonation and nonlinguistic tone sequence analogs (Nicholson et al., 2003). In this case, however, the damage was in the right parietal cortex and this may have disrupted the ability to extract pitch patterns in both domains, rather than causing a problem in remembering these patterns (cf. Griffiths et al., 1997). It is also worth noting that IR was retested on the materials of Patel et al. approximately 10 years after the original study and showed a virtually identical pattern of performance. Thus her condition is very stable (Lochy & Peretz, personal communication, 2004).

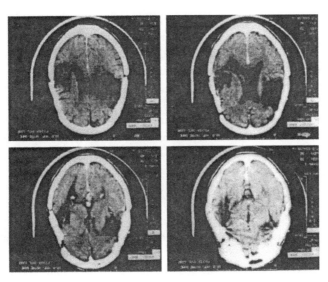

Figure 4.17 (a) Transverse CT scans of the amusic individual IR. Note that the right side of the brain is shown on the left of each image, per radiological convention. Scans proceed superiorly in 10-mm increments, in the order top left, top right, bottom left, and bottom right. The scans show bilateral temporal and right inferior frontal lobe damage (see Patel, Peretz, et al., 1998, for details).

refers to severe problems with music perception and production that cannot be attributed to hearing loss, lack of exposure to music, or any obvious nonmusical social or cognitive impairments. As mentioned in section 4.1.1, musically tone-deaf individuals (henceforth mTDIs) are typically unaware when music, including their own singing, is off-key. For example, they have difficulty detecting out-of-key notes in novel melodies, a task that most individuals (even those with no musical training) find quite easy (Ayotte et al., 2002). They also have difficulty discriminating and recognizing melodies without lyrics, even melodies that are quite common in their culture.

It is important to distinguish true mTD from the "tone deafness" label that people sometimes apply to themselves. In survey studies, about 15% of people self-define as tone deaf (Cuddy et al., 2005). Research reveals that many such people are in fact referring to their poor singing skills, even if they have a keen ear for music and show no music perception deficits (Sloboda et al., 2005). Lack of singing ability in such individuals may simply reflect a lack of training, which could presumably be ameliorated by guided practice. It is also important to distinguish mTD (which appears to have its roots in pitch perception deficits, as discussed below) from a less commonly reported disorder in which musical sounds lose their normal timbral qualities, being heard, for example, as "the banging of pots and pans" (cf. Sacks, 2007, for descriptions of such cases).

An important fact about mTD is that it is not due to lack of exposure to music, as many mTDIs report having music lessons in childhood and/or coming from musical households (Peretz & Hyde, 2003). Furthermore, research on twins suggests that there are specific genes that put one at risk for this condition (Drayna et al., 2001). Thus it makes sense that most mTDIs report having their condition for as long as they can remember. Indeed, one oft-heard story is that an mTDI first discovered his or her problem in childhood, when a choir teacher in school asked them to stop singing and simply move their lips to the music. Until that time, he or she was unaware of any musical problem.

Although the existence of mTD has been noted for over a hundred years (Allen, 1878), systematic research on this phenomenon is a relatively recent endeavor (e.g., Peretz et al., 2002; Ayotte et al., 2002; Peretz & Hyde, 2003; Foxton et al., 2004). Research in this area is poised to grow rapidly, because mTDIs are estimated to comprise about 4% of the population (Kalmus & Fry, 1980) and are thus easier to locate and work with than acquired amusics.

For the current purposes, the significance of mTD is that it manifests as a highly selective deficit for music, with no readily apparent consequences for other cognitive abilities (though see Douglas and Bilkey, 2007). Indeed, mTDIs may excel in other domains: Their ranks include numerous famous individuals, including the Nobel-prize–winning economist Milton Friedman. This makes mTD particularly attractive for the comparative study of speech and music perception. Returning to the topic at hand, what is known about musical versus spoken melodic contour perception in mTD?

In one relevant study, Ayotte et al. (2002) tested mTDIs for their ability to discriminate between sentences that differed only in intonation, and to discriminate between nonlinguistic tone sequences created from the intonation patterns of the sentences. (The tone sequences were created using the methods of Patel, Peretz, et al., 1998, described in the previous section.) In contrast to the earlier findings of Patel, Peretz, et al., which had focused on acquired amusia, Ayotte et al. found a dramatic dissociation between performance on the sentences and their nonlinguistic analogs. Specifically, mTDIs had no difficulty discriminating between sentences differing in intonation, but had substantial difficulty discriminating between the corresponding tone sequences. Controls, in contrast, performed equally well in both domains. This suggests a dissociation between melodic contour processing in speech and music, with normal speech intonation processing but impaired musical melodic contour processing.

How can the dissociation reported by Ayotte et al. (2002) be explained? Psychophysical research with mTDIs has revealed that they have deficits in detecting fine-grained pitch changes. For example Hyde and Peretz (2004) had mTDIs listen to sequences of 5 high-pitched piano tones (C6, which has a fundamental frequency of 1046 Hz), the fourth of which could differ in pitch from the others. The listeners had to indicate if the sequence contained a pitch change or not. To reach a criterion of 75% correct, mTDIs needed a pitch change of

1/2 semitone. Controls, in contrast, were nearly 100% correct for the small-est pitch change used: 1/4 semitone. Furthermore, mTDIs did not perform as well as controls until the pitch change was 2 semitones. Based on such find-ings, Peretz and Hyde (2003) suggested that pitch contrasts in the sentences used by Ayotte et al. (2002) were coarser than in the tone sequences, and were thus large enough to overcome the mTDIs' deficits in pitch change detection. This was a reasonable suggestion, as the process of converting F0 contours to tones used by Patel, Peretz, et al. (1998) involved converting the dynami-cally changing pitch within each syllable to a single pitch near the mean F0 of the syllable, thus compressing the overall amount of pitch variation in a sentence. Peretz and Hyde's suggestion also led to a testable prediction: namely, if the nonlinguistic tone sequences followed the original F0 contours exactly, then tone-deaf individuals should be able to discriminate them without diffi-culty. Patel, Foxton, and Griffiths (2005) tested this idea, using a population of mTDIs from the United Kingdom. The stimuli were based on an English version of the prosody-music battery, and concentrated on focus-shift pairs in language and their nonlinguistic tone analogs.

Patel, Foxton, and Griffiths (2005) made two types of nonlinguistic analogs from the focus-shift pairs. The first type was the same as used previously, in other words, each syllable was replaced by a tone of fixed pitch set to the Hz value midway between the maximum and minimum F0 values within that syl-lable. These were referred to as the "discrete pitch" analogs. In the other (new) type of analog, each tone's pitch exactly followed the F0 contour within the syl-lable, gliding up and/or down just as the F0 did: These were referred to as the "gliding pitch" analogs. In both types of sequences, tone onsets occurred at the vowel onset times of corresponding syllables, and tone offsets were determined by the offset of F0 within each syllable. Thus each tone sequence had the same temporal rhythm as the syllables in the parent sentence. All tones had a funda-mental and several harmonics, giving the analogs a clarinet-like quality (Sound Examples 4.10a–f). The three types of stimuli (speech, discrete pitch analogs, and gliding pitch analogs) were presented in separate blocks, and scoring of performance was based on percentage of hits minus percentage of false alarms, in accordance with the procedure of Ayotte et al. (2002).[18] Figure 4.18 shows results on the three tasks.

Consistent with the findings of Ayotte et al. (2002), tone-deaf individuals were significantly better at discriminating sentences based on intonation than they were at discriminating discrete-pitch analogs of the intonation contours (cf. Ayotte et al., 2002, Figure 3). Surprisingly, however, tone-deaf individuals also had difficulty discriminating gliding-pitch analogs that exactly mimicked

---

[18] A hit was defined as a *different* configuration pair that was classified as different, whereas a false alarm was defined as a *same* configuration pair classified as different.

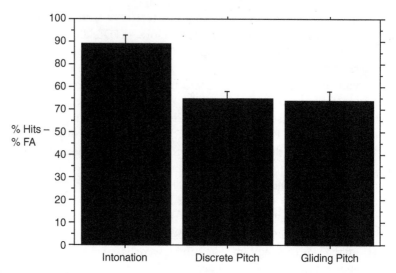

Figure 4.18 Performance of musically tone-deaf individuals on discrimination of three types of pitch patterns: intonation contours in speech, nonlinguistic analogs of intonation contours based on discrete pitches, and nonlinguistic analogs of intonation contours based on gliding pitch movements that exactly replicate the pitch pattern of intonation. The vertical axis shows percentage of hits minus percentage of false alarms. Error bars show 1 standard error. From Patel, Foxton, & Griffiths, 2005.

the intonation patterns of the sentences. In fact, performance on the discrete and gliding pitch analogs was indistinguishable, and performance on the gliding pitch analogs was significantly worse than on the sentences.

These findings are particularly striking in light of certain psychophysical findings by Foxton et al. (2004) with these same mTDIs. Foxton et al. examined thresholds for detecting a pitch change between two successively presented pure tones. In one condition ("segmented pitch-change detection"), the tones were separated by a short silent interval. In another condition ("gliding pitch-change detection"), this interval was filled by a linear frequency ramp that bridged the pitch difference between the tones. For the mTDIs in the study of Patel, Foxton, and Griffiths (2005), the threshold for pitch-change detection was significantly smaller when pitches were connected by an intervening glide than when they were separated by a silent interval (threshold = 0.21 st for gliding pitch change, versus 0.56 st for segmented pitch change, based on 75% correct discrimination).

Thus not only do mTDIs have difficulty discriminating gliding-pitch analogs of intonation, they have these difficulties *despite* the fact that they have substantially smaller thresholds for detecting pitch changes in gliding-pitch patterns than in segmented pitch patterns. It therefore appears that the relatively normal intonation perception of mTDIs cannot be explained by the idea that intonation uses coarse pitch contrasts that exceed their psychophysical thresholds for pitch-change detection.

Clearly, a hypothesis is needed that can account for the normal performance of mTDIs in discriminating spoken intonation contours versus their impaired performance in discriminating the same contours extracted from a phonetic context. In the following section, I propose one such hypothesis, based on the idea that melodic contour perception in speech and music does in fact rely on common neural circuitry.

The Melodic Contour Deafness Hypothesis

Prima facie, the finding of Patel, Foxton, and Griffiths (2005) seems to be good evidence for the modularity of contour processing (Peretz & Coltheart, 2003) because pitch contours in speech are discriminated better than the same contours extracted from speech. There is another possibility, however, as explored in this section. I call this the "melodic contour deafness hypothesis." This hypothesis proposes that mTDIs have equivalent problems in judging the *direction* of pitch change in speech and music, but that intonation perception is largely robust to this problem, whereas music perception is not. Before discussing how this hypothesis can account for the dissociations observed in the study of Patel, Foxton, and Griffiths (2005), it is worth delving into the findings that motivated the development of this hypothesis.

One such finding was the discovery that some mTDIs do in fact have problems with intonation perception in language. Specifically, Lochy et al. (2004; cf. Patel, Wong, et al., in press) tested a group of mTDIs using the sentence stimuli of Patel, Peretz, et al., (1998), and found that some had deficits in same/different discrimination of linguistic statement-question pairs. That is, when asked to tell whether two sentences were acoustically identical or not, they had difficulty when one sentence was a question and the other was a statement, a task that control participants found easy. In contrast, they did well when the two sentences were members of a focus-shift pair, in which emphasis (as signaled by pitch movement) was on a different word in each sentence (cf. two subsections back for examples of a statement-question and a focus-shift pair). The critical difference between these tasks is that the statement-question task requires discriminating the *direction* of pitch movement on the same word (up versus down), whereas the focus-shift task simply requires detecting a salient pitch movement within a sentence, because different words bear the large movement in the two members of a focus-shift pair. That is, sensitivity to the direction of pitch movement is irrelevant to the focus-shift task: As long as one can detect a pitch change, and can remember that this change happened on the same or different words in the two sentences, one can solve the task.

Another finding that motivated the melodic contour deafness hypothesis was the discovery that mTDIs have marked deficits in nonlinguistic tasks that require the perception of pitch direction. Figure 4.19 shows thresholds for 75% correct performance on three types of tasks: segmented pitch-change detection, gliding pitch-change detection, and pitch-direction judgments (Foxton et al., 2004).[19]

The first two tasks are simple pitch-change detection tasks, and were described in the previous section. The third task involves judging pitch direction: Listeners hear two pairs of pure tones and decide in which pair the pitch goes up. (Pitch always goes down in one pair and up in the other. In both pairs, tones are connected by a glide.) Note the dramatic difference between mTDIs and controls on this latter task: Their thresholds are about 20 times higher than those of controls, compared to thresholds that are 2 or 3 times worse than controls in terms of pitch-change detection.

The data of Lochy et al. (2004) and Foxton et al. (2004) suggest that mTDIs have problems with pitch-direction perception in both speech and nonlinguistic sounds. If the melodic contour deafness hypothesis is correct, then a common processing deficit for pitch direction underlies these deficits, but speech intonation perception is largely robust to this deficit, whereas music perception is not.

Why would intonation perception be robust to the deficit? One reason is that in intonation languages such as English (in which pitch does not distinguish lexical items, as it does in tone languages), the direction of a pitch change is seldom crucial to understanding. For example, if a pitch movement is used to signal focus on a word, it may matter little to a listener if the movement is upward or downward, as long as it is salient and detectable. Although the direction of pitch movement *is* important for distinguishing statements from questions, there are often redundant syntactic, semantic, or contextual cues to indicate whether an utterance is a question or not. Hence a pitch direction deficit in speech may be largely asymptomatic, revealing itself only in controlled situations in which pitch direction is crucial to the task and redundant sources of information are suppressed. A second reason that intonation perception may be robust to a pitch-direction deficit is that such a deficit is not all-or-none, but a matter of degree. Recall from Figure 4.19 that the direction deficit is defined by an elevated *threshold* for accurate detection of pitch direction. In the study of Foxton et al. (2004), mTDIs succeeded on the pitch-direction task when pitch movements were significantly above their threshold.

Hence the key question is how the size of *linguistically relevant* pitch movements in speech compares to the pitch direction thresholds of mTDIs. Consulting Figure 4.19, it can be seen that the average pitch-direction threshold for mTDIs is a little above 2 semitones. How does this compare to the size of rising or falling pitch accents in English (e.g., L+H* movements in autosegmental-metrical theory)? Existing research on intonation suggests that 2 semitones is

---

[19] Data presented in Figures 4.19 and 4.20 were kindly provided by Jessica Foxton. The data come from the same set of participants doing different perceptual tasks. Two outliers have been excluded from the analysis (one amusic and one control).

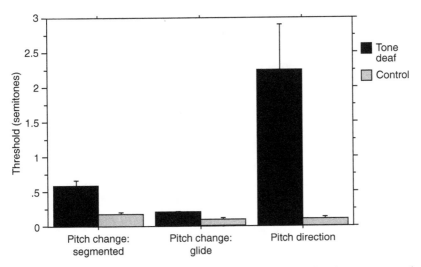

Figure 4.19 Performance of tone-deaf individuals on three kinds of pitch perception tasks: segmented pitch-change detection, gliding pitch-change detection, and pitch-direction detection. Error bars show 1 standard error. Data from the study by Foxton et al. (2004).

near the low end of the spectrum for rising or falling pitch accents in speech (e.g., Xu & Xu, 2005; Arvaniti & Garding, in press). In other words, most linguistically relevant pitch movements are likely to be in excess of the pitch-direction thresholds of mTDIs.[20] However, circumstances may arise in which an individual with a large threshold hears a linguistically relevant pitch movement below their threshold, and cannot determine its direction. Such a circumstance may explain the cases found by Lochy et al. (2004), who could not discriminate questions from statements.

Turning to music, why would music perception be so severely affected by a pitch direction deficit? As noted earlier in this chapter (section 4.5.1), musical melodies are dominated by small pitch intervals of 2 semitones or less in size. Note that this is below the average pitch-direction threshold of mTDIs. This suggests that mTDIs often cannot tell if a musical melody is going up or down in pitch. This degraded perception of musical melodic contour would make it very difficult to gauge crucial aspects of melodic structure such as motivic similarity and contrast. Furthermore, without an accurate mental representation

---

[20] Interestingly, in Mandarin, the rising and falling lexical tones appear to have a lower limit of about 2 semitones in connected speech (Xu, 1994, 1999), suggesting that these tones will exceed the pitch direction thresholds of most mTDIs. If this lower limit is representative for tone languages generally, it would suggest that mTD should have little consequence for speech perception in such languages under ordinary circumstances.

of melodic contour, there would be no developmental framework for learning musical intervals (Dowling, 1978). Hence mTDIs would never acquire the normal tonal schemata for music perception, which might explain why they fail to detect off-key ("sour") notes in music.

How can the melodic contour deafness hypothesis account for the dissociations observed in the study of Patel, Foxton, and Griffiths (2005)? Consider the focus-shift questions used in the speech intonation task. In such sentences, the salient pitch movement is on a different word (as noted earlier in this section). Thus, a same/different task with such sentences can be solved with a "semantic recoding strategy," in other words, by simply listening for a word with a salient pitch movement in each sentence, and then deciding if these words are the same or different. If the intonation contours are separated from their lexical context, however, as in the discrete-pitch and gliding-pitch analogs of intonation, then this strategy is no longer possible and success depends on remembering the patterns of ups and downs of pitch over time. Hence a problem in perceiving pitch direction could disrupt this task.

An important question about the melodic contour deafness hypothesis concerns its proposed neural foundation. In this regard, it is interesting to examine the relationship between mTDIs problems with pitch direction and their problems with simple pitch-change detection. Figure 4.20 shows thresholds for pitch-change detection versus pitch-direction detection for 12 mTDIs. As can be seen, the pitch-change detection thresholds do not predict pitch-direction thresholds.

This suggests an independent pitch-direction deficit. There are reasons to believe that such a deficit could arise from abnormalities in right auditory cortex. Research on patients with surgical excisions of temporal lobe regions has revealed that individuals with excisions of right secondary auditory cortex (lateral Heschl's gyrus) have pronounced deficits in judging pitch direction, even though their thresholds for simple pitch-change detection are normal. In contrast, patients with comparable excisions of left auditory cortex show no such direction deficits (Johnsrude et al., 2000). Evidence supporting a link between pitch-direction detection and melodic contour perception is the fact that both are disrupted by lesions to right auditory cortex (Johnsrude et al., 2000; Liégeois-Chauvel et al., 1998).

Neurophysiological research on animals also supports a right-hemisphere basis for coding of pitch direction (Wetzel et al., 1998), and suggests that direction sensitivity may arise from patterns of lateral inhibition among cortical neurons (Shamma et al., 1993; Ohl et al., 2000; cf. Rauschecker et al., 1998a, 1998b). Indeed, asymmetric lateral inhibition has been successfully used to give cells pitch-direction sensitivity in computational models of auditory cortex (e.g., Husain et al., 2004). In these models, direction sensitivity emerges from specific anatomical patterns of inhibitory connections between neighboring cells in tonotopic maps.

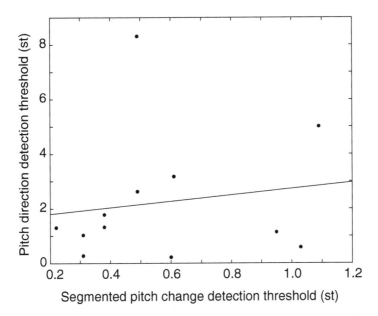

Figure 4.20 The relationship between performance on the segmented pitch-change detection task and the pitch-direction detection task for 12 musically tone-deaf individuals.
The best fitting regression line is shown. The severity of the pitch-direction deficit is not
predicted by the severity of the pitch-change detection deficit. Equation for regression
line: Direction threshold = 1.16 * change threshold + 1.57 (r^2 = 0.02, p = .65).

Thus one plausible hypothesis for the etiology of the pitch-direction deficits
in mTDIs is abnormal wiring of inhibitory connections in tonotopic maps of
right secondary auditory cortex. This miswiring may occur early in development due to genetic factors (Drayna et al., 2001). Such miswiring may not
be detectable using macro-imaging methods such as MRI, and may require
cellular-level investigations (e.g., postmortem histology) or electrophysiological techniques (cf. Peretz et al., 2005). Interestingly, in-vivo structural brain
imaging has revealed that mTDIs have a neural anomaly in the right cerebral
hemisphere (Hyde et al., 2006). However, the anomaly is in a region of right
inferior frontal cortex, which is thought to be involved in short-term memory
for pitch patterns. The anomaly consists of a decrease in white matter tissue
(i.e., the fibers that connect nerve cells rather than nerve cell bodies themselves).
At the moment, it is not known whether the anomaly is inborn or if it arises
in development due to anomalous connections between right frontal regions
and auditory cortex, particularly because both gray and white matter patterns
in the frontal cortices develop well into adolescence (Toga et al., 2006). For
example, a problem in perceiving melodic contour (arising in auditory cortex)
may lead to the underdevelopment of normal musical memory skills, because it

would disrupt recognition of motivic similarity across time, a very basic aspect of melody perception that depends on short-term memory for pitch patterns (cf. section 4.2.5). A pitch-memory deficit might explain why mTDIs have deficits in discriminating the melodic contour of two short melodies even when the steps between pitches are large, and hence presumably above their pitch-change detection and pitch-direction detection thresholds (Foxton et al., 2004).

Taking a step back, the significance of the melodic contour deafness hypothesis is that it suggests that a behavioral dissociation between music and speech perception in everyday life may disguise a neural commonality in the processing of spoken and musical melodies. In other words, a behavioral dissociation is not necessarily the same as a neural dissociation: A nondomain-specific deficit can give rise to domain-specific problems because of the different demands that each domain places on the ability in question.

4.6 Conclusion

The linguist Dwight Bolinger once commented that "since intonation is synonymous with speech melody, and melody is a term borrowed from music, it is natural to wonder what connection there may be between music and intonation" (Bolinger, 1985:28). Although this connection has interested scholars for hundreds of years, empirical comparisons of musical and spoken melody are a recent endeavor. This chapter has shown that despite important differences between the melodic systems of the two domains (such as the use of pitch interval categories, a regular beat, and a tonal center in musical melodies), there are numerous points of contact between musical and linguistic melody in terms of structure and processing. For example, the statistics of pitch patterning in a composer's native language can be reflected in his or her instrumental music. Furthermore, neuropsychological research indicates that melodic contours in speech and music may be processed in an overlapping way in the brain. These and other findings suggest that musical and spoken melody are in fact more closely related than has generally been believed, and invite further research aimed at refining our understanding of the relations between these two types of melody.

Appendix

This is an appendix for section 4.1.2.

To convert a value in Hz to the semitone scale (st) on the y-axis of the prosogram:

$$st = 12 * \log_2(X), \text{ where } X \text{ is the value in Hz.}$$

To convert a st value along the y-axis of a prosogram to Hz:

$$Hz = 2^{(X/12)}, \text{ where } X \text{ is the value in st.}$$

Syntax

5

Syntax

5.1 Introduction

The comparison of linguistic and musical syntax is a topic that has generated both warm enthusiasm and cool skepticism. The former reaction is illustrated by a set of lectures given by Leonard Bernstein at Harvard in 1973, later published as *The Unanswered Question* (1976). Bernstein, who had long been interested in the analysis of musical structure and meaning (Bernstein, 1959), found inspiration in the generative linguistic theory of Noam Chomsky (1972) and set out to analyze the grammar of Western tonal music in a linguistic framework. As part of his presentation, Bernstein made comparisons between linguistic and musical syntax. Although his musical knowledge and personal charisma make his lectures well worth watching, the details of his exposition were not persuasive to scholars in either linguistics or music. Keiler (1978) has enumerated several of the problems with Bernstein's approach, which include rather strained analogies between linguistic parts of speech such as nouns and verbs and particular musical elements such as motives and rhythms.

Nevertheless, Bernstein's efforts had an important effect on language-music studies. As a result of his lectures, a seminar on music and linguistics was organized at MIT in the fall of 1974, and two of the participants (the musicologist Fred Lerdahl and the linguist Ray Jackendoff) ultimately produced one of the most influential books in music cognition, *A Generative Theory of Tonal Music* (1983). The use of the term "generative" in their title refers to the use of formal procedures to generate a structural description of a given musical piece. This description focuses on four types of structural relations a listener perceives when hearing music. Two of these relations concern rhythm: grouping structure and metrical structure (cf. Chapter 3). The other two relations are more abstract, and concern hierarchies in the relative structural importance of tones ("time-span reduction") and in the patterning of tension and relaxation over time ("prolongation reduction"). Although Lerdahl and Jackendoff adapted the tools of generative grammar to analyze music (cf. Sundberg & Lindblom, 1976), they did not focus on comparisons of linguistic and musical syntax.

Indeed, they were skeptical of such comparisons, noting that "pointing out superficial analogies between music and language, with or without the help of generative grammar, is an old and largely futile game" (p. 5). In support of their skepticism, they point out specific differences between the two syntactic systems, including the lack of musical equivalents for linguistic parts of speech such as nouns and verbs, and differences in the way linguistic and musical "syntactic trees" are constructed (cf. section 5.3.1 below).

Despite Lerdahl and Jackendoff's skepticism, comparisons between linguistic and musical syntax have continued to fascinate scholars. Theoretical treatments of the issue include work by musicologists and linguists (e.g., Swain, 1997; Horton, 2001; Tojo et al., 2006; Pesetsky, 2007; Rohrmeier, 2007). It is fair to say, however, that for each theorist who approaches the topic with enthusiasm, there is another who sounds a note of warning (e.g., Powers, 1980; Feld, 1974). A particularly fascinating example of this dialectic concerns two articles on Javanese gamelan music by leading ethnomusicological scholars (Becker & Becker, 1979, 1983), the first enthusiastically analyzing the grammar of this music in a linguistic framework and the second (by the same authors a few years later) rejecting this original approach as an exercise in empty formalisms yielding little new insight.

Theoretical comparisons between linguistic and musical syntax will no doubt continue for many years to come, with voices on both sides of the issue. In the past few years, however, something new has happened: Empirical studies of this topic have started to emerge in cognitive neuroscience. The appeal of this topic for modern brain science is easy to understand. Linguistic syntax is emblematic of the special abilities of the human mind and has been claimed to engage "domain-specific" cognitive mechanisms (i.e., mechanisms unique to language; see Fodor, 1983). The presence of a second syntactic system in the human mind naturally leads to the question of the relation between them. Are they mentally isolated, modular systems, or might there be cognitive and neural overlap?

This chapter is divided into three parts. The first provides background on musical syntax. The second part discusses formal differences and similarities between musical and linguistic syntax. The final part discusses what neuroscience has revealed about musical-linguistic syntactic relations in the brain. As we shall see, there is evidence for significant neural overlap in syntactic processing in the two domains. Furthermore, exploring the nature of this overlap provides a novel way to explore the cognitive and neural foundations of human syntactic abilities.

Before embarking, it is worth addressing the question, what is "musical syntax?" because this term may mean different things to different scholars. In this chapter, syntax in music (just as in language) refers to the principles governing the combination of discrete structural elements into sequences. The vast majority of the world's music is syntactic, meaning that one can identify both perceptually discrete elements (such as tones with distinct pitches or drum sounds with distinct timbres) and norms for the combination of these elements into sequences. These norms are not "rules" that musicians must obey. On the contrary, composers and performers can and do purposely contravene these norms for artistic purposes. However, such departures are meaningful precisely because there *are* norms against which they operate. The cognitive significance of the norms is that they become internalized by listeners, who develop expectations that influence how they hear music. Thus the study of syntax deals not only with structural principles but also with the resulting implicit knowledge a listener uses to organize musical sounds into coherent patterns.

As with language, the syntax of music varies across cultures and historical eras. Unlike language, however, in which a number of important syntactic features are shared by all human languages (Van Valin, 2001), syntactic universals in music appear to be limited to a few very general features such as the organization of pitch in terms of musical scales with (typically) 5 to 7 tones per octave (cf. Chapter 2). Such universals hardly provide a basis for a detailed comparison of linguistic and musical syntax.[1] This lack of syntactic unity in human music should not be surprising. Unlike language, music is not constrained to transmit a certain kind of information, so that the range of sonic structures considered "music" by at least some people reflects the vast and ever-growing diversity of human aesthetic creativity and interest.

Meaningful comparison of linguistic and musical syntax thus requires focus on the music of a particular period and style. I have chosen to focus on Western European tonal music (or "tonal music" for short), a music that flourished between about 1650 and 1900 and whose syntactic conventions have been influential since that time. (In this chapter, the term "tonality" is sometimes used as a shorthand term for these conventions.) For example, most of the music heard in Europe and the Americas today is tonal music. Another reason to focus on this tradition is that of all known musical systems, it is the most extensively studied from both a theoretical and an empirical perspective (e.g., Krumhansl, 1990; Lerdahl, 2001).

5.2 The Structural Richness of Musical Syntax

Does musical syntax really merit comparison with linguistic syntax? The simple fact that a nonlinguistic system is syntactic does not guarantee an interesting comparison with language. For example, the songs of the swamp sparrow

---

[1] I am dealing here with "substantive universals" of musical syntax: structural patterns that appear in most if not all widespread musical cultures. A different approach to the notion of musical universals is to consider the cognitive universals underlying music processing (cf. Lerdahl & Jackendoff, 1983; Jackendoff, 2002:75).

Melospiza georgiana are made up of a few acoustically discrete elements ("notes"), and different geographic populations order these notes in different ways to form larger chunks ("syllables") that are repeated in time to create a song (Figure 5.1).

Elegant experiments have shown that these syntactic differences are learned and are meaningful to the birds. Indeed, they serve as the basis of geographic song "dialects" that the birds use in identifying potential competitors or mates (Balaban, 1988; cf. Thompson & Bakery, 1993). Yet such a system can hardly sustain a meaningful comparison with linguistic syntax. Linguistic syntax is remarkable for its structural richness, attaining a level of complexity that sets it apart from any known nonhuman communication system.

One aspect of this richness is multilayered organization. There are principles for the formation of words from meaningful subunits, or "morphemes" (such as the use of the suffix "-ed" in English to form the regular past tense), for the formation of phrases from words (such as noun phrases and prepositional phrases), and for the formation of sentences from phrases. Furthermore, sentence formation includes principles of recursive structure (such as embedding

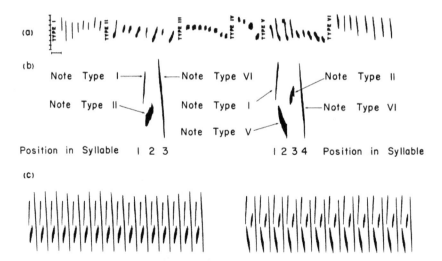

Figure 5.1 Swamp sparrow song organization. (a) Examples of the six categories of minimal acoustic elements (notes) that make up swamp sparrow songs. Scale at the left represents frequency (1–8KHz); time scale bar on the bottom is 100 ms. (b) From two to six (most commonly three or four) notes are put together to form syllables. Two syllables from two different New York songs are shown. Birds in a given geographic location have preferences for placing certain notes in certain positions in a syllable; this constitutes the syntax of a song. (c) Swamp sparrow syllables are repeated to form a ~2-sec song. The two songs depicted here consist of repetitions of the two syllables detailed in (b). From Balaban, 1988.

one noun phrase within another) that appear to set human language apart from nonhuman animal communication systems (Hauser et al., 2002; though see Gentner et al., 2006).

Another aspect of the structural richness of linguistic syntax is the strong relationship between syntax and meaning, so that changes in the order of words (and/or the identity of grammatical morphemes) can greatly alter the meaning of an utterance. For example, "The man with the thin cane saw the girl" means something quite different from "The thin girl with the cane saw the man." Peter Marler (2000) has pointed out that this aspect of human syntax sets it apart from other vertebrate syntactic systems such as bird song and whale song, in which the meaning of the sequence is not intricately related to the order in which the elements occur. Instead, current evidence suggests that these nonhuman vocal displays always mean the same thing: territorial warning and sexual advertisement. In these simple syntactic systems, the order of the elements simply identifies the caller as a member of a particular species or group.

A third and very important aspect of the richness of linguistic syntax is the fact that words can take on abstract grammatical functions (such as subject, direct object, and indirect object) that are determined by their context and structural relations rather than by inherent properties of the words themselves (Jackendoff, 2002). For example, there is nothing about the word "cat" that makes it a subject, object, or indirect object, yet in a sentence context it can take on one of these functions, and as a consequence trigger syntactic phenomena at other locations such as subject-verb agreement for number.

The next four sections discuss the syntax of tonal music, illustrating that musical structure has many of the key features that make linguistic syntax so rich.

5.2.1 Multiple Levels of Organization

Like language, tonal music has syntactic principles at multiple levels. The following sections focus on three levels of pitch organization. As background, recall from Chapter 2 that the basic pitch materials of tonal music are drawn in an orderly way from the continuum of physical frequencies. Specifically, each octave (doubling in frequency) contains 12 tones such that the frequency ratio between each tone and the tone below it is constant. This basic ratio, called the semitone, is about 6%, equal to the pitch distance between an adjacent black and white key on a piano. Also recall from Chapter 2 that tonal music exhibits octave equivalence, whereby pitches whose fundamental frequencies are related by a 2/1 ratio are perceived as highly similar in pitch and are thus given the same letter name or *pitch class* irrespective of the octave in which they occur. These 12 pitch classes are given letter names: A, A♯, B, C, C♯, D, D♯, E, F, F♯, G, G♯, in which ♯ = "sharp" (or equivalently, A, B♭, B, C, D♭, D, E♭, E, F, G♭, G, A♭ in which ♭ = "flat"). The octave in which a note occurs is indicated by a number after its pitch class name, for example, 220 Hz corresponds to A3, whereas 440 Hz is A4.

Scale Structure

The most basic level of syntactic organization of pitch concerns musical scales (cf. Chapter 2, section 2.2.2 for background on musical scales). In tonal music the pitches played at any given moment are not uniformly distributed across the 12 possible pitch classes per octave but are instead constrained by a musical scale, a subset of 7 tones (or "scale degrees") per octave with an asymmetric pattern of pitch spacing ("intervals") between them. One such scale (the C major scale) is shown in Figure 5.2.

As noted in Chapter 4 (section 4.2.6, which should be read as background for this section), in a musical context, the different scale tones take on different roles in the fabric of the music, with one tone being the structurally most central and stable (the "tonic"). The use of one pitch as a tonal center is not restricted to Western European tonal music, but appears repeatedly in diverse musical traditions. This suggests that the organization of pitch around a tonic may be congenial to the human mind, perhaps reflecting the utility of psychological reference points in organizing mental categories[2] (Rosch, 1975; Krumhansl, 1979; cf. Justus & Hutsler, 2005).

An interesting aspect of scale structure in tonal music is that listeners' intuitions of the stability of scale degrees is not simply binary, with the tonic being stable and all other tones being equally less stable. Instead, empirical evidence suggests that there is a hierarchy of stability. An important aspect of this hierarchy is the contrast in stability between the tonic and its neighboring scale tones (scale degrees 2 and 7), which creates a psychological pull toward the tonal center. This is reflected in the music-theoretic names for the 2nd and 7th scale degrees: The second is called the "supertonic" (i.e., the tone just above the tonic), and the seventh is known as the "leading tone" (i.e., the tone that leads to the tonic). In an early set of studies, Robert Francès (1988) provided evidence for the "pull to the tonic" by demonstrating that listeners were less sensitive to upward mistunings of the leading tone when it was in an ascending melodic context, in other words, when the mistuning brought it closer to the tonic.

Another approach to the mental representation of scale structure concerns the perceived relatedness (or mental distance) between different tones in a scale. Krumhansl (1979) explored this issue using a paradigm in which listeners first

---

[2] By including the notion of a tonal hierarchy in the concept of "scale," I am using the term "scale" to include what Dowling (1978) has called "mode" in his discussion of scale structure in music.

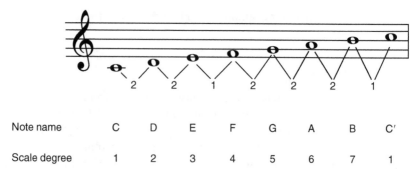

Figure 5.2 The C-major musical scale. The small numerals between the notes on the musical staff indicate the size of pitch intervals in semitones. (2 st = a major second, 1 st = a minor second.) The interval pattern [2 2 1 2 2 2 1] defines a major scale. C′ is the pitch one octave above C. Modified from Cuddy et al., 1981.

heard a tonal context (e.g., an ascending or descending C major scale) and then heard two comparison tones from the scale. The task was to judge how closely related the first tone was to the second tone in the tonal system suggested by the context. The results of this task were analyzed using multidimensional scaling. This technique translates judgments of relatedness into a spatial display so that the closer the perceived relatedness, the closer the elements are in the resulting graph. The three-dimensional solution for the similarity ratings is shown in Figure 5.3.

As can be seen, scale degrees 1, 3, and 5 of the C major scale (C, E, and G) are perceived as closely related, whereas the remaining scale tones are less closely related, and nonscale tones are distantly related. One very notable feature of this figure is the large distance that separates tones that are adjacent in frequency, such as C and C♯. This contrast between the physical and psychological proximity of pitches is likely to be part of what animates tonal music.

Listeners appear to be quite sensitive to scale structure in tonal music, as evidenced by the familiar phenomenon of the "sour note," as discussed in Chapter 4, section 4.2.6. At what age does this sensitivity emerge? Trainor and Trehub (1992) examined 8-month-old infants' and nonmusician adults' ability to detect two types of changes in a repeating 10-note melody. (The melody was transposed on each repetition, so the task involved discerning a change in pitch *relationships* rather than simply detecting an absolute pitch change.) In both cases, one note in the middle of the melody was changed: In one case, it was raised by four semitones, but remained within the scale of the melody; in another case, it was raised by just one semitone, but now departed from the scale of the melody. Thus the two changes cleverly pitted physical distance against scale membership. Infants detected both kinds of changes equally well.

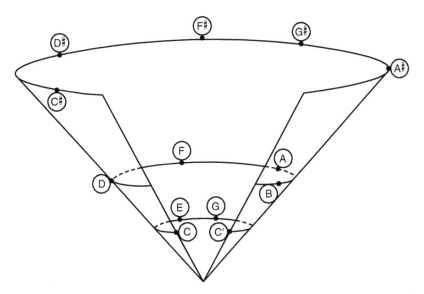

Figure 5.3 Geometrical representation of perceived similarity between musical pitches in a tonal context. The data are oriented toward the C major scale, in which C serves as the tonic. C' is the pitch one octave above C. From Krumhansl, 1979.

Adults performed better than infants overall, but crucially, they detected the change that violated scale structure significantly better than the within-scale change, even though the former change was a smaller physical change than the latter. This reflects the fact that for the adults the nonscale tone "popped out" as a sour note. These results show that the infants had not yet developed an implicit knowledge of scale structure, as one might expect. It is interesting to note that infants *have* already started acquiring learned sound categories for language at 10 months (e.g., the vowels of their native language; Kuhl et al., 1992), which may reflect the greater amount of linguistic versus musical input that infants have experienced by that age.

What is the earliest age that sensitivity to scale membership can be demonstrated? In a follow-up study using a very similar paradigm, Trainor and Trehub (1994) showed that 5-year-old children with no formal training in music detected out-of-scale melodic alterations better than within-scale alterations, even though the former changes were physically smaller than the latter.[3] This naturally raises the question of the ontogeny of scale-membership sensitivity

[3] It should be noted that in this study, melodies were not presented in transposition, because in the same-different task the children tended to respond "different" to transpositional changes.

between 10 months and 5 years. Because behavioral tests with young children can be difficult, it may be preferable to use event-related brain potentials (ERPs) in such studies. ERPs do not require a behavioral response from the listener, and distinct ERP responses to out-of-scale notes have been observed in adults (e.g., Besson & Faïta, 1995).

Chord Structure

A very important aspect of tonal music's syntax is the simultaneous combination of scale tones into chords, creating harmony. Chords are formed in principled ways: basic "triads" are built from scale degrees separated by musical thirds, in other words, by a distance of two scale steps. Because of the asymmetric interval structure of Western scales, a distance of two scale steps can correspond to a distance of either three or four semitones, in other words, to a minor or major third. For example, in the C major scale (cf. Figure 5.2), the chord C-E-G consists of a major third between C and E and a minor third between E and G, whereas D-F-A consists of a minor third between D and F and a major third between F and A. These two chords represent "major" and "minor" triads, respectively. As shown in Figure 5.4, building triads from a major scale results in three major triads (built on scale degrees, 1, 4, and 5), three minor triads (built on scale degrees 2, 3, and 6), and one "diminished" triad in which both intervals are minor thirds (built on scale degree 7).

In chordal syntax, one tone of each chord acts as its "root" or structurally most significant pitch. This is the lowest note in each triad in Figure 5.4, and is the note that gives the chord its name as well as its Roman numeral harmonic label. For example, in Figure 5.4, the chord with a root of E (the

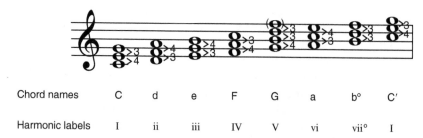

Chord names	C	d	e	F	G	a	b°	C′
Harmonic labels	I	ii	iii	IV	V	vi	vii°	I

Figure 5.4 Basic triadic chords of the C-major musical scale. Small numbers between the notes of a given chord indicate the interval in semitones between notes. Major, minor, and diminished chords are indicated in the "chord names" and "harmonic labels" lines by fonts: uppercase = major, lower case = minor, lower case with "°" superscript = diminished. The musical note in parentheses at the top of the V chord, if included in the chord, creates a seventh chord (V7, or G7 in this case). Modified from Cuddy et al., 1981.

3rd scale degree) is an E-minor chord (E-G-B), with a harmonic label of "iii." (The use of a lower case roman numeral indicates that this chord is a minor chord.) Similarly, in Figure 5.4, the chord with a root of G (the 5th scale degree) is a G major chord (G-B-D), with a harmonic label of V. (The use of an upper case roman numeral indicates that this chord is a major chord.) Even when the notes of a triad occur in a different vertical ordering, the root and harmonic label remain the same, and the chord is treated as having the same basic harmonic status. Thus C-E-G and G-E-C both have C as the root and harmonically labeled as "I"; the latter is simply considered an "inversion" of the C-E-G chord.

Chord syntax also includes principles for modifying triads with additional tones. For example, one very common modification is to add a fourth tone to a triad to convert it to a "seventh" chord, so called because the added tone is seven scale steps above the root of the chord. For example, in a C major scale, the chord G-B-D-F would be a seventh chord built on the root G, or G7 (cf. Figure 5.4), and its harmonic label would be V7. Seventh chords play an important role in chord progressions, by implying forward motion toward a point of rest that has not yet been reached.

The above discussion of chord syntax concerns the "vertical" organization of tones in music. Another important aspect of chord syntax concerns the "horizontal" patterning of chords in time. In tonal music, there are norms for how chords follow one another (Piston, 1987; Huron, 2006), and these norms play a role in governing the sense of progress and closure in musical phrases. A prime example of this is the "cadence," a harmonic resting point in music. An "authentic cadence" involves movement from a V chord (or a V7 chord) to a I chord and leads to a sense of repose. Moving beyond this simple two-chord progression, some longer chord progressions can be identified as prototypical in tonal music, such as I-V-I, I-IV-V-I, I-ii-V-I, and so on. One of the governing patterns behind these progressions is the "cycle of fifths" for chords, a sequence in which the roots of successive chords are related by descending fifths. In its entirety, the progression is I-IV-vii°-iii-vi-ii-V-I. Smith and Melara (1990) have shown that even musical novices are sensitive to syntactic prototypicality in chord progressions, showing that implicit knowledge of these progressions is widespread among listeners.

Chord sequences are also important in melody perception, in which the chords are implied by important melody tones rather than explicitly played as simultaneities of tones (cf. Chapter 4, section 4.2.8). Listeners are sensitive to this implied harmony. Cuddy et al. (1981) have shown that melodic sequences that imply prototypical chord sequences are better remembered than other sequences. Furthermore, Trainor and Trehub (1994) have shown that musically unselected adults are more sensitive to melodic changes that violate the implied harmony than to physically larger changes that remain within the implied harmony (cf. Holleran et al., 1995).

Like the tones of the scale, different chords built on the 7 different scale degrees are not equal players in musical contexts. Instead, one chord (the tonic chord, built on the 1st scale degree) is the most central, followed by the dominant chord (built on the 5th scale degree) and the subdominant chord (built on the 4th scale degree). Informal evidence for the structural importance of the tonic, subdominant, and dominant chords (harmonically labeled as I, IV, and V chords) comes from the fact that many popular and folk songs can be played using just these three chords as the underlying harmony. More formal evidence comes from a study by Krumhansl et al. (1982) in which a musical context (an ascending scale) was followed by two target chords. Listeners were asked to judge how well the second chord followed the first in the context of the preceding scale. The judgments were then subject to multidimensional scaling in order to represent perceived relatedness as spatial proximity. Figure 5.5 shows the multidimensional scaling solution, and reveals that chords I, IV, and V form a central cluster around which the other chords are arrayed.

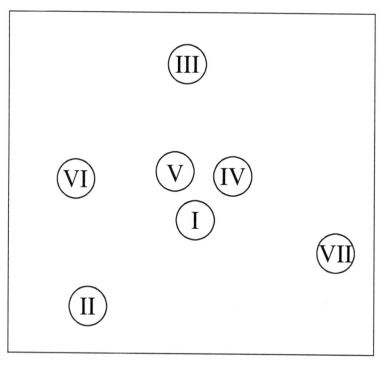

Figure 5.5 Psychological relatedness of different chords in a musical context. Chords are indicated by their harmonic labels, with uppercase Roman numerals used in a generic fashion (i.e., major, minor, and diminished chords are not distinguished). From Krumhansl et al., 1982.

Key Structure

A scale and its tonal hierarchy, plus its system of chords and chord relations, defines a "key" or tonal region in Western European music. Because there are 12 pitch classes in tonal music, each of which can serve as the tonic of a scale, and because there are two commonly used scale structures (major and minor), there are 24 keys in tonal music. Keys are named for their principal note and their scale structure, for example, C major, B minor. Thus keys and scales are named in a similar way, which may be one reason that people sometimes confuse the two.

A great deal of tonal music moves between keys during the course of a composition. These "modulations" of key allow a composer to explore different tonal regions and add diversity to the tonal journey outlined by a piece. Part of the syntax of tonal music is the pattern of key movement in music, which is far from a random walk between the 24 possible keys. Instead, modulations tend to occur between related keys, in which relatedness is defined in particular ways. Major keys are considered closely related if they share many of their basic scale tones. For example, the notes of the C major scale (C, D, E, F, G, A, B, C) and the G major scale (G, A, B, C, D, E, F♯, G) differ only in terms of one pitch class. (Recall that a major scale is obtained by starting on one note and choosing subsequent tones according to the major scale interval pattern [2 2 1 2 2 2 1].) Generalizing this relationship, any two keys whose 1st scale degrees are separated by a musical fifth are closely related, because their scales share all but one pitch class. This pattern of relations can be represented as a "circle of fifths" for major keys (Figure 5.6).

Music theory also suggests that each major key is also closely related to two different minor keys. One is the "relative minor," which shares the same notes of the scale but has a different tonic. For example, A-minor (A, B, C, D, E, F, G, A) is the relative minor of C major, because it has all the same pitch

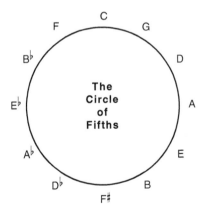

Figure 5.6 The circle of fifths for major keys. Each key is represented by a letter standing for its tonic. Keys that are adjacent on the circle share all but one pitch class.

classes. (Recall that the minor scale is obtained by starting on one note and choosing subsequent notes by following the minor-scale interval pattern of [2 1 2 2 1 2 2].) The other minor key related to a given major key is the "parallel minor," which shares the same tonic but has different scale tones. Thus C-minor (C, D, E♭, F, G, A♭, B♭, C) is the parallel minor of C major.

One way to represent this pattern of relationship among musical keys is via a geometric diagram in which psychological distance between keys is reflected by spatial distance. One such diagram, proposed by Krumhansl and Kessler (1982) on the basis of perceptual experiments, is shown in Figure 5.7. An important aspect of this two-dimensional diagram is that the left and right edges are equivalent, as are the top and bottom edges. That is, the map is actually an unfolded version of a shape that is circular in both dimensions (a torus), reflecting the circular nature of perceived key relations.

An interesting form of evidence for implicit knowledge of key distances comes from experiments in which listeners hear a melody followed by a transposed version of the same melody and must judge whether the two melodies are the same or different. A number of researchers have found that performance on this task is better if the melody is transposed to nearby versus a distant key (e.g., Cuddy

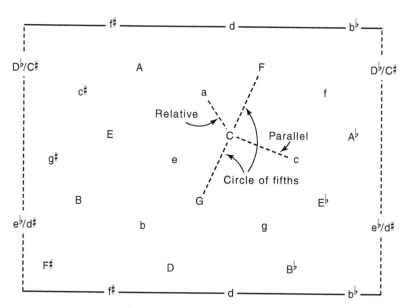

Figure 5.7 A map of psychological distances between musical keys. Major keys are indicated by uppercase letters and minor keys by lowercase letters. Dashed lines extending from the key of C major indicate related keys: two adjacent major keys along the circle of fifths (G and F; cf. Figure 5.6) and two related minor keys (see text for details). Modified from Krumhansl & Kessler, 1982.

et al., 1981; Trainor & Trehub, 1993; cf. Thompson & Cuddy, 1992). There is also neural evidence for implicit knowledge of key structure. When listening to a chord sequence in a particular key, an "alien" chord from a distant key produces a larger P600 (an event-related brain potential elicited by structural incongruity) than an alien chord from a nearby key, even when both chords contain the same number of out-of-key notes (Patel, Gibson, et al., 1998). Janata et al. (2002) have also provided evidence for maps of key distance in the brain, using the technique of functional magnetic resonance imaging (fMRI).

5.2.2 The Hierarchical Structure of Sequences

One of the principal features of linguistic syntax is that relationships between words are not simply based on nearest neighbor relations. For example, consider the sentence, "The girl who kissed the boy opened the door." Although the sentence contains the sequence of words "the boy opened the door," a speaker of English knows that the boy did not do the opening. This is because words are not interpreted in a simple left-to-right fashion, but via their combination into phrases and the combination of phrases into sentences. Figure 5.8 shows a syntactic tree diagram for this sentence specifying the hierarchical organization of words in relation to each other.

As with language, structural relations in tonal music are not merely based on adjacency. Instead, events are organized in a hierarchical fashion. The structure

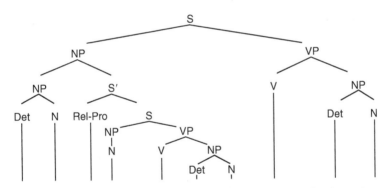

The girl who$_i$ e$_i$ kissed the boy opened the door

Figure 5.8 The hierarchical syntactic structure of an English sentence. (S = sentence; NP = noun phrase, VP = verb phrase, S′ = sentence modifier [relative clause], N = noun; V = verb; Det = determiner; Rel-Pro = relative pronoun.) Within the clause, the relative pronoun "who" is referred to as a filler and is interpreted as the actor for the verb "kissed." This relationship is identified by the presence of a coindexed empty element e$_i$ in the subject position of the relative clause. Modified from Patel, 2003b.

of these hierarchies is a major focus of modern cognitively oriented music theory, as exemplified by Lerdahl and Jackendoff's generative theory of tonal music (GTTM). Figure 5.9 shows a hierarchical structure for the tones in a musical passage according to GTTM. The details of this syntactic tree will be explained in the next section. For now, two conceptual points need to be made. First, this type of hierarchy is an "event hierarchy," which describes structural relations in a particular sequence of music. This must be clearly distinguished from the "pitch hierarchies" described in previous sections, which concern overall, atemporal aspects of the tonal musical style, for example, the fact that scale degree 1 is the most structurally stable tone in the scale (Bharucha, 1984a). Pitch hierarchies are only one factor that influences the construction of event hierarchies. The second point is that music theory posits two types of event hierarchies for musical sequences, describing different kinds of structural relations between musical events (Lerdahl & Jackendoff, 1983; cf. Jackendoff & Lerdahl, 2006). These will be discussed in turn below.

Musical Event Hierarchies I: Structure and Ornamentation

The concept that some pitches serve to elaborate or ornament others is central to Western European music theory (see, e.g., the theories of Schenker, 1969; Meyer, 1973; and Lerdahl & Jackendoff, 1983; cf. Cook, 1987a). The ability to recognize a familiar tune in a richly ornamented jazz version, or more generally, the ability to hear one passage as an elaborated version of another, implies that not all events in a musical sequence are perceived as equally important. Instead, some events are heard as more important than others. Note that calling some pitches "ornamental" is not meant to imply that they are aesthetically more or less important than other pitches. Rather, the distinction is meant to capture the fact that not all pitches are equal in forming the mental gist of a musical sequence. It is also worth noting that the concept of melodic elaboration is not unique to Western European tonal music (cf. Chapter 4, section 4.2.7).

One particularly clear treatment of event hierarchies of structure and ornamentation is Lerdahl and Jackendoff's theory of "time-span reduction." The tree in Figure 5.9a is a time-span reduction of two phrases of a musical melody, showing the hierarchy of structural importance for the tones in this passage. Shorter branches terminate on less important pitches, whereas longer branches terminate on more important pitches.[4]

---

[4] The oval shape in the right part of the tree is meant to indicate that the short motif that projects upward to it from the left (the first four notes of the second phrase, C-C-G-G) is subordinate to both branches touched by the oval, not just the left branch (cf. Lerdahl & Jackendoff, 1983:138). This subtlety is not essential for the current discussion.

Construction of such a tree requires decisions about which pitches are more structural than others; these decisions are influenced by tonal hierarchies, but also take rhythmic and motivic information into account. The use of a tree structure to indicate structure versus ornament (rather than a simple binary scheme whereby each pitch is either structural or ornamental) is based on the hypothesis that music is organized into structural levels, so that a pitch that is structural at one level may be ornamental at a deeper level. Thus taking a cross section of the tree at any particular height leaves one with the dominant events at that level (cf. Figure 5.9b). The trees are thus meant to model an experienced listener's intuitions about levels of relative structural importance of tones.

Although the notion of structure versus ornament is deeply ingrained in theories of tonal syntax, empirical studies of this issue have been relatively rare. One important study was conducted by Large et al. (1995), who examined pianist's improvised variations on children's melodies, such as the one shown in Figure 5.9. The pianists began by playing a melody from notation, and then produced five simple improvisations on the same melody. Large et al. reasoned that the structural importance of a pitch would be reflected in the number of times it was preserved in the same relative location across the variations. Consistent with this idea, the authors found substantial variation in the extent to which different pitches were retained across improvisations, suggesting that the pianists had a notion of the structural skeleton of the melody. The pattern of pitch retention could be accounted for largely on the basis of the pitch hierarchy of different scale degrees in combination with note duration and degree of metrical accent on a given note (all of which are incorporated in Lerdahl and Jackendoff's time-span reduction). Thus in these melodies, a typical "elaboration" pitch was one that occurred on a scale degree of low tonal stability, was of short duration, and was not aligned with an accented beat.

Large et al.'s study provides insights on elaboration in music performance, but leaves open the question of the *perception* of elaboration relations by listeners. Ideally, one would like a measure of the perceived structural importance of each pitch in a sequence, resulting in a tone-by-tone profile that could be analyzed in a quantitative fashion. Such measurements are difficult to make in practice, however, and creative approaches are needed in this area. One relevant study is that of Bharucha (1984b), who used a memory experiment to show that the salience of a tonally unstable note was influenced by its serial position relative to the following note. Specifically, Bharucha demonstrated that an unstable note that is immediately followed by a tonally stable pitch neighbor (e.g., B-C in a C-major context) is less prominent/detectable than an unstable note that is not "anchored" in this way. It is as if the stable tone subordinates the preceding tone as a local ornament and makes it less conspicuous than if

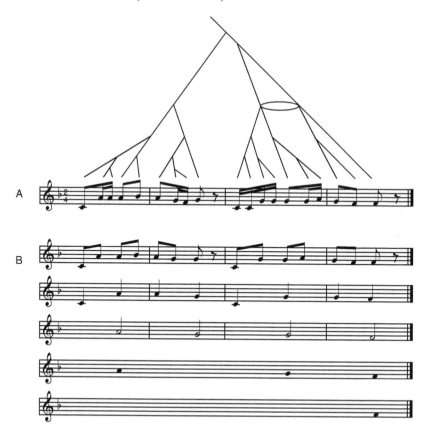

Figure 5.9 (A) A time-span reduction of the first two phrases of the children's song "Hush Little Baby." Shorter branches terminate on less important pitches, whereas longer branches terminate on more important pitches. (B) The lower staves show the dominant events at successively higher levels of tree structure. Modified from Large et al., 1995.

that same tone were inserted randomly into the sequence. This suggests that the tonal hierarchy is involved in perceived elaboration relations in music. There is clearly room for more work in this area, however, aimed at generating a note-by-note metric of the perceived structural importance of events in musical sequences.

Musical Event Hierarchies II: Tension and Resolution

Central to the experience of tonal music is a listener's sense of tension and resolution as a piece unfolds in time (Swain, 1997). Lerdahl and Jackendoff

(1983) refer to this aspect of music as "the incessant breathing in and out of music . . . [whose perception] is at the very heart of musical understanding" (pp. 123, 179). The notion of tension is related to the sense of mobility or openness (i.e., a sense that the music must continue), whereas resolution is associated with repose or rest. Although tension can be conveyed by surface features of music such as loudness and tempo, a very important component of tension in tonal music is the harmonic structure of a piece, in other words, its underlying sequence of chords and keys. These contribute to the pattern of "tonal tension" that arises from relations between harmonic elements in a structured cognitive space.

Lerdahl and Jackendoff devote a major component of their GTTM to the description of tension and relaxation, and propose that tension is organized in a hierarchical fashion. That is, they seek to capture the intuition that local tensing and relaxing motions are embedded in larger scale ones. The formalism they develop to represent the patterning of tension and relaxation is a tree-like structure that they refer to as a "prolongation reduction." An example of a prolongation reduction is given in Figure 5.10 (cf. Sound Example 5.1).

In this type of tree, right branching indicates an increase in tension and left branching a decrease in tension (i.e., a relaxation). Thus in Figure 5.10, the tree indicates that the first chord locally relaxes into the second, whereas the second

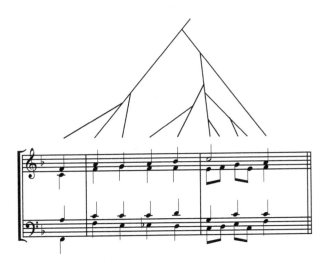

Figure 5.10 A prolongation reduction of a phrase from a composition by J. S. Bach (*Christus, der ist mein Leben*). In this type of tree, right branching indicates an increase in tension and left branching a decrease in tension (i.e., a relaxation). The tree shows how local tensing and relaxing motions are embedded in larger scale ones. Modified from Lerdahl, 2001:32.

chord locally tenses into the third. The fourth chord (the point of maximum tension in the phrase) is the first event originating from a right branch that attaches high up in the tree, and represents an increase in tension at a larger level. Following this chord, local relaxations into chords 5 and 6 are followed by local tensing movements before a more global relaxation, indicated by the left branch connecting chord 6 and the final chord. Note that the construction of trees such as that of Figure 5.10 relies on time-span reduction but is not determined by it: The two kinds of trees can organize the musical surface in different ways (see Lerdahl & Jackendoff, 1983, Chs. 5–9 for details). Thus prolongation reduction is another kind of event hierarchy that relates events (typically chords) to each other in ways that are more complex than simple nearest-neighbor relations.

Evidence that tension is actually perceived in a hierarchical fashion comes from studies in which listeners rate perceived tension as they listen to musical passages (Krumhansl, 1996). Such empirically measured "tension profiles" can then be compared to predictions based on numerical models of tonal tension based on computing psychological distances between pitches, chords, and keys. One such model is discussed in section 5.4.3 (subsection on tonal pitch space theory). The tonal pitch space (TPS) model can generate predictions based on hierarchical versus purely sequential analyses of tension-relaxation relationships, so that one can determine which type of structure better fits the empirical data. Research in this area has produced apparently contradictory evidence, with some studies favoring a purely sequential structure of perceived tension-relaxation patterns, whereas other studies support a hierarchical structure. Closer examination of these studies suggests these differences may arise from different paradigms used to collect tension ratings. For example, in Bigand and Parncutt's (1999) study, listeners heard increasingly long fragments of chord sequences and made tension ratings at the end of each fragment. This "stop-tension" task has the advantage of temporal precision, but suffers from an unnatural listening situation that may encourage local rather than global listening. Indeed, Bigand and Parncutt found that the tension profiles of their listeners were well modeled using local harmonic structure (especially cadences), with a negligible contribution of hierarchical structure. In contrast, research using a "continuous-tension" task, in which a listener moves a slider while listening to an ongoing piece, has provided evidence for hierarchical structure in perceived tension patterns (Lerdahl & Krumhansl, 2007; Smith & Cuddy, 2003). Thus there is evidence that musical tension and relaxation is in fact organized in a hierarchical fashion, though more work is needed in this area.[5]

---

[5] One important direction for future research using TPS is to design musical sequences in which predictions based on purely sequential relations are very different from predictions based on hierarchical relations (cf. Smith & Cuddy, 2003). It would be particularly interesting to determine if some listeners hear more sequentially, whereas others hear more hierarchically, and if this reflects the degree of musical training.

Order and Meaning

As noted earlier in this chapter, there is a strong link between syntax and meaning in language: Changing the order of elements can result in a sequence with very different meaning. This stands in contrast to other vertebrate communication systems such as bird song and whale song, in which there is no evidence for a rich relation between the order of elements and the meaning of the message (Marler, 2000). Turning to human music, if the pattern of tension and resolution in music is taken as one kind of musical meaning, then it is clear that changing the order of musical elements (e.g., rearranging chord sequences) will have a strong impact on meaning via its influence on tension-relaxation patterns. Of course, there is much more to say about musical meaning in relation to language (cf. Chapter 6). The key point here is that musical syntax, like linguistic syntax, exhibits a strong structure-meaning link.

5.2.3 Context Dependent Structural Functions

It is evident from the discussion above that tonal music has a rich syntax, but one important issue has not yet been addressed. To what extent does this syntax reflect abstract cognitive relationships between sounds, versus psychoacoustic relationships? Put another way, are syntactic relationships in tonal music merely a natural outcome of the psychoacoustic facts of sound, such as the overtone series and the smoothness or roughness of certain frequency intervals between tones? (Cf. Chapter 2 for a review of the overtone series and the sensory qualities of different frequency intervals.) If so, this would imply that tonal syntax lacks the abstractness of linguistic syntax, because psychological relations between elements reflect physical properties of sounds rather than purely conventional structural relations (cf. Bigand et al., 2006).

The search for a physical basis for tonal syntax dates back to the theorist Rameau (1722), and has had strong advocates ever since. Its appeal is understandable, in that it links music perception to a more basic level of sound perception. The advocates of this view in the last century include Bernstein (1976), who argued that the overtone series provides the foundation for musical scales and for the existence of a tonal center in music. More recently, Parncutt (1989) has provided a sophisticated quantitative analyses of harmony that seeks to understand structural relations between chords in tonal music on the basis of their psychoacoustic properties (see also Huron & Parncutt, 1993; Leman, 1995; Parncutt & Bregman, 2000).

Debates between "physicalist" and "cognitivist" views of musical syntax have existed for some time. For example, the culturally widespread importance of the octave and fifth in musical systems is likely due to universal acoustic/ auditory mechanisms (cf. Chapter 2). On the other hand, in a review of Bernstein's *The Unanswered Question,* Jackendoff (1977) points out that the match between the natural overtone series and the details of musical scales (particularly

pentatonic scales) is actually not that good, and there are cultures in which musical scales have little relationship to the overtone series, yet whose music still
has a tonal center. Back on the physicalist side, Leman (2000) has shown that
some of Krumhansl's probe-tone ratings can be accounted for on the basis of a
particular model of auditory short-term memory. Back on the cognitivist side,
research on the perception of chord relations that has directly pitted predictions based on psychoacoustics against those based on conventional harmonic
relations has found evidence for the latter (Tekman & Bharucha, 1998; Bigand
et al., 2003). There is little doubt that this debate will continue. At the current
time, the evidence suggests that Western European musical tonality is not a
simple byproduct of psychoacoustics, but is not a blatant contradiction of it either. That is, the psychoacoustic properties of musical sounds appear to provide
a "necessary but insufficient" basis for tonal syntax (Lerdahl, 2001; cf. Koelsch
et al., 2007, for relevant neural data).

   One strong piece of evidence for a cognitivist view of tonal syntax is that
certain psychological properties of musical elements derive from their context
and structural relations rather than from their intrinsic physical features. One
such a property is the "harmonic function" of different chords. The harmonic
function of a chord refers to the structural role it plays in a particular key. For
example, consider the two chords G-B-D and C-E-G. In the key of C major,
these chords play the role of a V chord and a I chord, respectively, whereas in
the key of G major, they play the role of a I chord and a IV chord. The different
feeling conveyed by these different functions is illustrated by Sound Examples
5.2a and 5.2b, in which these two chords form the final chords of sequences in
C major and G major, respectively. In the former case, the two chords form an
authentic cadence (V-I), and bring the phrase to a musical conclusion. In the
second case, the same two chords (and thus physically identical sound waves)
act as a I-IV progression and leave the phrase sounding unfinished. Numerous studies have shown that musically untrained listeners are sensitive to this
syntactic difference. For example, they react more quickly and accurately in
judging whether the final chord is mistuned when it functions as a I chord than
when it functions as a IV chord (Bigand & Pineau, 1997; Tillmann et al., 1998),
and show different brain responses to the same chord when it functions in these
two distinct ways (Regnault et al., 2001; cf. Poulin-Charronnat et al., 2006).
Bigand et al. (2001) have used such "harmonic priming" experiments to show
that the difference between chord functions even influences linguistic processes.
They constructed sequences in which chord progressions were sung in four-part
harmony, with each chord corresponding to a different nonsense syllable. The
listeners' task was simply to indicate if the final syllable contained the phoneme
/i/ or /u/. The correct responses of both musicians and nonmusicians were faster
when the final chord functioned as a I chord rather than as a IV chord.

   Evidence for an even broader level of abstraction regarding harmonic function
comes from research examining chord perception in isolation versus in musical

contexts. This work suggests that physically *different* chords are difficult to tell apart in a musical context if they have a similar harmonic function (in the sense of providing a similar prediction for a subsequent chord). Specifically, it has been shown that listeners can easily distinguish a IV chord from a II⁶ chord in isolation.[6] Yet the same listeners find it very difficult to distinguish a I-IV-V chord sequence from a I-II⁶-V sequence (Hutchins, 2003). This is likely due to the fact that it is quite common for the IV or II⁶ chord to function in a similar way in tonal music, in other words, as a preparation for a V chord. (Theorists refer to the function played by the IV or II⁶ chord in this context as the "subdominant function," named after the IV chord, which is the prototypical chord fulfilling this function; cf. Lerdahl & Jackendoff, 1983:192.) A crucial control condition in this study demonstrated that listeners could distinguish a V from a III⁶ chord both in isolation and in a musical context (I-V-I vs. I-III⁶-I), though the difference between these chords is akin to that between the IV and II⁶ chords. Importantly, the V and III⁶ chords are not functionally similar in tonal music in terms of predicting a following chord. (For similar evidence on the influence of tonal functions in melody perception, see Cuddy & Lyons, 1981.)

5.2.4 Some Final Comments on Musical Syntax

From the preceding discussion, it is clear that musical syntax is structurally complex, suggesting that it can sustain a meaningful comparison with linguistic syntax. Before embarking on such a comparison, it is worth making three final points about musical syntax.

First, syntax allows music to achieve perceptual coherence based on contrast rather than on similarity. A defining feature of music perception is hearing sounds in significant relation to one another rather than as a succession of isolated events (Sloboda, 1985). The most pervasive type of relationship used in music is similarity, such as the similarity created via the repetition or variation of a melodic phrase, or via the similarity of a theme to a stock of musical themes known in a culture (cf. Gjerdingen, 2007). Syntactic organization complements similarity-based coherence by creating coherent patterns based on contrast. For example, a chord progression involves the sequential use of different chords, yet these differences articulate a coherent journey, such as from repose to tension and back to repose. Musical syntax also creates coherence via hierarchical contrasts. For example, by hearing the difference between structural and ornamental tones, a listener can extract the gist of a musical sequence and recognize

---

[6] The superscript 6 refers to the fact that the standard II chord, in other words, D-F-A in C major, is played in an "inverted" form such that the F is the lowest note. Chord inversions are common in tonal music.

its similarity to (or contrast with) other passages in the same musical idiom. As suggested by this latter example, much of the richness of tonal music comes from the way that contrast-based and similarity-based cognitive processes interact in forming perceptually coherent patterns.

Second, although the different levels of syntactic organization of music have been described independently above (e.g., scales, chords, and keys), there is a good deal of interaction between levels. For example, for an experienced listener, even one or two chords can suggest a key, and a melody of single tones can suggest an underlying chord structure. Specifying the precise nature of interlevel interactions has been the focus of various models of tonal perception. For example, in one model suggested by Bharucha (1987), tones, chords, and keys are represented as nodes in different layers of an artificial neural network, and activity at one level can propagate to other levels according the to the pattern of interlevel connectivity (cf. Tillmann et al., 2000). This model has been able to account for the results of harmonic priming experiments that show how a chord's processing is influenced by its harmonic relation to preceding chords (Bigand et al., 1999). Another artificial neural network model that addresses the relations between syntactic levels involves a self-organizing map that is used to model how a sense of key develops and shifts over time as a sequence of musical chords is heard (Toiviainen & Krumhansl, 2003).

Third, a very important issue about tonal syntax concerns the relationship between its acquisition during development and its application during perception. Statistical research suggests that pitch hierarchies among scale tones and chords reflect the relative frequency of different notes and chords in tonal music (Krumhansl, 1990). Thus there is reason to believe that the acquisition of tonal syntax reflects the statistics of a particular musical environment. However, once a musical syntax is acquired, it can be activated by patterns that do not themselves conform to the global statistics that helped form the syntactic knowledge. For example, Bigand et al. (2003) found that listeners reacted more quickly and accurately to mistunings of the final chord of a sequence when it functioned as a I chord versus a IV chord (cf. section 5.2.3 above), even when the preceding chords had more instances of IV chords than I chords. Thus cognitive factors, namely the structural centrality of the I chord in a musical key, prevailed over the frequency of the IV chord in influencing perception and behavior. This provides strong evidence for a syntactic knowledge system that influences how we hear our musical world.

5.3 Formal Differences and Similarities Between Musical and Linguistic Syntax

The preceding sections provide the background for comparing linguistic and musical syntax in formal terms. Such a comparison is meaningful because language and music are rich syntactic systems that are not trivial variants of one another. Formal similarities between the systems are best appreciated in light of a clear understanding of formal differences, to which I turn first.

5.3.1 Formal Differences

Perhaps the most obvious difference between syntax in the two domains is the presence of grammatical categories in language, such as nouns, verbs, and adjectives, that have no counterparts in music. The attempt to find musical analogs for such categories is a trap that Bernstein fell into in *The Unanswered Question,* and is part of what Lerdahl and Jackendoff correctly labeled as "an old and largely futile game." Another example of uniquely linguistic syntactic entities are the linguistic grammatical functions that words play in sentences, in other words, subject, direct object, and indirect object (Jackendoff, 2002). Searching for direct musical equivalents of such functions is a misguided enterprise.

Beyond these differences in category identity, the hierarchical organization of grammatical categories in sequences also shows important differences in the two domains. Syntactic trees in language, such as that in Figure 5.8, convey the relationship of constituency: A determiner plus a noun is a noun phrase, a noun phrase plus a verb phrase is a sentence, and so forth. Syntactic trees in music, such as that in Figures 5.9 and 5.10, are not constituent trees. In the case of structure-elaboration trees (time-span reduction trees in GTTM), the branches of the tree join in ways that indicate which events are more structurally important. In tension-relaxation trees (prolongation-reduction trees in GTTM), the branching pattern indicates whether an event represents a tensing or a relaxing movement in relation to another event.[7]

Another difference between linguistic and musical syntax concerns long-distance dependencies. Such relations, such as between "girl" and "opened" in Figure 5.8, are ubiquitous in language and every normal listener can be assumed to perceive them (Chomsky, 1965). In contrast, the long-distance relations posited by musical syntax, such as the relations embodied in tension-relaxation trees (Figure 5.10), cannot simply be assumed to be perceived and are better viewed as hypotheses subject to empirical test, for example, using the tension-rating experiments described in section 5.2.2 (subsection on tension and resolution). Put another way, a particular sequence of notes or chords does not

---

[7] In GTTM, there is a kind of pseudoconstituency in prolongation-reduction trees, in that nodes in a tree have a distinct syntactic identity as a progression, a weak prolongation, or a strong prolongation (Lerdahl & Jackendoff, 1983:182). However, even in these cases, the chords are not really in a constituent relationship in a linguistic sense, in that one cannot define a priori what the grammatical categories of a constituent must be.

constrain perceived dependencies to the same degree as a particular sequence of words, suggesting that words have more intricate syntactic features built into them than do notes or chords. (For example, the mental representation of a verb is thought to include its syntactic category and thematic role information, in addition to its semantic meaning; cf. Levelt, 1999.)

One final formal difference that can be mentioned concerns the role of syntactic ambiguity in the two domains. In language, syntactic ambiguity is generally eschewed by the cognitive system, which seeks to arrive at a single structural analysis for a sentence. For example, in the sentence "The fireman left the building with the large sign," most individuals will parse the sentence so that "the large sign" is a modifier of "the building" rather than of "the fireman," even though the sentence is structurally ambiguous. In contrast, there is much greater tolerance for syntactic ambiguity in music. Krumhansl (1992) notes that "a chord may be heard simultaneously in its multiple roles in different keys, with the effect that modulations between closely related keys are easily assimilated. The role of a chord need never be disambiguated" (p. 199). Examples of such "pivot chords" abound in tonal music, and show that music not only tolerates syntactic ambiguity, it exploits it for aesthetic ends.

5.3.2 Formal Similarities: Hierarchical Structure

Having reviewed several important formal differences between musical and linguistic syntax, we can now turn to similarities. As reviewed in section 5.2.1, one similarity is the existence of multiple levels of organization. In language, there are syntactic principles that guide how basic lexical subunits (morphemes) are combined to form words, how words are combined to form phrases, and how phrases are combined to form sentences. In music, there are syntactic principles that govern how tones combine to form chords, how chords combine to form chord progressions, and how the resulting keys or tonal areas are regulated in terms of structured movement from one to another. In both domains, this multilayered organization allows the mind to accomplish a remarkable feat: A linear sequence of elements is perceived in terms of hierarchical relations that convey organized patterns of meaning. In language, one meaning supported by syntax is "who did what to whom," in other words, the conceptual structure of reference and predication in sentences. In music, one meaning supported by syntax is the pattern of tension and resolution experienced as music unfolds in time.

As noted earlier, the hierarchical organization of linguistic and musical syntactic structures follows different principles. Specifically, linguistic syntactic trees embody constituent structure, whereas musical syntactic trees do not (cf. section 5.3.1). Nevertheless, some interesting parallels exist between linguistic and musical syntactic trees at an abstract level, particularly between linguistic trees and prolongation-reduction trees in GTTM. First, just as each node of a linguistic tree terminates on a linguistic grammatical category (e.g., noun, verb, preposition), each node of a prolongation-reduction tree terminates on musical grammatical category: a chord assigned to a particular harmonic function in a given key (e.g., I, IV). That is, in both cases the tree structures relate grammatical categories in a hierarchical fashion, and in both cases the same grammatical categories can be filled by different members of the same category. That is, one can have the same sentence structure with different words, and the same harmonic structure with different chords (such as chords in different inversions, or if the key is changed, an entirely different set of chords). Note that in making this comparison, there is no claim for a direct correspondence between categories in the two domains (e.g., between tonic chords and nouns).

One final similarity regarding hierarchical syntactic relations in language and music bears mention, namely the shared capacity for recursive syntactic structure. In language, phrases can be embedded within phrases of the same type, for example, in Figure 5.8 the noun phrase "the boy" is embedded within the larger noun phrase "the girl who kissed the boy." In music, small-scale patterns of tension and relaxation can be embedded in larger tension-relaxation patterns of identical geometry but of a longer timescale (see Lerdahl & Jackendoff, 1983:207, for an example). Recursive syntactic structure has been proposed as a feature that distinguishes human language from nonhuman communication systems (Hauser et al., 2002; though see Gentner et al., 2006). If this is the case, then human music, no less than human language, is fundamentally different from animal acoustic displays such as bird song and whale song.

5.3.3 Formal Similarities: Logical Structure

Although the previous section dealt with hierarchical structure, this section is concerned with nonhierarchical aspects of "logical structure" of syntax in the two domains. For example, both domains recognize a distinction between "structural" and "elaborative" elements in sequences. In language, elaborative elements take the form of modifiers such as adjectives and adverbs. In tonal music, as discussed in a previous section, elaborative elements are identified on the basis of relative importance in the tonal hierarchy, together with rhythmic and motivic information. Although the means for distinguishing structure from elaboration are quite different in language and music, in both domains this conceptual distinction plays a role in organizing communicative sequences.

Another parallel in logical structure concerns grammatical functions in language and music. In the syntax of language, such functions include subject, object, and indirect object. These are logical functions that words take on with respect to other words in a sentence context, rather than being inherent properties of isolated words. The evidence that such a level of organization exists is that there are a number of grammatical principles that refer to these functions, such as verb agreement, which requires agreement between a subject or an object and its verb (Jackendoff, 2002:149). Tonal music also has a system of grammatical functions, discussed as "harmonic functions" in section 5.2.3 above. Such functions pertain to the structural role a chord plays in a particular key. As noted in that section, the harmonic function of a chord derives from the its context and its relation to other chords rather than to intrinsic properties of the chord itself. Typically, three such functions are recognized: tonic, subdominant, and dominant, prototypically instantiated by the I, IV, and V chords of a key, respectively. The same chord (e.g., C-E-G) can be a tonic chord in one key but a dominant or subdominant chord other keys, and empirical research shows that listeners are quite sensitive to this functional difference, as discussed in section 5.2.3. (Note that the tonic function is not limited to major chords: In minor keys, the tonic function is played by a minor chord, e.g., A-C-E in A minor; Krumhansl et al., 1982.) Conversely, two distinct chords in the same key—for example, a IV chord and a II⁶ chord—can have the same harmonic function by virtue of the way in which they are used (cf. section 5.2.3).[8] The salient point is that a chord's harmonic function is a psychological property derived from its relation to other chords. Thus music, like language, has a system of context-dependent grammatical functions that are part of the logical structure of communicative sequences. There is, of course, no claim for any mapping between functions in the two domains, for example, between subjects in language and tonics in music.

As an aside, readers may be curious why the number of harmonic functions in music has generally been recognized as three, when there are seven distinct chord categories in any key. This theory is based on the idea that chords whose roots are separated by a musical fifth or a musical second (e.g., I and V, or I and ii) are functionally different, whereas chords whose roots are separated by a musical third (e.g., I and vi, or ii and IV) are functionally similar (Dalhaus, 1990:58) The philosophical basis of this theory lies in the work of the 19th-century music theorist Hugo Riemann, who related the different chord functions to three different logical aspects of thought: thesis (tonic), antithesis (subdominant), and synthesis (dominant; Dalhaus, 1990:51–52). As noted by Dalhaus,

---

[8] This discussion of harmonic functions in music highlights the need to make a clear conceptual distinction between the names of chords based on the scale tones on which they are built and the more abstract harmonic functions that chords fulfill. Unfortunately, music theory terminology is confusing in this regard, in that the same terms (such as tonic, dominant, and subdominant) are used to refer to chords on the basis of their tonal constituents and on the basis of their harmonic functions. One way to avoid this confusion would be to call chords by their Roman numeral names (e.g., a IV chord) when referring to their inner tone structure and by verbal labels (e.g., "subdominant") when referring to their functions.

Riemann's basic thesis was "that the act of listening to music is not a passive sufferance of the effects of sound on the organ of hearing, but is much more a highly developed application of the logical functions of the human mind." Thus Riemann arrived at the notion of three distinct functions without any reference to linguistic grammatical relations.

5.3.4 Formal Differences and Similarities: Summary

The above sections have confirmed that there are important differences between linguistic and musical syntax, but have also shown that these differences need not prevent the recognition and exploration of formal similarities between syntax in the two domains. The key to successful comparison is to avoid the pitfall of looking for musical analogies of linguistic syntactic entities and relations, such as nouns, verbs, and the constituent structure of linguistic syntactic trees. Once this pitfall is avoided, one can recognize interesting similarities at a more abstract level, in what one might call the "syntactic architecture" of linguistic and musical sequences. These include the existence of multiple levels of combinatorial organization, hierarchical (and recursive) structuring between elements in sequences, grammatical categories that can be filled by different physical entities, relationships of structure versus elaboration, and context-dependent grammatical functions involving interdependent relations between elements. These similarities are interesting because they suggest basic principles of syntactic organization employed by the human mind.

5.4 Neural Resources for Syntactic Integration as a Key Link

The past decade has seen the birth of a new approach to music-language syntactic relations, based on empirical research in cognitive neuroscience. A primary motivation for this work has been a debate over the extent to which linguistic syntactic operations are "modular," conducted by a cognitive subsystem dedicated to linguistic function and largely independent of other forms of brain processing (Fodor, 1983; Elman et al., 1996). Music provides an ideal case for testing this claim. As we have seen, musical and linguistic syntax are rich systems that are not trivial variants of one another. Are musical and linguistic syntax neurally independent, or is there significant overlap? Any significant overlap would serve as compelling evidence in the debate over modularity. Furthermore, exploring this overlap could provide novel insights into fundamental syntactic operations in the human brain.

Although the prospect of overlap is stimulating, evidence from neuroscience long seemed to disfavor it. Specifically, neuropsychology provided well-documented cases of dissociations between musical and linguistic syntactic abilities. For example, individuals with normal speech and language abilities may show impaired perception of musical tonality following brain damage or due to a lifelong condition of musical tone-deafness (amusia without aphasia; Peretz, 1993; Peretz et al., 1994; Ayotte et al., 2000; Ayotte et al., 2002). Conversely, there are persons with severe language impairments following brain damage but with spared musical syntactic abilities (aphasia without amusia; e.g., Luria et al., 1965). This double dissociation between amusia and aphasia has led to strong claims about the independence of music and language in the brain. For example, Marin and Perry (1999) state that "these cases of total dissociation are of particular interest because they decisively contradict the hypothesis that language and music share common neural substrates" (p. 665). Similarly, Peretz and colleagues have used such dissociations to argue for a highly modular view of musical tonality processing (Peretz & Coltheart, 2003; Peretz, 2006).

As we shall see, there are reasons to doubt that this view is correct. One reason concerns neuroimaging evidence from healthy individuals processing syntactic relations in music and language. This evidence suggests far more neural overlap than one would expect based on dissociations in brain-damaged cases. Another reason concerns the nature of the evidence for aphasia without amusia, as discussed in the next section. These two factors have led to a reevaluation of syntactic relations between music and language in the brain. One outcome of this reevaluation is the hypothesis that the two domains have distinct and domain-specific syntactic representations (e.g., chords vs. words), but that they share neural resources for activating and integrating these representations during syntactic processing (Patel, 2003b). This "shared syntactic integration resource hypothesis" (SSIRH) is explained in more detail in section 5.4.3. For now, suffice it to say that the SSIRH can account for the apparent contradiction between neuropsychology and neuroimaging, and that it suggests a deep connection between musical and linguistic syntax in the brain.

The remainder of section 5.4 is divided into four parts. The first part reviews some of the classical evidence for neural dissociations between musical and linguistic syntax. The second part discusses neuroimaging research that contradicts this traditional picture. The third part discusses the use of cognitive theory to resolve the apparent paradox between neuropsychology and neuroimaging, and introduces the SSIRH. The fourth part discusses predictions of the SSIRH and how these predictions are faring in empirical research.

5.4.1 Neuropsychology and Dissociation

There is good evidence that musical syntactic deficits can exist in the absence of linguistic difficulties. An exemplary case for this is provided by the patient G.L., investigated by Peretz and colleagues (Peretz, 1993; Peretz et al., 1994). G.L. had bilateral temporal lobe damage, with infarctions on both sides of the brain due to strokes. This is a rare neurological occurrence, but is not infrequent among cases of acquired amusia. In G.L.'s case, primary auditory cortex was spared, but there was damage to rostral superior temporal gyri, which encompasses several auditory association areas (Peretz et al., 1994; cf. Tramo et al., 1990). G.L. was a well-educated individual who had been an avid music listener, though he had no formal musical training. Ten years after his brain damage, G.L. was referred for neuropsychological testing because of persistent problems with music perception. Peretz and colleagues administered a large battery of tests to study the nature of G.L.'s musical deficits, ranging from simple pitch discrimination to melody discrimination and tests for sensitivity to tonality. G.L. could discriminate changes between single pitches and was sensitive to differences in melodic contour in short melodies. He also showed some residual sensitivity to patterns of pitch intervals (e.g., in tests involving discrimination of melodies with the same contour but different intervals). What was most striking about his case, however, was his complete absence of sensitivity to tonality. For example, G.L. was given a probe-tone task in which a few notes (which establish a musical key) were followed by a target tone. The task was to rate the how well the target fit with the preceding context (cf. Cuddy & Badertscher, 1987; and Chapter 4, section 4.2.6, for background on probe-tone studies). Normal controls showed the standard effect of tonality: Tones from the key were rated higher than out-of-key tones. G.L., in contrast, showed no such effect, and tended to base his judgments on the pitch distance between the penultimate and final tone. He also failed to show an advantage for tonal versus atonal melodies in short-term memory tasks, in contrast to controls. Additional experiments showed that his problems could not be accounted for by a general auditory memory deficit. Most importantly for the current purposes, G.L. scored in the normal range on standardized aphasia tests, showing that he had no linguistic syntactic deficit.

G.L. is one of a handful of well-documented cases of acquired amusia. Cases of musical tone-deafness or congenital amusia are much more common (cf. Chapter 4, section 4.5.2, second subsection, for background on musical tone deafness). For example, Ayotte et al. (2002) presented a group study of 11 such individuals. These were well-educated persons with no other neurological or psychiatric problems, whose tone deafness could not be attributed to lack of exposure to music (indeed, all had music lessons in childhood). When tested, all showed a variety of musical deficits. Crucially, all failed a melodic sour-note detection task, which is a simple test of musical syntactic abilities. Normal individuals enculturated in Western music find this an easy task, even if they have had no formal musical training,

Acquired and congenital amusia thus provide compelling evidence that musical syntax can be disrupted without associated linguistic syntactic deficits. What about the reverse condition? The relevant evidence comes from cases of aphasia without amusia. The most often-cited case is that of the Russian composer Vissarion Shebalin (1902–1963). Shebalin attracted the interest of the famous neuropsychologist A. R. Luria (Luria et al., 1965), who commented that "the relationship of the two kinds of acoustic processes, namely verbal and musical, constitutes one of the most interesting problems of cortical neurology" (p. 288). Shebalin suffered two strokes in his left hemisphere, affecting the temporal and parietal regions. After the second stroke, he had severe difficulties in comprehending and producing language. Shebalin died 4 years after this second stroke, but in those few years he composed at least nine new pieces, including a symphony hailed by the Soviet composer Shostakovich as a "brilliant creative work" (p. 292).

Shebalin's case is not unique. Tzortzis et al. (2000, Table 4) list six published cases of aphasia without amusia, and report a seventh case in their own paper. However, Tzortzis et al. also point out a crucial fact about these cases: They are all professional musicians. Indeed, most cases represent composers or conductors, individuals with an extraordinarily high degree of musical training and achievement. (Note that this stands in sharp contrast to case studies of amusia without aphasia, which typically involve nonmusicians.) The question, then, is whether findings based on highly trained musicians can be generalized to ordinary individuals. There are reasons to suspect that the answer to this question is "no." Research on neural plasticity has revealed that the brains of professional musicians differ from those of nonmusicians in a variety of ways, including increased gray matter density in specific regions of frontal cortex and increased corpus callosum size (Schlaug et al., 1995; Gaser & Schlaug, 2003). This suggests that generalizations about language-music relations in aphasia cannot be drawn on the basis of case studies of professional musicians. To conclusively show a double dissociation between amusia and aphasia, one needs evidence of aphasia without amusia in nonmusicians. Peretz and colleagues (2004) have argued that such cases exist, but closer examination of their cited cases reveals that these individuals suffered from a phenomenon known as "pure word deafness." Although pure word deafness is sometimes referred to as a form of aphasia, it is in fact an auditory agnosia. An individual with pure word deafness can no longer understand spoken material but can understand and/or produce language in other modalities (i.e., writing). This is qualitatively different from true aphasia, which is a deficit of core language functions that cuts across modalities (Caplan, 1992).

The relevant point for the current discussion is that there has not been a convincing demonstration of a double dissociation between musical and linguistic syntactic abilities in ordinary individuals with brain damage. Indeed, as discussed later, new evidence from aphasia (in nonmusicians) points to an *association* between linguistic and musical syntactic disorders. Furthermore, the phenomenon of musical tone deafness, in which otherwise normal individuals exhibit musical syntactic deficits, is largely irrelevant to the question of music-language syntactic relations, as we shall see. Before discussing these issues, however, it is important to review some of the neuroimaging evidence that challenged the idea of separate processing for linguistic and musical syntax in the human brain.

5.4.2 Neuroimaging and Overlap

One of the first studies to compare brain responses to linguistic and musical syntactic processing in the same set of individuals was that of Patel, Gibson, et al. (1998). This study was inspired by two earlier lines of work. First, research on brain responses to harmonic incongruities in music, such as an out-of-key note at the end of a melodic sequence (Besson & Faïta, 1995), had revealed that these incongruities elicited a positive-going event-related brain potential (ERP). This positive ERP stood in sharp contrast to the commonly observed negative-going ERP associated with semantic anomalies in language (the N400, which peaks about 400 ms after the onset of a semantically incongruous word, such as the word "dog" in "I take my coffee with cream and dog"; Kutas & Hillyard, 1984). The second line of research concerned brain responses to syntactic (rather than semantic) incongruities in language (Osterhout & Holcomb, 1992, 1993; Hagoort et al., 1993). This research has revealed that when a word disrupted the syntactic form of a sentence, a positive-going ERP was generated. This ERP was referred to as the P600, because it peaked about 600 ms after the onset of the incongruous word (e.g., after the onset of "was" in "The broker hoped to sell the stock was sent to jail").[9]

The question asked by Patel, Gibson, et al. (1998) was whether harmonically incongruous chords within chord sequences would generate P600s akin to those elicited by syntactically incongruous words in sentences. If so, then this would suggest that some aspect of syntactic processing was shared between the two domains.

Before discussing this study in more detail, it is worth making an important point about the N400 and P600. These ERPs have been most often studied in the context of incongruities (semantic or syntactic), but it is a mistake to think they are therefore simply "error signals" emitted by the brain due to surprise, attention switching, and so forth. Crucially, both of these ERPs can be elicited in sentences without any semantic or syntactic errors. For example, if ERPs are measured to each word of the sentences "The girl put the sweet in her mouth after the lesson"

---

[9] The fact that the P600 peaks after the N400 does not necessarily mean that semantic operations precede syntactic ones. ERPs are an indirect measure of brain activity that are especially sensitive to locally synchronous activity patterns. Although one can infer from ERPs that processing occurs no *later* than a certain time, one cannot infer from ERPs how early processing begins, because it is always possible that relevant processing commences before one sees the ERP, but is not synchronous enough to be detected.

and "The girl put the sweet in her pocket after the lesson," a comparison of the ERP at "pocket" versus "mouth" reveals an N400 to the former word (Hagoort, et al., 1999). This reflects the fact that "pocket" is a less semantically predictable word than "mouth" given the context up to that point. The N400 is thus a sensitive measure of semantic integration in language.

Similarly, the P600 can be elicited without any syntactic error (cf. Kaan et al., 2000; Gouvea et al., submitted). For example, if the word "to" is compared in the sentences "The broker hoped to sell the stock" and "The broker persuaded to sell the stock was sent to jail," a P600 is observed to "to" in the latter sentence, even though it is a perfectly grammatical sentence (Osterhout & Holcomb, 1992). This is because in the former sentence, the verb "hoped" unambiguously requires a sentential complement, so that "to" is structurally allowed. In the latter sentence, however, when the word "persuaded" is first encountered, a simple active-verb interpretation is possible and tends to be preferred (e.g., "The broker persuaded his client to sell his shares"). This interpretation does not permit the attachment of a constituent beginning with "to." As a consequence, there is some syntactic integration difficulty at "to," although it soon becomes obvious that the verb "persuaded" is actually functioning as a reduced relative clause (i.e., "The broker who was persuaded . . ."), and sentence understanding proceeds apace. Thus although frank anomalies are often used to elicit the N400 and P600, it is important to note that this is simply a matter of expediency rather than of necessity.

Returning to our study (Patel, Gibson, et al., 1998), we constructed sentences in which a target phrase was either easy, difficult, or impossible to integrate with the preceding syntactic context, such as the following:

(5.1a) Some of the senators had promoted *an old idea* of justice.

(5.1b) Some of the senators endorsed promoted *an old idea* of justice.

(5.1c) Some of the senators endorsed the promoted *an old idea* of justice.

The syntactic structure of sentence 5.1b is considerably more complex than that of 5.1a, as shown in Figure 5.11 (Note that in sentence 5.1b, the verb "endorsed" has the same type of ambiguity as the verb "persuaded" in the discussion above.)

Thus in sentence 5.1b, the target phrase should be more difficult to integrate with the preceding structure than in 5.1a. In contrast to sentences 5.1a and 5.1b, which are grammatical sentences, 5.1c is ungrammatical, making the target impossible to integrate with the previous context.

We also constructed sequences of 7–12 chords in which a target chord within the middle part of the phrase was designed to vary in its ease of integration with the prior context. We based our musical design principles on previous research showing that listeners were sensitive to key distance in music. Thus the target chord was either the tonic chord of the key of the sequence, or the tonic chord of a nearby or distant key. "Nearby" and "distant" were defined using the

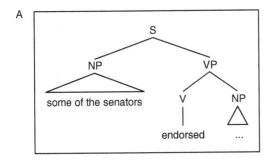

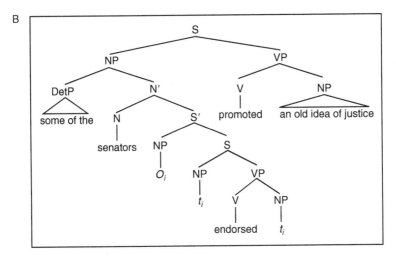

Figure 5.11 Syntactic structures for the simple and complex sentences in the study of Patel, Gibson et al. (1998). Most symbols are explained in the caption of Figure 5.8; N' = noun phrase projection, O = operator, t = trace. The sentence in (B) is substantially more complex than the sentence in (A) because the verb "endorsed" functions as a reduced relative clause (i.e., "some of the senators who were endorsed . . .").

circle of fifths for major keys: A nearby key was three counterclockwise steps away on the circle of fifths, and a distant key was five counterclockwise steps away (Figure 5.12).

For example, if the chord sequence was in the key of C major, then the target chords were: C major (C-E-G), E-flat major (E♭-G-B♭), or D-flat major (D♭-F-A♭). This design had the advantage that the two out-of-key chords had the same number of out-of-key notes relative to C major, so that differences in harmonic incongruity could not be attributed to differences in the number of out-of-key notes within the chords.

Two other aspects of the chord sequences bear mention. First, the target chord always occurred after a dominant (V or V7), and was thus always in

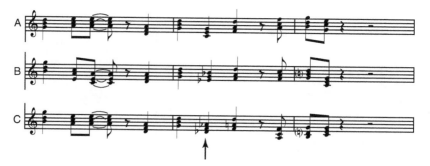

Figure 5.12 Example chord sequences from Patel, Gibson et al.'s (1998) study. The position of the target chord is indicated by the arrow. (A) The target chord is the tonic of the key of the phrase (a C major chord in this case, as the phrase is in the key of C). (B) The target chord is the tonic of a nearby key (E-flat major). (C) The target chord is the tonic of a distant key (D-flat major). Nearby and distant keys are defined as three versus five counterclockwise steps away from key of the phrase on the circle of fifths for keys (cf. Figure 5.6). Note that each stimulus has the same chord progression but differs slightly in terms of the inversion of chords before and after the target (though the two chords before and one chord after the target are held constant).

a specific harmonic context. Second, the chord sequences were composed in a popular, rather than a classical style: They sound like musical jingles rather than like traditional four-part harmony (Sound Examples 5.3a–c). Thus for both language and music, we used syntactic principles to construct sequences with varying degrees of syntactic incongruity. A single group of 15 musically trained listeners heard numerous linguistic and musical sequences like those shown above, and for each sequence, judged whether it sounded normal or structurally odd (we chose to work with musically trained listeners because we wanted to ensure sensitivity to musical syntax). ERPs to the target phrases in language were compared to ERPs to the target chords in music. The primary result of interest was that incongruities in both domains elicited P600s, and that these ERPs were statistically indistinguishable in amplitude and scalp distribution at both the moderate and strong levels of incongruity (Figure 5.13 shows ERPs to linguistic and musical targets at the strong level of incongruity.) This demonstrated that the P600 was not a signature of a language-specific syntactic process. Patel et al. suggested that the P600 may reflect domain-general structural integration processes in both domains (I return to this point in section 5.4.3, subsection "Reconciling the Paradox").

What can be said about the underlying neural source of the P600s in this study? Both the linguistic and musical P600s were maximal over temporal/posterior regions of the brain, but it is difficult to make any conclusions about the precise location of their underlying sources on this basis. This is because

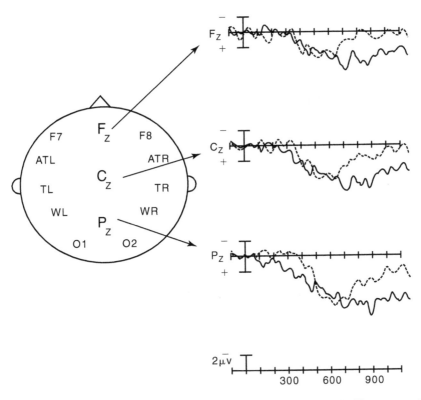

Figure 5.13 Traces show ERPs to linguistic (solid line) and musical (dashed line) syntactic incongruities from three electrodes along the middle of the head (Fz = front; Cz = vertex; Pz = back). (The schematic on the left side of the figure shows the electrode positions as if looking down on the head from above.) The ERP responses are highly similar in the vicinity of 600 ms. The continued positivity of the linguistic P600 beyond 600 ms is due to the continuing ungrammaticality of the sentence beyond this point. See Patel, Gibson et al., 1998, for details.

the ERP technique has excellent time resolution but poor spatial resolution. One thing that can be said with confidence, however, is that the generators of the P600 are unlikely to be strongly lateralized, as the ERP was symmetric across the left and right sides of the brain. (We also observed an unexpected and highly lateralized right anterior-temporal negativity elicited by out-of-key chords, which peaked at about 350 ms posttarget-onset. See Patel, Gibson, et al., 1998, for discussion, and Koelsch and Mulder, 2002, for a similar finding using more naturalistic musical materials and nonmusician listeners.)

Subsequent work on musical syntactic processing has supported the case for syntactic overlap between language and music by showing that musical syntactic processing activates "language" areas of the brain. Maess et al. (2001)

provided evidence from MEG that an early right anterior negativity (ERAN) associated with harmonic processing in music originates in a left frontal brain area known as Broca's area and its right hemisphere homologue (cf. Koelsch & Siebel, 2005). An fMRI study of harmonic processing (Tillmann et al., 2003; cf. Tillmann, 2005) also reported activation of these areas, and a second such study (Koelsch et al., 2002) implicated both Broca's and Wernicke's areas in musical harmonic processing (cf. Levitin & Menon, 2003; Brown et al., 2006).

These findings from neuroimaging, which point to overlap between linguistic and musical syntax in the brain, stand in sharp contrast to the evidence for music-language dissociations provided by neuropsychology (cf. section 5.4.1). Any attempt to understand the neural relationship of musical and linguistic syntax must come to terms with this paradox. One such attempt, based on cognitive theory in psycholinguistics and music cognition, was offered by Patel (2003b). An updated version of this approach is offered in the next section.

5.4.3 Using Cognitive Theory to Resolve the Paradox

Cognitive theories of language and music suggest that the mental representations of linguistic and musical syntax are quite different. For example, as discussed in section 5.3.1, one very important difference between syntax in language and music is that language has universal grammatical categories (such as nouns and verbs) and grammatical functions (subject, direct object, and indirect object) that are unique to language. Furthermore, the perception of long-distance syntactic dependencies is much more constrained by linguistic structure than by musical structure. In music, proposed hierarchical patterns (such as that in Figure 5.10) are best viewed as hypotheses subject to empirical test.

These observations suggest that the overlap in linguistic and musical syntax is not at the level of representation. Thus one way to break the paradox outlined above is to propose a conceptual distinction between syntactic representation and syntactic processing. This can be understood as the distinction between long-term structural knowledge in a domain (i.e., in associative networks that store knowledge of words and chords) and operations conducted on that knowledge for the purpose of building coherent percepts. A key idea of this approach is that some of the processes involved in syntactic comprehension rely on brain areas separate from the those areas in which syntactic representations reside. Such "dual system" approaches have been proposed by several researchers concerned with the neurolinguistics of syntax. For example, Caplan and Waters (1999) have suggested that frontal areas of the brain support a special working memory system for linguistic syntactic operations, and Ullman (2001) has suggested that frontal areas contain a symbol-manipulation system for linguistic syntax. The approach taken here is a dual system approach, but does not propose that linguistic and musical syntax share a special memory system or symbol manipulation system. Instead, a hypothesis for what is shared by linguistic and musical syntactic processing is derived from comparison of cognitive theories of syntactic processing in the two domains.

Before introducing these theories, two related points should be made. First, there are theoretical approaches to linguistic syntax that reject a separation between representation and processing, and artificial neural network ("connectionist") models in which syntactic representation and processing occur in the same network (MacDonald & Christiansen, 2002), and thus by implication in the same brain areas. Second, the theories considered below are by no means the only theories of syntactic processing in language and music. They were chosen because of their strong empirical basis and because they show a remarkable point of convergence.

Syntactic Processing in Language I: Dependency Locality Theory

Gibson's dependency locality theory (DLT; Gibson, 1998, 2000) was developed to account for differences in the perceived complexity of grammatical sentences and for preferences in the interpretation of syntactically ambiguous sentences. DLT posits that linguistic sentence comprehension involves two distinct components, each of which consumes neural resources. One component is structural storage, which involves keeping track of predicted syntactic categories as a sentence is perceived in time (e.g., when a noun is encountered, a verb is predicted in order to form a complete clause). The other component is structural integration, in other words, connecting each incoming word to a prior word on which it depends in the sentence structure. A basic premise of this theory is that the cost of integration is influenced by locality: Cost increases with the distance between the new element and the site of integration. Distance is measured as the number of new "discourse referents" (nouns and verbs) since the site of integration. Thus DLT uses a linear measure of distance rather than a hierarchical one (e.g., based on counting nodes in a syntactic tree), and thus does not depend on the details of any particular phrase structure theory.

To illustrate DLT's approach, consider the relationship between the words *reporter* and *sent* in the sentences:

(5.2a) The reporter who sent the photographer to the editor hoped for a story.

(5.2b) The reporter who the photographer sent to the editor hoped for a story.

In sentence 5.2a, when "sent" is reached, integration with its dependent "reporter" is relatively easy because the words are nearly adjacent in the sentence. In sentence 5.2b, however, the integration between "sent" and "reporter" (now the object of the verb) is more difficult, because it must cross an intervening noun phrase, "the photographer."[10] A strength of this theory is its ability to provide numerical predictions of the processing (storage plus integration) cost at each word in a sentence. Figure 5.14 illustrates the numerical accounting system for integration cost using the example sentences given above.[11]

The numerical predictions of DLT can be empirically tested in reading time experiments in which the amount of time spent viewing each word of a sentence on a computer screen is quantified. The assumption of such experiments is that longer reading time is a reflection of greater processing cost. DLT has been supported by empirical research on sentence processing in English and other languages (e.g., Warren & Gibson, 2002; Grodner & Gibson, 2005). The relevant aspect of the theory for the current purpose is the idea that mentally connecting distant elements require more resources.[12]

Syntactic Processing in Language II: Expectancy Theory

DLT provides one account of syntactic integration difficulty in language, namely, due to distance between an incoming word and its prior dependent word. A different theoretical perspective suggests that syntactic integration difficulty is associated with how well a word fits a perceiver's syntactic expectations at that point. The underlying assumption of this view is that at each

---

[10] Technically, the integration is between "sent" and an empty-category object that is coindexed with the pronoun "who."

[11] For those interested in detail, the distance between "The" and "reporter" is 1 because one new discourse referent ("reporter") has been introduced since the site of integration on "The." The distance between "reporter" and "who" is 0 because no new discourse referents have been introduced by "who," and so forth. The critical difference between the sentences concerns the integration of "sent" into the existing sentence structure. In the upper sentence (which has a subject-extracted relative clause), "sent" has one integration (with "who") with a distance of 1. In the lower sentence (which has an object-extracted relative clause), "sent" has two integrations (with "photographer" and "who"), the former having a distance of 1 and the latter having a distance of 2. This results in a total integration cost of 3 for "sent" in the lower sentence.

[12] Gibson recognizes that equating integration cost with linear distance is a simplification. Other factors which may influence the integration cost of a word include the complexity and contextual plausibility of structural integrations that have taken place between the incoming word and its site of integration (cf. Gibson, 2000), and potential interference among items in the intervening region, including the incoming word (cf. Gordon et al., 2001). Furthermore, integration cost may reach an asymptote after a few intervening new discourse referents rather than remaining a linear function of distance. Nevertheless, equating cost with linear distance provides a good starting point and performs well in predicting behavioral data such as reading time data in sentence processing experiments.

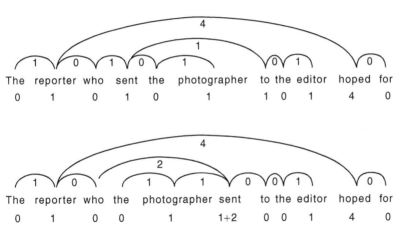

Figure 5.14 Example of distance computation in DLT. Links between dependent words are shown by curved lines, and the distances associated with each link are shown by the integers below the curved line. The number below each word shows the total distance of that word from its prior dependent words. The total distance is used as a measure of the integration cost for that word. Combining integration costs with storage costs (not shown) yields a total processing cost for each word, which can be compared to empirical data from reading time experiments.

point during sentence comprehension, a perceiver has specific expectations for upcoming syntactic categories of words (Narayanan & Jurafsky, 1998, 2002; Hale, 2001; Levy, in press; cf. Lau et al., 2006, for neural data). These expectations reflect structural analyses of the sentence currently being considered by the parsing mechanism. When a word is encountered that does not match the most favored analysis, resources must be reallocated in order to change the preferred structural interpretation. Such an explanation can account for a number of different sentence processing effects, including difficulty caused by "garden-path" sentences in which a comprehender encounters a syntactically unexpected word, such as "to" in "The broker persuaded to sell the stock was sent to jail" (cf. section 5.4.2)

The expectancy theory of syntactic processing has old roots (Marslen-Wilson, 1975; cf. Jurafsky, 2003 for a historical perspective) but has only recently begun to be systematically investigated using psycholinguistic methods. Notably, the approach can successfully account for sentence processing effects not predicted by DLT. For example, Jaeger et al. (2005, described in Levy, in press) had participants read sentences that varied in the size of an embedded relative clause (marked by brackets below):

(5.3a) The player [that the coach met at 8 o'clock] bought the house . . .

(5.3b) The player [that the coach met by the river at 8 o'clock] bought the house . . .

(5.3c) The player [that the coach met near the gym by the river at 8 o'clock] bought the house . . .

According to DLT, the verb "bought" should be harder to integrate with its prior dependent ("player") as the size of the intervening relative clause increases. In fact, precisely the opposite pattern of results was found: Reading times on "bought" became *shorter* as the size of the relative clause increased. Expectancy theory predicts this result, because as each additional modifying phrase occurs within the relative clause, a main verb ("bought," in this case) becomes more expected. This in turn likely reflects experience with the statistics of language, in which short relative clauses are more common than long ones (as confirmed by Jaeger et al.'s measurements of corpus statistics). For other studies supporting expectancy theory, see Konieczny (2000), and Vasishth and Lewis (2006).

Notably, however, there are cases in which DLT makes more accurate predictions than expectancy theory. For example, in the example sentences in the previous subsection, when "sent" is encountered in sentence 5.2b, its grammatical category (noun) is highly expected, yet the word is still difficult to integrate due to its distance from "reporter." Hence at the current time, it appears that DLT and expectancy theory are successful in different circumstances, meaning that work is needed to reconcile these two theories. (For one recent framework that seeks to unify distance-based effects and expectancy-based effects, see Lewis et al., 2006.) For the current purposes, however, the relevant point is that both DLT and expectancy theory posit that difficult syntactic integrations consume processing resources used in building structural representations of sentences.

Syntactic Processing in Music: Tonal Pitch Space Theory

Lerdahl's (2001) tonal pitch space (TPS) theory concerns the perception of pitch in a musical context. It builds on the empirical findings about the perceived relations between scale tones, chords, and keys outlined in section 5.2.1, and illustrated in Figures 5.3, 5.5, and 5.7. The main formalism used to represent these relations is a "basic space" organized as a hierarchy of pitch alphabets (based on Deutsch & Feroe, 1981). Figure 5.15 shows a basic-space representation of a C major chord in the context of the C major key.

As noted by Lerdahl, "Each level of the space elaborates into less stable pitch classes at the next [lower] level; conversely, the more stable pitch classes at one level continue on to the next [upper] level. The structure is asymmetrical and represents the diatonic scale and the triad directly" (p. 48). The basic space provides a mechanism for computing the psychological distance between any two musical chords in a sequence. The algorithm for computing distance involves measuring how much one has to shift a chord's representation in the basic space to transform it into another chord. The details of this algorithm are beyond the

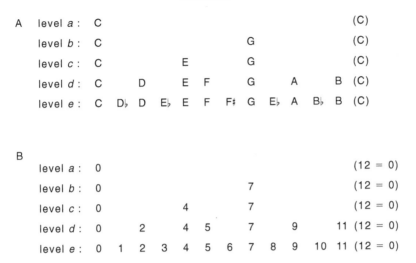

A   level *a* :   C   (C)

   level *b* :   C   G   (C)

   level *c* :   C   E   G   (C)

   level *d* :   C   D   E F   G   A   B (C)

   level *e* :   C D♭ D E♭ E F F♯ G E♭ A B♭ B (C)

B

   level *a* :   0   (12 = 0)

   level *b* :   0   7   (12 = 0)

   level *c* :   0   4   7   (12 = 0)

   level *d* :   0   2   4 5   7   9   11 (12 = 0)

   level *e* :   0 1   2 3   4 5 6   7 8   9 10 11 (12 = 0)

Figure 5.15 Lerdahl's basic space for representing musical chords in a manner that incorporates multiple levels of pitch structure. Panel (A) shows the representation of a C major triad in the context of the C major key, and panel (B) shows the same in a numerical format. The basic space provides a mechanism for measuring distances between chords in a manner that reflects the tripartite psychological distances of pitch classes, chords, and keys. From Lerdahl, 2001.

scope of this book (see Lerdahl, 2001 for details); what is important is that the basic space provides an algebraic method for computing chord distances in a manner that incorporates the tripartite distances of pitch classes, chords, and keys, and yields a single distance value that can be expressed as an integer.

TPS also provides a method for deriving tree structures such as that in Figure 5.10, which serve as a hypothesis for the perceived dependencies between chords. Using the tree structure, one computes the distance of each chord from the chord to which it attaches in the tree, with the added stipulation that a chord "inherits" distances from the chords under which it is embedded. Thus each chord is associated with a numerical distance value from another chord. This distance plays an important role in predicting the perceived ebb and flow of tension in musical sequences, with the basic idea being that tension increases with tonal distance between chords. For example, when a chord is introduced from a new key area, tension increases (cf. Steinbeis et al., 2006). The numerical predictions of TPS can be compared to tension profiles produced by listeners who rate perceived tension over time in musical passages (cf. section 5.2.2, second subsection). Such experiments have provided support for TPS, and suggest that listeners do in fact hear relations between chords in a hierarchical rather than a purely sequential manner (Lerdahl & Krumhansl, 2007).

It is important to note, however, that the essential feature of TPS for the current purposes is not the tree structures it proposes. This is because one cannot simply assume that listeners hear long-distance harmonic relations in music, so that such tree structures are best viewed as hypotheses subject to empirical test, as previously mentioned (cf. section 5.3.1). Instead, the essential feature of TPS is that chord relations are perceived in terms of distances in a structured cognitive space of pitch classes, chords, and keys. Such harmonic distances apply even when chords are heard in a purely sequential way, so that each chord's harmonic distance is computed from the immediately preceding chord (cf. section 5.2.2, second subsection). It is this notion of distance-based syntactic processing that provides a key link to language processing, as discussed in the next section.

Convergence Between Syntactic Processing in Language and Music

We have seen that words can be difficult to integrate syntactically into sentences when they are distant from their dependents or when they are syntactically unexpected. In both cases, resources are consumed as part of constructing the structural interpretation of a sentence. In DLT, distant integrations are costly because they require reactivating a prior dependent word whose activation has decayed in proportion to the distance between the words. In expectancy theory, unexpected syntactic categories are costly because they require changing the preferred structural interpretation of a sentence, which amounts to boosting the activation of a structure that previously had a low activation level. In other words, both language theories posit that difficult integrations arise from activating low-activation items.

In music, as in language, a listener is continuously involved in building a structural interpretation of a sequence, including a sense of the local key.[13] I hypothesize that when building a sense of key, a harmonically unexpected note or chord creates a processing cost due to its tonal distance (in the sense of TPS) from the current musical context. This cost arises because the incoming note or chord has a low activation level in the associative networks that store information about chord relationships (cf. Bharucha, 1987; Tillmann et al., 2000), yet its representation must be rapidly and selectively activated in order for it to be integrated with the existing context. In other words, harmonic distance translates into processing cost due to the need to activate a low-activation item. (Note that according to this idea, harmonically unexpected notes or chords are precisely those that are harmonically distant from the local key, because listeners tend to expect chords from the local key; cf. Schmuckler, 1989; Huron, 2006.)

---

[13] Having a sense of key permits tones to be perceived in terms of varying degrees of stability, which contributes strongly to the dynamic perceptual quality of music.

Overlap in the syntactic processing of language and music can thus be conceived of as overlap in the neural areas and operations that provide the resources for difficult syntactic integrations, an idea termed the "shared syntactic integration resource hypothesis" (SSIRH). According to the SSIRH, the brain networks providing the resources for syntactic integration are "resource networks" that serve to rapidly and selectively bring low-activation items in "representation networks" up to the activation threshold needed for integration to take place (Figure 5.16).

The neural location of the hypothesized overlapping resource networks for language and music is an important question that does not yet have a firm answer. One idea consistent with current research on language processing is that they are in frontal brain regions that do not themselves contain syntactic representations but that provide resources for computations in posterior regions where syntactic representations reside (Haarmann & Kolk, 1991; Kaan & Swaab, 2002). Defining the neural locus of overlap will require within-subjects comparative studies of language and music using techniques that localize brain activity, such as fMRI. For example, if independent linguistic and musical tasks are designed with two distinct levels of syntactic integration demands within

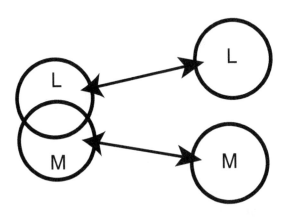

Resource networks   Representation networks

Figure 5.16 Schematic diagram of the functional relationship between linguistic and musical syntactic processing. L = language, M = music. The diagram represents the hypothesis that linguistic and musical syntactic representations are stored in distinct brain networks, whereas there is overlap in the networks which provide neural resources for the activation of stored syntactic representations. Arrows indicate functional connections between networks. Note that the circles do not necessarily imply highly focal brain areas. For example, linguistic and musical representation networks could extend across a number of brain regions, or exist as functionally segregated networks within the same brain regions.

them, one could search for brain regions that show increased activation as a function of integration cost in *both* language and music (a technique known as "cognitive conjunction" neuroimaging; Price & Friston, 1997). These regions would be strong candidates for the overlapping resource networks proposed by the SSIRH.

Reconciling the Paradox

One appeal of the SSIRH is that it can reconcile the apparent contradiction between neuroimaging and neuropsychology described earlier in this section. With respect to neuroimaging, the SSIRH is consistent with the findings of Patel, Gibson, et al. (1998) under the assumption that the P600 reflects syntactic integration processes that take place in posterior/temporal brain regions (cf. Kaan et al., 2000). It is also consistent with localization studies that find that musical harmonic processing activates frontal language areas (Koelsch et al., 2002; Tillmann et al., 2003) under the view that these anterior loci house the resource networks that serve to activate representations in posterior regions. (It should be noted, however, that the precise localization of overlapping resource networks requires a within-subjects design comparing language and music, cf. above.)

With respect to neuropsychology, the SSIRH proposes that the reported dissociations between musical and linguistic syntactic processing in acquired amusia are due to damage to domain-specific representations of musical syntax (e.g., long-term knowledge of harmonic relations), rather than a problem with syntactic integration processes. Consistent with this idea, most such cases have been associated with damage to superior temporal gyri (Peretz, 1993; Peretz et al., 1994; Patel, Peretz, et al., 1998; Ayotte et al., 2000), which are likely to be important in the long-term representation of harmonic knowledge. The SSIRH also proposes that musico-linguistic syntactic dissociations in musical tone deafness (congenital amusia) are due to a developmental failure to form cognitive representations of musical pitch (Krumhansl, 1990). Consistent with this idea, research by Peretz and Hyde (2003) and Foxton et al. (2004) has revealed that congenital amusics have basic psychophysical deficits in pitch discrimination and in judging the direction of pitch changes. As discussed in section 4.5.2 (subsection "The Melodic Contour Deafness Hypothesis"), these problems likely prevent such individuals from forming normal cognitive representations of musical scale, chord, and key structure. Without such representations, there is no basis on which musical syntactic processes can operate. This is the reason why musical tone deafness is largely irrelevant to the study of music-language syntactic relations, as alluded to in section 5.4.1.

How can the SSIRH account for reports of aphasia without amusia, for example, a stroke that results in severe language impairment but spared musical abilities? As discussed in section 5.4.1, such reports often focus on case studies of individuals with extraordinary musical abilities, and may not be relevant to music processing in the larger population. Furthermore, most reports of aphasia without amusia are seriously out of date. For example, in Marin and Perry's (1999) review of 13 cases, many cases were from the 1800s, and the most recent was from 1987. Needless to say, none contain any systematic tests of musical syntactic processing—e.g., harmonic processing of chords—in individuals with well-defined linguistic syntactic processing deficits. In fact, it is striking that there are no modern studies of harmonic processing in aphasia, despite suggestive older research (Francès et al., 1973). This is an area that merits careful study, and is a crucial testing ground for SSIRH, as discussed in the next section.

5.4.4 Predictions of a Shared-Resource Hypothesis

A principal motivation for developing the SSIRH was to generate predictions to guide future research into the relation of linguistic and musical syntactic processing. One salient prediction regards the interaction of musical and linguistic syntactic processing. In particular, because the SSIRH proposes that linguistic and musical syntactic integration rely on common neural resources, and because syntactic processing resources are limited (Gibson, 2000), it predicts that tasks that combine linguistic and musical syntactic integration will show interference between the two. In particular, the SSIRH predicts that integrating distant harmonic elements will interfere with concurrent difficult syntactic integration in language. This idea can be tested in paradigms in which a harmonic and a linguistic sequence are presented together and the influence of harmonic structure on syntactic processing in language is studied. Several relevant studies are discussed in the following subsection.

A second prediction made by the SSIRH regards aphasia. Several language researchers have argued that syntactic comprehension deficits in Broca's aphasia can be due to disruption of processes that activate and integrate linguistic representations in posterior language areas, rather than damage to these representations per se (Kolk & Friederici, 1985; Haarmann & Kolk, 1991; Swaab, Brown, & Hagoort, 1998; Kaan & Swaab, 2002). For these aphasics, the SSIRH predicts that syntactic comprehension deficits in language will be related to harmonic processing deficits in music. Relevant evidence is discussed in the second subsection below.

Interference Between Linguistic and Musical
Syntactic Processing

If music and language draw on a common pool of limited resources for syntactic processing, then one should observe interference between concurrent difficult musical and linguistic syntactic integrations. Testing this prediction requires experiments in which music and language are presented together. Although a number of past studies have paired linguistic and harmonic manipulations, they have largely focused on the relationship between musical harmonic processing and linguistic *semantic* processing. What is notable about these studies is that they either find a lack of interaction in processing (Besson et al., 1998; Bonnel et al., 2001) or report an interaction that is likely due to nonspecific factors having to do with attention (Poulin-Charonnat et al., 2005). These studies are briefly reviewed next as background for studies motivated by the SSIRH.

STUDIES EXAMINING THE INTERACTION BETWEEN LINGUISTIC SEMANTICS AND MUSICAL SYNTAX   Besson et al. (1998) and Bonnel et al. (2001) had participants listen to sung sentences in which the final word of the sentence was either semantically normal or anomalous, and sung on an in-key or out-of-key note. Besson et al. found that the language semantic violations gave rise to a negative-going ERP (N400), whereas the out-of-key notes gave rise to a late positive ERP, and that a simple additive model predicted the data for combined semantic/music syntactic violations quite well. Bonnel et al. had listeners either perform a single task (judge incongruity of final word or note) or a dual task (judge incongruity of both), and found that the dual task did not result in a decrease in performance compared to the single-task conditions. Thus both studies supported the independence of linguistic semantic versus musical syntactic processing.

Poulin-Charonnat et al. (2005), in contrast, did find an interaction between musical syntactic processing and linguistic semantic processing. They employed the harmonic priming paradigm, using chord sequences of the type introduced in section 5.2.3 (cf. Sound Example 5.2). Recall that these sequences are constructed so that the first six chords establish a musical context that determines the harmonic function of the last two chords. These two chords, which are physically identical in both contexts, form a V-I progression (a perfect cadence) in one context but a I-IV progression in the other. This leads to a sense of closure in the former context but not the latter.

To combine music and language, the chord sequences were sung (in four-part harmony) with one syllable per chord. The words formed sentences in which the final word was semantically either expected or unexpected. For example, the sentence "The giraffe had a very long . . ." could end either with "neck" (the expected ending) or "foot" (an unexpected ending). Participants were asked to listen to each sequence and decide if the last word was a real word or a nonsense word (in half the cases, the last word was in fact a nonsense word such as "sneck"). The focus of interest was on reaction times to real words. Based on standard psycholinguistic research, a faster RT was predicted for semantically expected versus unexpected words, reflecting semantic priming. The question of interest was whether this semantic priming effect would be modulated by the harmonic function of the final chord (I vs. IV, i.e., tonic vs. subdominant). Indeed, this is what was found. In particular, the RT difference between the expected and unexpected word was diminished when the final chord functioned as a subdominant chord. This result was obtained even for participants without musical training, showing that musical and linguistic processing interacted even in nonmusicians.

This study showed that a musical syntactic manipulation influenced linguistic semantic processing. However, the authors suggested that this effect might be mediated by general attentional mechanisms rather than by shared processing resources between language and music. Specifically, they proposed that the harmonic manipulation influenced linguistic semantics because the different chord endings affected the listeners' attention to the final word/chord in different ways. For example, ending a chord sequence on a IV chord might draw attention to the music (because it sounds incomplete) and thus distract from language processing. This interpretation is supported by a study by Escoffier and Tillmann (2006), who combined harmonic-priming chord sequences with geometric visual patterns rather than with words (one pattern per chord), and showed that ending on a IV chord (vs. a I chord) slowed the speed of processing of the target pattern at the end of the sequence. Thus ending a sequence on a IV chord appears to have a nonspecific influence on the speed of responding to various kinds of stimuli (cf. Bigand et al., 2001).

The study of Poulin-Charronnat et al. raises an important issue for work on music-language syntactic interactions. Specifically, such work should control for indirect effects of music on language due to general attentional mechanisms (e.g., via the use of nonharmonic but attention-getting auditory manipulations in music).

STUDIES EXAMINING THE INTERACTION BETWEEN LINGUISTIC AND MUSICAL SYNTAX We now turn to studies motivated by the SSIRH that combine musical harmonic manipulations with linguistic syntactic manipulations. Currently three such studies exist, one neural study (by Koelsch et al., 2005) and two behavioral studies (Fedorenko et al., 2009; Slevc et al., 2009).

Koelsch et al. (2005) conducted an ERP study in which short sentences were presented simultaneously with musical chords, with one chord per word (words were presented visually and in succession, at a rate of about 2 words per second). In some sentences, the final word created a grammatical violation via a gender disagreement. (The sentences were in German, in which many nouns are marked for gender. An example of a gender violation used in this study is: Er trinkt den kühlen Bier, "He drinks the$_{masculine}$ cool$_{masculine}$ beer$_{neuter}$.") This final word violates a syntactic expectancy in language (cf. section 5.4.3, subsection on expectancy theory in language). The chord sequences were designed to strongly invoke a particular key, and the final chord could be either the tonic chord of that key or a (harmonically unexpected) out-of-key chord from a distant key (i.e., a D-flat major chord at the end of a C major sequence).[14] The participants (all nonmusicians) were instructed to ignore the music and simply judge if the last word of the sentence was linguistically correct.

Koelsch et al. focused on early ERP negativities elicited by syntactically incongruous words and chords. Previous research on language or music alone had shown that the linguistic syntactic incongruities were associated with a left anterior negativity (LAN), whereas the musical incongruities were associated with an early right anterior negativity (ERAN; Gunter et al., 2000; Koelsch et al., 2000; Friederici, 2002). (Note that the degree of lateralization is stronger for the LAN than for the ERAN. While the ERAN is strongest over the right anterior hemisphere, it can be clearly observed over the left anterior hemisphere.) For their combined language-music stimuli, Koelsch et al. found that when sentences ended grammatically but with an out-of-key chord, a normal ERAN was produced. Similarly, when chord sequences ended normally but were accompanied by a syntactically incongruous word, a normal LAN was produced. The question of interest was how these brain responses would interact when a sequence had simultaneous syntactic incongruities in language and music.

The key finding was that the brain responses were not simply additive. Instead, there was an interaction: The LAN to syntactically incongruous words was significantly *smaller* when these words were accompanied by an out-of-key chord, as if the processes underlying the LAN and ERAN were competing for similar neural resources. In a control experiment for general attentional effects, Koelsch et al. showed that the LAN was not influenced by a simple auditory oddball paradigm involving physically deviant tones on the last word in a sentence. Thus the study supports the prediction that tasks that combine linguistic and musical syntactic integration will show interference between the two processes.

Turning to the behavioral study of Fedorenko et al. (2009), these researchers combined music and language using sung sentences. Linguistic syntactic integration difficulty was manipulated via the distance between dependent words. In sentence 5.4a below, the relative clause "that met the spy" contains only local integrations (cf. section 5.4.3, subsection on dependency locality theory). In sentence 5.4b, the relative clause "that the spy met" contains a nonlocal integration of "met" with "that," known to be more difficult to process (e.g., King & Just, 1991).

(5.4a) The cop that met the <u>spy</u> wrote a book about the case.

(5.4b) The cop that the spy <u>met</u> wrote a book about the case.

---

[14] This chord is also known as a Neapolitan 6th chord, and in longer musical contexts (i.e., in which it is not the final chord) it can function as a substitution for the subdominant chord.

The sentences were sung to melodies that did or did not contain an out-of-key note on the last word of the relative clause (underlined above). All the words in the sentences were monosyllabic, so that each word corresponded to one note. A control condition was included for an attention-getting but nonharmonically deviant musical event: a 10 dB increase in volume on the last word of the relative clause. After each sentence, participants were asked a comprehension question, and accuracy was assumed to reflect processing difficulty.

The results revealed an interaction between musical and linguistic processing: Comprehension accuracy was lower for sentences with distant versus local syntactic integrations (as expected), but crucially, this difference was larger when melodies contained an out-of-key note. The control condition (loud note) did not produce this effect: The difference between the two sentence types was of the same size as that in the conditions that did not contain an out-of-key note. These results suggest that some aspect of structural integration in language and music relies on shared processing resources.

The final study described here, by Slevc et al. (2009), manipulated linguistic syntactic integration difficulty via structural expectancy (cf. section 5.4.3, subsection on expectancy theory in language), and also directly compared the influence of musical harmonic manipulations on linguistic syntactic versus semantic processing. In this study, participants read sentences phrase by phrase on a computer screen. They controlled the timing of phrases by pushing a button to get the next phrase. In such studies, the amount of time spent viewing a phrase is assumed the reflect the amount of processing difficulty associated with that phrase. This "self-paced reading" paradigm has been much used in psycholinguistic research. The novel aspect of Slevc et al.'s study was that each phrase was accompanied by a chord so that the entire sentence made a coherent, Bach-style chord progression.

The sentences contained either a linguistic syntactic or semantic manipulation. In the syntactic manipulation, sentences like 5.5a included either a full or reduced sentence complement clause, achieved by including or omitting the word "that." In sentence 5.5a, for example, omitting "that" results in the reduced complement clause "the hypothesis was being studied in his lab." (Note: the vertical slashes in 5.5a and 5.5b below indicate the individual phrases used in the self-paced reading experiment.) In this case, when readers first encounter the phrase "the hypothesis", they tend to interpret it as the direct object of "confirmed," which causes syntactic integration difficulty when "was" is encountered, as this signals that "the hypothesis" is actually the subject of an embedded clause. In other words, the omission of "that" creates a "garden path" sentence with localized processing difficulty (on "was") due to violation of a syntactic expectancy. In the semantic manipulation, sentences like 5.5b included either a semantically consistent or anomalous word, thereby confirming or violating a semantic expectancy. The chord played during the critical word (underlined below) was either harmonically in-key or out-of-key. (Out-of-key chords were drawn from keys 3–5 steps away on the circle of fifths from the key of the phrase.) Because out-of-key chords are harmonically unexpected, the experiment crossed syntactic or semantic expectancy in language with harmonic expectancy in music. The dependent variable of interest was the reading time for the critical word.

> (5.5a) The scientist | wearing | thick glasses | confirmed (that) | the hypothesis | <u>was</u> | being | studied | in his lab.

> (5.5b) The boss | warned | the mailman | to watch | for angry | <u>dogs/pigs</u> | when | delivering | the mail.

The main finding was a significant three-way interaction between linguistic manipulation type (syntactic or semantic), linguistic expectancy, and musical expectancy. That is, syntactically and semantically unexpected words were read more slowly than their expected counterparts; a simultaneous out-of-key chord caused substantial additional slowdown for syntactically unexpected words, but not for semantically unexpected words. Thus, processing a harmonically unexpected chord interfered with the processing of syntactic, but not semantic, relations in language. Once again, these results support the claim that neural resources are shared between linguistic and musical syntactic processing.

Taken together, the three studies reviewed above point to shared neural resources underlying linguistic and musical syntactic processing. They also suggest that studies examining concurrent processing of language and music, which have been relatively rare to date, are a promising area for exploring issues of modularity in both domains.

Musical Syntactic Deficits in Aphasia

Remarkably, there has been virtually no work on musical syntactic processing in aphasia in modern cognitive neuroscience. This is particularly striking because an early study by Francès et al. (1973) suggested that aphasic individuals with linguistic comprehension disorders also have a deficit in the perception of musical tonality. The researchers studied a large group of aphasics and had them judge whether two short, isochronous melodies were the same or different. The melodies were either tonal or atonal. Under these circumstances, normal participants (even those with no musical training) show superior performance on the tonal stimuli. Aphasics failed to show this tonal superiority effect, leading the authors to suggest that the perception of tonality "seems to engage pre-established circuits existing in the language area" (p. 133).

This idea has lain fallow for decades, with no further studies of tonality perception in aphasia. Why might this be? Good tools for testing linguistic comprehension in aphasia and for probing the perception of tonal relations have long been available, yet no one has attempted to replicate or extend these results. This is made even more puzzling by the fact that the findings of Francès et al. were somewhat clouded by methodological issues, and naturally called for further work (cf. Peretz, 1993). It is likely that the absence of research on this topic reflects the emphasis on dissociations between aphasia and amusia (cf. section 5.4.1). However, given the caveats about such dissociations raised in section 5.4.1, and the predictions of SSIRH, it is clearly time to revisit this issue.

Patel, Iversen, Wassenaar, and Hagoort (2008) recently examined musical and linguistic syntactic processing in a population of 12 Broca's aphasics (none of whom had been a professional musician). Broca's aphasia is a type of aphasia in which individuals have marked difficulty with sentence production, though their speech comprehension often seems quite good. In fact, careful testing often reveals linguistic syntactic comprehension deficits. To check whether the aphasics we studied had such deficits, we employed a standard psycholinguistic test for syntactic comprehension. This "sentence-picture matching task" involves listening to one sentence at a time and then pointing to the corresponding picture on a sheet with four different pictures. Sentences varied across five levels of syntactic complexity. For example, a sentence with an intermediate level of complexity (level 3) was the passive structure: "The girl on the chair is greeted by the man" (Figure 5.17).

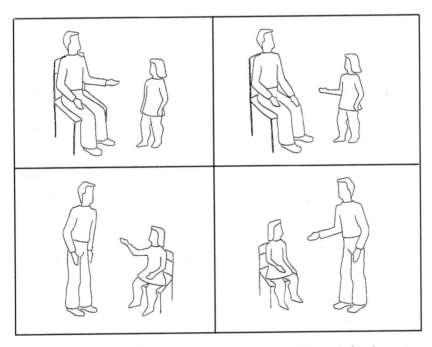

Figure 5.17 Example panel from the sentence-picture matching task for the sentence: "The girl on the chair is greeted by the man."

Determining who did what to whom in such sentences relies on syntactic information (e.g., simple word-order heuristics such as "first noun = agent" do not work). The aphasics performed significantly worse than controls on this test, which established that they did indeed have a syntactic comprehension deficit in language. They were therefore an appropriate population for studying relations between linguistic and musical syntactic deficits.

To test music and language in a comparable fashion, we had the aphasics (and matched controls) perform acceptability judgments on musical and linguistic sequences. The linguistic sequences were sentences ($n = 120$): Half contained either a syntactic or a semantic error. For example, the sentence "The sailors call for the captain and **demands** a fine bottle of rum" contains a syntactic agreement error, whereas "Anne scratched her name with her **tomato** on the wooden door" is semantically anomalous. We tested both syntax and semantics in order to determine if musical syntactic abilities were specifically related to linguistic syntax. The musical sequences were chord sequences ($n = 60$): Half contained an out-of-key chord, violating the musical syntax (harmony) of the phrase. The musical task was thus comparable to a sour-note detection task, though it used chords instead of a melody of single tones. (The chord sequences were taken from Patel, Gibson, et al.'s 1998 ERP study, and represented the "in-key" and "distant-key" conditions—cf. section 5.4.2 for background on these stimuli, and Figure 5.12 for an example.) We also had the aphasics and controls do an experiment involving same/different discrimination of short melodies, to check if they had any auditory short-term memory problems for musical material.

All aphasics had left-hemisphere lesions, though the locations were variable and did not always include Broca's area. Such variability is well known from studies of Broca's aphasia (Willmes & Poeck, 1993; Caplan et al., 1996) and precluded us from addressing issues of localization. We focused instead on cognitive relations between music and language based on performance on tasks in both domains.

Two aphasics and one control performed poorly on the melodic same/different task, and were excluded from further analysis; the remaining aphasics and controls did not differ in their performance on the melodic task, indicating that the groups were matched on basic perception of tone sequences. Turning to the main results, the primary finding of interest was that the aphasics performed significantly worse than controls on detecting harmonic anomalies in chord sequences, indicating a deficit in the processing of musical tonality (Figure 5.18).

They also showed a severe deficit on the linguistic syntactic task, and an impairment on the linguistic semantic task, though this just escaped statistical significance. Figure 5.19 shows the data in a different way, permitting the performance of individuals on the music task to be compared to their performance on the two language tasks.

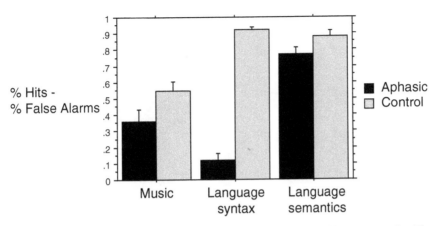

Figure 5.18 Performance of aphasics and controls on musical and linguistic tasks. The vertical axis shows percentage of hits minus percentage of false alarms in detecting harmonic, linguistic syntactic, and linguistic semantic anomalies. Error bars show 1 standard error.

As can be seen, there is a good deal of overlap between aphasics and controls on the music task, suggesting that linguistic agrammatism was associated with a relatively mild impairment of tonality perception in this group. Indeed, the fact that most aphasics score within the normal range on the music syntax test raises a question. Is the observed aphasic group deficit in tonality perception simply due to a few individuals with lesions that affect separate brain areas involved in language and music (and hence who score poorly in both domains)? Or is the lower performance of the aphasics as a group indicative of some systematic degradation in their perception of tonality, related to linguistic agrammatism? One way to address this question is to look at the correlation between performance on the music task and the language syntax task. For the aphasics, the simple correlation was not significant, but interestingly, when the controls were included in the correlation (via a multiple regression analysis), performance on the music syntax task was a significant predictor of performance on the language syntactic task. This points to some process common to language and music syntax that operates in both the controls and the aphasics, though at a degraded level in the aphasics. Notably, when the same type of multiple regression analysis was conducted on music syntax versus language semantics, performance on the music task did not predict linguistic performance. Hence the putative shared process appears to link music syntax to language syntax rather than to language semantics.

Although the above study employed explicit judgments of tonality, it is also important to test musical syntactic abilities using implicit tasks. This is because research by Tillmann (2005) has shown that individuals with music syntactic

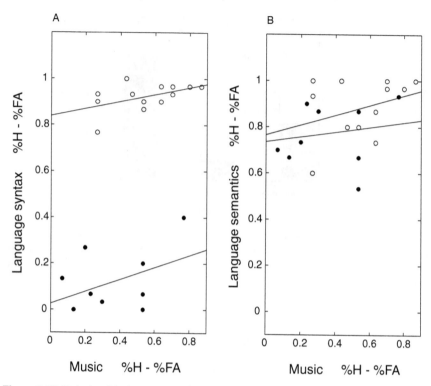

Figure 5.19 Relationship between performance on musical and linguistic tasks for aphasics (black dots) and controls (open circles). Separate best-fitting regression lines are shown for aphasics and controls. (A) shows relations between performance on the music task and the language syntax task, and (B) shows relations between performance on the music task and the language semantics task.

deficits in explicit tasks can nevertheless show implicit access to musical syntactic knowledge. The task we used to tap implicit syntactic abilities is harmonic priming (Bharucha & Stoeckig, 1986). Harmonic priming is a well-studied paradigm in music cognition that tests the influence of a preceding harmonic context on the processing of a target chord (cf. sections 5.2.3 and 5.2.4). Much research has shown that a target chord is processed more rapidly and accurately if it is harmonically close to (vs. distant from) the tonal center created by the prime (Bigand & Pineau 1997; Tillmann et al., 1998; Bigand et al., 1999; Justus & Bharucha, 2001; Tillmann & Bigand, 2001). Importantly, this advantage is due not simply to the psychoacoustic similarity of context and target, but to their distance in a structured cognitive space of chords and keys (Bharucha & Stoeckig, 1987; Tekman & Bharucha, 1998; Bigand et al., 2003). The harmonic priming effect thus indicates implicit knowledge of syntactic conventions in tonal music, and has been repeatedly demonstrated in nonmusician listeners in Western cultures (e.g., Bigand et al., 2003).

Patel, Iversen, and colleagues (2008) studied harmonic priming in Broca's aphasia using a second group of 9 Broca's aphasics (cf. Patel, 2005). (As in the first study, we first established that the aphasics had a syntactic comprehension deficit using the sentence-picture matching task. As in that study, all aphasics had left hemisphere lesions, but these did not always include Broca's area.) We used the original two-chord version of the harmonic priming task, with a single chord serving as the prime (Bharucha & Stoeckig, 1986). Prime and target were 1 s long each, separated by 50 ms. This places minimal demands on attention and memory and is thus suitable for use with aphasics. The harmonic distance between prime and target was regulated by the circle of fifths for musical keys: Harmonically close versus distant targets were two versus four steps clockwise steps away from the prime on the circle, respectively. This directly pits conventional harmonic distance against psychoacoustic similarity, because the distant target shares a common tone with the prime (Tekman & Bharucha, 1998; Figure 5.20).

The participants' task was to judge whether the second chord was tuned or mistuned (on 50% of the trials, it was mistuned by flattening one note in the chord). The main focus of interest, however, was the reaction time (RT) to

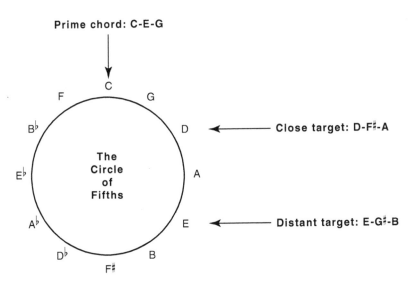

Figure 5.20 Example of prime and target chords for the harmonic priming task. All chords were major chords, being the principal chord of a key from the circle of fifths. In this case, the prime is a C major chord. The close target is a D major chord, and the distant target is an E major chord.

well-tuned targets as a function of their harmonic distance from the prime. A faster RT to close versus distant chords is evidence of harmonic priming. (Prior to doing the priming study, the aphasics completed two short experiments that showed that they could discriminate tuned from mistuned chords and did not have auditory short-term memory deficits.)

The results were clear. Controls showed normal harmonic priming, with faster reaction times to harmonically close versus distant well-tuned targets. Aphasics, however, failed to show a priming effect, and even showed a nonsignificant trend to be faster on distant targets, suggestive of responses driven by psychoacoustic similarity rather than by harmonic knowledge (Figure 5.21).

Thus aphasics with syntactic comprehension problems in language seem to have problems activating the implicit knowledge of harmonic relations that Western nonmusicians normally exhibit. Importantly, this deficit is not a generalized consequence of brain damage, because there are cases of individuals with bilateral cortical lesions who show normal harmonic priming (Tramo et al., 1990; Tillmann, 2005).

Together, these two aphasia studies point to a connection between linguistic and musical syntactic processing. The results are consistent with the SSIRH,

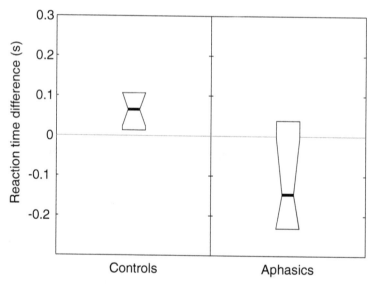

Figure 5.21 Box plots for RT difference to harmonically distant versus close targets. Data are for correct responses to tuned targets. The horizontal line in each box indicates the median value, the slanted box edges indicate confidence intervals, and the upper and lower bounds of the box indicate interquartile ranges. Absolute mean RTs for controls (s.e. in parentheses): close targets .99 (.07) s, distant targets 1.05 (.06) s. Aphasics: close targets 1.68 (.22) s, distant targets 1.63 (.17) s.

which suggests that music and language share neural resources for activating domain-specific representations during syntactic processing. A deficiency in these resources appears to influence both music and language. From the standpoint of neurolinguistics, this supports a "processing view" of syntactic disorders in aphasia, that is, a general problem activating stored syntactic representations (e.g., verbs together with their lexical category and thematic role information), rather than a disruption of these representations (Kolk & Friederici, 1985; Haarmann & Kolk, 1991; Kolk, 1998; Swaab et al., 1998; Kaan & Swaab, 2002). From the standpoint of music cognition, the results are notable in suggesting that left hemisphere language circuits play a role in musical syntactic processing in nonprofessional musicians. Future work seeking to determine the importance of particular left hemisphere circuits to music processing will need to employ aphasics with more tightly controlled lesion profiles. It will be interesting to know if aphasics with a more uniform lesion profile (e.g., agrammatic aphasics with left frontal brain damage) would show even stronger links between performance on language and music tasks than found in the current experiments, which employed aphasics with rather variable lesion profiles.

From a broader perspective, the above results indicate that it is time to re-awaken the study of music syntactic processing in aphasia, a topic that has experienced a 30-year hiatus since the pioneering work of Francès et al. (1973). Parallel studies of music and language offer a novel way to explore the nature of aphasic processing deficits (cf. Racette et al., 2006). Such research has clinical implications, and raises the intriguing possibility that it may ultimately be possible to model linguistic and musical syntactic deficits in aphasia in a common computational framework (cf. Tillmann et al., 2000; McNellis & Blumstein, 2001).

5.5 Conclusion

Roughly 30 years ago, Leonard Bernstein's provocative lectures at Harvard sparked interest in cognitive comparisons between musical and linguistic syntax. Although his own ideas on the subject have not stood the test of time, his intuition of an important link is now being supported by modern research in cognitive neuroscience. This research suggests that although musical and linguistic syntax have distinct and domain-specific syntactic representations, there is overlap in the neural resources that serve to activate and integrate these representations during syntactic processing (the "shared syntactic integration resource hypothesis" [SSIRH]). Exploring this overlap is exciting because it provides a novel way to illuminate the neural foundations of syntax in both domains.

This chapter has attempted to illustrate that comparative research on musical and linguistic syntax should be grounded in a solid understanding of the important differences between the two systems. Understanding these differences need not deter comparative research. On the contrary, they should guide such research past the pitfalls that trapped earlier thinkers (including Bernstein). Once these traps are avoided, a large and fertile field for investigation is reached, a field that has only just begun to be explored. Such explorations are likely to be the most fruitful when they are hypothesis-driven and based on empirically grounded cognitive theory in the two domains. If this can be achieved, then the power of the comparative method in biology can be brought to bear on the human mind's remarkable capacity for syntax.

Chapter 6
Meaning

6

Meaning

Note: Throughout this chapter, "language" refers to the ordinary language of everyday communication, not poetry, philosophy, or other specialized forms of discourse. "Music" refers to instrumental music—music without words—unless otherwise stated. The reasons for comparing instrumental music to ordinary language are rooted in cognitive science, and are discussed in Chapter 1.

6.1 Introduction

The relationship between linguistic and musical meaning has a paradoxical character. On the one hand, consider the much-cited remark of Claude Lévi-Strauss that music is "the only language with the contradictory attributes of being at once intelligible and untranslatable"[1] (Lévi-Strauss, 1964:18). That is, although it is possible to translate between any two human languages with reasonable fidelity,[2] it makes little sense to think of translating music into language (e.g., a Mozart symphony into words), or music into music (e.g., a Beethoven chamber music piece into a Javanese gamelan work) and expect that the meaning of the original material would be preserved.

On the other hand, music crosses cultural boundaries more easily than language does. That is, it is possible to encounter music from another culture and to take to it very quickly.[3] (In contrast, listening to speech in a novel foreign

---

[1] It should be noted that Hanslick (1854) made a similar observation more than 100 years earlier, in *The Beautiful in Music:* "In music there is both meaning and logical sequence, but in a musical sense; it is a language we speak and understand, but which we are unable to translate" (p. 50).

[2] I am speaking of ordinary day-to-day language, not poetry, and so forth. For ordinary language, the key point is that any natural language X can be translated into any other natural language Y well enough to convey the gist of the sentences in X. Of course, each language contains within its grammar and vocabulary a different way of looking at the world (Genter & Goldin-Meadow, 2003), so that no translation is ever perfect.

language is unlikely to sustain one's interest for long unless one has studied the language.) I have had this experience with several kinds of music, including Japanese koto music and Javanese gamelan music. In each case, I heard things in the music that I had never heard before, and felt compelled to return to the music to experience the new thoughts and feelings it inspired.

How can these apparently contradictory facts about music and language be explained? Let us first consider the issue of the translatability of language versus music. At a very general level, one can view different languages as different ways of achieving the same thing: the transmission of certain basic types of meanings between individuals. For example, all languages allow speakers (1) to make propositions, in other words, to refer to specific entities or concepts (such as "cousin" or "justice") and to predicate things about them, (2) to express wishes and ask questions, and (3) to make metalinguistic statements, such as "In my language we do not have a word that means the exactly the same thing as 'justice' in your language" (Hermerén, 1988).

Music does not bear these kinds of meanings. Furthermore, ethnomusicological research suggests it is unlikely that different musics are different ways of transmitting *any* basic, common set of meanings (Becker, 1986). Even within the confines of Western culture, the diversity of music belies simplistic ideas such as "musical meaning is always about X," in which X represents any single concept. Consider, for example, the assertion that the meaning of instrumental music is "always about emotion." Asserting that emotion is the sine qua non of musical meaning is problematic, because there are cases in which a listener can find music meaningful as a brilliant play of form without any salient sense of emotion (my own response to Bach fugues falls in this category).

6.1.1 Music and Translation

Broadening the view from Western music to the diversity of human cultures, it is difficult if not impossible to assign a universal set of meanings to music. This is why music, unlike language, cannot be translated without significantly changing the meaning of the original material. Consider the example given above of a Beethoven chamber music piece versus a Javanese gamelan piece. Let us assume for the sake of argument that these pieces are comparable in terms of the size of the musical ensemble (i.e., number of musicians and instruments). Let us further assume that these pieces are heard in Europe and Indonesia, respectively, by communities of knowledgeable listeners who know little about the music of other cultures. What would it mean to try to "translate" the Beethoven piece into a gamelan piece or vice versa? Of course, one could

---

[3] I have no empirical data to support this claim other than my own experience, but I doubt that I am unique. See Holst (1962) for an informal description of Indian children coming to appreciate Western classical music after an initial aversive reaction.

transfer certain surface features: The Western orchestra could play the Javanese melodies and the gamelan could play the Beethoven melodies. Yet even here there would be challenges, such as differences in musical scales and a loss of the original timbres and textures. Unlike with language, these sonic changes due to translation are not merely incidental to meaning. The meaning of the Beethoven piece is intimately tied to the particular sounds used to create it—the scales and their attendant harmonies, the timbre of the string instruments, and so forth—and the same can be said of the gamelan piece. Furthermore, even if a highly talented composer managed to create a Western piece that captured some of the features of gamelan music, this is no guarantee that the European audience hearing the "translated gamelan" would experience meanings at all similar to the Indonesian audience hearing real gamelan music (and vice versa), because of differences in listening habits, culture, and context. The difficulties of musical translation can be contrasted to the comparative ease of translating between language and having both audiences derive similar meanings from the resulting translations (e.g., translating an Indonesian news broadcast into German).

Having discussed the difficulty of musical translation, let us now consider the seemingly paradoxical observation that music can be more readily appreciated across cultural boundaries than language when there is no translation, in other words, when the listener hears foreign sounds of which they have little or no previous experience. Of course, it is by no means guaranteed that a listener from one culture will appreciate the music of another. However, the salient fact is that such a thing *can* occur. Thus the relevant question is "How is this possible?" One idea is that appreciation of foreign music is purely sensual: Unfamiliar timbres may "tickle the ear," but there is no real sense of the music's structure or significance. In this view, the foreign music is simply experienced as a pleasant and somewhat evocative sonic goulash. There are empirical reasons to treat this view with skepticism, because research has shown that listeners unfamiliar with a new music are nevertheless sensitive to the statistical distributions of tones within the music, and can infer some structural relations on this basis (Castellano et al., 1984; Kessler et al., 1984; Oram & Cuddy, 1995; Krumhansl et al., 1999, 2000).

Another possible basis for cross-cultural appreciation of music is that one hears sonic relationships based on one's own culture-specific listening habits. For example, one might hear rhythmic groups and melodic motives, though these may not correspond to the groups and motives heard by a native listener (Ayari & McAdams, 2003). In Javanese gamelan music, this can happen when a Western listener parses a rhythmically strong event as the "downbeat" or beginning of a rhythmic pattern, when native listeners hear it as the end of the pattern. The key point, however, is that even though one's parsing of the music may be "wrong" from the standpoint of a cultural insider, one may nevertheless find the music rewarding because one perceives patterns and sensibilities that are not just trivial variants of those known from one's native music.

Finally, one may actually perceive musical relations in a manner resembling that of a native listener. This could occur because certain patterns occur in both one's native music and in the new music, such as a steady beat or the tendency for a structural "gap" in a melody to be "filled" by subsequent notes (Meyer, 1973; cf. Krumhansl et al., 2000). Intuitively, however, it seems unlikely that naïve listening will yield results similar to culturally informed listening, especially if one considers more complex structural relations and the cultural significance of musical phenomena.

Let us focus on one explanation offered above, namely the idea that one can perceive structure and significance in unfamiliar music even if one's parsing of the music is not the same as a native listener's. The fact that this can occur suggests that there is an aspect of musical meaning that is purely formal. That is, unlike language, music can have meaning for a listener simply because of its perceived sonic logic, without knowledge of the context that gave rise to the music or of an insider's understanding of its cultural significance (Rothstein, 1996).

Thus music can have the paradoxical properties of being untranslatable yet at times still able to cross cultural boundaries without translation. *In both of these respects, musical meaning is quite unlike linguistic meaning.* Is it therefore the case that linguistic and musical meaning are incommensurate, and that comparative empirical research is unlikely to be fruitful? Not at all. As we shall see, certain aspects of the relationship between linguistic and musical meaning can be studied in an empirical fashion. Such comparative studies are worthwhile because they can contribute to the ongoing scholarly dialogue about musical versus linguistic meaning, and can help shed light on human cognitive and neural function.

6.1.2 What Does One Mean by "Meaning"?

Any systematic comparison of meaning in music and language presupposes that one has a clear idea of what one means by linguistic and musical "meaning." On the linguistic side, it may come as a surprise to some readers that there is considerable debate over what linguistic meaning is and how it is constituted (Langacker, 1988; Partee, 1995). For the purposes of this book, we will not delve into these debates and will treat linguistic meaning in a fairly elementary way. Linguistic meaning can be broadly divided into two areas: semantics and pragmatics. Semantics concerns how words and sentences reflect reality or our mental representation of reality, and its units of analysis are propositions. Pragmatics concerns how listeners add contextual information to sentences and draw inferences about what has been said (Jaszczolt, 2002). Most comparative discussions of linguistic and musical meaning focus on semantics, though as we shall see in section 6.3.2, it may ultimately prove more fruitful to focus on pragmatics.

What of musical meaning? The introduction of this chapter discussed musical meaning without defining it, leaving the definition to the reader's intuition. For scientific research, however, this is unsatisfactory. A natural place to turn for help in defining musical meaning is the work of music theorists and philosophers of aesthetics, who have written (and continue to write) a great deal on the topic (e.g., Meyer, 1956; Cooke, 1959; Coker, 1972; Rantala et al., 1988; Kivy, 1990; 2002; Nattiez, 1990; Davies, 1994; 2003; Cumming, 2000; Monelle, 2000; Koopman & Davies, 2001; Kramer, 2002; Zbikowski, 2002, among many other books and articles). No consensus has emerged from these writings for a definition of musical meaning, although several positions have been clearly articulated and carefully argued. Broadly speaking, these positions can be arrayed along a conceptual axis with regard to how specific versus general the term "meaning" is taken to be. An example of a position with a very specific view is that of the philosopher Kivy (2002), who argues that "meaning" should be reserved for the linguistic sense of reference and predication. In this view, music does not have meaning. Indeed, Kivy (personal communication) argues that music "cannot even be meaningless," because music does not have the *possibility* of being meaningful in this linguistic sense. In this view, asking whether music has meaning is like asking whether a rock is dead: It is a "category error." (The concept of "dead" does not apply to rocks because only things that are alive have the possibility of being dead.) Kivy readily acknowledges that music can have "significance" and "logic" (in syntactic terms), and that music can express emotion. In rejecting the notion of musical meaning, he is taking a highly specific view of "meaning," perhaps in order to avoid diluting the term to the point at which it ceases to make useful distinctions in discussing the varieties of human thought.

At the other end of the spectrum, the music theorist and ethnomusicologist Jean-Jacques Nattiez has argued for an inclusive use of the term "meaning." Nattiez (1990) considers meaning to be signification in the broadest semiotic sense: Meaning exists when perception of an object/event brings something to mind other than the object/event itself. Implicit in this view is the notion that language should not be taken as the model of signification in general (Nattiez, 2003). Also implicit is the idea that meaning is not a property of an object/event, because the same object/event can be meaningful or meaningless in different circumstances, depending on whether it brings something else to mind (cf. Meyer, 1956:34). That is, "meaning" is inherently a dynamic, relational process. I would add to Nattiez's view the idea that meaning admits of degrees, related to the number and complexity of things brought to mind. For example, in some circumstances, the sound of a piano piece may mean nothing more to a listener than "my neighbor is practicing," whereas in other circumstances, the same piece may engage the same listener's mind in intricate mentations related to musical structure, emotion, and so forth.

From the standpoint of comparative research on language and music, both Kivy's and Nattiez's positions are interesting. The first position focuses our attention on meaning as semantic reference, and leads us to ask what the closest musical analog of this might be. As we shall see in section 6.3.1, recent research in cognitive neuroscience is pertinent to this issue. The second view encourages us to think about the variety of ways in which musical elements bring other things to mind. In the spirit of the second approach, section 6.2 provides a brief taxonomy of musical meaning, to explore the different ways in which music can be meaningful. This is followed by a section on linguistic meaning in relation to music, which discusses linguistic semantics and pragmatics. The final section of the chapter explores the expression and appraisal of emotion as a key link between spoken language and music.

6.2 A Brief Taxonomy of Musical Meaning

The following is a brief review of 11 types of musical meaning that have been discussed by scholars of music. This is not an exhaustive list, but it touches on many of the major areas of discussion and serves to illustrate the breadth of meanings conveyed by instrumental music. The list is arranged such that more "intramusical" meanings are discussed first: Meanings become more and more "extramusical" (relating to things outside the music) as one moves down the list. The focus is on Western European music unless otherwise stated, and comparisons with linguistic meaning are made whenever possible.

It should be noted that an interesting line of research on musical meaning concerns the study of film music, which is not reviewed here because our focus is on purely instrumental music (see Cohen, 2001, and Tagg & Clarida, 2003, for research on this topic).

6.2.1 The Structural Interconnection of Musical Elements

The purest form of intramusical meaning exists when musical elements bring other musical elements to mind. The prototypical example of this is musical expectation, when heard elements bring other, expected elements to mind (Meyer, 1956). This is illustrated by the "gap-fill" pattern discussed by Meyer (1956, 1973), in which a large interval in a melody (a "gap") leads to an expectation for successive pitches that will "fill" this interval by traversing the gapped space in small steps (cf. Huron, 2006:84–85).

Expectations in music can come from multiple sources. Some expectations are thought to be based on auditory universals related to Gestalt properties of audition (cf. Narmour, 1990), such as an overall expectation for small pitch intervals. Expectations also arise via learning of style-specific aspects of music, such as the chord progressions typical of Western tonal music (cf. Chapter 5), and from piece-specific regularities, such as the realization that a particular antecedent phrase is answered by a particular consequent phrase in the current piece. In each of these cases, the type of meaning generated is music-internal: It refers to nothing outside of the music itself. Meyer (1956) has called this form of meaning "embodied" meaning, which exists when a stimulus "indicates or implies events or consequences that are of the same kind as the stimulus itself" (p. 35). Meyer contrasted this with "designative" meaning, which exists when a stimulus "indicates events or consequences which are different from itself in kind, as when a word designates or points to an object which is not itself a word" (p. 35). Following Meyer, different scholars have used different terms to refer the same basic distinction, for example, Nattiez's (1990) "intrinsic versus extrinsic referring," and Jakobson's (1971) "introversive versus extroversive semiosis." I will use the terms "intramusical" and "extramusical," because "embodied" has a specific connotation in modern cognitive neuroscience that is distinct from what Meyer intended.

A focus on intramusical meaning is a characteristic of the "absolutist" or "formalist" approach to musical aesthetics. As noted above, expectation is an important processes in creating formal meaning. Kivy (2002:78) suggests another process, analogous to a game of hide and seek, whereby a listener seeks to identify previously heard themes, which may be more or less disguised via their embedding in larger musical textures. Although expectation is a forward-directed process in which current musical elements bring future ones to mind, musical "hide and seek" is a recollective process in which current elements bring past elements back to mind. In both cases, meaning exists because the mind reaches out beyond the present moment to make contact with other musical elements in the imagination or in memory.

A forerunner of the absolutist position was Eduard Hanslick, whose short and influential book *The Beautiful in Music* (1854) argued that the study of musical aesthetics should be rooted in musical structure, and not in the emotions of listeners (which he argued were quite capricious). Hanslick proposed that "the essence of music is sound in motion," and offered the analogy of a kaleidoscope in describing musical beauty:

> When young, we have probably all been delighted with the ever-changing tints and forms of a kaleidoscope. Now, music is a kind of kaleidoscope, though its forms can be appreciated only by an infinitely higher ideation. It brings forth a profusion of beautiful tints and forms, now sharply contrasted and now almost imperceptibly graduated; all logically connected with each other, yet all novel in their effect; forming, as it were, a complete and self-subsistent whole, free from all alien admixture. (p. 48)

Hanslick's analogy of music as ever-shifting and self-contained forms nicely captures a formalist view of music. There is a flaw in his analogy, however, that leads to an interesting psychological question for the formalist position. In a kaleidoscope, the successive patterns are not really logically connected: One pattern merely follows another without any sense of progress or direction (Kivy, 2002:62–63). In contrast, a sense of logical connectedness in music is central to the formalist approach to musical meaning. Formalist theories often posit structural relations at time scales ranging from a few adjacent notes to thousands of notes, in other words, up to time scales spanning an entire piece (which can take many tens of minutes to perform). Human cognition is known for its limited capacity to remember and process information in short-term memory, raising the question of the relevance of large-scale form to intramusical meaning from a listener's perspective.

Whether large-scale relations are in fact part of a listener's apprehension of a music has been the focus of an interesting line of empirical research. One early and influential study in this vein is that of Cook (1987b), who focused on an aspect of structure known as "tonal closure." Tonal closure exists when music starts and ends in the same key, and is characteristic of most of the music in the Western European tradition. Music theorists have posited that departure from the initial key of a piece contributes to musical tension, and that this component of tension is not resolved until the home key is reached again (e.g., Schenker, 1979; Lerdahl & Jackendoff, 1983). This idea naturally predicts that listeners should distinguish between pieces that start and end in the same key versus in different keys, perhaps preferring the former as sounding more coherent or aesthetically satisfying. Cook tested this idea by transposing the final section of a number of classical piano pieces to a different key, so that the starting and ending key were different. Undergraduate music students heard the original and manipulated pieces and were asked to rate them on four aesthetic scales, including "coherence" and "sense of completion."

Cook found that only for the shortest piece (1 minute in length) did the listeners rate the original piece higher than the altered one. Cook notes that because most classical pieces are considerably longer than 1 minute, theories of large-scale tonal unity might not be relevant to a listener's perceptual experience. Cook wisely points out that this does not mean that such theories are musically irrelevant; they may help reveal how composers' designed their work, thus addressing the piece's *conceptual* structure (rather than its *perceptual* structure). What is notable, however, in both Cook's study and subsequent studies that have manipulated musical form by scrambling the order of sections in a piece, is the lack of sensitivity to large-scale structure, *even in highly trained musicians* (e.g., Karno & Konečni, 1992; Deliège et al., 1996; Tillmann & Bigand, 1996; Marvin & Brinkman, 1999). At least one philosopher who favors a formal approach to music has argued that the structural relations we apprehend in music are much more localized in time than has been generally assumed (Levinson, 1997), perhaps limited to about 1 minute in duration (see Tan & Spackman, 2005 for some relevant empirical data)

From the standpoint of comparison with language, these studies of musical manipulation are quite interesting, because doing comparable experiments with language would likely produce quite a different result. For example, imagine taking a magazine article that requires tens of minutes to read, scrambling the order of the paragraphs or sections, and then asking readers to judge whether the original or scrambled version is more coherent. There is little doubt that readers would favor the original. This suggests that unless sequences have the qualities of semantic reference and predication, the mind can forge only structural relations within such sequences over a rather limited timescale.[4]

As described so far, the absolutist position is quite "cold," focusing only on structure and devoid of any discussion of music's expressiveness or of the dynamic feelings it engenders. For many people, these latter aspects are fundamental to musical meaning. Absolutists recognize the importance of emotion in music, and have found different ways of making a link to emotion. Meyer (1956) argues that music creates emotion in a listener when an expectation is not fulfilled. Because this type of affect is inextricably intertwined with expectation, it can be considered a part of intramusical meaning (p. 39). That is, Meyer's emotion is a type of musical affect reflecting a transient arousal due to a dynamic process, and is not the same as emotion in the everyday sense of the term (e.g., happiness, sadness), because it lacks a positive or negative valence (though it may receive a post hoc interpretation in terms of valence). As we shall see in section 6.2.3, this view has found interesting support in empirical studies of music and emotion.

A related way of reconciling formalism and emotion is to focus on the feelings of tension and resolution that music engenders. A formalist could argue that these feelings are part of intramusical meaning, because they do not depend on mental connection to concepts or phenomena in the outside world, growing instead out of music-internal factors such as harmonic syntax (cf. Chapter 5 for an extended discussion of musical syntax and tension, including empirical studies). Jackendoff (1991) argues that these feelings are an important part of musical affect. Once again, it is worth noting that this form of affect is unlike everyday emotions: It is a dynamic feeling that is essentially unvalenced (Sloboda, 1998).

A different approach to linking formalism and emotion is taken by Kivy (1980, 2002) and Davies (1980, 1994), who argue that music is capable of expressing everyday human emotions (such as happiness, sadness) by virtue of its form. The details of the link between form and emotion will be explored

---

[4] People can perceive structural coherence in at least one type of nonlinguistic sequence over long timescales, namely in films without words. However, this reflects the perceived coherence of the story, which has a strong semantic component.

in the next section; for the moment, the relevant point is that this approach effectively treats emotion as an extramusical issue, because music somehow brings to mind the emotions of everyday human life.

6.2.2 *The Expression of Emotion*

Any scientific discussion of emotion and music requires a conceptual distinction between the expression of emotion by music and the experience of emotion by listeners. The former refers to the affective qualities of a musical piece as judged by a listener (i.e., the "mood" projected by the music), whereas the latter refers to a listener's own emotional reaction to music. The crucial point is these are distinct phenomena (cf. Juslin & Laukka, 2004). It is quite possible, for example, for a listener to judge a piece as "sounding sad" but to have no emotional reaction to it. This section deals with the expression of emotion by music, and the next section deals with the experience of emotion by listeners.

Contemporary scientific studies of musical expression typically take the following form. Listeners are presented with pieces of instrumental music and are asked to select from a list of a few simple emotional categories—such as happiness, sadness, anger, and fear—the one that best captures the emotions expressed by each piece (Gabrielsson & Juslin, 1996; Krumhansl, 1997; Balkwill & Thompson, 1999; Peretz, Gagnon, et al., 1998; Peretz, 2001). Listeners may also be asked to give a numerical rating of how strongly the piece expresses the chosen emotion or other emotions. The experimenter chooses pieces that they feel exemplify these different categories, or use pieces in which a performer was explicitly instructed to play in a manner that expresses one of the basic emotions. (They may also create pieces by manipulating musical parameters of existing pieces, such as tempo or mode [major/minor].) Experiments of this sort, using music from Western European tradition, have found broad agreement among listeners in judging expressive qualities in music (see Gabrielsson & Lindström, 2001, for a thorough review). Indeed, when the categories are restricted to just two (e.g., happy vs. sad) and the stimuli are chosen appropriately, adults can reliably judge affect after hearing less than a second of music (Peretz, Gagnon, et al., 1998, cf. Bigand et al., 2005), and children can make reliable affective judgments of extended passages by the age of 5 or 6 (Gerardi & Gerken, 1995; Dalla Bella et al., 2001).

Although the consistency of affective judgments in such studies is impressive, one might object that research that focuses on only a few emotion categories is not very realistic in terms of the affective subtleties of music. One way to address this problem is to offer listeners a greater range of emotion terms to choose from. Hevner (1936, 1937) set an important precedent in this regard: She had a list of nearly 70 adjectives that listeners could check to indicate the affective characteristics of a piece. She arranged these adjectives into eight clusters to create an "adjective circle" in which relatedness between clusters was reflected by distance along the circle (Figure 6.1).

Gregory and Varney (1996) also used an extensive list, and showed that listeners chose different adjectives for different types of music, rather than using the same basic adjectives for all music (cf. Nielzén & Cesarec, 1981). Perhaps the best way to simultaneously give listeners freedom of choice while also constraining choices to some degree (to facilitate empirical analysis) is to conduct a preliminary study in which listeners supply their own adjectives, and then to conduct a second experiment using rating scales based on frequently chosen adjectives (cf. Gregory, 1995).

There is another reason to be cautious about studies that offer listeners only a few simple emotion terms to describe music. Musicologists who have studied expression in a serious way often suggest affective categories that are more nuanced than simple labels such as "happy" and "sad." For example, in his widely read book *The Language of Music*, Cooke (1959) argued that composers of Western European tonal music shared a "vocabulary" of 16 musical figures that expressed different types of affect. For example, he argued that the pattern 5-6-5 in minor (in which the numbers indicate scale degrees) gives "the effect of a burst of anguish. This is the most widely used of all terms of musical language: one can hardly find a page of 'grief' music by any tonal composer of any period without encountering it several times" (p. 146). Cooke supported this claim with examples from a 14th-century Belgian *chanson*, from the "Virgin's Cradle Song" by Byrd, from Mozart's *Don Giovanni*, Beethoven's *Fidelio*, and so forth. This example illustrates Cooke's general approach of identifying a musical figure and then presenting an impressive array of examples over historical time, expressing (according to Cooke) similar affective meaning.

Cooke felt that the affective associations of his "basic emotional vocabulary" were rooted in the tonal properties of the figures (their particular intervals and harmonic implications), and that they became conventional and widely understood by both composers and listeners via centuries of consistent use in tonal music. One perceptual study with modern listeners has failed to support Cooke's hypothesis (Gabriel, 1978), though it should be noted that this study may have not have been an entirely fair test due to methodological issues (Sloboda, 1985:62–64). Although Cooke's ideas have been a favorite target of criticism by many philosophers and music theorists, it remains an open question the extent to which Western European listeners would agree on the emotions expressed by the musical figures he investigated.[5] For the moment, however, the salient point is that Cooke is an example of a thoughtful humanist who has

---

[5] Indeed, some of Cooke's writing leads quite naturally into specific and interesting empirical hypotheses (see especially 1959: Ch. 4).

VI
bright
cheerful
gay
happy
joyous
merry

VII
agitated
dramatic
exciting
exhilarated
impetuous
passionate
restless
sensational
soaring
triumphant

V
delicate
fanciful
graceful
humorous
light
playful
quaint
sprightly
whimsical

VIII
emphatic
exalting
majestic
martial
ponderous
robust
vigorous

IV
calm
leisurely
lyrical
quiet
satisfying
serene
soothing
tranquil

I
awe-inspiring
dignified
lofty
sacred
serious
sober
solemn
spiritual

III
dreamy
longing
plaintive
pleading
sentimental
tender
yearning
yielding

II
dark
depressing
doleful
frustrated
gloomy
heavy
melancholy
mournful
pathetic
sad
tragic

Figure 6.1 The Hevner adjective circle. The underlined term in each cluster was chosen by Hevner as a key term, broadly representing the adjectives in each cluster. From Gabrielsson & Lindström, 2001, and Farnsworth, 1954.

studied musical expression and finds that far more than four or five basic terms are needed to adequately describe the emotions expressed by music.

Although recognizing the limitations of studies of expression based on just a few predetermined emotional categories, we will focus on such studies here because they have been the most sophisticated in terms of analyzing cues to musical expressiveness. That is, they have simplified one problem (the number of emotional categories) in order to focus efforts on another complex problem: the relation between perceived expressiveness and specific acoustic properties. This has allowed good progress to be made, and one hopes that future work will expand the number of categories so that research can be both conceptually and technically sophisticated.

Some of the cues that have proven to be important in the perception of musical expression are tempo, pitch register, and timbre (see Box 6.1 and references in Balkwill & Thompson, 1999, p. 48, and cf. Gabrielsson & Lindström, 2001, Table 10.2 for more detail). For example, music with a fast tempo, high average pitch, and bright timbre is much more likely to be identified as expressing "happiness" than "sadness," and vice versa. In contrast to these cues, which do not depend on the particular tonal structure of Western music, other affectively relevant cues do reflect the peculiarities of the Western European musical system. The most obvious of these is the conventional link between major keys and positive emotions, and minor keys and negative emotions, a link to which even very young children in Western culture are sensitive (Gerardi & Gerken, 1995). One important point, emphasized by Gabrielsson and Lindström (2001), is that the influence of any given factor depends on what other factors are present, and a good deal more work is needed to study how factors interact in the perception of expressive qualities.

Demonstrating that there are reliable links between particular musical cues and judgments of musical mood is an important step in the scientific study of musical expressiveness, but it is just the first step. From a cognitive perspective, two questions are especially salient. First, what is the mental basis for each observed link? Second, how universal are these links across musical cultures?

In answering the first question, one obvious candidate is speech. Listeners are quite good at judging the affective qualities of a voice, in other words, judging the mood it expresses independent of the lexical meanings of the words. There is a sizable body of research on the acoustic cues to vocal affect, and some of the findings are quite parallel to those found in research on perception of musical affect (Johnstone & Scherer, 2000). For example, tempo and average pitch height are important cues to affect in both speech and music: Sad voices and musical passages are likely to be slower and lower pitched than happy ones. The link between cues to emotion in speech and music has been the focus of research effort in recent years, and will be discussed in more detail in section 6.5.1. For now, suffice it to say that language may be one important source of music's expressive power.

Box 6.1 Some Cues Associated With Judgments of Musical Expressiveness in Western European Tonal Music

Tempo	Melodic contour	Harmonic complexity
Melodic complexity	Rhythmic complexity	Articulation
Dynamics	Consonance/dissonance	Pitch register
Pitch range	Timbre	Key (major/minor)

Source: Adapted from Balkwill & Thompson, 1999.

There are, of course, other possible bases for links between acoustic cues and perceived expression. Both Kivy (1980) and Davies (1980), for example, suggest that musical patterns can resemble the physical bearing or movements of people in different emotional states. Thus, for example, slow, sagging musical themes might get their expressive power from the way they resemble the physical movements of a depressed person (cf. Clynes, 1977, Damasio, 2003). According to this view, certain cues are experienced as expressive simply by virtue of their resemblance to human bearings or expressions. Davies (2003:181) offers the analogy of the face of a basset hound, which is often perceived as expressive of sadness not because the dog itself is sad, but because its physiognomy resembles in some ways the visage of a sad person.

In addition to links with vocal affect and body image, another possible source of expressiveness in music is a metaphorical relation between structure and emotion. For example, empirical research has shown that simple melodic structure is often linked with judgments of happiness, and complex structure with judgments of sadness, at least in Western listeners (Nielzén & Cesarec, 1981; Balkwill & Thompson, 1999). It is difficult to relate these facets of music to vocal affect or to aspects of human comportment. They may instead reflect a form of metaphorical understanding whereby happiness is considered a simpler mental state, whereas sadness is considered more complex and multifaceted (as intimated in the famous opening line of Tolstoy's *Anna Karenina*).

The second question posed above, about the universality of links between particular cues and particular emotions, is actually two independent questions. First, do the emotional categories that have been proposed for Western European tonal music apply cross-culturally? Second, if other cultures can be found in which it makes sense to talk about music expressing sadness, happiness, and so forth, how consistent is the mapping between musical cues and perceived affect? For example, might one find a culture in which slow tempi are associated with happy music and fast tempi with sad music? With regard to the first question, it is known that non-Western musical traditions exist that posit that instrumental music can have expressive qualities. One well-studied case is that of Indian classical music, in which different ragas (musical compositions characterized by a particular scale, tonal hierarchy, and melodic gestures) are claimed to express different characteristic moods, or "rasas" (Becker, 2001). Another case is Javanese gamelan music, which also recognizes that different compositions can have quite different affective content. Recently, Benamou (2003) conducted an interesting comparative analysis of affective terms applied to Western versus Javanese music by experts within each culture. For Western music, he took the eight key terms from Hevner's adjective circle, such as "dignified," "sad," "serene," (see Figure 6.1). For Javanese music, he proposed a set of six Javanese affect terms derived from field work with musical experts in Java. In some cases, there was a fairly good semantic mapping between Western and Javanese affect terms: For example, the Javanese musical affect terms "regu" and "sedih" include "dignified" and "sadness" in their connotations, respectively. In other cases, however, terms did not map from one culture to another in a straightforward way. Benamou's work alerts us to the fact that one cannot simply assume that musical affective categories are uniform across cultures. Only those affective categories shared by different cultures are appropriate for addressing the consistency of the link between musical cues and musical expressiveness.

Fortunately, such affective categories do exist and have been the focus of cross-cultural research on cues to expression. One such line of research has been pioneered by Balkwill and colleagues, based on fieldwork in multiple countries and on perceptual experiments. For example, Balkwill and Thompson (1999) examined Western listeners' perception of mood in Indian ragas. These listeners had no knowledge of Indian classical music, and heard 12 ragas that were meant to express four different emotions according to the Indian rasa system: hasya (joy), karuna (sadness), raudra (anger), and shanta (peace). The ragas were performed on sitar or flute (i.e., there was no vocal component). For each raga, listeners rated which emotion was expressed the most strongly, and then gave a numerical rating of how strongly each of the four emotions was expressed in that raga. They also rated each piece for tempo, rhythmic complexity, melodic complexity, and pitch range. The results revealed that listeners could identify the intended emotion when it was joy, sadness, or anger, even though they were naive with respect to the Indian classical tradition. Using correlation and regression techniques, Balkwill and Thompson showed that ratings of joy were associated with fast tempo and low melodic complexity, ratings of sadness were associated with slow tempo and high melodic complexity, and ratings of anger were related to timbre: Listeners were more likely to identify the "harder" timbre of the sitar (a stringed instrument) with anger than the softer timbre of the flute.

Balkwill and Thompson (1999) argue for a distinction between "psychophysical" and "culture-specific" cues to musical expressiveness. They regard their findings as evidence for the cross-cultural nature of psychophysical cues to expression. In contrast, sensitivity to culture-specific cues presumably requires enculturation in a particular tonal system. This would predict, for example, that the affective quality of the major/minor distinction in Western music is evident only to those who have grown up listening to this music and who have formed associations between these modes and expressive content (e.g., via hearing songs in which words with affective content are paired with music). As noted above, a link with affective cues in speech might be one reason that certain musical cues to affect are perceived in a consistent way across cultures. This topic is discussed in more detail in section 6.5.

6.2.3 The Experience of Emotion

Some of the oldest written observations about music concern its power over the emotions. More than 2,000 years ago, Plato claimed in *The Republic* that melodies in different modes aroused different emotions, and argued that this was such a strong influence on moral development that society should ban certain forms of music (cf. Holloway, 2001). Many other writers have affirmed music's emotional power, and there is ample evidence for the importance of emotion in the musical experience of many contemporary listeners (Juslin & Sloboda, 2001). To take just one example, psychological studies of music's role in everyday life reveal that listening to music is often used as a way of regulating mood (Denora, 1999; Sloboda & O'Neill, 2001). Given the pervasive link between music and emotional response, it may come as a surprise that the scientific study of this topic is a relatively young endeavor. Undoubtedly, one reason for this is the challenge of measuring emotion in a quantitative and reliable fashion: Emotions associated with music may not have any obvious behavioral consequence, can be fleeting and hard to categorize, and can vary substantially between individuals listening to the same music. Although these challenges make the empirical study of musical emotion difficult, they do not make it impossible, as evidenced by a growing stream of publications from researchers who have sought creative ways of tapping into the moment-by-moment emotional experience of listeners.

In this brief section, it is impossible to provide a thorough review of empirical studies of emotion in music (see Juslin & Sloboda, 2001). Hence I focus instead on one question of cognitive interest: Are the emotions experienced during music listening the same as the everyday emotions of human life (e.g., happiness, sadness, anger), or does music elicit emotions that do not fit neatly into the preestablished everyday categories (cf. Scherer, 2004)? To answer this question, one needs to first provide a list of everyday emotions, in other words, emotions that are part of the normal business of living life, and whose basic role in human existence is attested by their presence cross-culturally. Emotion researchers have offered different lists based on different criteria (though it should be noted that some researchers are critical of the idea of basic emotions altogether, for example, Ortony & Turner, 1990). Based on universal facial expressions, Ekman et al. (1987) have proposed the following list: anger, disgust, fear, joy, sadness, and surprise. Other researchers have included emotions such as shame, tenderness, and guilt in their lists. For the purposes of this section, I will take happiness, sadness, anger, and fear as basic human emotions. Can music elicit these emotions? How can one determine scientifically if in fact a listener is experiencing these emotions?[6]

In a relevant study, Krumhansl (1997) had participants listen to six 3-minute instrumental musical excerpts chosen to represent sadness, fear, or happiness. (For example, Albinoni's *Adagio in G minor* was used for sadness, Mussorgsky's *Night on Bare Mountain* for fear, and Vivaldi's "La Primavera" from *The Four Seasons* for happiness.) One group of participants listened to all pieces and rated them for sadness; another group rated all pieces for happiness, and a third group rated the pieces for fear. Crucially, participants were instructed to judge their own emotional reactions to the pieces, not the emotion expressed by the music. They indicated how strongly they felt the target emotion in a continuous fashion by moving a slider on a computer screen while listening. Krumhansl found that the musical selections did produce the intended emotions according to participant ratings.

In addition to this behavioral study, Krumhansl also conducted a physiological study in which a separate group of participants listened to the same pieces but gave no behavioral responses. Instead, a dozen different aspects of their physiology were monitored during music listening, including cardiac interbeat interval, respiration depth, and skin conductance. Many of these measures reflected the amount of activation of the autonomic (sympathetic) nervous system. Furthermore, physiological parameters changed depending on the dominant emotion (e.g., cardiac interbeat interval was lowest—i.e., heartbeat was fastest—for the happy excerpts), and these changes were fairly (but not totally) consistent with physiological changes associated with emotions elicited in other, nonmusical contexts using dynamic media, such as film and radio plays (cf. Nyklíček et al., 1997). Overall, Krumhansl's results suggest that everyday emotions can be aroused by instrumental music, and raise interesting questions about the psychological mechanisms by which this takes place. In particular, although it is known that music can express different emotions via the use of specific cues (cf. section 6.2.2), why does this lead people to respond with a similar emotion (vs. a "distanced" perception of mood)? Does the reaction reflect something about human capacity for empathy? Or is it an example of contagion, in other words, the passive spreading of an affective response (cf. Provine, 1992)?

---

[6] Based on extensive firsthand cross-cultural research, Becker (2001, 2004) argues that the precise emotions experienced during musical listening appear to vary from culture to culture, being subject to social and contextual forces. Although acknowledging this point, I focus here on basic emotions that arguably appear in every human society, though they may be culturally inflected.

Accepting that music can elicit everyday emotions, is it also possible to demonstrate that there are musical emotions that are not simple counterparts of
the emotions of everyday life? Such a view has been proposed by a number of
philosophers, including Susanne Langer (1942), who argues that "a composer
not only indicates, but *articulates* subtle complexes of feeling that language
cannot name, let alone set forth" (p. 222). More recently, Raffman (1993) has
also argued for "ineffable" musical feelings, related to the flow of tension and
resolution in music.[7] Psychologists have also been concerned with the possibility that musical emotions are not adequately captured by the few categories
typically employed in nonmusical emotion research. Scherer (2004) has cau-
tioned about the dangers of forcing musical emotion judgments into a "corset
of a pre-established set of categories" (p. 240). Other psychologists and musicologists have argued that although music can evoke everyday emotions, there
is another aspect to musical emotion that is more personal and complex, and
perhaps ultimately more important. This is listeners' active use of music in a
process of "emotional construction," in other words, in creating an emotional
stance that helps define their attitude toward aspects of their own life (Denora,
2001; Sloboda & Juslin, 2001, cf. Cook & Dibben, 2001). This "constructive"
view of musical emotion is relatively young and presents significant challenges
for empirical research, but is worthy of the effort.

Is there any scientific evidence that music can evoke emotions distinct from
everyday emotions? Consider, for example, the sense of admiration or wonder evoked by a hearing a musical work of great beauty. Intuitively, these
emotions certainly seem different from the everyday emotions we experience
when listening to speech (cf. Davies, 2002; Gabrielsson & Lindström Wik,
2003). Although providing a scientific basis for this intuition is difficult, there
is a related phenomenon that may offer some support for emotions induced
by music but not by ordinary speech. This concerns a physiological response
known as "chills" or "shivers down the spine," which many people have experienced when listening to music. (Music is among the most common source
of chills, but people can also get chills to other stimuli experienced as deeply
moving, including visual and literary art; Goldstein, 1980.) Sloboda (1991)
conducted a survey of 83 listeners, about half of whom were trained musicians, examining the occurrence of chills and other physiological responses
to music. A substantial number of respondents had experienced chills, including to purely instrumental pieces. Sloboda asked the participants to identify
as accurately as they could the particular pieces and passages in which chills

---

[7] Although I have cited 20th-century thinkers here, the idea of music-specific emotions
dates further back. Herbert Spencer (1857), for example, argued that "music not only
. . . strongly excites our more familiar feelings, but also produces feelings we never had
before—arouses dormant sentiments of which we had not conceived the possibility and
do not know the meaning" (p. 404).

or other responses occurred. The participants were often able to locate quite precisely those regions associated with physiological responses (interestingly, these responses were often noted to occur quite reliably, in other words, without habituation even after dozens of listenings). Via musical analysis, Sloboda was able to show that there was a relationship between musical structure and physiological response. Chills, for example, were often associated with sudden changes in harmony, which can be regarded as a violation of expectancy (Meyer, 1956).[8]

Chills are interesting because they are clearly an emotional response, but they do not resemble the everyday emotions such as happiness or sadness. Everyday emotions are generally recognized as having at least two psychological dimensions: a dimension of valence (positive vs. negative) and a dimension of arousal (more vs. less aroused; Russell, 1989). Chills can perhaps be interpreted as a transient increase in arousal, but they do not seem to have any intrinsic valence (i.e., they can occur with "happy" or "sad" music, suggesting that any interpretation in terms of valence is post hoc and context dependent).[9] Furthermore, chills are not normally a physiological concomitant of everyday emotions, as evidenced by the fact that some perfectly normal people do not experience them at all (Goldstein, 1980).

One scientific way to study whether chills are distinct from everyday emotions is to determine if brain responses to chills engage different brain regions than responses to emotions such as happiness and sadness. Blood and Zatorre (2001) conducted a neural study of chills in which listeners heard self-selected, chill-inducing instrumental music while brain activity in different regions was measured with positron emission tomography (PET). (The occurrence of chills was confirmed by physiological measures such as heart rate and respiration.) The brain regions where activity was positively correlated with chills included deep brain structures associated with reward and motivation, including the ventral striatum and dorsal midbrain (cf. Menon & Levitin, 2005). These same areas are known to be active in response to other biologically rewarding stimuli, including food and sex, and to be targeted by certain drugs of abuse. These fascinating findings revealed that music can engage evolutionarily ancient brain structures normally involved in biologically vital functions. Unfortunately, Blood and Zatorre did not also measure brain responses to "everyday emotions" elicited by music, so that no direct comparison of brain areas associated with chills versus everyday emotions is currently available. However, there is

---

[8] Sloboda (1991) also found that tears were associated with (among other things) harmonic movements through the chordal circle of fifths to the tonic. This is interesting because it is an example of an emotional response associated with a *confirmation* of expectancy.

[9] Even if chills are considered a form of arousal, it is an unusual form of arousal compared to everyday emotions, because they are so transient.

now a good deal of work on the neural correlates of everyday emotions (e.g., Damasio, 1994, 2003; LeDoux, 1996; Panksepp, 1998; Lane & Nadel, 2000), and an experiment involving a direct comparison of the type envisioned here should be possible.

Let us assume for the moment that chills are neurally distinct from everyday emotions, as seems likely. What would this imply with regard to the relationship between language and music? As noted in the previous section, listeners are sensitive to the affective qualities of the voice (independent of semantic content), but the types of affect expressible by the voice seem to be limited to everyday emotions such as happiness and anger. Thus although speech may be able to elicit an affective response from a listener (e.g., via empathy), it is not clear if it can elicit a response equivalent to "chills." (The semantic *content* of speech, in combination with affective/rhetorical qualities of the voice, can lead to chills. For example, many people report getting chills when listening to the famous "I Have a Dream" speech by Martin Luther King, Jr. However, here we are discussing the affective qualities of the voice independent of the lexical meaning of the words.)[10] If the sound of ordinary speech cannot evoke chills, this would imply that musical sounds can evoke emotions that speech sounds cannot.

6.2.4 *Motion*

One remarkable and oft-noted property of music is its ability to evoke a sense of motion in a listener (Zohar & Granot, 2006). One example of this is our tendency to synchronize to a musical beat, a response that appears to be uniquely human (cf. Chapters 3 and 7). However, even music without a strong beat can bring to mind a sense of motion. Clarke (2001) discusses this aspect of music in the framework of an "ecological" approach to sound, whereby sounds are perceived as specifying properties of their sources. (This framework is based on J. J. Gibson's [1979] approach to the psychology of vision; cf. Bregman, 1990; Windsor, 2000; Dibben, 2001; Clarke, 2005.) Clarke (2001) argues that because sounds in everyday life specify (among other things) the motional characteristics of their sources, "it is inevitable that musical sounds will also specify movements and gestures, both the real movements and gestures of their actual physical production…and also the fictional movements and gestures of the

---

[10] Sometimes people say "his/her voice gives me the chills," but I suspect that by this they mean that they find a particular voice unsettling in a general way. If they are in fact referring to the kind of chills under discussion here, it is most likely to be due to emotional associations with a particular person rather than a response to the sound structure of the voice per se. Indeed, "chills via association" can occur in music as well, as noted by Goldstein (1980), when music reminds a listener of an emotionally charged event or person from their past.

virtual environment" (p. 222). As one example, Clarke points to a particular orchestral crescendo on Alban Berg's opera *Wozzeck,* in which the combination of a constant pitch with a continuous change in timbre and dynamics yields an auditory sense of "looming," suggestive of an immanent collision (cf. Seifritz et al., 2002).

Clarke suggests that music can evoke two kinds of motion: a sense of self-motion (as emphasized by Todd, 1999, who appeals to neurophysiological arguments) and a sense of external objects moving in relation to the self or to one another (cf. Friberg & Sundberg, 1999; Honing, 2005). One appealing aspect of Clarke's ideas is his concern with empirical validation. For example, he points out that one way to test whether musical motion is a perceptual (vs. a metaphorical) phenomenon is to see if it interferes with tasks that require the perception or production of actual motion.

It is interesting to note that within speech science, there is also a theory inspired by ecological acoustics. "Direct realist theory" (Fowler, 1986; Fowler et al., 2003) claims that the objects of speech perception are not acoustic events but phonetically structured articulatory gestures that underlie acoustic signals. Thus the notion of sound as a medium for the perception of movement is shared by theories of speech and music perception, though it should be noted that the link between sound and perceived movement is subject to a fair amount of controversy in speech science (e.g., Diehl et al., 2004).

6.2.5 Tone Painting

"Tone painting" or "sound painting" refers to the musical imitation of natural phenomena. These can include environmental sounds, animal sounds, or human sounds. Examples of the former two categories are found in Beethoven's *Symphony No. 6* ("Pastoral"). In the second movement, the songs of the nightingale and cuckoo are represented by flute and clarinet melodies, and in the fourth movement a furious thunderstorm is depicted using all the sonic resources of the orchestra. An example of an imitation of a human sound is the "sighing figure" used by many composers, including Mozart in his *Fantasia in D minor, K.397.*

With tone painting, composers are purposefully trying to bring something to mind that lies outside the realm of music. However, as noted by many theorists, skillful tone painting is never just a simple imitation of natural sounds: The musical components must also make sense in the larger structural framework of a piece. Tone painting that lacks this musical sensitivity typically arouses the ire of critics. Langer (1942) cites one 18th-century critic (Hüller) as complaining that "Our intermezzi...are full of fantastic imitations and silly tricks. There one can hear clocks striking, ducks jabbering, frogs quacking, and pretty soon one will be able to hear fleas sneezing and grass growing" (p. 220).

6.2.6 Musical Topics

According to Ratner (1980), "From its contacts with worship, poetry, drama, entertainment, dance, ceremony, the military, the hunt, and the life of the lower classes, music in the early 18th century developed a thesaurus of *characteristic figures,* which formed a rich legacy for classic composers" (p. 9). Ratner designated these figures "topics," a term meant to capture the idea that they were subjects for musical discourse. Ratner identified a number of topics, including dance forms, hunt music, and the pastoral topic. He argued, for example, that the dance form of the minuet "symbolized the social life of the elegant world, [whereas] the march reminded the listener of authority" (p. 16). Pastoral topics were simple melodies (e.g., characteristic of the music of shepherds), and presumably called to mind ideas of innocence and a connection to nature. The idea of topic has proved fruitful for music theorists (see, for example, Gjerdingen, 2007; Agawu, 1991; Monelle, 2000; Hatten, 2004), and has also attracted attention from cognitive psychologists of music. Krumhansl (1998) conducted a perceptual study of topics in which listeners heard a string quintet by Mozart (or a string quartet by Beethoven) and provided real-time judgments on one of three continuous scales: memorability, openness (a sense that the music must continue), and emotion. Krumhansl compared these responses to a detailed analysis of topics in these pieces by Agawu (1991), who identified 14 topics in the Mozart piece and 8 in the Beethoven (Figure 6.2).

Krumhansl found that the perceptual responses were correlated with the timing of the topics in the music. For example, in the Mozart piece, the "Pastoral" and "Sturm und Drang" (storm and stress) topics were associated with openness and memorability, likely due to the fact that these topics frequently occurred at the beginning of major sections or subsections in the music.

It is noteworthy that Krumhansl's subjects were unfamiliar with the musical pieces, and many had little musical training (in fact, the results of the study showed no effect of musical expertise). Presumably, for her listeners the topics did not bring to mind their original cultural associations. In other words, modern listeners likely did not activate the meanings that a knowledgeable 18th-century listener might have activated. Nevertheless, Krumhansl's study suggests that the topics still play a role in the psychological experience of the piece.

What is the significance of "topic theory" from the standpoint of language-music comparisons? Krumhansl suggests that there may be a parallel between topical structure in music and language. In both of the pieces she studied, different topics were repeated at various delays, which she argues "seems compatible with Chafe's (1994) notion that topics within conversations can be maintained for a time in a semiactive state, ready to be reactivated later" (p. 134). That is, discourse analysis suggests that a process of reactivating semiactive information

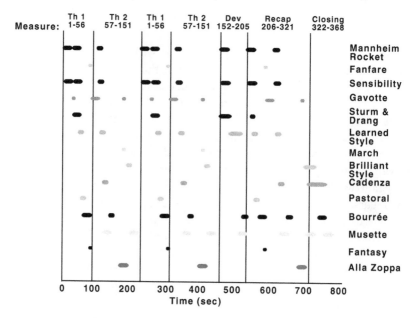

Figure 6.2. An analysis of topics in a Mozart string quintet. From Krumhansl, 1998. Th1 = Theme 1, Th2 = Theme 2, Dev = Development, Recap = Recapitulation.

is basic to human linguistic discourse; Krumhansl suggests that via the use of topics, instrumental music may play on this process in artful ways. This idea may help explain the intuition of certain musically sensitive people that the sound of a string quintet or quartet is somehow reminiscent of a well-wrought "conversation" between several individuals.

Another form of musical topic, the leitmotif, is also relevant to language-music comparisons. A leitmotif is a musical figure used in association with a particular character, situation, or idea, permitting a composer to use music to bring something nonmusical to mind. Because leitmotifs are primarily used in opera or film (in which an association can be formed between by juxtaposing music with characters and situations), they will not be discussed further here, because our focus is on purely instrumental music. They are discussed further in the cognitive and neural section.

6.2.7 Social Associations

Instrumental music does not exist in a vacuum. Different types of instrumental music (e.g., "classical" music vs. bluegrass) are associated with different cultures, contexts, and classes of people. Music can bring these social associations to mind, and empirical research has shown that this aspect of musical meaning can influence behavior. This research includes studies of how consumers behave in the presence of different kinds of background music. In one study, Areni and Kim (1993) played classical music versus Top 40 selections in a wine shop, and found that customers bought more expensive wine when classical music was played. In another study, North et al. (1999) played French versus German folk music on alternate days in the wine section of a supermarket. (The French music was mainly accordion music, and the German music was played by a Bierkeller [beer-hall] band, primarily on brass instruments.) They arranged the French and German wines on adjacent shelves, marked by national flags to help clue the shoppers to the origin of the wines. They found that on "French music days," the French wines outsold the German wines, and vice versa.

Another form of social association in instrumental music is the linking of music to ethnic or group identity. For example, Stokes (1994, cited in Gregory, 1997) "describes the boundary between 'Irish' and 'British' identities in Northern Ireland as being patrolled and enforced by musicians. The parades of Protestant Orangemen with fife and drum bands define the central city space in Belfast as the domain of the Ulster Protestants and of British rule. On the other hand 'Irish traditional' music, which is often considered 'Catholic' music, is widely played in bars and clubs, and defines the Catholic areas of the city" (p. 131).

In language, speech sounds are also associated with different cultures, contexts and classes of people via the perception of a speaker's accent. (Note that accent is distinct from dialect: The former refers to a particular way of pronunciation, whereas the latter refers to a language variant distinguished by pronunciation, vocabulary, and sentence structure.) Sociolinguists have demonstrated that a speaker's accent can influence a listener's beliefs about a speaker's educational background, ethnic identity, and so forth (Honey, 1989; cf. Labov, 1966; Docherty & Foulkes, 1999). Thus a tendency to link sound with social associations appears to be shared by language and music.

6.2.8 Imagery and Narrative

It is informally attested that listening to instrumental music can evoke mental imagery of nonmusical phenomena, such as scenes from nature or "half forgotten thoughts of persons, places, and experiences" (Meyer, 1956:256). There is also informal evidence that listening can give rise to forms of narrative thought, for example, a sense that a particular piece of music reflected "the feeling of a heroic struggle triumphantly resolved" (Sloboda, 1985:59). Indeed, one early tradition of interpretive writing about instrumental music was based on the idea that instrumental music was a kind of "wordless drama" (Kivy, 2002). These suggestions have recently been supported by empirical research in which listeners were asked to listen to short orchestral pieces (e.g., Elgar's "Theme" from the *Enigma Variations*) and to draw something that visually described what they were hearing (Tan & Kelly, 2004). Participants also wrote a short essay to explain the drawing they made. Musicians tended to create abstract (nonpictorial) representations that focused on structural aspects such as repetition and theme structure, whereas nonmusicians were much more likely to draw images or stories, often with salient affective content.

Although there is no obvious connection between music and language in terms of imagery, it does seem plausible that a "narrative tendency" in music perception is related to our constant trafficking in coherent linguistic narratives, whereby sound structure is used to infer a sequence of logically connected events in the world, linked by cause and effect.

6.2.9 Association With Life Experience

If a particular piece or style of music is heard during an important episode in one's life, that music can take on a special, personal meaning via the memories it evokes. Typically, these sorts of associations revolve around songs (which have a verbal narrative element), but there are also documented cases of instrumental music being a powerful vehicle for "taking one back in time," in other words, leading to vivid recall of what one was thinking and feeling at a particular point in life (Denora, 2001; Sloboda et al., 2001).

6.2.10 Creating or Transforming the Self

Sociologists and ethnomusicologists have helped draw attention to the use of music to *construct* (vs. express) self-identity (Becker, 2001; Denora, 2001, Seeger, 1987). In this view, listening to music is not simply a matter of experiencing one's everyday emotions or the worldview one already has, it is a way of changing one's psychological space, and an "opportunity to be temporarily be another kind of person than one's ordinary, everyday self" (Becker, 2001:142). In Western culture, these aspects of music seem to be particularly important to adolescents, for whom music can be part of the processes of identity formation. For example, North et al. (2000) found that British boys' primary stated reason for listening to music was not to regulate mood but to create an impression on others, *even though the majority of respondents said that they listened to music on their own.* Thus the music seemed to be playing a role in construction of identity. Of course, songs probably formed the bulk of the music listened to by these boys, meaning that the identity-forming process is really a product of both language and music. One wonders if instrumental music can be as strong a force in identity formation as can music with words.

Although the construction of identity is a process that unfolds over years, in certain circumstances, music can play a key role in rapidly transforming the sense of self via an altered states of consciousness known as trance (Becker, 2001, 2004). Trance occurs in many cultures, for example, among Sufi mystics in Iran, ritual dancers in Bali, and Pentecostal Christians in America. Although some skeptics regard trance as a form of fakery, cross-cultural similarities in trance behavior suggest that trancers really are in an altered neurophysiological state. Such commonalities include difficulty remembering what happened during the trance and a greatly increased pain threshold during the trance (i.e., amnesia and analgesia). Furthermore, extensive and careful fieldwork with trancers in different cultures makes it seem very likely that the phenomenon in question is psychologically real (Becker, 2004; cf. Penman & Becker, submitted), a view supported by recent preliminary electroencephalographic (EEG) from Balinese dancers during a trance ceremony (Oohashi et al., 2002). In this pioneering study, the researchers used an EEG telemetry system and compared the brain waves of a dancer who went into trance versus two other dancers who did not, and found a markedly different pattern of brain waves in the former individual (increased power in the theta and alpha bands).

Although music plays an important role in trance, its relationship to trance is complex, and there is no evidence that music can put a listener in a trance without the right context and the listener's implicit consent. The music is typically part of a larger ritual event that includes words (e.g., the words of Sufi or Pentecostal songs or of Balinese drama), suggesting that rapid psychological transformation involves the use of both language and music. Once again, one wonders if instrumental music alone could have a comparable effect.

6.2.11 Musical Structure and Cultural Concepts

The final form of musical meaning discussed in this taxonomy is the most abstract, and the most speculative from the standpoint of the psychological experience of music. This is the relationship between musical structure and extramusical cultural concepts, a link that has been posited by ethnomusicologists as part of the meaning of music in a social context. An example of this type of meaning is provided by the analysis of Javanese gamelan music by Becker and Becker (1981; see also Becker, 1979). These authors note that gamelan music is structured by cyclic melodic patterns (played by different instruments) embedded within each other. The patterns proceed at different rates and thus create a cyclic patterns of predictable coincidences as the different parts come together at certain points in time. They argue that these patterns are conceptually similar to Javanese calendrical cycles. In Java a day is described by its position within five different calendric cycles moving at different rates. The cyclic coincidences that emerge are culturally important, because they make certain days auspicious and other days hazardous. Becker and Becker write:

> The iconicity of sounding gongs [i.e., gamelan music] with calendars (and other systems within the culture) is one of the devices whereby they resonate with import beyond themselves. Coincidence, or simultaneous occurrence, is a central source

of both meaning and power in traditional Javanese culture. Coincidings in calendars and in music both represent events to be analyzed and scrutinized because of the importance of the concept which lies behind both. *Kebetulan*, "coincidence" in Indonesian, and *kebeneran* in Javanese both derive from root words meaning "truth," *betel/bener*. As pitches coincide at important structural points in gamelan music, so certain days coincide to mark important moments in one's personal life. One might say that gamelan music is an idea made audible and tactile (one hears with one's skin as well as one's ears). (p. 210)

It might interest the reader to know that Becker and Becker find further evidence for this link between culture and art in the structure of shadow-puppet plays, which are also built around cycles and coincidences (between different plot lines) rather than around a unified causal sequence leading to a climax.

Although this is but one example, analyses of this sort are widespread in the ethnomusicological literature. Western European instrumental music can be analyzed in this framework as well, by asking what aspects of its culture are reflected in its structure. One could argue, for example, that the sense of harmonic progression that is so valued in Western musical chord syntax reflects a Western cultural obsession with progress and transformation. There may be truth in such observations, but from a psychological perspective, the relevant question is whether metaphorical connections between music and culture play any role in musical meaning as experienced by individual listeners. Presumably, the sound of a gamelan does not bring calendars to mind for Javanese listeners, and chord progressions do not provoke thoughts of the industrial revolution in Western listeners. Nevertheless, there may be an indirect psychological influence in simply making the music of one's culture sound "natural," in other words, somehow fitting with the general conceptual framework with which one is familiar.

Does this sort of relationship have any analog in language? Clearly, language reflects cultural concepts via its vocabulary (though see Pullum's classic 1991 essay, "The Great Eskimo Vocabulary Hoax" for a word of caution), but it seems unlikely that linguistic structures (e.g., syntax, or discourse structure) reflect aspects of culture.[11] This is sensible, because musical structure is the result of conscious choices made by individuals, whereas linguistic structure emerges from the interplay of cognitive factors with the distributed forces of language change. The link between complex sonic structures and specific cultural concepts may be unique to the domain of music.

---

[11] There are interesting studies of how language structure can influence the perception of nonlinguistic phenomena in the world (Genter & Goldin-Meadow, 2003; Casasanto, in press), but this is a different topic. I am aware of only one case in which it has been argued that a culture's linguistic syntactic system reflects a particular cultural belief system (Everett, 2005).

6.3 Linguistic Meaning in Relation to Music

Discussions of music's relation to linguistic meaning often focus on semantics, and on the question of how instrumental music can be meaningful when it lacks propositional content. Note that this question assumes that "meaning" is equivalent to semantic meaning in language. If "meaning" is construed in this way, then comparisons of linguistic and musical meaning must address how close music can come to being semantically meaningful. Indeed, research in cognitive science and neuroscience has attempted to do just that (discussed in section 6.3.1 below). I believe there is another, potentially more fruitful way to compare linguistic and musical meaning, however. Recall from section 6.1.2 that linguistic meaning can be broadly divided into two distinct areas: semantics and pragmatics. Pragmatics refers to the study of how listeners add contextual information to semantic structure and how they draw inferences about what has been said. The relationship of musical meaning to linguistic pragmatics is virtually unexplored. Yet as discussed in section 6.3.2 below, this relationship may be a promising area for future investigation.

6.3.1 Music and Semantics

Recall from section 6.1.2 that one philosophical approach to the question of musical meaning is to hold fast to the idea that "meaning" indicates semantic reference and predication, and to therefore deny that music has meaning, or "can even be meaningless" (Kivy, 2002). In this view, any discussion of "meaning" in music commits a philosophical category error. This is certainly a minority position, because music theorists and philosophers continue to produce a steady stream of publications on "musical meaning," treating "meaning" in a broader sense than Kivy allows (cf. section 6.2). Nevertheless, Kivy's position is interesting because it is clearly articulated and provokes the following question: Is it categorically true that music lacks a semantic component, or is the situation more subtle and complex? Might music at times engage semantic processing, using cognitive and neural operations that overlap with those involved in language? In this section, I will focus on semantic reference (rather than predication), because comparative empirical data exist on this issue.

Let us begin our discussion with the following thought experiment. Choose the most talented composers living today, and give each of them a list of 50 common nouns or verbs (e.g., "school," "eye," "know"). Ask them to write a passage of instrumental music for each word that conveys the sense of the word in the clearest possible way. Then, tell a group of listeners that they are going to hear a series of musical passages, each of which is meant to convey a common noun or verb. After each passage, have the listeners write down what they think the word is (or choose it from a list of the 50 words used). Needless to say, it is extremely unlikely that the listeners will arrive at the words that the composers intended. This thought experiment demonstrates that music lacks the kind of arbitrary, specific semantic reference that is fundamental to language.

However, lacking specificity of semantic reference is not the same as being utterly devoid of referential power. Let me offer the following conceptual distinction: Instrumental music lacks specific semantic *content,* but it can at times suggest semantic *concepts.* Furthermore, it can do this with some consistency in terms of the concepts activated in the minds of listeners within a culture. The evidence for this view is empirical, and is reviewed in the following two sections.

The Semantics of Leitmotifs

In his operas, Richard Wagner constructed compact musical units designed to suggest extramusical meanings such as a particular character, situation, or idea. These leitmotifs were woven into the music for dramatic effect, sometimes complementing the scene and at other times serving to bring characters, and so forth, to mind when they were not part of the current scene. Although leitmotifs are most commonly discussed with reference to Wagner's music, it is important to note that they are not limited to his music. Film music often employs the leitmotif technique. Many people who saw the 1970s film sensation, *Jaws,* for example, remember the menacing theme that indicated the presence of the great white shark (cf. Cross, submitted, for an interesting discussion of musical meaning in relation to this famous leitmotif).

Leitmotifs provide an opportunity to study the semantic properties of music because they are designed to have referential qualities. Specifically, one can present these musical units to listeners previously unfamiliar with them, and ask the listeners to indicate the semantic associations that the units suggest. One such study has been conducted by Hacohen and Wagner (1997), focusing on nine leitmotifs from Wagner's *Ring* cycle, listed in Box 6.2. The selected leitmotifs were 7–13 seconds long and purely instrumental, and onomatopoeic leitmotifs such as the "storm" motive were avoided.

One interesting feature of Hacohen and Wagner's study was that it took place in Israel, where there was a historical ban on playing Wagner's music in concert halls or on the radio due to its association with the Nazi regime. Thus the researchers had unique access to a population of students familiar with Western European tonal music but with little or no exposure to Wagner.

Box 6.2 Wagnerian Leitmotifs Studied by Hacohen and Wagner (1997)

Curse	Valhalla	Fire
Death	Hunding (a character)	Love
Frustration	Sleep	Fate

Box 6.3 Semantic Scales Used by Hacohen and Wagner (1997)

Joy-sadness	Strength-weakness	Dignity-humility
Hope-despair	Impetuosity-restraint	Kindness-cruelty
Natural-supernatural		

In the first part of their study, 174 listeners were presented with the motifs and asked to rate them on seven semantic scales, shown in Box 6.3. None of the scales had names that were similar to the topics of the leitmotifs. In addition, each leitmotif was rated for how much it made the listener feel "liking" or "disliking."

Statistical analyses of the results revealed that most leitmotifs fell into one of three clusters, a "friendly" cluster, a "violent" cluster, and a "dreary" cluster, shown in Figure 6.3. As is evident from the figure, there was much consistency within clusters in terms of the semantic profiles of the leitmotifs, and each cluster even featured a pair of "synonyms," in other words, two leitmotifs with a highly similar semantic profile (love-sleep, curse-Hunding, and death-frustration). It is interesting that most of the concepts represented in the semantic scales are affective (e.g., joy-sadness), pseudoaffective (e.g., strength-weakness, which can be seen as analogous to the "activity" dimension of a two-dimensional emotion space of valence and activity, cf. section 6.2.3), or "personality"-like (e.g., impetuosity-restraint), suggesting that listeners perceive leitmotifs in terms of a "persona" (cf. Watt and Ash, 1998).

Although these results are interesting, they are a somewhat weak test of music's power to evoke semantic concepts, because they provide concepts in the form of semantic scales and simply ask listeners to rate them. A stronger test would be to allow listeners to choose concepts without any constraints. Fortunately, Hacohen and Wagner conducted a second experiment relevant to this issue. They asked 102 of their participants to listen to each leitmotif, imagine that it was the musical theme of a film, and then to give the film a name. No constraints or preestablished categories were given. An example of the result is shown in Figure 6.4, which gives 16 of the 75 titles produced for the "fire" motif (note that this motif did not fit into any of the three clusters in the semantic scale method).

Figure 6.4 is arranged in a "modular" fashion, with actions or events in one column, agents of the action in another column, and so forth. The figure shows a fair degree of overlap in the gist of the titles provided, as well as some diversity within this commonality. Using this "film-naming" technique, Hacohen and Wagner found a remarkable amount of consistency for each leitmotif, though only the "love" and "death" motives were given titles that matched the original ones.

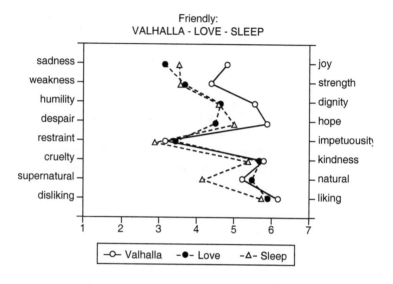

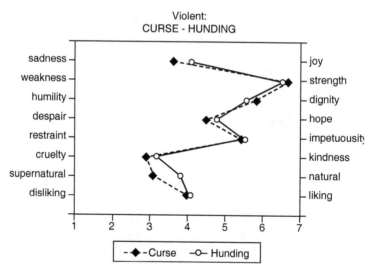

Figure 6.3 Semantic profiles of Wagnerian Leitmotifs, from Hacohen & Wagner, 1997. The numbers along the x-axes represent how much a given leitmotif expresses one of two opposite semantic concepts, in which 1 represents strong expression of the concept on the left of the scale (e.g., sadness), 7 represents strong expression of the concept on the right of the scale (e.g., joy), and 4 is neutral.

continued

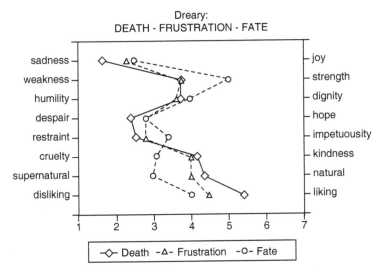

Figure 6.3, *continued*

They also found two other interesting things. First the film-naming technique differentiated between leitmotifs that emerged as synonymous in the semantic scale technique. For example, for the love-sleep pair, they found that titles associated with "love" emphasized the interpersonal aspect, whereas titles associated with "sleep" emphasized scenery (tranquil images of nature) and atmosphere (mystery). This demonstrates that studies of musical semantics should not rely solely on ratings using preestablished semantic scales, but should also study the results of free association. The second interesting finding was that certain topics never appeared in the titles, such as religious, historical, urban, or domestic concepts. Hacohen and Wagner argue that this is consistent with the mythological, pagan, and ahistorical character of the *Ring*.

Neural Evidence That Music Can Evoke Semantic Concepts

An innovative study of semantic reference in music has been conducted by Koelsch and colleagues, using event-related potentials (ERPs; Koelsch et al., 2004). The question they sought to address was whether unfamiliar, purely instrumental music (taken from Western European classical music) could suggest semantic concepts to a listener. Koelsch et al. tested this idea using a neural signature of linguistic semantic processing known as the N400. The N400 is an ERP produced in response to a word, whether presented in isolation or in a sentence context. (The name "N400" reflects the fact that it is a negative-going potential with an amplitude maximum approximately 400 ms after the onset of a word.) The amplitude of the N400 is modulated by the semantic

A Short Map of the Fire Motif

Action or Event		Agent			Place	Affect
Animated Movement	Celebration	Legendary, Magical, Animals, Many	Legendary, Magical, Single (s)	Creatures of Nature	Country-side/ Magic	Pleasant Affect
The dance		of the fairies			in the forest	
The race		of the angels				
		of the horses				
The dance		of the muses				
The dance		of the stars				
The dance		of the witches				
The dance		of the devils				
		of the dolls				
	The wedding		of the marionette			
The adventures			of Peter Pan			
The dance		of the Hobbits				
		In the Guzmeks'			forest	
The escape		of the dwarfs				
The war against		the cockroaches				
The flight		of the fireflies				
The dizziness				of Nature		
The dance			of the lovers			before the tragedy A moment of happiness

Figure 6.4 Some titles associated with the "fire" motif in the study of Hacohen & Wagner, 1997.

fit between a word and its context. For example, the N400 to the final word in the sentence "the pizza was too hot to cry" is significantly larger than the N400 to the final word in the sentence "the pizza was too hot to eat" (Kutas & Hillyard, 1984). Although this "N400 effect" has been most extensively studied using frank semantic anomalies such as this one, it is important to note that the N400 effect does not require an anomaly. As discussed in Chapter 5, the N400 effect can be observed when comparing sentences in which words are simply more or less predicted from a semantic standpoint. For example, when the sentences "The girl put the sweet in her mouth after the lesson" and "The girl put the sweet in her pocket after the lesson" are compared, an N400 effect occurs for "pocket" versus "mouth" (Hagoort et al., 1999). This reflects the fact that "pocket" is a less semantically probable word than "mouth" given the context up to that word. The N400 is thus a sensitive measure of semantic integration in language, and is thought to reflect processes that relate incoming words to the semantic representation generated by the preceding context.[12]

Koelsch et al. exploited the N400 effect to test whether music can suggest semantic concepts. Listeners heard short musical excerpts[13] taken from the classical music repertoire, each of which was followed by a visually presented noun (which could be concrete, e.g., "pearls" or abstract, e.g., "illusion"). The particular pairing of musical excerpts and target words was chosen based on a separate behavioral study in which listeners rated the semantic relatedness of musical excerpts and words. The bases for the relatedness judgments were rather diverse. In some cases, the basis seemed metaphorical. For example, a musical excerpt judged as a good semantic fit for the word "wideness" had large pitch intervals and consonant harmonies, whereas a musical excerpt judged as a bad semantic fit for "wideness" had narrow pitch intervals and dissonant harmonies. In other cases, the match/mismatch was based on iconic resemblance between the music and the word. For example, the word "sigh" was matched with an excerpt in which the melody moved in a way that suggested the intonation of a sigh, whereas it was mismatched with an excerpt that suggested the angry intonation of a fight. Yet another way in which matches/mismatches were achieved was by conventional association of the type one might associate with film music. For example, "caravan" was matched with an exotic, Middle Eastern sounding excerpt, and mismatched with an excerpt that suggested rapid movement and a European pastoral setting.

Koelsch et al. found an N400 effect for words following semantically mismatched versus matched musical excerpts. This effect was quantitatively similar to the N400 effect seen when these same words followed semantically mismatched versus matched linguistic sentences, and occurred even when listeners were not required to make any explicit judgment about the relatedness of the excerpt and the target. Furthermore, source localization techniques suggested that the N400s to words following linguistic versus musical contexts came from similar regions of the brain: the posterior portion of the middle temporal gyrus, bilaterally (Figure 6.5). The authors argue that this indicates the ability of music to activate semantic concepts with some specificity.

Koelsch et al.'s findings raise interesting questions. First of all, it is evident that in this study the types of associations between musical excerpts and target words

---

[12] Note that this context can be as little as a single word. That is, if words are presented in pairs, and the degree of semantic relatedness between them is manipulated, an N400 effect will be observed to words that are semantically less related to their context words. Thus elicitation of the N400 effect does not require linguistic propositions.

[13] The stimuli can be heard at http://www.stefan-koelsch.de/ by following the links to the Koelsch et al. 2004 article.

A   **Language**

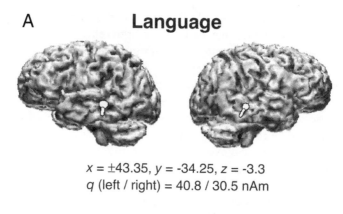

$x = \pm43.35, y = -34.25, z = -3.3$
q (left / right) = 40.8 / 30.5 nAm

B   **Music**

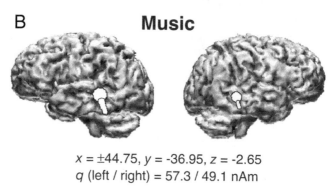

$x = \pm44.75, y = -36.95, z = -2.65$
q (left / right) = 57.3 / 49.1 nAm

Figure 6.5 Neural generators of the N400 effect elicited by target words that were semantically unrelated to preceding sentences (A), or to preceding instrumental musical excerpts (B). The estimated neural generators (shown as white dipole sources in the temporal lobes) did not differ between the language and the music conditions (x-, y-, and z-coordinates refer to standard stereotaxic space, dipole moments [q] in nanoamperes). Adapted from Koelsch et al., 2004.

are rather heterogeneous. For example, conventional associations between Middle Eastern music and images of caravans are much less abstract than analogies between pitch intervals/consonance and the spatial concept of "wideness," and both are different from the iconic resemblance between music and meaning represented by the excerpt of a musical "sigh." Thus it would be interesting to examine Koelsch et al.'s stimuli in detail and develop a taxonomy of ways in which the musical excerpts conveyed semantic meanings. If sufficient new stimuli could be generated for each category of this taxonomy, one could do ERP studies to see which types of association most strongly drive the N400 effect. Presumably it is these associations that are truly activating semantic concepts.

Taking a step back, although the study of Koelsch et al. suggests that music can activate certain semantic concepts, it by no means shows that music has a semantic system on par with language. First of all, the specificity of semantic concepts activated by music is likely to be much lower (and much more variable between individual listeners) than activated by language. Secondly, there is no evidence that music has semantic compositionality, in other words, a system for expressing complex semantic meanings via structured combinations of constituents (Partee, 1995). What Koelsch's study shows is that the claim that music is absolutely devoid of semantic meaning (cf. Kivy, 2002) is too strong: The semantic boundary between music and language is not categorical, but graded.

Before closing this section, it is worth noting the interesting fact that to date there are no published studies showing that music alone can elicit an N400. Although there have been many experiments examining brain responses to incongruous notes or chords in both familiar and unfamiliar music (starting with the pioneering work of Besson & Macar, 1987), none have found an N400. A study showing that music alone (i.e., both as context and target) can produce an N400 would be of considerable interest, because it would inform both the study of "musical semantics" and the study of the cognitive basis of the N400 ERP component (cf. Miranda & Ullman, in press). In this regard, it is worth noting that out-of-key chords at the ends of chord sequences can elicit a late negativity peaking around 500 ms after the onset of the chord (e.g., the "N5" reported by Koelsch et al., 2000; cf. Johnston, 1994), but the timing and scalp distribution of this component indicates that it is not the same as the linguistic N400. One way to investigate whether this late negativity shares any neural mechanisms with the N400 is to do ERP experiments that combine sentences with chord sequences, so that semantic incongruities occur at the same time as out-of-key chords (cf. Steinbeis & Koelsch, in press). If the brain signals come from independent processes, then they should combine in an additive fashion, whereas if they draw on similar neural mechanisms, they should interact (cf. Chapter 5, section 5.4.4, subsection "Interference Between Linguistic and Musical Syntactic Processing" for an example of this strategy applied to syntactic processing).

6.3.2 Music and Pragmatics

The meaning a person derives in listening to language is more than just the meaning of individual words and sentences. For example, each sentence in example 6.1 below is perfectly well formed and meaningful, but a listener would likely judge the passage incoherent in terms of its meaning as a discourse.

(6.1) The father saw his son pick up his toy chainsaw. Seashells are often shiny on the inside. John likes peas.

In contrast, the sentences in 6.2 are likely to be perceived as coherent.

(6.2) The father saw his son pick up his toy chainsaw. The boy pretended to cut down a tree, but didn't touch the delicate flowers growing in the garden. Mom was pleased.

The perceived coherence of 6.2 illustrates some often unappreciated facts about deriving meaning from discourse. First, it involves assuming unstated information (e.g., that "the boy" in the second sentence is the same individual as "the son" in the first sentence; that "mom" is the mother of that same boy; that "mom" is the wife of the father). Second, it also involves drawing inferences about what was said (e.g., that mom was pleased because the boy didn't cut down her flowers). Language users are so accustomed to adding contextual information and making inferences that they are generally unaware that such processes are taking place. Nevertheless, establishing discourse coherence is central to language understanding. As noted by Kehler (2004), "just as hearers attempt to recover the implicit syntactic structure of a string of words to compute sentence meaning, they attempt to recover the implicit coherence structure of a series of utterances to compute discourse meaning" (p. 243).

The study of how listeners add contextual information to semantic structure and how they draw inferences about what has been said is called pragmatics. Linguists distinguish pragmatics from semantics: The latter focuses on the meanings of words and propositions, whereas the former focuses on how hearers recover a speaker's intended meaning based on contextual information and inferencing (Jaszczolt, 2002). A central concern for research in pragmatics is establishing the types of conceptual connections a listener makes between utterances. As with most areas of research in linguistics, there are multiple theories regarding this issue. For the purposes of this book, I will focus on one particular theory that is notable for its concern with psychological plausibility. (It is also notable for its success in accounting for linguistic phenomena that are difficult to explain in other frameworks, though there is not space here to go into this aspect.)

This is the theory of Kehler (2002). Drawing on the philosophical work of David Hume in his 1748 *Enquiry Concerning Human Understanding*, Kehler's theory posits that there are three broad types of connections that listeners make between utterances: resemblance, cause-effect, and contiguity. Importantly, Hume's ideas were not developed in the context of the study of linguistic discourse, but as part of a philosophical investigation of the types of "connections among ideas" that humans can appreciate. Thus central to Kehler's theory is the idea that coherence relations in language are instantiations of more basic cognitive processes that humans apply in order to make sense of sequences of events. (Kehler shares this perspective with several other linguists, including Hobbs, 1990, who first drew attention to the fact that discourse coherence relations could be classified according to Hume's system.) Specifically, the different categories are thought to represent three basic ways in which human minds draws inferences. Resemblance relations are based on the ability to reason analogically, categorizing events and seeing correspondences between them. Cause-effect relations are based on drawing a path of implication between events. Contiguity relations are based on understanding that events happen in a certain order, and reflects knowledge about the sequence in which things happen under ordinary circumstances.

Cognitive Aspects of Discourse Coherence

If there are general cognitive processes underlying the perception of coherence in linguistic discourse, might these same processes apply to the perception of coherence in music? That is, do common mental mechanisms apply in the interpretation of coherence relations in language and music? One reason that this question is sensible is that as with language, the perception of coherence in music requires more than the recognition of independent, well-formed musical segments: It requires that connections be perceived between the segments, connections that link the segments into a larger, organized whole. Of course, this begs the question of what the musical "segments" in question are. In the case of language, an obvious candidate for a discourse segment is a clause, though other possibilities exist (see Wolf & Gibson, 2005). In music, defining the relevant segments is not so straightforward. In particular, if one wants to segment music into nonoverlapping units for the purpose of studying coherence relations, how big should these units be? Short motifs? Middle-length phrases? Long themes? Entire sections? For the sake of argument, I will assume that the relevant level for ordinary musical listening is likely to involve fairly short units, perhaps on the order of musical phrases or themes (cf. Levinson, 1997).

We can now pose our question more pointedly: Do coherence relations between clauses in linguistic discourse have analogs to coherence relations between phrases and themes in musical discourse? In order to address this question, let us examine some specific coherence relations posited by linguistic theory, using Kehler (2002) as a source. In the category of "resemblance" Kehler lists six relations, three of which are of interest from the standpoint of comparative language-music research: parallelism (similarity), contrast, and elaboration. Linguistic examples of these relations are given in examples 6.3–6.5, respectively. (All examples below are adapted from Wolf and Gibson, 2005. Brackets indicate discourse segments.)

(6.3) [There is a an oboe leaning on the black music stand.] [There is another oboe leaning on the gray music stand.]

(6.4) [John liked salsa music,] [but Susan liked reggae.]

(6.5) [A new concert series was launched this week.] [The "Stravinsky retrospective" is scheduled to last until December.]

Abstracting away from the semantic content of these sentences, each sentence exemplifies a coherence relation recognized by musicologists as basic to music. A musical phrase/theme can be recognizably similar to another phrase/theme, provide a contrast to it, or elaborate it.

Turning to the category of "cause-effect," Kehler identifies four coherence relations, two of which are of interest to comparative research: "result" and "violated expectation." Examples of these are given in examples 6.6 and 6.7.

(6.6) [There was bad weather at the airport,] [and so our flight got delayed].

(6.7) [The weather was nice,] [but our flight got delayed].

Again, one must abstract away from semantics to see the relationship to music. Recall that cause-effect relations concern the process of drawing a path of implication between discourse segments. The notion that musical events can be related by implication or expectation to other events is fundamental to Western music theory (e.g., Meyer, 1956; Narmour, 1990). These forces are particularly strongly at play in the perception of harmonic chord sequences, in which chord progressions create coherence via the contrast between earlier chords (which set up expectations) and subsequent chords (which either fulfill or deny these expectations). Thus it is perfectly congruent with what we know about music to think of musical segments as fulfilling or violating expectations created by previous segments.

In the final category used by Kehler, "contiguity," there is only one coherence relation. Kehler refers to this relation as "occasion," but the notion of "temporal sequence" (used by Wolf & Gibson, 2005) is a subset of this and is adequate for our current purposes. An example is given in 6.8.

(6.8) [Roger took a bath.] [He went to bed].

Part of what makes 6.8 coherent is one's world knowledge that these events typically occur in a given order. Does this relation have any parallel in music? The most likely parallel is a listener's knowledge of specific musical forms in which a succession of themes or patterns occurs in a particular order, not because of any intrinsic internal logic but simply because that is the order that the culture has specified (cf. Meyer, 1956:128).

If one accepts that there are overlapping coherence relations between language and music, as suggested by the previous paragraphs, how is one to transform this observation into comparative empirical research? One promising direction is suggested by the work of Wolf and Gibson (2005). These researchers have developed an annotation system for coherence relations in text, based largely on the relations suggested by Hobbs (1985) and Kehler (2002). Their system has eight relations, shown in Table 6.1. I have indicated those relations with putative musical parallels with an "M." (Note that Wolf and Gibson's cause-effect relation is akin to Kehler's "result.")

The annotation system of Wolf and Gibson involves segmenting a text into discourse segments (clauses), grouping topically related segments together, and then determining coherence relations between segments. These relations are

Table 6.1 Coherence Relations Between Discourse Segments

Similarity	M
Contrast	M
Elaboration	M
Cause-effect	M
Violated expectation	M
Temporal sequence	M
Condition (e.g., "if…then")	
Attribution (e.g., "he said")	

Source: Adapted from Wolf & Gibson, 2005.

diagrammed as arcs between discourse segments. For example, the text shown in 6.9 is segmented into discourse segments, indicated by the numbers 1–4:

(6.9)

1. Susan wanted to buy some tomatoes
2. and she also tried to find some basil
3. because her recipe asked for these ingredients.
4. The basil would probably be quite expensive at this time of the year.

The coherence relations between these segments are indicated in Figure 6.6.

Wolf and Gibson derive this example analysis as follows. "There is a *similarity* relation between 1 and 2; 1 and 2 both describe shopping for grocery items. There is a *cause-effect* relation between 3 and 1–2; 3 describes the cause for the shopping described by 1 and 2. There is an *elaboration* relation between 4 and 2; 4 provides details about the basil in 2" (pp. 265–266).

Wolf and Gibson trained two annotators in their system and had each independently annotate 135 texts (the texts had an average of 61 discourse segments and 545 words each). They found good agreement between the annotators (~90%), and went on to make several interesting observations. One of these was that there were many instances of "crossed dependencies" (e.g., the crossing of the "ce" and "elab" lines in Figure 6.6), in other words, dependencies that are not well captured by the traditional nested hierarchical tree structures used to analyze syntax. This suggests that coherence relations have a different mental organization than syntactic structures. Another finding was that certain relations are much more common than others. For example, "elaboration" was a very frequent relation, accounting for almost 50% of relations, whereas violated expectation was quite rare, accounting for about 2% of relations. Of course, data from more annotators and texts are needed, but even these preliminary findings are quite intriguing from a cognitive standpoint.

From the standpoint of comparative language-music research, Wolf and Gibson's system is of interest because it produces coherence structure graphs (such as that in Figure 6.6) that are abstracted away from specific semantic content, and whose topology can be studied from a purely formal standpoint using principles of graph theory (Wilson, 1985). That is, one can quantify aspects of graph architecture. For example, one can quantify the mean "in-degree" of all segments (i.e., the mean number of incoming connections to a segment), the mean arc length associated with different coherence relations, and so forth. The resulting numbers provide a quantitative characterization of linguistic discourse structure.

Because so many of the relations used by Wolf and Gibson have analogs in music (Table 6.1), one can imagine conducting similar analyses of musical pieces, resulting in graphs comparable to that in Figure 6.6. One could then quantify the topology of these graphs using the same measures as applied to linguistic coherence graphs, and then examine similarities and differences between the architecture of linguistic and musical discourse in a quantitative framework. It would be very interesting to know, for example, if musical pieces that generated graphs quantitatively similar to linguistic graphs were perceived as more perceptually coherent than musical pieces with topological patterns very different from linguistic patterns. Were this the case, one might argue that not only are similar cognitive principles at play in organizing the flow of meaning in linguistic and musical discourse, but that the patterning of this flow is shaped by similar forces (e.g., perhaps by limited processing resources).

Neural Aspects of Discourse Coherence

Just as there are brain regions that are critical to linguistic syntax and semantics, it seems reasonable to expect that there are brain regions critical to the inferencing processes involved in linguistic discourse comprehension, in other words, processes that connect individual segments into a larger, meaningful whole. Where do these brain regions reside? There is a good deal of evidence from neuropsychology that these regions are in the right cerebral hemisphere, possibly in homologs of left hemisphere language areas (Beeman, 1993, 1998). For example, in an influential early study, Brownell et al. (1986) presented

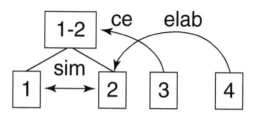

Figure 6.6 Coherence relations between segments of a short discourse (example 6.9 in the text). In this diagram, "sim" = "similar," "ce" = "cause-effect," and "elab" = elaboration. From Wolf & Gibson, 2005.

right-hemisphere-damaged patients and normal individuals with the simplest form of connected discourse: pairs of sentences. Participants were instructed to try to think of the sentences as a complete story, and were then asked true/false questions about the story. An example sentence pair and its associated questions are given in examples 6.10 and 6.11:

(6.10) Barbara became too bored to finish the history book. She had already spent five years writing it.

(6.11)

Correct inference question:	Barbara became bored writing a history book.
Incorrect inference question:	Reading the history book bored Barbara.
Incorrect factual question (first sentence):	Barbara grew tired of watching movies.
Correct factual question (second sentence):	She had been writing it for five years.

The factual questions were included as a control condition to test for simple memory abilities. Both normal individuals and patients had greater difficulty with the inference questions than the factual questions, but the critical result was that the right-hemisphere-damaged patients had a significantly greater discrepancy between performance on the inference questions and fact questions. Of course, because Brownell et al. did not test patients with left-hemisphere damage, their result could not rule out the effect of brain damage per se (vs. damage localized to the right hemisphere). Subsequent work on more patients has provided evidence, however, that the right hemisphere has a special role to play in linguistic inferencing processes (see Beeman, 1998, for a review). Functional neuroimaging work with normal individuals has been less conclusive regarding hemispheric laterality, with some studies favoring a strong right-hemisphere laterality (e.g., Mason & Just, 2004), and others favoring the involvement of regions on both sides of the brain (e.g., Kuperberg et al., 2006).

In the previous subsection, parallels were suggested between the mental processes underlying the perception of discourse coherence in language and music. One way to address whether these parallels actually reflect common neural processing is to test patients with problems with linguistic inferencing on musical tasks that probe the perception of coherence relations in music. For example, one could use the "scrambled music" method, in which musical pieces are divided into short segments that are locally coherent (e.g., musical phrases/themes) and the order of these segments is rearranged (e.g., using the method and stimuli of Lalitte & Bigand, 2006, cf. section 6.2.1). One could then elicit judgments of musical coherence as a function of the amount of scrambling. (As with the Brownell et al. study, it would be important to have control conditions that test for memory problems.) Would patients with linguistic inferencing problems be relatively insensitive to musical scrambling compared to normal controls? If so, this would suggest commonalities in the mental processes underlying perception of coherence relations in language and music.

6.4 Interlude: Linguistic and Musical Meaning in Song

As with the rest of this book, the focus of this chapter is on the relationship between spoken language and instrumental music. Nevertheless, it is worth touching briefly on song, in which musical and linguistic meanings intertwine. One simple form of this interplay is "word painting," which is related to tone painting (cf. section 6.2.5). With word painting, a composer can try to musically complement the meaning of words by using tonal patterns that iconically reflect some aspect of word meaning. For example, in the first phrase of the spiritual "Swing Low, Sweet Chariot," the melody takes a downward leap (of 4 semitones) from "swing" to "low," thus using pitch movement to reflect the idea of something sweeping downward to earth, whereas the second phrase "comin' for to carry me home" has a rising pitch contour, reflecting an ascent to heaven. Another example of word painting, this time from rock music, is the opening chord of the Beatles' song "A Hard Day's Night." This chord is based on a normal, harmonious-sounding G major triad, in other words, the notes G-B-D (the tonic triad of the opening key of the song), but with two additional tones added: a C (the 4th degree of the scale), and F-natural (which is not in the scale of G major, and is thus highly unstable; cf. Chapter 5). The combination of B and C in the chord creates a dissonance, and this together with the unstable F-natural gives this chord a jarring quality that reflects the disorientation of going beyond one's limits (Stevens, 2002:52), complementing the meaning of the song's title (which is its opening line).

Music can go beyond word painting to create meanings that intertwine with linguistic meaning in a more sophisticated fashion. For example, aspects of harmonic syntax can be used to imply meanings that either complement or contradict the meaning of a text (Cone, 1974; Youens, 1991; and see especially Zbikowski, 1999 for a modern music-theoretic approach to text-music interactions inspired by cognitive science). This is because harmonic syntax can articulate points of tension and resolution (i.e., instability vs. stability), and points of openness and closure. For example, in the Bach chorale "Aus tiefer Noth schrei ich zu dir" (based on Psalm 130), the emotional climax occurs in the third line, when the speaker asks, "If you, O Lord, kept a record of sins, O Lord, who could stand?" This is the only question in the psalm (which ends several lines later), but it seems that Bach focuses on this line in creating the harmonic setting. The original melody of the chorale predates Bach and is tonally centered on E. Nevertheless, Bach incorporates this melody into a harmonic setting that is tonally centered on A minor, thus making the E and its associated chord serve the function of the dominant (V). In tonal music, the V chord conveys a sense of incompleteness because points of musical closure are often indicated by a movement from V to I, in other words, by a cadence (I is the tonic chord of a key; cf. Chapter 5). Remarkably, Bach ends the chorale on an E major chord, so that the chorale does not conclude with a cadence but is left harmonically open, emblematic of a question in wait of a response. Thus by using harmony, Bach has picked out a part of the psalm's semantic meaning and spiritual significance, and given it a musical voice.

Although the interplay of linguistic and musical meaning in songs has been fertile ground for music theorists, there has been little empirical research in this area. Most of the existing work simply asks whether listeners find lyrics more meaningful when they are embedded in their original musical context, the answer typically being "yes" (Galizio & Hendrick, 1972; Iverson et al., 1989; Stratton & Zalanowski, 1994). Thompson & Russo (2004) conducted a study of this sort with interesting results. They used hit songs from the 1970s that were unfamiliar to their undergraduate participants. The lyrics were presented as spoken or as sung with a musical accompaniment. In one experiment, participants rated the extent to which the lyrics conveyed a happy or sad message. In a second experiment, listeners heard both unfamiliar and familiar songs and rated the meaningfulness of the song lyrics. (These ratings reflected the extent to which the lyrics were perceived as "informative, artful, novel, generating strong and multiple associations, and are persuasive.") In a third experiment, separate groups of listeners rated the meaningfulness of unfamiliar lyrics/songs after just one exposure or after five exposures. The repeated exposure group heard the songs in the background while they read magazines or books.

In the first experiment, Thompson and Russo found that the musical context influenced the perceived affective valence of lyrics. For example, the lyrics of Paul Simon's "Kodachrome," which are rather wistful, were rated as expressing significantly more positive affect when heard in the context of their musical accompaniment, which is quite upbeat.[14] In their second study, they found that the lyrics of familiar songs were judged as more meaningful when accompanied by music, but (somewhat surprisingly) the lyrics of unfamiliar songs were not. In the final study, they found that repeated background exposure to songs led to higher ratings of the meaningfulness of the associated lyrics. Together, the results of experiments 2 and 3 suggest that mere familiarity with music leads listeners to believe that music enhances the meaning of lyrics. It is as if music is semiotically protean, and via repeated association with a text comes to enhance its meaning.

---

[14] I happen to be familiar with this song, both as a listener and a performer, and I would argue that part of its affective power comes from the *contrast* between the wistful lyrics and the bright music, which captures something about the complex, polyvalent affect associated with memory of one's youth.

All of the above studies examine the relationship between musical and linguistic meaning via a rather gross manipulation: the presence or absence of music. Drawing on the insights of music theorists, it may be more interesting for future studies to manipulate the musical structure associated with a given text and to ask if listeners show any sensitivity to the relation of linguistic and musical semiosis (e.g., via judgments of the meaningfulness of the lyrics, using measures of type employed by Thompson and Russo). For example, one could present the Bach chorale "Aus tiefer Noth schrei ich zu dir" with a different harmonization, full of conclusive cadences, or to set the lyrics of "Kodachrome" to more somber music, so that it lacks the tension between wistful lyrics and an upbeat accompaniment. If listeners who were not familiar with the original songs judge the lyrics as more meaningful in the original (vs. altered) contexts, this would provide evidence that the details of musical structure are contributing to the meaningfulness of the song.

6.5 The Expression and Appraisal of Emotion as a Key Link

Of the different points of contact between musical and linguistic meaning discussed in this chapter, one stands out as particularly promising. This is the link between musical and vocal cues to affect (first discussed in section 6.2.2). The idea that there may be such a link has a long history. Philosophers and theorists as far back as Plato have speculated that part of music's expressive power lies in acoustic cues related to the sounds of emotive voices (Kivy, 2002). Such a view is sensible because there is a relationship between vocal affect and "musical" aspects of speech such as pitch, tempo, loudness, and timbre (voice quality; Ladd et al., 1985; Johnstone & Scherer, 1999; 2000). Over the years there have been a number of suggestions by music researchers about parallels between musical and vocal affect. For example, in a cross-cultural study of lullabies, including African, Native American, Samoan, and Ukrainian material, Unyk et al. (1992) examined which structural features best predicted Western adults' ability to judge whether a song from another culture was a lullaby. The researchers found that accuracy of lullaby judgments was predicted by the percentage of descending intervals in the melodies. They related this fact to Fernald's (1992) observation that descending pitch contours dominate in infant-directed speech used to soothe infants (whereas ascending contours dominate in infant-directed speech used to arouse infants). Another interesting link between musical and vocal affect was proposed by Cohen (1971), who focused on the rules of counterpoint in the vocal music of the Renaissance composer Palestrina (1525/6–1594). Cohen argues that many of these rules act to suppress sudden changes in volume, pitch, or rhythm, thus making the music similar to the prosody of "unexcited speech." She notes, "The rules served an ideal of calm, religious expression, which satisfied the reforms introduced by the Council of Trent: that the vocal expressions in all ceremonies 'may reach tranquilly into the ears and hearts of those who hear them...'" (p. 109).

Observations such as those of Unyk et al. and Cohen are thought-provoking and call for empirical research on the relation between acoustic cues to vocal and musical affect. Fortunately there has been a surge of research in this area, as discussed below.

6.5.1 Acoustic Cues to Emotion in Speech and Music

Perceptual research has revealed that listeners are good at decoding basic emotions (such as happiness, sadness, anger, and fear) from the sound of a voice, even when the words spoken are emotionally neutral or semantically unintelligible, as in speech in a foreign language (Johnstone & Scherer 2000; Scherer et al., 2001; Thompson & Balkwill, 2006).[15] This suggests cross-cultural commonalities in the acoustic cues to different emotions in speech, perhaps reflecting the physiological effects of emotion on the vocal apparatus, as first suggested by Herbert Spencer (1857). Spencer also argued that these cues played a role in musical expression, based on the idea that song employs intensified versions of the affective cues used in speech. Since Spencer's time, the idea of a parallel between affective cues in speech and music has been explored by several modern researchers (e.g., Sundberg, 1982; Scherer, 1995).

In a landmark study, Juslin and Laukka (2003) conducted a comprehensive review of 104 studies of vocal expression and 41 studies of music performance (about half of these studies focused on vocal music, and the other half on instrumental music). They found that in both domains, listeners were fairly accurate in judging the emotion intended by a speaker or performer uttering/performing a given spoken/musical passage, when the emotions portrayed were limited to five basic categories: happiness, sadness, anger, fear, and tenderness. This naturally raises the question of the relationship between the acoustic cues used by listeners in judging emotion in emotional prosody versus music performance. Juslin and Laukka found substantial overlap in the acoustic cues used to convey basic emotions in speech and music. Some of the cross-modal similarities are listed in Table 6.2.

---

[15] Thompson and Balkwill's (2006) study is notable for including non-Western languages. English listeners were able to identify happiness, sadness, anger, and fear in semantically neutral sentences at above-chance levels in five languages (including Japanese and Tagalog), though they showed an in-group advantage for English sentences and lower recognition rates in Japanese and Chinese sentences. This suggests subtle cultural differences in vocal affect that merit further study (cf. Elfenbein & Ambady, 2003).

Table 6.2 Shared Acoustic Cues for Emotions in Speech and Music

Summary of Cross-Modal Patterns of Acoustic Cues for Discrete Emotions

Emotion	Acoustic Cues (Vocal Expression/Music Performance)
Anger	Fast speech rate/tempo, high voice intensity/sound level, much voice intensity/sound level variability, much high-frequency energy, high F0/pitch level, much F0/pitch variability, rising F0/pitch contour, fast voice onsets/tone attacks, and microstructural irregularity
Fear	Fast speech rate/tempo, low voice intensity/sound level (except in panic fear), much voice intensity/sound level variability, little high-frequency energy, high F0/pitch level, little F0/pitch variability, rising F0/pitch contour, and a lot of microstructural irregularity
Happiness	Fast speech rate/tempo, medium-high voice intensity/sound level, medium high-frequency energy, high F0/pitch level, much F0/pitch variability, rising F0/pitch contour, fast voice onsets/tone attacks, and very little microstructural regularity
Sadness	Slow speech rate/tempo, low voice intensity/sound level, little voice intensity/sound level variability, little high-frequency energy, low F0/pitch level, little F0/pitch variability, falling F0/pitch contour, slow voice onsets/tone attacks, and microstructural irregularity
Tenderness	Slow speech rate/tempo, low voice intensity/sound level, little voice intensity/sound level variability, little high-frequency energy, low F0/pitch level, little F0/pitch variability, falling F0/pitch contour, slow voice onsets/tone attacks, and microstructural regularity

Note: F0 = Fundamental frequency.

Source: From Juslin & Laukka, 2003.

Juslin and Laukka note that in both domains, cues are used probabilistically and continuously, so that cues are not perfectly reliable but have to be combined. Furthermore, evidence suggests that the cues are combined in an additive fashion (with little cue interaction), and that there is a certain amount of "cue trading" in musical expression reflecting the exigencies of particular instruments. (For example, if a performer cannot vary timbre to express anger, s/he compensates by varying loudness a bit more.)

Given these similarities between speech and music, Juslin and Laukka put forth the interesting hypothesis that many musical instruments are processed by the brain as "superexpressive voices." That is, even though most musical instruments do not sound like voices from a phenomenological standpoint, they can nevertheless engage emotion perception modules in the brain because they contain enough speech-like acoustic features to trigger these modules. According to this view, "the emotion perception modules do not recognize the difference between vocal expressions and other acoustic expressions and therefore react in much the same way (e.g., registering anger) as long as certain cues (e.g., high speed, loud dynamics, rough timbre) are present in the stimulus" (p. 803). This perspective is interesting because it leads to specific predictions about neural dissociations, discussed later in this section.

One criticism of the majority of studies reviewed by Juslin and Laukka is that their musical circumstances were rather artificial, consisting of a single musician who has been instructed to play a given musical passage with the intent to convey different emotions such as happiness, sadness, anger, and so forth. One might object that such studies have little to do with emotions in real music, and simply lead a performer to imitate whatever acoustic cues to the emotion are most familiar to them (e.g., cues from speech). Thus, in future work, it may be preferable to restrict analyses to more naturalistic musical stimuli, such as those employed by Krumhansl in her psychophysiological study of musical emotion (cf. section 6.2.3). Another important source of data would be from comparative ethnomusicology, especially from studies in which listeners from one culture attempt to identify the emotions in naturalistic but unfamiliar musical excerpts taken from another culture. When cross-cultural identification is successful, then acoustic cues can be examined to determine if any cues are related to the cues in affective speech prosody (cf. the research of Balkwill and colleagues discussed in section 6.2.2).

6.5.2 Neural Aspects of Auditory Affect Perception

One way to test whether music engages brain mechanisms normally used to decode affective prosody in language (Juslin & Laukka, 2003) is to examine the neural relationship of affect perception in speech and music. This issue can be approached in two ways. First, one can use functional neuroimaging to examine patterns of activity in healthy brains. Research on the perception of emotional prosody has implicated regions in the right hemisphere including right inferior frontal regions (George et al., 1996; Imaizumi et al., 1997; Buchanan et al., 2000). There is some inconsistency in the localization results, however, and evidence that many brain regions (both cortical and subcortical) are involved (Peretz, 2001). There are also a few studies of the neural correlates of affect perception in music (e.g., Blood et al., 1999; Schmidt & Trainor, 2001; cf. Trainor & Schmidt, 2003), although once again the results have been variable in terms of localization and hemispheric asymmetry (see Peretz, 2001, for a review).

Some of this variability may be due to differences in methodology. For example, Blood et al. (1999). examined brain correlates of the perceived pleasantness or unpleasantness of music based on changing degrees of dissonance and found that most activation was in the right hemisphere (e.g., in right parahippocampal gyrus and precuneus, though there was bilateral orbitofrontal cortex). In contrast, Schmidt and Trainor (2001) used music expressing joy, happiness, sadness, or fear and found hemispheric asymmetries in brain responses (as measured by

EEG), with greater left frontal activity for positive emotions and greater right frontal activity for negative emotions. Thus at this time, one cannot state with any confidence whether the brain regions associated with vocal and musical affect perception overlap or not. However, the question is quite amenable to empirical analysis, using a within-subjects design and linguistic and musical stimuli designed to be expressive of similar basic emotions.

Besides neuroimaging, there is another approach to the study of the neural relationship of spoken versus musical affect. This is to focus on individuals who have difficulty judging the affective quality of speech following brain damage. The syndrome of receptive "affective aprosodia" has been known for some time (Ross, 1981). Such individuals have difficulty discriminating emotion in speech (and sometimes in faces) due to brain damage, despite relative preservation of other linguistic abilities (Ross, 2000). No single brain locus of this disorder has emerged: It appears that both hemispheres are involved in recognizing emotional prosody, though right inferior frontal regions appear to be particularly important (Adolphs et al., 2002; Charbonneau et al., 2002). To date, no studies have been published of these individuals' ability to perceive emotional expression in music. Such studies are clearly called for, because they would provide an important test of the Juslin and Laukka's hypothesis that the brain treats instruments as "superexpressive voices."

6.5.3 Cross-Domain Influences

Another way to test if music and speech engage common mechanisms for affect perception is to examine transfer effects from one domain to the other. Thompson et al. (2004) have done just this, by studying whether musical training improves the ability to discriminate between different emotions expressed by the voice. At first glance, such a facilitation seems unlikely. The ability to discriminate vocal emotions would seem to be a basic biological function, important enough to survival that evolution would make the brain learn this discrimination with minimum experience, so that training in music or any other domain would make little difference to performance. On the other hand, if discrimination abilities for speech affect are related to the amount of experience with emotional voices, and if there are important similarities in acoustic cues to emotion in speech and music (as suggested in section 6.5.1), then one might expect that musical training would improve vocal affective discrimination skills. In Thompson et al.'s study, musically trained and untrained English-speaking adults listened to emotional sentences in their own language or in a foreign language (Tagalog, a language of the Philippines) and attempted to classify them into one of four basic categories: happiness, sadness, anger, and fear. The researchers found that musical training did improve the ability to identify certain emotions, particularly sadness and fear. Particularly notable was an effect of training on the ability to discriminate emotions in Tagalog: This was the first evidence that musical training enhances sensitivity to vocal emotions in a foreign language.

Of course, it is possible that individuals who seek out musical training are already more sensitive to vocal affect in general. As an attempt to get around this "causal directionality" problem, Thompson et al. (2004) conducted another experiment in which 6-year-old children were assigned to groups that took 1 year of music lessons (keyboard or singing), drama lessons, or no lessons. Prior to starting the lessons, the children were equivalent in terms of IQ and academic achievement on a number of different psychological tests. At the end of the year, the children were tested for their ability to discriminate vocal affect, using a slightly simplified procedure in which they either had to discriminate between happy and sad or between angry and frightened. The researchers found that discrimination of happy/sad vocal affect was so good across groups that no differences could be observed (a "ceiling" effect). However, the fear/anger discrimination performance levels were lower, and here significant group differences did emerge. Specifically, children who had keyboard lessons or drama lessons did significantly better than children with no lessons. That children who studied keyboard did as well as children who studied drama (in which vocal affect is an explicit target of training) is particularly interesting, and Thompson et al. suggest that this transfer effect may reflect overlapping processes in decoding emotional meaning in music and speech prosody (specifically, processes that associate pitch and temporal patterns with emotion).[16]

6.5.4 Emotion in Speech and Music:
Future Directions

The preceding three sections show that the empirical comparative study of emotional expression (and perception) in music and speech is off to a good start and has interesting avenues to explore, for example, the perception of musical affect in patients with affective aprosodia. This section touches on some issues likely to prove important to future work. One of these concerns is the number of dimensions used to describe emotions engendered by speech and music. As discussed in section 6.2.3, psychological studies often describe emotions in terms of two distinct dimensions, one corresponding to valence (positive vs. negative) and one to activity (low vs. high). It may be that two dimensions are too few. Indeed, in a study comparing acoustic cues to affect in music and speech, Ilie and Thompson (2006) needed three dimensions to capture patterns in their data, whereas a study of vocal affect by Laukka et al. (2005) used four dimensions. Scherer (2004) also feels that two-dimensional descriptions

---

[16] Alternatively, it may be that musical training increases raw sensitivity to pitch variation in speech (cf. Magne et al., 2006; Wong et al., 2007), and that this is partly responsible for the observed transfer effect.

of musical emotion are too simple, and may be low-dimensional projections of high-dimensional emotional qualia.

A second issue for future work concerns differences in the way acoustic cues map onto emotions in speech and music. Comparative speech-music research has mostly emphasized cross-domain similarities, but differences exist and are likely to prove informative for cognitive issues. For example, Ilie and Thompson (2006) found that manipulations of pitch height had opposite effects on the perceived valence of speech and music: Higher pitched speech (but lower pitched music) was associated with more positive valence.

A final issue concerns timbre. Although much research on affect in speech and music has focused on tempo, intensity, and pitch contours, the role of timbre (or "voice quality" in speech) in conveying affect has been less explored, perhaps because it is harder to measure. Yet timbre may be crucial for affect expression and perception (cf. Ladd et al., 1985). Note, for example, how similar anger and happiness are in Table 6.2 in terms of acoustic cues relating to rate, intensity, and pitch patterns. Timbral cues are thus likely to be very important in distinguishing these emotions. There can be little doubt that timbre is also important in conveying affect in music (cf. Bigand et al., 2005). (An informal demonstration is provided by listening to a musical theme as performed by an orchestra, with all of its attendant sound color, and as performed by a solo piano. These two passages contain the same rhythm and melody, but can have a very different affective impact. The difference is in the timbre.) Separate brain imaging studies of spoken voice versus instrumental music perception (using fMRI) have implicated overlapping regions in the superior temporal sulcus in vocal versus musical timbre analysis (Belin et al., 2000; Menon et al., 2002, cf. Chartrand & Belin, 2006). However, these regions appear not to overlap completely, consistent with the observation that the perception of musical (vs. voice) timbre can be selectively impaired in neurological cases (cf. Sacks, 2007). Hence it may be that vocal versus musical sounds are first analyzed for timbre by specialized brain regions, and that the resulting timbral information is then handled by common circuits in terms of mapping onto emotional qualities.

6.6 Conclusion

At first glance, it seems that linguistic and musical meaning are largely incommensurate. Indeed, if one restricts "meaning" to semantic reference and predication, then music and language have little in common (though perhaps more than suspected, as suggested by recent cognitive and neural research). The approach taken here is to adopt a broader view of meaning, inspired by Nattiez's semiotic research on music (1990). In this view, meaning exists when perception of an object/event brings something to mind other than the object/event itself. This definition stimulates systematic thinking about the *variety* of ways in which music can be meaningful, which in turn refines the discussion of how musical and linguistic meaning are similar or different. When one takes this perspective, many interesting topics for cross-domain research come to the fore, including the expression and appraisal of emotion, the cognitive relations that make a linguistic or musical discourse coherent, and the combination of linguistic and musical meaning in song. Comparative research on music and language can help illuminate the diversity of ways in which our mind derives meaning from structured acoustic sequences.

Chapter 7
_____

Evolution

7

Evolution

7.1 Introduction

From an evolutionary standpoint, language and music are peculiar phenomena, because they appear in only one species: *Homo sapiens.* The closest that nonhuman animals have come to language has been in studies in which pygmy chimpanzees learn a simple vocabulary and syntax based on interactions with humans (Savage-Rumbaugh et al., 1998, cf. Herman & Uyeyama, 1999; Pepperberg, 2002). Although these results are fascinating and important, these animals show no evidence of a language-like communicative system in the wild, based on either vocal or gestural signals (Tomasello, 2003). Furthermore, even the most precocious language-trained apes, who may acquire a few hundred words, are far surpassed by ordinary human children, who learn thousands of words and complex grammatical structures in the first few years of life. Finally, no nonhuman primate has ever been successfully trained to speak, despite numerous efforts (Fitch, 2000). Language, as we commonly understand the term, is the sole province of humans.

What of music? Initially it may seem that music is not unique to humans, because many species produce "songs" that strike us as musical (Baptista & Keister, 2005). Songbirds and certain whales (e.g., humpbacks) are notable singers, and in some species, such as the European nightingale (*Luscinia megarhynchos*), an individual singer can have hundreds of songs involving recombination of discrete elements in different sequences (Payne, 2000; Slater, 2000). Furthermore, songbirds and singing whales are not born knowing their song, but like humans, learn by listening to adults.

Closer inspection of the biology of bird and whale song, however, reveals several important differences from human music, a few of which are listed here (cf. Cross, 2001; Hauser & McDermott, 2003). First, songs are typically produced by males, who use them to attract mates and/or warn competing males off of territories (Catchpole and Slater, 1995). Second, hormonal and neural changes (stimulated by photoperiod) play an important role in determining seasonal peaks in avian singing (e.g., Dloniak & Deviche, 2001). This suggests that song is not a volitional aesthetic act but a biologically mediated reproductive behavior. Third, although it is true that many species learn their songs, there appear to be strong constraints on learning. Research by Marler and colleagues has shown that juvenile birds learn their own species' song much more readily and accurately than songs of other species (Marler, 1997, 1999; Whaling, 2000). Of course, there are constraints on human musical learning as well. Due to cognitive capacity limits, for example, no child would accurately learn melodies built from a scale using 35 notes per octave (Miller, 1956; cf. Chapter 2). The constraints on human musical learning appear to be much weaker than on bird song learning, however, as evidenced by the great diversity of human music compared to the songs of any given bird species. Finally, and perhaps most importantly, the structural diversity of animal songs is not associated with an equal diversity of meanings. On the contrary, animal songs always advertise the same set of things, including readiness to mate, territorial warnings, and social status (Marler, 2000; cf. Chapter 5 of this book). Thus the fact that English uses the term "song" for the acoustic displays of certain animals should not mislead us into thinking that animals make or appreciate music in the sense that humans do.[1]

Given the universality and uniqueness of language and music in our species, it is clear that these abilities reflect changes in the brain that have taken place since our lineage's divergence from our common ancestor with chimpanzees about 6 million years ago (Carroll, 2003). Thus one can accurately say that language and music evolved in the human lineage. However, this sense of "evolved" is not very meaningful from a biological standpoint. The ability to make and control fire is also universal and unique to human cultures, and one could therefore say that fire making "evolved" in the human lineage. Yet few would dispute that the control of fire was an invention based on human ingenuity, not something that was itself a target of evolutionary forces. Thus a more biologically meaningful question is, to what extent have human bodies and brains been shaped by natural selection for language? Similarly, to what extent have human bodies and brains been shaped by natural selection for music? These questions are the main focus of this chapter.

The example of fire making teaches us that when we see a universal and unique human trait, we cannot simply assume that it has been a direct target of selection. In fact, from a scientific perspective it is better (because it assumes less) to take the null hypothesis that the trait in question *has not* been a direct target of selection. One can then ask if there is enough evidence to reject this hypothesis. The two main sections of this chapter address this question for language and music. Section 7.2 argues that there is enough evidence to reject this

---

[1] Whether or not animals can be trained to produce or appreciate music is dealt with later in this chapter.

hypothesis in the case of language, whereas section 7.3 argues the opposite for music. That is, section 7.3 reviews a variety of relevant research and concludes that there is as yet no compelling evidence that music represents an evolutionary adaptation. Section 7.4 asks, "If music is not an evolutionary adaptation, then why is it universal?" The final section discusses an area of research area likely to prove crucial to future debates over the evolutionary status of music, namely beat-based rhythmic processing.

Before embarking, it is worth discussing two phenomena that may seem to be prima facie evidence of natural selection for music. The first involves the existence of individuals with selective deficits in music perception due to brain damage, in other words, with "acquired selective amusia" (e.g., Peretz, 1993; Peretz & Coltheart, 2003). For example, such individuals may be unable to recognize familiar melodies or to spot out-of-key ("sour") notes in novel melodies, despite the fact that they were previously quite musical and still seem normal in other ways. The existence of such individuals shows that parts of the brain have become specialized for music. It is sometimes thought that this "modularity" indicates that natural selection has shaped parts of the brain to carry out musical functions. In fact, the modularity of music processing in adults is orthogonal to the issue of selection for musical abilities. This is because modules can be a product of development, rather than reflecting innately specified brain specialization. An instructive phenomenon in this regard is orthographic alexia: a specific deficit for reading printed letters due to brain damage. Because written language is a recent human invention in evolutionary terms, we can be confident that specific brain areas have not been shaped by natural selection for reading printed script. Nevertheless, both neuropsychological and neuroimaging studies have shown that there are areas in the occipitotemporal region of the left hemisphere that are specialized for recognizing alphabetic letters in literate individuals (Cohen et al., 2002; cf. Stewart et al., 2003; Hébert & Cuddy, 2006). In this case, the areas are in a part of the brain ordinarily involved in object recognition. This is a powerful demonstration of "progressive modularization" during development (Karmiloff-Smith, 1992; Booth et al., 2001) and shows why selective deficits of music are largely irrelevant to evolutionary arguments.

A second phenomenon that might seem to suggest natural selection for music concerns the role of genes in musical ability. Musical "tone deafness" is estimated to occur in about 4% of the population (Kalmus & Fry, 1980). It is not due to hearing loss or lack of exposure to music, or to any social or affective abnormality. In fact, musically tone-deaf individuals can appear perfectly normal in every other way, except for a striking difficulty with music that they have often had for as long as they can remember (Ayotte et al., 2002; Foxton et al., 2004). For example, they cannot hear when music is out of tune (including their own singing voice) and cannot recognize what should be very familiar melodies in their culture unless the words are provided. In 1980 Kalmus and

Fry noted that tone deafness tends to run in families. A more recent study found that identical twins (who share 100% of their genes) resemble each other more closely on tests of tone deafness than do fraternal twins (who share only 50% of their genes on average). These findings suggest that there is a specific gene (or genes) that puts one at risk for this disorder (Drayna et al., 2001). To some, this might suggest that there are "genes for music," and that therefore music was a target of natural selection. Although we will delve into the genetics of music and language later in this chapter, for now suffice it to say that tone deafness provides no evidence for genes that are specifically involved in musical abilities.[2] On the contrary, current evidence suggests that tone-deaf individuals have rather basic deficits with pitch perception that impact their musical abilities because music places much more stringent demands on pitch perception than does any other domain (cf. Chapter 4, section 4.5.2).

Thus there is no simple, cut-and-dried evidence that music has been the focus of natural selection. The question of selection's role in human musical abilities requires careful investigation. The approach taken here is to compare music and language in this regard.

7.2 Language and Natural Selection

Have human bodies and brains been shaped by natural selection for language? Before delving into details, it is worth clarifying what is meant by "natural selection for language." Clearly, people are not born knowing their native tongue: They learn the sonic and structural patterns of their native language in childhood. Thus "natural selection for language" really refers to selection for the ability to acquire language. From an evolutionary perspective, what we want to know is whether selection has played a direct role in shaping the mechanisms of language acquisition. Those who favor a direct role for selection can be termed "language adaptationists." For example, Pinker and Jackendoff (2005) argue that language acquisition involves a set of cognitive and neural specializations tailored by evolution to this rich communicative system. In their view, the selective pressure behind language evolution was the adaptive value of expressing and understanding complex propositions.[3]

An alternative view proposes that there has been no direct selection for language. Instead, selection acted to create certain unique social-cognitive learning

---

[2] The genetics of absolute pitch and its relevance to evolutionary arguments are dealt with later in this chapter, in section 7.3.4.

[3] There are of course alternative proposals for the selective pressure behind language, including the idea that language originally served to facilitate bonding in social groups that were too large for traditional primate grooming strategies (Dunbar, 2003). The precise selective pressures behind language evolution are not the focus here.

abilities in humans, such as "shared intentionality," the capacity and drive for shared goals and joint attention. According to Tomasello et al. (2005), this transforms individual cognition into cultural cognition, lays the foundation for imitation and instructed learning, and permits the invention of a cooperative communication system based on symbols. In this view, humans used their special social-cognitive abilities to *construct* language. Tomasello and other "language constructivists" offer a very different picture of language evolution than language adaptationists, and have presented some cogent criticisms of the adaptationist position (cf. Tomasello, 1995; Elman, 1999). One interesting corollary of the constructivist viewpoint is the notion that our brains are not biologically different from those of our most recent prelinguistic ancestors. This is because language is a seen as a social construct. A useful analogy is to chess playing. Chess playing is a complex cognitive ability that is unique to our species, but which has certainly not been the target of natural selection. Although some of the cognitive abilities used in chess may have been direct targets of selection, these abilities were not shaped by selection *for* chess nor are they specific to it (cf. Sober, 1984). The key conceptual point here is that natural selection has played only an *indirect* role in shaping our chess-playing abilities.

Thus the debate between language adaptationists and language constructivists can thus be seen as a debate between scholars who believe in a direct versus an indirect role for natural selection in shaping human linguistic abilities. There are also well-articulated positions that do not fall neatly into either category: For example, Deacon (1997) has argued that language and the human brain have acted as selective forces on each other via a process of coevolution. For those interested in the range of current thinking on language evolution (which is broad and growing rapidly), there are several useful books and review articles to consult (e.g., Christiansen & Kirby, 2003a, 2003b). The main point is that there is a lively debate over the extent to which human bodies and brains have been directly shaped by selection for language. What follows is a list of 10 lines of evidence that I find the most compelling in favor of a direct role for natural selection in the evolution of language.

7.2.1 Babbling

One of the most striking aspects of language development is babbling: Around the age of 7 months, babies begin to produce nonsense syllables such as /ba/ and /da/ in repetitive sequences (Locke, 1993). Babbling likely helps babies learn the relationship between oral movements and auditory outcomes, in other words, to tune the perceptual-motor skills they will use in acquiring their species' communication system. Babbling is evidence that selection has acted on language acquisition because its emergence is spontaneous, and not simply an imitation of adult speech. A key piece of evidence in this regard is that deaf babies produce vocal babbles even though they have no experience with the speech of others (Oller & Eilers, 1988). Thus the onset of babbling appears to reflect the maturation of neural mechanisms for vocal learning.[4] This view is further supported by experimental studies of songbirds, who, like humans, learn to produce complex acoustic signals for communication. Young birds go through a babbling stage (called "subsong") during which they produce immature versions of the elements of adults' song (Doupe & Kuhl, 1999). Furthermore, they babble even if deafened at birth (Marler, 1999). Thus babbling appears to be evolution's way of kick-starting the vocal learning process.

Interestingly, in the human case, the mechanisms underlying babbling are not bound to speech. Deaf babies exposed to sign language will babble with their hands, producing nonreferential signs in reduplicated sequences (e.g., the sign language equivalent of "bababa"; Petitto & Marentette, 1991; Petitto et al., 2001, 2004). Emmorey (2002) has suggested that babbling thus represents the maturation of a mechanism that maps between motor output and sensory input, and guides humans toward the discovery of the phonological structure of language, whether spoken or signed.

7.2.2 Anatomy of the Human Vocal Tract

Compared to other primates, humans have an unusual vocal tract: The larynx sits much lower in the throat due to a gradual anatomical descent between about 3 months and 3 years of age (Fitch, 2000).[5] The low position of the larynx in humans has a biological cost. In other primates, the larynx connects with the nasal passages, allowing simultaneous swallowing and breathing. In contrast, humans risk choking each time they ingest food. Lieberman and colleagues (1969; cf. Lieberman, 1984) were the first to suggest that this special aspect of human anatomy was related to the evolution of language. Lieberman argued that a lowered larynx increases the range and discriminability of speech sounds because it gives the tongue room to move both vertically and horizontally in the vocal tract, allowing for a more distinctive palette of formant patterns (formants are discussed in Chapter 2). This has been a fertile hypothesis, leading to a good deal of research and debate (Ohala, 1984; Fitch 2000; cf. Ménard et al., 2004). As of today, it is still a viable idea and points

---

[4] Of course, once babbling has commenced, it is quickly influenced by environmental input. For example, hearing babies begin to show signs of the influence of their native language's intonation in their first year (Whalen et al., 1991), and the quantity and complexity of babbling is modulated by social feedback from their caregiver (Goldstein et al., 2003).

[5] A second, smaller descent occurs in males at puberty (Fitch & Giedd, 1999). See Ohala (1984) for a discussion of the evolutionary significance of this difference between the sexes.

to a direct role for natural selection in shaping the human body for speech and thus for language.[6]

7.2.3 Vocal Learning

Vocal learning refers to learning to produce vocal signals based on auditory experience and sensory feedback. This ability seems commonplace to us because every child exhibits it as part of learning to speak. An evolutionary perspective, however, reveals that vocal learning is an uncommon trait, having arisen in only a few groups of animals (including songbirds, parrots, and cetaceans; cf. Fitch, 2006; Merker, 2005). Notably, humans are unique among primates in exhibiting complex vocal learning (Egnor & Hauser, 2004). Even language-trained apes are poor at imitating spoken words, and rely instead on visual symbols to communicate.[7] The neural substrates of vocal learning in humans are not well understood, but this difference between humans and other primates is almost certainly part of an ensemble of characteristics (including babbling and a modified vocal tract) shaped by natural selection to favor children's acquisition of a complex acoustic communication system.

7.2.4 Precocious Learning of Linguistic Sound Structure

The phonemes and syllables of human languages are acoustically complex entities, and infants seem to come into the world prepared to learn about them. By 6 months of age, they start to show evidence of learning the particular vowel sounds of their language (Kuhl et al., 1992). Soon thereafter, they lose sensitivity to certain phonetic contrasts that do not occur in their language, and gain sensitivity for other, difficult phonetic contrasts in their native tongue (Werker & Tees, 1984; 1999; Polka et al., 2001). That is, infants come into the world with open ears suited to the sounds of any human language, but soon begin to "hear with an accent" in ways that favor their native tongue. Infants also show an impressive ability to recognize the equivalence of a speech sound (such as a particular vowel or a syllable) across differences in speaker, gender, and speech rate, a task that has proven difficult for even very powerful computers (e.g., Kuhl, 1979, 2004).

---

[6] Note that although language does not require speech (as evidenced by the fact that sign languages are full human languages; Klima & Bellugi, 1979; Emmorey, 2002), speech is a primary channel for language and thus morphological specializations for speech are also evidence of selection for language.

[7] Gibbons are great apes well known for their impressive singing and their male-female duets, but in contrast to songbirds, they do not appear to learn their song (Geissmann, 2000).

Complementing these perceptual skills are skills at sound production. Speaking involves regulating the airstream while producing rapid and temporally overlapping gestures with multiple articulators (Stevens, 1998). Children largely master these complex motor skills by the age of 3 or 4, producing speech that is not only fluent and highly intelligible but that has many of the subtleties of their native language (e.g., context-dependent phonological modifications, which contribute to native accent). These abilities stand in sharp contrast to other motor skills of 3- to 4-year-olds, such as their ability to throw and catch objects with accuracy.

Of course, perception and production of speech are intimately linked in learning. One fact that suggests a role for selection in shaping learning mechanisms is the exquisite sensitivity of vocal development to perceptual experience in this domain. For example, even casually overhearing a language before the age of 6 can have an influence on one's production of phonemes from that language as an adult. Au et al. (2002; see also Knightly et al., 2003) found that American college students who had overheard informal Spanish for a few years before the age of 6 produced word-initial stop consonants such as /p/ and /k/ in a manner identical to native speakers when asked to produce Spanish sentences.[8] In contrast, a control group without casual childhood exposure produced these sounds in a manner more characteristic of native English speakers. Interestingly, the two groups performed no differently on tasks that involved making grammatical judgments about Spanish, showing that the casual-exposure group did not simply know Spanish better in any explicit sense. Thus the speech-learning system seems specially prepared to put perceptual experience to work in shaping production abilities (cf. Oh et al., 2003 for a replication and extension of this work based on Korean).

The field of infant speech perception is a dynamic research area with evolving theories and ongoing debates (e.g., Kuhl, 2004; Werker & Curtin, 2005), but there is consensus on the following fact: Humans are precocious learners of the sound structure of language, achieving complex perceptual and production skills at a very young age. This suggests that natural selection has shaped the mechanisms of speech acquisition.

7.2.5 Critical Periods for Language Acquisition

A critical period or sensitive period is a time window when developmental processes are especially sensitive to environmental input. Input (or lack of it) during this time can have a profound effect on the ultimate level of adult ability in specific areas. Vocal development in songbirds is a well-studied case in biology.

---

[8] The dependent measure was voice-onset time (VOT), the time between the release of a stop consonant to the onset of voicing for the vowel.

If birds who learn their song (e.g., baby swamp sparrows) are not permitted to hear the song of an adult before a certain age, they will never acquire full proficiency in their species' song, even if given unlimited exposure later in life (Marler, 1999). The mechanisms behind critical periods are still a matter of debate. One idea is that the rate of neural proliferation (e.g., as measured by synaptic density) in specific brain areas is under biological control, with gradual reduction over time due to internal factors (Huttenlocher, 2002). Critical periods are suggestive of mechanisms shaped by natural selection to favor early acquisition of ethologically important abilities.

In an influential book, Lennenberg (1967) proposed that humans have a critical period for language acquisition that ends at puberty. Of course (and thankfully), one cannot test this idea with the kind of deprivation experiments done with songbirds. There are a few cases of language-deprived children (e.g., Curtiss, 1977), but the confounding effects of social trauma make these cases hard to interpret (Rymer, 1993). At the present time, the best evidence for a critical period for language comes from studies of second-language learning and from research on sign language. In the former category, Johnson and Newport (1989) studied Chinese and Korean immigrants to the United States, examining their proficiency in English as a function of the age at which they entered the country (overall number of years of exposure to English was matched across groups). They found strong effects of age of exposure on grammatical abilities. One might argue that this is due not to any biological mechanism, but simply to the fact that older individuals have a better developed native language, which interfered more with the acquisition of a new language. This concern is mitigated by studies of sign language acquisition. Mayberry and colleagues (Mayberry and Eichen, 1991, Mayberry and Lock, 2003) have shown that when sign language input is delayed in individuals with no other language, there is a significant impact on adult grammatical skills and on the ability to acquire a second language later in life.[9]

7.2.6 Commonalities of Structure and Development in Spoken and Signed Language

Although there is little doubt that speech is the biologically given channel for human language, it is a remarkable fact that individuals can communicate linguistically without sound, by using sign language. It is important to note that true sign languages such as American Sign Language (ASL) and British Sign

---

[9] Studies of the critical period have shown that although age of exposure to language has a salient influence on grammar and on phonology (i.e., "native accent"; Piske et al., 2001), it does not have a pronounced effect on the acquisition of vocabulary (Newport, 2002). Thus the critical period for language appears to influence the formal, combinatorial aspects of language more than the semantic aspects.

Language (BSL) are not merely spoken language translated into gesture (e.g., finger-spelled English). Instead, they are distinct human languages with structural patterns that can be quite different from the surrounding spoken language (Klima & Bellugi, 1979; Emmorey, 2002). Thus for example, although American and British English are mutually intelligible, ASL and BSL are not.

Cognitive research has revealed that sign and spoken languages share the basic ingredients of human language: phonology, morphology, syntax and semantics, and that deaf children exposed to sign from an early age acquire these aspects of language in ways quite parallel to hearing children (Emmorey, 2002). Furthermore, studies of sign language aphasia and modern neuroimaging techniques have revealed that despite its visuospatial modality, sign language relies on many of the same left hemisphere brain areas as spoken language (see Emmorey 2002, Ch. 9 for an overview). I shall have more to say about sign language in section 7.2.8 below. For now, suffice it so say that the fact that language can "jump modalities" is a powerful testament to the human drive for language, suggesting a role for natural selection in shaping the language acquisition process.

7.2.7 Robustness of Language Acquisition

All normal infants exposed to language rapidly develop a complex set of linguistic production and perception skills, as evidenced by the linguistic abilities of 3- to 4-year-olds. An interesting question about this process concerns the variability in the quality and quantity of linguistic input received by infants and young children. In one of the few published studies that measured language input to the infant over an extended period, van de Weijer (1998) recorded most of what a single Dutch infant heard during its waking hours between 6 and 9 months of age. In analyzing a subset of this data (18 days), he found that the infant heard about 2.5 hours of speech per day, of which about 25% was directed at the infant (i.e., about 37 minutes per day, on average). This seems surprisingly small, and is no doubt less than some infants receive (i.e., those alone at home with a talkative caregiver). Yet it may be far more than babies receive in some cultures, in which it is claimed that adults barely talk to prelingual infants (e.g., the Kaluli of Papua New Guinea; see Schieffelin, 1985). Unfortunately, we lack data on the range of linguistic input to infants who subsequently develop normal language. I suspect, however, that this range is quite large (even within Western culture). If this proves to be true, then the robustness of language acquisition suggests that natural selection has shaped both a strong predisposition to learn language and the mechanisms to learn it quickly, even from minimal input.

In making this point, I do not wish to suggest that variability in experience does not matter to language development. On the contrary, there is good evidence for a relationship between the richness and complexity of linguistic input and a child's own vocabulary acquisition, use of complex syntax, and so forth (Huttenlocher et al., 1991; Hart & Risley, 1995). However, the key point is that these relations build on a basic set of abilities that appear to develop with remarkable robustness.

7.2.8 Adding Complexity to Impoverished Linguistic Input

Over the past 25 years, linguists have had an unprecedented opportunity to document the birth of a new language, created by a deaf community in Nicaragua. The history of this community is interesting. Before the 1970s, deaf Nicaraguans were mostly isolated from each other, and communicated with their hearing families using gestures that showed only the rudiments of language and that varied widely from one person to the next ("home sign" systems; Goldin-Meadow, 1982; Coppola, 2002). However, in 1977, a special school for deaf children was founded in Managua, and its student body grew rapidly. Although the teachers focused on lip reading and speaking Spanish (with little success), the deaf children used gestures to communicate among themselves, and began a process of language development in which each new cohort of children learns from the previous cohort. Research on this community has produced a remarkable finding: As the language develops, it is becoming increasingly grammaticalized, and this change is being driven *by the children*. That is, the second cohort did not just reproduce the language of the first cohort; they changed it as they learned it. For example, they systematized the use of spatial locations to signal grammatical relationships, enabling the expression of long-distance dependencies between words (Senghas & Coppola, 2001). They also showed a strong preference for breaking holistic gestures into discrete components and arranging these in sequences (Senghas et al., 2004). These findings complement earlier work on the emergence of structure in spoken Creole languages (Bickerton, 1984; Holm, 2000), but provide an even stronger case for mental predispositions for language learning, because the Nicaraguan children had no access to adults who spoke a fully developed language. That is, unlike most cultural systems, in which the structures used by adults are more organized and systematic than those used by children, Nicaraguan Sign Language illustrates a case in which children are creating the more systematic patterns. This is suggestive of learning predispositions that have been shaped by natural selection (cf. Sandler et al., 2005).

7.2.9 Fixation of a Language-Relevant Gene

Recent years have seen the discovery of a single-gene mutation in humans that has a strong influence on speech and language. When one copy of this gene (known as FOXP2) is damaged, individuals show a range of problems with speech and language, including deficits in oral movements (which extend to complex nonspeech gestures), difficulty in manipulating phonemes, and problems with grammar and lexical judgments (see Marcus & Fisher, 2003 for an overview). These individuals also have nonlinguistic deficits (Alcock et al., 2000a,b), but importantly, they do not simply suffer from an overall intellectual deficit: Verbal abilities are more impaired than nonverbal abilities, with some individuals having nonverbal abilities in the normal IQ range.

FOXP2 is not unique to humans. It occurs in many other species, including chimpanzees, birds, and crocodiles. However, the exact DNA sequence of human FOXP2 differs from other species, and shows almost no variation within *Homo sapiens*. Quantitative analysis of this variability suggests that this gene has been a target of selection in human evolution, and was fixed (i.e., became universal) in its current form within the past 200,000 years (Enard et al., 2002).

FOXP2 is discussed further in section 7.3.4, where we will delve into more mechanistic details about this gene and its role in brain and language. For the moment, the relevant point is that the extremely low variability in the DNA sequence of human FOXP2 suggests that this language-relevant gene has been a target of natural selection.

7.2.10 Biological Cost of Failure to Acquire Language

If a trait has been directly shaped by natural selection, this by necessity means the trait conferred an evolutionary advantage in terms of survival and reproductive success. Thus if an existing member of a species fails to develop the trait, that individual is likely to bear a significant biological cost. For example, a little brown bat (*Myotis lucifugus*) that cannot echolocate is likely to have much lower survival and reproduction rate than one that can. With bats, one can do an experiment to test this idea (e.g., by plugging the bat's ears from birth). With humans, we thankfully cannot do language-deprivation studies, but it seems highly likely that a human being without language abilities would be at a severe disadvantage in terms of survival and reproduction in any human society, past or present.

7.2.11 Other Evidence

The brief review above by no means exhausts the evidence that one could proffer in favor of a role for natural selection in language evolution. A few examples will suffice to illustrate this point. First, Deacon (1997) argues that the relative size of our frontal cortex is unusually large compared to other primates, and that this reflects selective pressure for specific cognitive operations underlying language. Second, MacLarnon and Hewitt (1999) report that regions of the spinal cord involved in supplying neurons for breath control are enlarged in *Homo ergaster (erectus)* and *Homo sapiens* relative to other primates and earlier hominids, and argue that this may reflect an adaptation for speech. Third, Conway and Christiansen (2001) review studies showing that humans outperform other primates in their ability to learn hierarchical sequences, and one could argue that this reflects selection for cognitive skills that are employed by language. Fourth, it is often claimed that universals of linguistic grammar are evidence for an innate knowledge of language. I have avoided these and other arguments because they are subject to a great deal of debate. For example, recent comparative analyses of primate frontal cortex suggest that human frontal cortex has not expanded much beyond what one would predict for a primate of our size (Semendeferi et al., 2002). With regard to increased breath control, Fitch (2000) has pointed out that this may have evolved for reasons other than language (e.g., prolonged running, cf. Bramble & Lieberman, 2004). Grammatical universals are the focus of an interesting controversy, with some researchers arguing that these are not built into our brains but result from the convergence of a number of forces, including human limits on sequential learning and the semiotic constraints that govern complex communication systems (e.g., Christiansen & Kirby 2003b and references therein; Deacon, 2003). Finally, evidence that humans are superior at learning hierarchical sequences may not reflect specific selection for language (for example, in principle this could arise via selection for music!).

The salient point, however, is that even if one eschews these contentious lines of evidence, there is still a solid basis for rejecting the null hypothesis for language evolution. That is, the combined weight of the evidence reviewed in sections 7.2.1 to 7.2.10 strongly favors the idea that human bodies and brains have been shaped by natural selection for language.

7.3 Music and Natural Selection

As noted in the introduction, the fact that music is a human universal is not evidence for a direct role of natural selection in the evolution of music. Nevertheless, music's universality, combined with its lack of an obvious survival value, has puzzled evolutionary thinkers since Darwin. In *The Descent of Man* (1871), Darwin remarked that our musical abilities "must be ranked among the most mysterious with which [humans are] endowed." Since Darwin's time, attitudes toward music and evolution have followed two main courses. One line of thought regards music as enjoyable byproduct of other cognitive skills. For example, William James said that a love of music was "a mere incidental peculiarity of the nervous system, with no teleological significance" (cited in Langer, 1942:210). This theme has been further developed in recent times by Pinker (1997) and others. In contrast, another line of thought favors the view that our musical abilities were a direct target of natural selection (e.g., Wallin et al., 2000; Balter, 2004; Mithen, 2005), an idea first proposed by Darwin (1871). Enthusiasm for this latter idea has spread rapidly, and there are a growing number of hypotheses about the possible adaptive roles of music in human evolution. A few of these are reviewed in section 7.3.1 below. As we shall see, each hypothesis has its problems, and it is likely that the original adaptive value of music (if any) will always be shrouded in mystery.

Thus a more promising approach to the study of music and evolution is to shift away from adaptationist conjectures to focus on factors that can be empirically studied in living organisms (cf. Fitch, 2006). For example, is there evidence that humans enter the world specifically prepared to learn about musical structures? Are there genes that have been shaped by selection for music? Are nonhuman animals capable of acquiring basic musical abilities? Analogous questions for language were behind the evidence reviewed in section 7.2 above. Ultimately, it is answers to these sorts of questions that will decide if the null hypothesis should be rejected (i.e., in the case of music, the hypothesis that humans have not been specifically shaped by evolution to be musical).

The purpose of this section is to examine the evidence for natural selections' role in directly shaping human musical abilities. To this end, music is first examined with regard to the 10 lines of evidence that were presented for language (in section 7.2 above). Following this, additional data from development, genetics, and animal studies are considered (in sections 7.3.3, 7.3.4, and 7.3.5). Prior to embarking on this survey however, it is worth describing a few adaptationist hypotheses about music, to give a flavor of some proposed functions of music in human evolution.

7.3.1 Adaptationist Hypotheses

Sexual Selection

Miller (2000), taking up an idea proposed by Darwin (1871), has argued that music is analogous to bird song in that it is a product of sexual selection (selection for traits that enhance the ability to successfully compete for mates). Miller sees music as a psychological adaptation that permitted males to perform complex courtship displays as part of competition for access to females. Presumably these displays conveyed various desirable mental and physical abilities to females. In support of his hypothesis, Miller claims that humans show a peak in their musical interests in adolescence, and that male musicians produce far more music (as measured by recorded output) than female musicians at this age.

This hypothesis has numerous difficulties. For example, sexual selection for male song production typically results in salient male-female differences in anatomy and/or behavior (e.g., among birds, whales, frogs, crickets), yet there is no evidence that human males and females differ in any substantial way in their music production or perception abilities (Huron, 2003). Another problem is that human music serves many roles both within and across cultures, including healing, mourning, celebrating, memorizing, and so forth (Cross, 2003). Courtship is only one of music's many functions, and there is no evidence that music is either necessary or sufficient for successful courtship across human cultures. A final difficulty with the idea is that the social patterns adduced by Miller as evidence for sexual selection can be explained by cultural factors, such as the importance of music in identity formation in adolescence (cf. Chapter 6) and male dominance in the control of the recording industry.

Mental and Social Development

A very different idea about music's adaptive value has been articulated by Cross (2003). Cross suggests that music plays an important role in mental development, in that it exercises and integrates a variety of cognitive and motor abilities and provides a safe medium for the exploration of social behavior. In other words, by promoting cognitive flexibility and social facility, music aids in the development of mind. Although this idea is appealing, it, too, encounters difficulties. If music were an important catalyst in mental development, then one would expect that individuals with congenital musical deficits would have detectable problems or delays in cognitive or social abilities. Yet this does not appear to be the case. About 4% of the population is estimated to be "tone-deaf," in other words, to have severe lifelong difficulties with music perception (cf. Chapter 4, section 4.5.2). This condition may result from genes that affect the auditory system (Kalmus & Fry, 1980; Drayna et al., 2001). At the current time, there is no evidence that tone-deaf individuals suffer from any serious nonmusical cognitive deficits or delays, or exhibit abnormal socialization of any sort (Ayotte et al., 2002). In fact, the tone-deaf can count numerous intellectually and socially prominent individuals among their ranks, including Milton Friedman (the Nobel Prize-winning economist) and Che Guevara (the charismatic Latin revolutionary). Thus although music may enrich the development of mind, it is does not appear to be necessary for normal mental development. This stands in contrast to language, because recent studies of an emerging language in Nicaragua suggest that language is necessary for the development of certain basic cognitive skills. One such skill is "false belief understanding," in other words, the ability to recognize that one's own thoughts and beliefs can be different from those of others, and /or mistaken (Pyers, 2006, cf. Section 7.2.8).

Social Cohesion

The final hypothesis discussed here concerns the role of music in promoting social cohesion among members of a group. Among the many different adaptationist conjectures about music, this is the most often heard and the one that attracts the most support. According to this hypothesis, music helped cement social bonds between members of ancestral human groups via its role in ritual and in group music making. The intuitive appeal of this idea is obvious. First, it does seem that a great deal of musical activity in contemporary small-scale cultures is social (Morley, 2003). Second, it is known that music can be a powerful force in mood regulation (Sloboda & O'Neill, 2001), suggesting that group music making could result in a shared mood state. Third, it seems plausible that a common mood state would enhance the subjective sense of a bond between individuals.

The social cohesion hypothesis occurs in various forms. One variant, proposed by Dunbar (2003), is that group singing resulted in endorphin release, thus mimicking the neural effects of physical grooming in primates (cf. Merker, 2000). (This forms part of Dunbar's larger argument that language evolved primarily to convey social information, thus allowing our hominid ancestors to replace physical grooming with "grooming at a distance" by means of verbal communication, and thus to achieve larger group size. Dunbar argues that group singing preceded the evolution of language.) Presumably this endorphin release would have some positive effect on social behavior, which in turn would have a payoff in terms of increased reproductive success (cf. Silk et al., 2003 for evidence of a link between sociability and reproductive success in primates).

Another variant of the social cohesion hypothesis focuses on the bond between mothers and infants. Trehub (2000, 2003a) and Dissanayake (2000), among others, have drawn attention to the role of music in mother-infant bonding. Trehub's work is especially notable for its empirical basis. She and her colleagues have done extensive research on lullabies across numerous cultures, identifying shared structural features such as simple structure and falling contours, which might serve to soothe the infant (e.g., Unyk et al., 1992; Trehub et al., 1993; Trehub & Trainor, 1998). Trehub and colleagues have also shown that maternal singing is attractive to infants: 6-month-olds look longer at audiovisual presentations of their own mother performing infant-directed singing versus infant-directed speech (Nakata & Trehub, 2004). In addition, this research team has examined cortisol in infant saliva (an indicator of arousal levels) before and after mothers spoke or sang to them. Cortisol levels dropped significantly after both types of stimuli, but stayed low for a longer period after infant-directed song than after infant-directed speech (Shenfield et al., 2003). Based on these and other data, Trehub has argued that maternal singing has an adaptive function, allowing female humans to soothe their babies without necessarily having to touch them (see Balter, 2004). This may have been an advantage to our ancestors because infant humans (unlike other infant primates) cannot cling to their mother's fur while the mother forages with both hands. Singing would have allowed mothers to put their infants down while foraging and still soothe them (cf. Falk, 2004a,b).

Although the social cohesion hypothesis is appealing, it, too, faces a number of challenges. First, the premise that music is primarily a social activity in small-scale cultures deserves critical scrutiny. It may be that most of the *obvious* music in these cultures is social, but there also may be a great deal of "covert music" as well, especially songs. By covert music, I mean music composed and performed discreetly for a very select audience (perhaps even only for oneself), because it represents an intimate statement of love, memory, loss, and so forth. A summer spent among the Wopkaimin of central Papua New Guinea, a tribal people who lived a stone-age hunter-horticulturalist lifestyle, alerted me to the fact that the amount of private, covert music can greatly outweigh the amount of social, overt music in small-scale cultures.

A more serious difficulty for the social cohesion hypothesis concerns one of its implications. If music were an adaptation to promote social bonding, then one would predict that biologically based social impairments would curtail responsiveness to music. Yet autistic children, who have pronounced deficits in social cognition, are sensitive to musical affect (Heaton et al., in press; cf. Allen et al., submitted). Furthermore, autistic individuals sometimes achieve musical abilities that are remarkable given their limited linguistic and other intellectual abilities (Rimland & Fein, 1988; Miller, 1989). Music thus does not appear to have an obligatory relationship to brain mechanisms involved in social behavior, as one might predict from the social cohesion hypothesis.

Finally, with regard to the mother-infant version of the social cohesion hypothesis, one may note that mothers have many ways of soothing their infants and bonding with them, and that musical interactions (although pleasing to mother and infant) may not be necessary for normal bonding or soothing to occur. The crucial weakness of this hypothesis is that there are at present no data to suggest that singing is needed for normal social or emotional development. (Those interested in studying this question could examine the social development of hearing infants with loving mothers who do not sing, perhaps including hearing children of deaf adults, or "CODAs.")[10]

7.3.2 Testing Music Against the Evidence Used for Language Evolution

How does music fare with regard to the 10 lines of evidence for natural selection's role in language evolution (reviewed in section 7.2)? Some of these lines of evidence would seem to apply equally well to music. For example, babbling, vocal learning, and the anatomy of the vocal tract could all reflect adaptations for an acoustic communication system that originally supported both language and vocal music (cf. Darwin, 1871; Mithen, 2005). It is thus ambiguous which

---

[10] "CODA" stands for "children of deaf adults," now a well-organized community. See http://www.coda-international.org.

domain (music or language) provided the relevant selective pressures for these features of human biology. Fixation of a relevant gene (FOXP2; section 7.2.9) is also ambiguous with regard to the source of selection pressure, because this gene appears to be involved in circuits that support both speech (articulation and syntax) and musical rhythm (cf. section 7.3.4 below). With regard to adding complexity to impoverished input (section 7.2.8), there are to my knowledge no relevant data to speak to this issue. Fortunately, there are relevant data with respect to the remaining lines of evidence, as reviewed below.

Rate of Learning of Musical Structure

Linguistic skills develop remarkably quickly. Even before the end of the first year of life, infants undergo perceptual changes that attune them to the relevant phonological contrasts in their native language, and by the age of 3 or 4, they are producing the highly complex phonological and grammatical patterns of fluent speech. Do humans also show precocious abilities when it comes to the perception or production of musical sound patterns?

One can address the question above by examining the development of an important aspect of musical cognition: sensitivity to tonality relations. This refers to sensitivity to the organized use of pitches in terms of scales, a tonal center, and so forth (cf. Chapter 5). (I focus here on Western European music, which has been the focus of more developmental research than any other tradition. It should be noted, though, that organized scales and the use of a tonal center are widespread in human music.). A very basic form of sensitivity to tonality is sensitivity to key membership in a sequence of notes. Normal adults with no musical training can readily spot "sour" notes in a melody, in other words, notes that violate the local key even though they are not odd in any physical sense (indeed, failure to detect sour notes is one symptom of musical "tone deafness" in adults; cf. Ayotte et al., 2002).

Current evidence suggests that sensitivity to key membership develops rather slowly in humans. Trainor and Trehub (1992) tested the ability of infants and adults to detect a change in a short, tonal melody that was repeated in the background.[11] Infants indicated their detection of a change by turning toward the loudspeaker on "change trials," for which they were reinforced by an animated toy. Half of the change trials contained a change of 4 semitones to one note, resulting in a new pitch that was still in key. On the other half of the change trials, the same note was changed by just 1 semitone, resulting in an out-of-key note. Thus the design cleverly pitted a large physical change against a smaller

---

[11] The melody was transposed on each repetition to one of three keys. The continuous transposition served to focus attention on relative rather than absolute pitch cues, and built on the fact that infants recognize the similarity of melodies presented in transposition (Cohen et al., 1987).

change that violated a learned tonal schema. The adults detected the out-of-key change better than the in-key change, whereas the infants detected both types of changes equally well (though their absolute level of performance was lower than the adults). This provided evidence that implicit knowledge of key membership is not in place by 8 months of age.

In a follow-up study of similar design, Trainor and Trehub (1994) showed that 5-year-olds were better at detecting out-of-key changes than in-key changes to melodies, though the children's discrimination performance was still only about half as good as adults' (cf. Costa-Giomi, 2003). Thus somewhere between 8 months and 5 years, children develop a sense of key membership, though the sense is still not as strong as in adults (cf. Davidson et al., 1981). Unfortunately, there is a paucity of research on the developmental time course of this ability between 8 months and 5 years. Dowling (1988) and colleagues conducted an experiment in which 3- to 5-year-old children heard tonal and atonal melodies matched for statistical properties such as average interval size (here "tonal" means all notes conformed to a single key). The task was to identify which melodies had "normal notes" and which had "odd notes." The children were divided into two groups based on how in tune their own spontaneous singing was. Dowling et al. found that 3-year-olds who sang more in tune could just barely discriminate tonal from atonal melodies (58% correct, in which chance performance was 50% correct). Three-year-olds who sang more out of tune did not discriminate the melodies.

Clearly, more work is warranted to study the development of sensitivity to key membership between 8 months and 5 years. Neural techniques such as ERPs are particularly promising for this purpose, because they do not require the child to make overt decisions about tonality (cf. Koelsch et al., 2003). The relevant neural work has yet to be done, however. The existing behavioral data suggests that sensitivity to key membership develops rather slowly in children. This stands in sharp contrast to language development, because ordinary 3- and 4-year-olds are adept at perceiving complex phonological and grammatical structures in language. This slower development of musical pitch perception may be one reason why children's singing is typically "out of tune" until about 5 years of age (Dowling, 1988). If musical pitch abilities had been the target of natural selection, one would expect accurate perception and production of musical pitch patterns to be learned far more quickly than the observed rate. The slow development is especially striking given that the music children hear (e.g., nursery songs) is especially strong in its tonal structure, with few out-of-key notes (Dowling, 1988).

One might object that sensitivity to key membership is actually quite a complex aspect of music, and that many other musically relevant abilities are in fact evident in young infants, such as sensitivity to melodic contour and an ability to discriminate consonant from dissonant sounds. However, it may be that these sensitivities are byproducts of attunement to speech or of general auditory processing principles (I return to this point in section 7.3.3, subsections on music and infancy). In contrast, sensitivity to key membership does not have any obvious relationship to nonmusical auditory functions, and is thus a more specific test of the development of musical abilities. Until good evidence appears showing rapid development of musical skills *that are not related to language or to general principles of auditory function,* there is no reason to reject the null hypothesis that music has not been a direct target of natural selection.

Critical Period Effects

As noted in section 7.2.5, a critical period or sensitive period is a time window when developmental processes are especially sensitive to environmental input. Input (or lack of it) during this time can have a profound effect on the ultimate level of adult ability in specific areas.

Is there a critical period for the acquisition of musical skills? One way to study this would be to conduct studies of musical ability in individuals who started to learn music at different ages, but who were matched for overall number of years of training. Such studies would be entirely parallel to the studies of second-language learning conducted by Newport and colleagues (cf. section 7.2.5.) Unfortunately such work has yet to be done (Trainor, 2005). If such studies indicate that early-onset learners are superior in their sensitivity to musical phonology (e.g., the perceptual categorization of sound elements such as intervals or chords; cf. Chapter 2) or musical syntax, this would favor a critical period hypothesis. However, even without doing these experiments, it seems that even if a critical period effect for music is found, the effect will be rather weak compared to language. One reason to suspect this is that some highly accomplished musicians did not start playing their instrument after the age of 10. (To take just one example, George Gershwin was introduced to the piano at 13.) In contrast, a child with no linguistic output until this age is unlikely to ever reach even a normal level of ability.

Some evidence for a disproportionate influence of early musical experience on the brain comes from modern structural neuroimaging, which allows one to study the neuroanatomy of healthy individuals. Bengtsson et al. (2005) used a special type of magnetic resonance imaging to examine white matter pathways in professional pianists.[12] (White matter refers to neural fibers that connect different parts of the brain.) They found that the amount of practice strongly correlated with the amount of white matter in specific neural regions, with the amount of childhood (vs. adolescent or adult) practice having the strongest predictive power in certain regions. Thus, for example, the amount of childhood practice correlated strongly with the amount of white matter in the posterior limb of the internal capsule, which carries descending fibers from the

---

[12] Diffusion tensor imaging (DTI).

motor cortex to the spinal cord, and which is important for independent finger movement. That is, even though there were significantly fewer practice hours in childhood than in adolescence or adulthood, the amount of practice during childhood was more predictive of the adult neuroanatomy of this region than the amount of practice during adolescence or adulthood.

Although this study indicates that early musical experience can have a disproportionate impact on the neuroanatomy of the motor system, it does not provide evidence of a critical period for cognitive abilities related to music. It is this latter issue that is more relevant for evolutionary issues (e.g., recall from section 7.2.5 how critical periods in language influenced phonology and syntax). There is, however, one aspect of musical cognition that shows a strong critical period effect, namely absolute pitch (AP). (Those unfamiliar with AP should consult section 7.3.4, subsection on absolute pitch, for an introduction.) It has been well documented that the prevalence of AP in musicians depends strongly on the age of onset of musical training. Specifically, it is very rare for individuals to have this ability if they began training after age 6 (Levitin & Zatorre, 2003). This is a provocative finding, given that the critical period for language acquisition is also thought to be around 6 or 7 years of age. However, AP is a rare trait, estimated to occur in 1 in 10,000 people, which means that AP is not necessary for the development of normal musical abilities. Furthermore, there is no evidence to suggest that people with AP are more musically gifted overall than non-AP musicians (e.g., in composition, creativity). Thus the critical period for AP is not evidence for a critical period for music acquisition. (See Trainor 2005 for a concise review of AP from a developmental perspective.)

To summarize, at the current time, there is no good evidence for a critical period in the acquisition of musical cognitive abilities (e.g., sensitivity to tonal syntax). Until such evidence is produced, the null hypothesis for the evolution of music is not challenged.

Robustness of Acquisition of Musical Abilities

Humans appear far more uniform in their linguistic than in their musical abilities. Although some normal people are certainly more fluent speakers or have keener ears for speech than do others, these variations seem minor compared to the range of musical abilities in normal people. Of course, empirical data on variation in abilities within both domains is needed to make a fair comparison. Ideally, such data would include tests designed to tap into implicit skills, in which explicit training in music is not a confounding variable (Bigand, 2003; Bigand et al., 2006).

Although such empirical comparative research has yet to be done, existing data do suggest a good deal of variability in musical abilities. To take just one example, consider the ability to tap in synchrony with a musical beat. This basic ability appears widespread, but in fact there are very few estimates for how common it is among randomly selected nonmusicians. Drake, Penel, and Bigand (2000) tested 18 individuals who had never taken music lessons or played an instrument. The participants were asked to listen to one piano piece at a time, and then tap in synchrony with the perceived beat on a second listening, a task that musically trained participants found very easy. Drake et al. used a very lenient measure of success at synchronization: All that was required was 10 consecutive taps that fell within a broad window surrounding the idealized beat location. Even with these lax criteria, they found that nonmusicians were unable to synchronize on over 10% of the trials. Thus it appears that the ability to tap to a beat may not be as universal as one might expect, though empirical data are needed to ascertain what percent of musically untrained individuals have this basic ability.

Another indicator that musical development is less robust than language development concerns the modality-uniqueness of music. The fact that human language can jump modalities from a sound-based system to a silent, sign-based system attests to the robustness of language acquisition mechanisms. If musical acquisition were equally robust, one might expect that deaf communities would create their own "sign music," in other words, a nonreferential but richly organized system of visual signs with discrete elements and principles of syntax, created and shared for aesthetic ends by an appreciative community. However, no such system exists (K. Emmorey, personal communication). Some deaf individuals do enjoy acoustic music via some residual hearing function and due the tactile sensations afforded by rhythm, but this is not the same as a sign-based form of music. Of course, one could argue that without basic auditory distinctions such as consonance and dissonance, music cannot "get off the ground." Yet such an argument has a post hoc flavor. In principle, the types of oppositions created by consonance and dissonance (e.g., sensations of roughness vs. smoothness) could have iconic parallels in visual symbols. Alternatively, "sign music" might be able to dispense with this opposition altogether, just as it dispenses with auditory distinctions that seem so central to spoken language (such as the basic distinction between vowels and consonants).

Overall, the current evidence suggests that the development of musical abilities is not nearly as robust as the development of linguistic abilities. This is consistent with the null hypothesis that there has been no specific selection for music in human evolution.

Biological Cost of Failure to Acquire Musical Abilities

As noted in section 7.2.10, traits that have been shaped by natural selection are by definition important to the survival and reproductive success of individuals. For example, adults without language would be at a serious disadvantage in human culture, whether one is speaking of our hunter-gatherer ancestors or of modern humans living in a complex technological setting. Is there any evidence that lack of musical abilities has a biological cost? Consider the case of musically tone-deaf individuals who are unable to do even very simple musical tasks such as recognize a familiar melody or spot a sour note in a novel melody. (Informal observation suggests that there may also be a population of individuals who are "rhythm deaf" and cannot keep a beat or do other basic rhythmic tasks.) Such individuals appear to bear no biological cost for their deficit, and there is no evidence that they are less successful reproducers than musically gifted individuals. This is consistent with the view that natural selection has not shaped our bodies and brain for specifically musical purposes.

7.3.3 Infant Studies: Are We "Born Musical"?

Section 7.3.2 showed that music does not fare well when compared to language with regard to several lines of evidence for natural selection. Those lines of evidence focused on how musical abilities develop in normal individuals. This section takes a different approach, and focuses on the musical abilities of infants. Proponents of the music-as-adaptation view often suggest that human babies are "born musical." It is certainly true that infants show very good auditory discrimination skills for frequency, pitch, timbre, and durational patterning (Fassbender, 1996; Pouthas, 1996). Furthermore, they show numerous more sophisticated abilities relevant to the development of musical skills, such as the ability to recognize the similarity of pitch patterns based on melodic contour independent of exact intervals sizes or overall pitch level, and to recognize the similarity of rhythms based on grouping structure independent of tempo. Furthermore, babies from Western cultures show a preference for consonant over dissonant intervals, superior encoding of certain pitch intervals such the perfect fifth, and a preference for infant-directed singing over infant-directed speech (see Trehub 2000, 2003b; and Trehub & Hannon, 2006, for reviews). To some, these findings suggest that evolution has specifically shaped humans to have the processing skills and predispositions needed to acquire mature musical abilities.

Although there is little doubt that infants have musically *relevant* traits, from an evolutionary standpoint the real question is whether they have innate predispositions or innate learning preferences that are *specific* to music (Justus & Hutsler, 2005; McDermott & Hauser, 2005). If instead these characteristics can be explained via other traits with a more obvious selective advantage (such as language), or as a byproduct of general auditory processing mechanisms, then they provide no evidence of selection for music. Furthermore, before this question of specificity is raised, one must have firm evidence that the predispositions or learning preferences really are innate and not due to experience. This is a nontrivial issue for infant studies, because auditory learning begins before birth (cf. section 7.3.3, subsection "Music and Infancy: Questions of Innateness"). Thus before discussing the auditory proclivities of human infants, it is worth giving two examples from animal studies that illustrate innate biases in perception. Both examples come from research on birds.

Innate Perceptual Predispositions: A Biological Example

Compelling evidence for innate perceptual predispositions comes from comparative work on baby domestic chickens and Japanese quails (henceforth chicks and quails). Park and Balaban (1991) housed chick and quail eggs in incubators in complete isolation from parental vocalizations. After hatching, birds were given a perceptual test in which they were placed in a chamber with speakers embedded in the left and right walls. Each speaker produced the maternal call of one of the two species (the maternal call is produced by a mother to draw baby birds to her, e.g., in case of danger). Each bird was exposed to equal numbers of maternal calls from the two species. Park and Balaban measured each bird's perceptual bias in terms of the amount of time it spent pushing against one wall or the other, and found that chicks and quails showed a significant preference to approach the calls of their own species.

A decade after this original study, Long et al. (2001) performed an impressive experiment that probed the neural basis of this preference. Using surgical techniques pioneered by Balaban et al. (1988), the researchers cut small holes in the eggs and operated on the embryos, transplanting different portions of the developing neural tube of quails into chicks. They then sealed up the eggs and housed them in incubators isolated from adult bird sounds. After hatching, they tested these chimeric birds for their perceptual preferences using the methods of Park and Balaban (1991). They found that when the transplant was in a specific region of the developing midbrain, the chimeras showed a preference for the quail maternal call. (They also showed that this was not due to the chimeras producing a quail-like call themselves.) Thus the scientists were able to transplant an inborn perceptual preference. Interestingly, subsequent work by these authors suggests that the transplanted region does not act as a simple "brain module" but has developmental effects on other regions of the brain, including the forebrain (Long et al., 2002). Thus the perceptual preference of a baby chicken or quail for its own species' maternal call may be the result of neural interactions among a number of brain regions.

These studies provide solid evidence for an innate perceptual predisposition. However, inborn predispositions are not the only form of innateness. Learning can also be guided by innate factors, as discussed in the next section.

Innate Learning Preferences: A Biological Example

Studies of songbirds provide good evidence for innate learning preferences in animals. It is well known that if a young white-crowned sparrow is not allowed to hear the song of an adult during an early portion of his life, it will never sing a normal song, but will produce instead a much simplified "isolate song" (Marler, 1970; cf. Zeigler & Marler, 2004). This fact has allowed biologists to explore how selective these birds are in terms of the songs that they will learn. One method that has been used to explore this question is to expose a young, male, white-crowned sparrow to songs of a variety of species (e.g., those that might occur in its natural habitat). Under these circumstances, the bird shows a strong predilection to learn the song of its own species (Marler & Peters, 1977). Furthermore, it has been demonstrated that this is not due to the inability to produce the songs of other species (Marler, 1991).

For neurobiologists, the key question is what acoustic cues and brain mechanisms mediate selective learning, and research on this issue is underway (e.g., Whaling et al., 1997). For our purposes, the relevant point is that evolution can provide animals with inborn learning preferences that do not depend on prior auditory experience with species-specific sound patterns. The innate learning preferences of white-crowned sparrows, like the innate perceptual predispositions of chicks and quails, are unquestionably the result of natural selection, because they are not a byproduct of any other trait and because they have a clear adaptive value.

Music and Infancy: Questions of Innateness

Box 7.1 summarizes a number of findings from human infant research that are often suggested as innate biases relevant to music (see references in Trehub 2000, 2003b, and in the following paragraph).

Box 7.1

1. Priority of contour over precise intervals in melody processing
2. Priority of relational temporal patterns over specific durations in rhythm processing
3. Sensitivity to Gestalt principles of auditory grouping
4. Better retention of pitch intervals with small-integer frequency ratios (e.g., the perfect fifth)
5. Better perception of pitch or rhythm deviations in melodies that exemplify Gestalt grouping principles
6. Hemispheric asymmetries for contour versus interval processing
7. Ability to elicit music-like modifications of adult speech ("motherese")
8. Preference for consonant over dissonant intervals
9. Superior processing of musical scales with unequal step sizes
10. Musicality of mother-infant interactions, particularly in the rhythmic structure of vocalization and movement
11. The existence of a specific genre of music for infants with cross-cultural similarities (e.g., lullabies)
12. Preference for infant-directed singing over infant-directed speech

The cumulative weight of these findings has led some researchers to speculate that human musical abilities have been a direct target of natural selection. There is a problem with this idea, however. Many of the findings (i.e., items 1–7 in Box 7.1) can be accounted for by biases related to speech processing or as a byproduct of general auditory processing, as explored in the next subsection (on issues of specificity). Let us briefly consider the remaining findings in turn. A preference for consonant over dissonant intervals and music has been repeatedly demonstrated in infants (e.g., Trainor, Tsang, & Cheung, 2002). Although intriguing, the role of prior experience in shaping this preference has been difficult to rule out: Infants have likely had significant exposure to music by the time they are tested (e.g., via lullabies, play songs), and this music almost certainly features many more consonant than dissonant intervals. This is a concern because research has established a link between mere exposure and preference for musical materials (e.g., Peretz, Gaudreau, et al., 1998). A strong test of an inborn preference for consonant versus dissonant intervals requires testing infants without previous musical exposure.

Fortunately, Masataka (2006) has conducted a study that comes close to this ideal. He tested 2-day-old infants of deaf and sign-language-proficient parents, who presumably had little prenatal exposure to the sounds of music and speech. Masataka examined looking times to a 30-second Mozart minuet in two versions: the original version and a dissonant version in which many of the intervals had been modified to be dissonant (Sound Example 7.1a, b; stimuli originally from Trainor & Heinmiller, 1998). The newborns showed a preference for the consonant version of the minuet, though the preference was very slight, which points to the need for replication. If this result can be shown to be robust, it would be important evidence in evolutionary debates over music, given the lack of such a preference in nonhuman primates (cf. section 7.3.5, subsection "Animals, Consonance, and Dissonance"). However, as noted by Masataka, even in his study population, it is impossible to rule out possible prenatal exposure to music in the ambient environment. This is a concern for any study of infant music cognition due to evidence for prenatal learning of musical patterns (as discussed in more detail later in this section). Thus at this time, whether humans have an inborn preference for consonant musical sounds is still an open question.

Turning to a bias for asymmetric musical scales (discussed in Chapter 2, section 2.2.2), this bias is actually not shown by adults, who perform no better on unfamiliar asymmetric than symmetric scales (Trehub et al., 1999). Thus the bias is rather weak and can be overruled by cultural factors. Even confining discussion to the infant data, it could be that that asymmetric patterns of pitch intervals provide listeners with a better sense of location in pitch space, just as it is easier to orient oneself in physical space in a room if the walls are of different lengths. That is, a music-specific cognitive principle may not be needed.

The musicality of mother-infant vocal interactions (e.g., Trevarthen; 1999, Longhi, 2003) is intriguing, especially because it is known that mother-infant interactions are subject to well-organized temporal contingencies (Tronick et al., 1978; Nadel et al., 1999). However, at the current time, we do not know whether mothers and infants interact in a musical fashion across cultures, because a limited number of cultures have been studied.

Lullabies have been documented across a wide range of cultures (Trehub, 2000) and have thus attracted attention in evolutionary studies (McDermott & Hauser, 2005). Lullabies also show a similarity of form and function across cultures (Unyk et al., 1992), which might lead one to suspect that infants are innately tuned to this specific musical form. However, this cross-cultural prevalence and similarity may simply reflect the fact that infants find vocalizations with certain characteristics (such as slow tempo and smooth, repetitive, falling pitch contours) to be soothing (cf. Papousek, 1996). Furthermore, infants usually find rituals comforting. Thus it may not be surprising that adults all over the world arrive at similarly structured musical rituals for the purpose of soothing infants.

Of all the items in Box 7.1, the preference for infant-directed singing over infant-directed speech is perhaps the most suggestive with regard to innate predispositions for music. Evidence for this comes from a study by Nakata and Trehub (2004), who conducted an experiment in which 6-month-old infants watched a video (with sound) of their own mother. One set of infants saw their mothers singing, whereas the other set saw them speaking. Both the speaking and the singing examples had been recorded during an initial visit to the lab in which the mother was recorded while either speaking or singing directly to her infant. When speaking, mothers naturally used infant-directed speech (or "motherese"). Infant-directed (ID) singing differs from ID speech in a number of ways, including slightly lower average pitch, more tightly controlled pitch variation (as expected, because singing involves moving between well-defined pitch levels), and slower tempo (Trainor et al., 1997; Trehub et al., 1997). The researchers found that infants looked significantly longer at videos of maternal song than of maternal speech. This is an interesting result because infants seem to be expressing a preference for music over speech, a somewhat surprising result if one believes that speech reflects biological adaptation but music does not.

The key question, however, is what is driving the longer looking time for videos of song versus speech. Perhaps the simplest explanation is simply a novelty preference, under the assumption that maternal singing is less commonly experienced by infants than maternal speech. Let us assume for the moment, however, that this is not the driving factor. It is known that ID singing is much more stereotyped than ID speech, being performed at nearly identical pitch levels and tempos on different occasions (Bergeson & Trehub, 2002). Thus song is a ritualized performance that infants may find compelling, in the same way they find other rituals (such as games like peek-a-boo) compelling. Alternatively, as suggested by Nakata and Trehub, ID singing may be preferred because infants perceive it as more emotive than ID speech (cf. Trainor et al., 1997, 2000). Thus their preference for music in this study could be an inborn preference for acoustic cues to positive affect, just as they prefer to listen to happy emotive speech than to affectively neutral speech (even when the former is adult-directed and the latter is infant-directed; Singh et al., 2002). A preference for positively affective vocal stimuli may also explain the finding that newborns prefer infant-directed over adult-directed singing, even when their parents are deaf and they thus had minimal exposure to singing before birth (Masataka, 1999; cf. Trainor et al., 1997).

If preference for ID song (vs. ID speech or adult-directed song) is driven by vocal cues to positive affect, this would predict that the preference would disappear if ID singing is done in a way that preserves the accuracy of the music but makes it affectively duller than the ID speech or adult-directed song. The basic point is that preference studies, if they are intended to address the question of innate predispositions for music, require careful controls. (It should be noted that Nakata and Trehub and Masataka did not design their study to address evolutionary issues.)

Thus at the current time, it appears that the case for music-specific innate biases is weak. However, it is possible that some compelling evidence will come to light in the future. To be convincing, however, future developmental studies of innate biases will have to address an issue that faces all current studies, in other words, the issue of prior exposure to music and the learning that accompanies it. What makes avian studies of innate biases so persuasive (cf. sections 7.3.3, first two subsections) is that they have rigorously excluded prior exposure as a possible variable in accounting for their results. Current research on infant music cognition is far from attaining this standard.

That being said, if it could be shown that auditory learning is minimal prior to the age at which most infant music perception studies are conducted (e.g., 6–8 months), then one might need not worry. Unfortunately, the data point in exactly the opposite direction. Unlike visual experience, auditory experience begins well before birth (Lecanuet, 1996). Humans begin responding to sound around 30 weeks' gestational age, and by the time of birth, they have already learned a good deal about their auditory environment. The has been demonstrated by studies of newborns tested using a method that allows them to indicate their auditory preferences by their rate of sucking on an artificial nipple (the "nonnutritive-sucking paradigm"; see Pouthas, 1996, for an introduction). This research has shown that newborns prefer their mother's voice to that of a stranger (DeCasper & Fifer, 1980), a story read by the mother during the last 6 weeks of pregnancy to a novel story (DeCasper and Spence, 1986), and their native language to a foreign language (Mehler et al., 1988; Moon et al., 1993). In each case, the preference could arise only through learning, in which prosodic patterns probably play an important role (DeCasper et al., 1994; Nazzi et al., 1998; Floccia et al., 2000).

The preferences of newborns for familiar auditory stimuli are not limited to speech. Hepper (1991) had one group of mothers listen to a particular tune once or twice a day throughout their pregnancy, whereas another group of mothers did not listen to this tune. Newborns from the prior group recognized the tune, as indicated by changes in heart rate, movement, and alertness upon hearing the tune after birth (the control group showed no such changes). To ascertain if the newborns were responding on the basis of the specific tune (or if prior exposure to music simply made them more responsive to music in general), Hepper conducted another study in which mothers listened to the same tune during pregnancy, but babies were tested with a different tune or a backward version of the original tune. In this case, the newborns did not show any sign of recognition. Hepper went on to show that selective response to the familiar tune could be observed even *before birth* (via ultrasound monitoring of fetal movement), at 36–37 weeks of gestational age. Hepper did a final study with 29- 30-week-old fetuses, showing that there was no evidence of tune recognition at this age.

Of course, if it can be shown that prenatal learning is limited to rhythm and melody in speech and music, then one could at least test newborns for preferences based on the spectral structure of isolated sounds, such as single syllables versus closely matched nonspeech (as in Vouloumanos & Werker's [2004] work with 2-month-olds), or such as consonant versus dissonant musical intervals (as Trainor, Tsang, and Cheung's [2002] work with 2-month-olds). A recent study of fetal auditory perception, however, suggests that fetal sound learning may not be limited to prosodic cues. Kisilevsky et al. (2003) presented 38-week-old fetuses with recordings of their own mother or another woman reading the same poem (each mothers' reading served as the "unfamiliar" voice for another fetus). Recordings were presented via a loudspeaker held above the abdomen. Fetal heart rate showed a sustained increased in response to the mother's voice, but a sustained decrease in response to the stranger's voice. This study is notable because the control condition was the same linguistic text produced by another speaker, which means that gross rhythmic and prosodic patterns were likely to be similar. More work is clearly called for, using Kisilevsky et al.'s paradigm with acoustic manipulations to determine which cues the fetus is using in discriminating its mother's voice from that of another woman (e.g., is it simply mean fundamental frequency, or is timbre also important?). The relevant point, however, is that by the time infants participate in early speech and music perception experiments (e.g., at 2 months of age), they have already learned a good deal about the sounds of their environment.

How then can one use infant studies to ask questions about processing predispositions? There are a number of ways in which this can be done. First, one can do cross-cultural experiments using musical material from another culture that is unfamiliar to the infants. This strategy has been employed by Lynch and colleagues, who have used the Javanese musical system to explore predispositions in the perception of musical scales (cf. Chapter 2, section 2.4.4), as well as by Hannon and Trehub, who used Balkan rhythms to study infants ability to detect temporal alterations in familiar versus unfamiliar metrical patterns (cf. this chapter's appendix). A related approach is to test infants from non-Western cultures on the perception of Western musical patterns. This would be a useful control for studies of Western infants that have shown a processing advantage for certain small-ratio pitch intervals, such at the perfect fifth (e.g., Schellenberg & Trehub, 1996; discussed in appendix 3 of Chapter 2). However, it is increasingly hard to find infants in other cultures who have not been exposed to Western music. It may be that the best approach for future cross-cultural research is to involve parents in studies of controlled exposure to music of different types. For example, it may be possible to convince some parents (particularly those from non-Western backgrounds) to listen exclusively to non-Western music at home, starting before birth and continuing until their infants participate in music perception experiments. These infants can then be compared to infants raised in homes exposed to Western music: Any commonalities that cannot be explained by similar musical input would be candidates for innate, music-relevant predispositions.

The idea of controlled-exposure studies can be extended further. At the current time, one cannot rule out the possibility that the precocious development of speech perception relative to music perception (cf. section 7.2.4 and 7.3.2, first subsection) is simply due to differences in amount of exposure (cf. McMullen & Saffran, 2004). For example, in van de Weijer's (1998) study, described in section 7.2.7 above, out of 18 days of an infant's life that were fully recorded and analyzed, the total amount of musical exposure amounted to no more than a few minutes (van de Weijer, personal communication). Of course, this is a study of a single infant and may not be representative. It seems almost certain, however, that most infants and children hear a great deal more speech than music, and that the amount of variability in music exposure across individuals is far greater than the amount of variability in speech exposure. Thus to really test whether speech perception is precocious compared to music perception, one should work with infants who have a large amount of musical exposure. For example, one could work with children of musicians or music teachers who practice/teach at home, or with babies who participate in infant music programs. (In the United States, infant music programs exist at the Eastman School of Music and at the University of South Carolina.)

Ultimately, comparing speech to musical development on a level playing field will require quantifying and equalizing the amount of linguistic versus musical input to infants over extended periods of time. This will require long-term recordings (of the type used by van de Weijer) and the cooperation of parents in order to give infants equal amounts of linguistic and musical input. For example, using modern computing technology to automatically classify spoken versus musical segments in digitized recordings (Scheirer & Slaney, 1997), parents could be given feedback at the end of each day on how much spoken versus musical input (in minutes) their child heard that day. They could then modify their home environment to try to equalize this amount of input (e.g., via singing, CDs, videos). One could even start this sort of input matching before birth, at the time the fetus begins to hear. Infants who have been exposed to matched amounts of speech and music could then be tested for a variety of linguistic and musical abilities. For example, one could use ERPs and behavioral experiments to probe the development of learned sound categories and syntactic knowledge in the two domains. The key question, of course, is whether the development of linguistic abilities will still outstrip the development of musical abilities when input is matched. If so, this would suggest that natural selection has not provided us with innate predispositions for learning music.[13]

In a sense, the experiment proposed above is simply an extended version of existing experiments on statistical learning. Such studies have shown that infants are adept at using distributional properties of the input (such as frequency of occurrence or co-occurrence of events) to form categories and infer structural properties of stimuli in both speech and music (e.g., Maye et al., 2002; Saffran et al., 1996; Saffran et al., 1999). These experiments involve controlled exposure to particular patterns, followed by tests to determine if statistical regularities in the input influence learning. These studies have the advantage of tight controllability, but they inevitably deal with infants that have had unmatched amounts of exposure to speech and music before coming into the laboratory. If one wants to address the evolutionary question of innate predispositions for music, then comparisons of music and language following a history of matched exposure provide an unparalleled, if logistically challenging, approach to this question.

Music and Infancy: Questions of Specificity

Although there is little doubt that infants have musically relevant abilities, the key question from an evolutionary standpoint is whether these reflect mechanisms shaped by selection for music, or whether they are a byproduct of mechanisms used in language comprehension or in general auditory processing (cf. Trehub & Hannon, 2006).

Several of the findings in Box 7.1 (i.e., items 1, 2, 6, and 7) can likely be accounted for via speech processing. The ability to recognize the similarity

---

[13] In making this suggestion, I am of course skimming over the thorny issue of how to match musical and linguistic input. Simply counting the number of minutes per day a child hears speech versus music may not be satisfactory, especially if the spoken input involves social interaction but the musical input is passively listening to CD, because social interaction facilitates learning of speech sounds in humans (Kuhl et al., 2003). However, I do not think this problem is insurmountable, particularly if one can work with music-loving parents who would enjoy musical interactions with their children. Musicians or music teachers who practice/work at home may be good candidates for such studies.

of pitch patterns based on melodic contours would be very useful in speech perception because infants must learn to recognize when an intonation contour is "the same" (e.g., has emphasis on the same word, or expresses a similar affect), whether spoken by males, females, or children. Similarly, sensitivity to temporal patterns independent of tempo (e.g., sensitivity to duration ratios between successive events) would be useful for dealing with variations in speech rate (Trehub, 2000). Hemispheric asymmetries in infants for contour versus interval could reflect early asymmetries in the grain at which pitch patterns are analyzed in the two hemispheres, which could once again be related to speech (e.g., brains could come prepared for processing pitch patterns at two levels of detail, a fine-grained level for lexical tones in tone languages versus a more global scale for prosodic contours). With regard to "motherese" (or more correctly, infant-directed speech, because fathers and older siblings do it, too), there is evidence that this special form of speech has numerous phonological benefits to the infant, including increased acoustic contrastiveness between vowels (which could facilitate the formation of vowel categories; Kuhl et al., 1997), and facilitating the learning of consonantal contrasts in polysyllabic words (Karzon, 1985). Furthermore, the distinct pitch sweeps that characterize this form of speech and that are so salient to the infant (Fernald & Kuhl, 1987) appear to play specific roles in modulating infant attention and arousal (Papousek et al., 1990; Papousek 1996). It can thus be explained without any reference to music.

Other findings in Box 7.1 (i.e., items 3, 4, and 5) can likely be accounted for as byproducts of general auditory processing. For example, sensitivity to Gestalt auditory patterns is likely due to mechanisms for assigning incoming sounds to distinct sources (Bregman, 1990), rather than having anything specifically to do with music. The superior processing of certain pitch intervals (e.g., the fifth) may reflect the way pitch is coded in the vertebrate nervous system (Tramo et al., 2003), which in turn could reflect the evolution of mechanisms for auditory object recognition (e.g., partials separated by a fifth may be more likely to come from a single object, because so many organisms make harmonic sounds). One way to test this idea is to see if similar biases exist in the auditory processing of nonhuman animals, for example, primates and birds (I will return to this topic in section 7.3.5).

Before concluding this section, it is useful to draw a conceptual distinction between two ways in which music and language can share developmental mechanisms. In one case, a mechanism specialized by evolution for language can be engaged by music whenever music employs structures or processes similar enough to language to activate these mechanisms. For example, the ability to form a system of learned sound categories in music—such as pitch intervals—may rely on mechanisms that enable the brain to learn the phonemic categories of speech (cf. Chapter 2, section 2.4). One might point out that there are dissociations of processing tonal and verbal material due to brain damage (e.g., "pure word deafness"), but such deficits simply show that the learned representations for musical and linguistic sound categories are stored in ways that allow for selective damage (for example, they may be stored in different brain areas). The learning mechanisms may still be the same. Evidence for overlap in learning mechanisms would come from associations between sound category learning in the two domains. For example, if performance in one domain predicts performance in the other, then this suggests common learning mechanisms (cf. Anvari et al., 2002; Slevc & Miyake, 2006). The second way in which music and language can share developmental mechanisms is if both draw on more general cognitive processes that are unique to neither language nor music. For example, general processes of analogical reasoning may be used in understanding discourse relations in both language and music (see Chapter 6, section 6.3.2).

7.3.4 Genetic Studies: What Is the Link Between Genetics and Music?

Discussions of genetics and music often revolve around the debate over innate musical talent (e.g., Howe et al., 1998; Winner, 1998), a debate that continues today with the added dimension of neuroimaging (Norton et al., 2005). Our concern here, however, is not with musical giftedness but with basic musical abilities, in other words, those musical abilities that are widespread in the population. At first blush, it may seem that any demonstration that genes influence such abilities would be evidence of natural selection for music. A moment's reflection, however, suggests otherwise. To take one example, there is a known single-gene mutation that has a profound influence on musical (vs. linguistic) ability, effectively disrupting music perception while leaving the potential for normal language processing intact. This is because the gene results in deafness (Lynch et al., 1997). Deaf individuals can have normal linguistic function (using sign language), but are excluded from pitch-related musical abilities. Thus although this gene influences music cognition, its existence obviously provides no evidence that music has been a direct target of natural selection.

Of course, we are not interested in such trivial cases, but the deafness example serves to highlight a key question for any study of gene-music relations, namely, *how specific is the link between genes and the trait of interest?* A related question is, *what are the mechanisms linking genes to the trait of interest?* For those interested in probing the links between genes, music, and evolution, these two questions must figure prominently in thinking about the relations between genetics and musical ability.

This section discusses two musical phenotypes that have attracted interest from geneticists. The first is musical tone deafness, which has been mentioned at various points throughout this chapter. Modern research on twins has suggested that specific genes put one at risk for this disorder. The second phenotype is absolute pitch (AP), defined here as the ability to accurately classify heard musical pitches into fine-grained categories (e.g., using the 12 note names of Western music, such as A and C♯) without any external reference. There is suggestive, though as yet not conclusive, evidence that genes play a role in determining which individuals have AP, and genetic studies are currently underway.

Can such studies help shed light on evolutionary issues? To put this question in the broader context of research on behavioral genetics, I will first discuss research on the genetics of language. This research helps highlight issues that studies of genetics and music must also face. It also contains an important lesson about the difference between popularized accounts of human gene-behavior links (which often imply simple one-to-one mappings between genes and high-level cognitive functions) and the complex reality that emerges when phenomena are studied in more detail.

An Example From Language

The example from language concerns a British family (the "KE" family) that provided the first clear link between a single gene and a developmental disorder of speech and language.[14] About half of the members of this family have a mutation in a gene on chromosome 7. This gene, which has been sequenced and is known as FOXP2, is subject to simple inheritance. It is an autosomal dominant, meaning that one damaged copy leads to the disorder.[15] An early description of the disorder focused on problems that affected family members have with grammar (Gopnik, 1990; cf. Gopnik & Crago, 1991), triggering a great deal of media attention and speculation about a "grammar gene." It is now clear, however, that affected members have a broad spectrum of speech and language deficits, including orofacial dyspraxia (i.e., problems controlling coordinated face and mouth movements), difficulties in distinguishing real words from nonwords, and difficulties manipulating phonemes (Vargha-Khadem et al., 1995; Alcock et al., 2000a; Watkins et al., 2002). Furthermore, although verbal IQ suffers more than nonverbal IQ in affected individuals, these individuals score lower than do unaffected family members on nonverbal IQ tests (on average; there is overlap in the distributions, with some affected members being in the normal range). Of special interest to researchers in music cognition, it has been demonstrated that affected members are as good as unaffected members on tests of musical pitch, but significantly worse on tests of musical rhythm (Alcock et al., 2000b). (From

---

[14] Another condition that could have been used to illustrate the complexity of human genotype-phenotype interactions in language abilities is Williams syndrome, which results from chance genetic deletion in a specific region of chromosome 7 (Bellugi & St. George, 2001; Karmiloff-Smith et al., 2003; Levitin et al., 2004).

[15] Like most other multicellular organisms, humans carry two copies of each gene, one per chromosome, except on portions of the male Y chromosome.

the standpoint of modern music cognition, Alcock used very simple tests of pitch and rhythm abilities; a great deal more remains to be done to characterize the musical abilities of affected vs. unaffected family members.)

Thus the notion that affected members of the KE family have a specific language deficit is untenable. This answers our first key question, "How specific is the link between genes and the trait of interest?" However, a negative answer to this question does not teach us much. What we would like to know is whether the spectrum of deficits seen in affected members can be attributed to a common underlying deficit. This leads immediately to our second key question, "What are the mechanisms linking genes to the trait of interest?" It is known that FOXP2 codes for a DNA-binding protein, and is therefore a gene that regulates other genes (see Marcus & Fisher, 2003 for a review). The gene occurs a wide variety of species, including chimpanzees, mice, birds, and crocodiles, and studies in other species are beginning to provide some clues about what FOXP2 does. In particular, studies of FOXP2 expression in birds that do versus do not learn their song suggest that FOXP2 expression in specific brain regions is related to learning of song sequences (Haesler et al., 2004; cf. Teramitsu et al., 2004).[16] Molecular biology research has shown that the basal ganglia are an important site for FOXP2 expression (Lai et al., 2003; Haesler et al., 2004). The basal ganglia are subcortical structures involved in motor control and sequencing, as well as in higher cognitive functions such a syntactic processing (DeLong, 2000; Kotz et al., 2003; Figure 7.1).

Structural brain imaging of the affected KE family members has revealed abnormalities in the basal ganglia, among other regions (Vargha-Khadem et al., 1998), and functional brain imaging reveals that the basal ganglia are among the regions that are underactivated during language tasks (Liégeois et al., 2003). Given the deficits that affected members have with complex temporal sequencing in both oral movements and in nonverbal musical rhythmic patterns, one wonders whether the underlying deficit is one of fine sequencing and timing. For example, one might imagine that FOXP2 somehow affects the temporal properties of neurons, which in turn influences neural network dynamics. Damage to this gene could thus make it difficult for networks to handle complex sequencing tasks. An important question is whether such deficits could influence the development of language abilities at multiple levels, from motor to cognitive. In fact, recent research and theorizing in neurolinguistics has

---

[16] Interestingly, the DNA sequence in the coding region of FOXP2 is very similar in avian learners and nonlearners (Webb & Zhang, 2005), even though the pattern of expression of this gene is very different in the brains of these two kinds of birds. This suggests that important evolutionary modifications to this gene occurred in its regulatory region rather than in its coding region. Regulatory changes may have influenced the timing and amount of the gene's expression during development, which had important effects on the functional properties of brain circuits in which it is expressed.

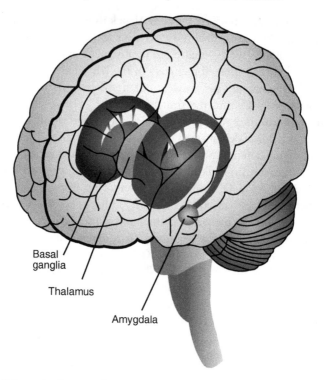

Basal
ganglia

Thalamus

Amygdala

Figure 7.1 Schematic diagram showing the location of the basal ganglia in the human brain. The basal ganglia are subcortical structures important to both language and music (cf. sections 7.3.4 and 7.5.3), and have reciprocal connections to large areas of the cerebral cortex. (The location of two other subcortical structures, the thalamus and the amygdala, are also shown for anatomical reference.)

implicated the basal ganglia in both motor and cognitive linguistic operations (Lieberman, 2000, Ch. 4). (As Lieberman notes, large parts of the basal ganglia project to nonmotor areas of cortex.)

In summary, studies of the KE family have helped scientists refine what they mean by a gene "for language." Although FOXP2 is crucial for the normal development of language, its effects are not specific to language. The real scientific question is thus about mechanism, in other words, in discovering the role this gene plays in the development of circuits involved in language processing. More generally, FOXP2 studies help us conceptualize the complex link between genes and behaviors. Rarely, if ever, is this a matter of simple one-to-one mappings between genes, neural circuits, and behaviors. Instead, the picture in Figure 7.2 is more representative of how biological systems work (Greenspan, 1995; 2004; Balaban, 2006).

The lesson for music is to be cautious about any report that a gene (or genes) has a specific effect on music. It is essential to ask what other abilities are also

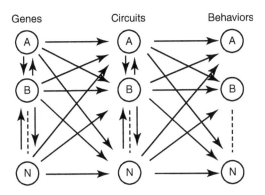

Figure 7.2 Conceptual diagram of the relations between genes, neural circuits, and behaviors. The mapping between genes and neural circuits, and between circuits and behaviors, tends to be many to many rather than one to one. Furthermore, there are important interactions between genes and between circuits. From Greenspan & Tully, 1994.

influenced and what mechanism leads to the observed effect. Only then can one address the evolutionary significance of the gene-behavior link. In the case of FOXP2, the lack of sequence variation in the human version of this gene suggests that this gene has been a target of selection. However, knowing what FOXP2 does profoundly influences our understanding of evolutionary issues. Thus, for example, if FOXP2 is involved in building circuits that do complex sequencing operations (both motor and cognitive), and if speech, language, and musical rhythm all draw on these operations, then any of these abilities could have been the target of selection. One must therefore rely on other evidence (such as the lack of biological cost for musical deficits) in order to decide which of these was a direct target of selection and which "came along for the ride."

Genetics and Musical Tone Deafness

In the late 1800s, Allen (1878) described an individual who could not recognize familiar melodies, carry a tune, or discriminate gross pitch changes in piano tones, though he was well educated and had received music lessons in childhood. Allen called this condition "note-deafness." Over 125 years later, musical tone deafness is receiving new research interest, with tools from modern cognitive science and neuroscience being brought to bear (Drayna et al., 2001; Ayotte et al., 2002; Foxton et al., 2004; Hyde et al., 2004). Ayotte et al. (2002) conducted a useful group study of individuals with musical tone deafness, which they term "congenital amusia." (Other researchers have used other terms, such as tune-deafness and dysmelodia. I prefer musical tone deafness and will use the acronyms mTD for "musical tone deafness" and mTDIs for "musically tone deaf individuals"). Ayotte et al. recruited mTDIs via advertisement, and selected those who had "(i) a high level of education, preferably university level, to exclude general learning disabilities or retardation; (ii) music lessons during childhood, to ensure exposure to music in a timely fashion; (iii) a history of musical failure that goes back as far as they could remember, to increase the likelihood that the disorder is inborn; and (iv) no previous neurological or psychiatric history to eliminate an obvious neuro-affective cause." The researchers tested the mTDIs on a variety of musical tasks, such as melody discrimination and tapping to a musical beat, and found severe impairments. One test in particular made a clean discrimination between mTDIs and control subjects. In this test, participants heard one brief melody at a time and indicated whether it contained a "wrong note" or not. (Wrong notes were out-of-key or "sour" notes created by a 1-semitone shift of an original note in a manner that preserved the melodic contour.) The mTDIs were severely impaired on this task, whether familiar or unfamiliar melodies were used (though like controls, they did better on familiar melodies). Ayotte et al. went on to show that mTD did indeed seem selective to music. Recognition of nonmusical sounds and perception of speech intonation, for example, appeared to be spared.

As noted earlier in this chapter, Kalmus and Fry (1980) showed that mTD tends to run in families, and a more recent study found that identical twins (who share 100% of their genes) resemble each other more closely on tests of tone deafness than do fraternal twins (who share only 50% of their genes on average). These findings suggest that there is a specific gene (or genes) that puts one at risk for this disorder (Drayna et al., 2001). Is this, then, evidence for a "music gene," which would imply a role for natural selection in the evolution of musical abilities?

Given what we have learned about the relation between genes and behavior in language, a key question is, how selective is the deficit to music? A number of studies (e.g., Hyde & Peretz, 2004; Foxton et al., 2004; Patel, Foxton, & Griffiths, 2005) have shown that mTDIs have basic problems in basic pitch-change detection and pitch-direction determination skills, outside of a musical context (see Chapter 4, section 4.5.2, subsection "Melodic Contour Perception in Musical Tone Deafness"). At present, we do not know which genes predispose individuals to mTD, or what mechanisms link the genes to the trait. However, for the sake of argument, let us assume that these genes are involved in the formation of auditory neural maps involved in pitch-change detection and pitch-direction discrimination, and that disruption of these genes leads to a slight change in patterns of connectivity between neurons in these maps during development. This in turn could lead to elevated thresholds for discerning when pitch changes and the direction in which it changes. Due to these elevated thresholds, individuals would receive a degraded version of the ambient musical input, so that normal cognitive representations of musical pitch would not develop (cf. Chapter 5). In contrast, speech intonation perception may be largely robust to this deficit, because most perceptually relevant pitch movements are above these thresholds (cf. Chapter 4, section 4.5.2, subsection "The Melodic Contour Deafness Hypothesis," for further discussion).

I suspect that just as with the case of language and FOXP2, genetic research on mTD will turn up a gene (or genes) that is not specific to musical ability but that is crucial for normal musical development. Only after the mechanism of the gene is understood can evolutionary questions be meaningfully asked. Given our current understanding of the basic pitch-processing deficits in mTD, however, it does not seem that this disorder and its genetic basis will provide any evidence that humans have been shaped by natural selection for music.

Genetics and Absolute Pitch

Few musical abilities appear as categorical in terms of presence versus absence as absolute pitch (AP), defined here as the ability to accurately classify heard pitches into fine-grained categories (e.g., using the 12 note names of Western music, such as A and C#) without any external reference. For example, a musician with AP (and trained in Western music) can effortlessly and rapidly call out the names (or "chroma") of individual pitches as they are heard: C-sharp, A-flat, G, and so forth. In contrast, non-AP musicians must rely on relative pitch to name notes, in other words, they must gauge the distance of the target pitch from some known standard, typically a much more effortful and error-prone endeavor. AP can seem an almost magical ability, particularly because AP musicians often recall making no special effort to acquire it. Little wonder, then, that AP is sometimes thought of as a gift that one simply gets from chance factors such as genes.

AP has been investigated for over 120 years (Stumpf, 1883) and has received much more research attention than musical tone deafness. Thus we know a good deal about the AP phenotype (see Takeuchi & Hulse, 1993; Ward, 1999; and Levitin & Rogers, 2005, for reviews). For example, it is known that AP musicians do not have better frequency resolution abilities than non-AP musicians (Hyde et al., 2004), and there is no evidence to suggest that AP possessors are superior musicians in general. (There are many great composers who did not have AP, such as Wagner and Stravinsky.) In fact, AP appears to have an elevated incidence in certain neurological disorders, such as blindness, Williams syndrome, and autism (Chin, 2003). Thus AP should not be confused with musical giftedness, though of course AP can be an asset to a musician.

Why is AP thought to have a relationship to genes? This supposition rests on two findings. First, Profita and Bidder (1988) reported familial aggregation of AP, a finding that has been replicated by subsequent work (Baharloo et al., 1998, 2000). Second, based on large surveys of music students in the United States, Gregersen and colleagues (1999, 2000) have shown that the incidence of AP is significantly higher in Asian students (Japanese, Korean, and Chinese) than in Western students (i.e.,~ 45% vs. 10% of music students who responded to the survey, though see Henthorn & Deutsch et al., 2007). The authors also found that Asians were more likely to engage in programs that encouraged the development of AP, but concluded that differences in training could not fully account for the asymmetries they observed.[17]

Of course, none of this is direct evidence that genes influence the development of AP, and work is currently underway to try and try to answer this question with certainty (Gitschier et al., 2004). It is evident, however, that even if genes do play a role in AP, environment also plays an very important role. Two salient environmental factors are the age of onset of musical training (cf. section 7.3.2) and type of musical training (Gregersen et al., 2000). AP may differ quite sharply from musical tone deafness in this respect, because the latter may be impervious to experience (Hyde & Peretz, 2004).

The rarity of the AP phenotype, and the fact that it is unnecessary for the development of normal musical ability, indicate that finding a genetic underpinning for AP would provide no evidence that humans have been shaped by natural selection for music. However, it may be that AP will prove an interesting model for studying genotype-phenotype interactions in humans (Zatorre, 2003). Future work in this area will benefit from finding creative ways to test for AP in nonmusicians. Although AP is usually demonstrated by being able to name pitches, the ability to remember and classify pitches should be conceptually distinguished from the ability to give them musical labels. For example, Ross et al. (2003) report AP-like abilities in a nonmusician in the context of a pitch perception task that usually separates AP from non-AP individuals. In this task, a listener hears one pitch (the target), a group of interpolated pitches, and then another pitch (the probe), and must decide if the probe and target are the same or not. Individuals with AP find this task easy, because they can simply compare their verbal labels for the target and probe. Individuals without AP find the task very difficult, because of the interfering effect of the interpolated tones on pitch memory (Deutsch, 1978). Ross found a young nonmusician who performed like AP individuals on this task, despite a lack of knowledge of the standard note names of the tones. (For another method that could be used to test AP in nonmusicians, see Weisman et al., 2004.)

The notion that some nonmusicians could have AP is bolstered by the fact that a simple form of AP based on memory for the absolute pitch of familiar tunes is widespread among nonmusicians (Levitin, 1994; Schellenberg & Trehub, 2003). Furthermore, non-AP musicians perform above chance on AP tests, suggesting that the distinction between AP and non-AP may not be as clear-cut as usually thought (Lockhead & Byrd, 1981; though it is difficult to rule out the use of relative pitch cues by non-AP musicians in these tests). Assuming for the

---

[17] Personally, I am not persuaded that differences in training have been ruled out. Even if Asian and Western students participate in the same training programs, there could be differences in attitudes about how much to practice and what skills to focus on during practice (e.g., due to differences in cultural background). I am grateful to Roger V. Burton for raising this point.

moment that the potential to acquire musical AP is widespread, the challenge for behavior genetics is to explain why AP develops in some individuals but not others even when environmental variables are matched (e.g., age of onset of musical training and type of training). For example, is this due to genes that influence the neural substrates of pitch perception (Zatorre, 2003), or to genes that influence "cognitive style" (Brown et al., 2003; Chin, 2003)? Although the behavior genetics of AP will doubtless prove an interesting enterprise, the relevant point here is that this research is orthogonal to the question of AP's relevance to evolutionary issues. As noted above, this relevance is basically nil.

7.3.5 Animal Studies: What Aspects of Musicality Are Shared With Other Animals?

The introduction of this chapter argued that animal communication, even when we term it "song," it not the same as music. However, whether or not animals exhibit musical predispositions akin to humans, or can learn specific aspects of human music, are interesting questions from an evolutionary standpoint. Because animals do not have music, whatever music-relevant behaviors they exhibit or can learn are clearly not a result of selection for music, but reflect more general aspects of auditory processing. Thus studies of animals can help shed light on what aspects of music processing are uniquely human and thus in need of evolutionary explanation (McDermott & Hauser, 2005).

Exactly this same strategy has been used with animal studies of speech and language. For example, early research by Kuhl and Miller (1975) showed that chinchillas exhibited categorical perception for certain speech sound contrasts (cf. Chapter 2, section 2.4.1), an ability that was previously thought be a uniquely human adaptation for speech perception. More recently, Hauser et al. (2001) have shown that cotton-top tamarin monkeys show statistical learning of syllable transition probabilities in a manner akin to human infants (Saffran et al., 1996; cf. Newport et al., 2004). In contrast, Fitch and Hauser (2004) showed that these same monkeys lack the ability to learn recursively structured sequences, a finding related to the hypothesis that recursion is a uniquely human ability related to language (cf. Hauser et al., 2002; but see Gentner et al., 2006, for data on birds that challenge this hypothesis).

In the following sections, I briefly review three areas of research on animals and music, and discuss the significance of this work to evolutionary issues. (These sections focus on pitch; a discussion of animal abilities with regard to musical rhythm is reserved for section 7.5.3.) Before embarking, it is worth noting that there is no shortage of anecdotal evidence for animal appreciation of music. Here is my favorite example, which came in a letter from a linguist in the summer of 2004:

> My late Irish setter responded most remarkably to radio broadcasts of chamber music by Beethoven and Schubert, though more to the works of Beethoven's

middle period than those of his late period (which I had preferred). In consequence I started listening more closely to the works of the middle period and came to appreciate them more than I previously had. It is relatively rare, I think, to have one's aesthetic sensibilities significantly enhanced by one's dog.

I'm sure there is no shortage of animal music stories (though perhaps none as charming as this one), but as the scientific adage goes, "the plural of anecdote is not data."

Animals, Absolute Pitch, and Relative Pitch

Research on animal pitch perception has revealed that absolute pitch is not a uniquely human ability. Indeed, it seems to be the preferred processing mode of several bird species (see Hulse et al., 1992 for a review). In these studies, various ways of testing AP have been devised that do not require verbal labels. In one study, Weisman et al. (2004) used a paradigm in which a frequency range of about 5,000 Hz was divided into eight equal-sized bands with five test tones per band. Birds (zebra finches and two other species) received positive reinforcement for responding to frequencies in four of the bands and negative reinforcement for responding to frequencies in the other bands. After training, birds showed extremely good discrimination, responding predominantly to tones in the positively reinforced regions. Thus they successfully classified heard pitches into fine-grained categories without an external reference, fulfilling our definition of AP. (Human nonmusicians were also trained using this procedure, with money as the reinforcement, but performed miserably on the task.) The significance of this finding is that it shows that AP does not depend on human-specific brain abilities, and is thus unlikely to reflect selection for music (cf. section 7.3.4, subsection "Genetics and Absolute Pitch").

As noted by McDermott and Hauser (2005), perhaps more remarkable than nonhuman animals' facility with AP is their lack of facility with relative pitch compared with humans'. Although animals can use relative pitch as a cue (e.g., to judge if a tone sequence is rising or falling independent of its absolute pitch range; Brosch et al., 2004), this often requires extensive training. This contrasts sharply with human perception. Even infants readily recognize the similarity of the same melodic contours in different pitch ranges (Trehub et al., 1984), and remember melodies based on patterns of relative rather than absolute pitch (Plantinga & Trainor, 2005). This suggests that natural selection may have modified the human auditory system to favor relative pitch processing, a modification that may have its origins in speech intonation perception (cf. section 7.3.3, subsection "Music and Infancy: Questions of Specificity").

Animals, Consonance, and Dissonance

Animal studies have shown that the ability to discriminate consonant from dissonant pitch intervals is not unique to humans. For example, Izumi (2000) trained Japanese macaques to discriminate the consonant interval of an octave from a dissonant major seventh, and then used a transfer test to show that the monkeys could generalize this discrimination to novel consonant versus dissonant intervals. (cf. Hulse et al., 1995) (Note that all studies discussed in this section involved simultaneous intervals constructed from complex tones, in other words, tones with a fundamental and upper harmonics. See Chapter 2, appendix 3 for background on consonance and dissonance in complex tones.) Izumi noted that because the monkey auditory system did not evolve for music appreciation, the ability to discriminate consonance from dissonance may reflect mechanisms of perceptual organization related to segregating incoming sounds into sources as part of auditory scene analysis (cf. Bregman, 1990). Further evidence that the perception of consonance versus dissonance is not unique to humans comes from neural research by Fishman and colleagues (2001), who have shown that consonant and dissonant intervals generate qualitatively different patterns of neural activity in monkey auditory cortex. Thus it is likely that our sense that certain intervals are inherently rougher sounding than others (or have a less unified sense of pitch) is not uniquely human, but is a result of general properties of the vertebrate auditory system.

Animals may be able to discriminate consonance from dissonance, but do they prefer one to the other? 2-month old human infants show a preference for consonant intervals (Trainor, Tsang, & Cheung, 2002), raising the question of whether this is a human-specific trait. McDermott and Hauser (2004) addressed this question with an elegant paradigm. They constructed a V-shaped maze in which each arm of the V contained a single concealed audio speaker. Each speaker produced a different sound. A cotton-top tamarin monkey was released into the maze, and depending on which arm it chose to sit in, it heard one or the other sound (the monkey was free to move back and forth between the two arms of the maze). McDermott and Hauser first used a loud and a soft noise to test their method. All monkeys spent most of their time on the side that played the soft noise, showing that the monkeys could use the maze to indicate a behavioral preference. The researchers then ran an experiment in which the two speakers played sequences of consonant or dissonant intervals (consonant intervals were the octave, fifth and fourth; dissonant were minor seconds, tritones, and minor ninths). This time, the monkeys showed no preference. The contrast between this finding and the preferences of 2-month-old humans suggests that preference for consonance may be uniquely human, raising the possibility that our auditory system has been shaped by selection for music.

A good deal more work is needed, however, before this conclusion could be reached. First, it would be important to replicate the primate findings with chimpanzees, who are much more closely related to humans than cotton-top tamarins (our last common ancestor with chimpanzees vs. tamarins was about 6 million vs. 40 million years ago). Second, it would be important to test animals that use learned, complex sounds in their communication, such as songbirds.

There is preliminary evidence that songbirds prefer consonant over dissonant sounds (Watanabe & Nemoto, 1998), which would indicate that this preference may be a byproduct of an auditory system adapted to a rich acoustic communication system. Finally, research on human infants would have to show that the preference for consonance was not due to prior exposure, by doing cross-cultural research or controlled-exposure studies (cf. section 7.3.3, subsection "Music and Infancy: Questions of Innateness"). If the difference between humans and other animals still persists after these more tightly controlled studies are conducted, then the burden will be on those who favor a nonadaptationist view of music to explain the origins of a human preference for consonance.

Animals and Tonality

There is abundant evidence that adults in Western culture show superior processing of tonal versus atonal melodies, in other words, melodies that follow the conventions of scale and key in Western music (cf. Chapter 5). Infants do not show this same asymmetry (e.g., Trainor & Trehub, 1992). They do, however, perform better at detecting changes in pitch patterns when those changes disrupt certain pitch intervals such as the perfect fifth (Schellenberg & Trehub, 1996). Young infants also show octave equivalence, treating tone sequences separated by an octave as similar (Demany & Armand, 1984). These findings, combined with the near universal use of the octave and fifth in organizing musical scales, suggest that certain pitch intervals have a favored status in human auditory processing, either due to innate properties of the auditory system or to early experience with harmonically structured sounds (such as speech, cf. Chapter 2, appendix 3). A question that naturally arises about these predispositions is whether they are limited to humans.

Wright et al. (2000) conducted a study in which two rhesus monkeys were tested to see if they treated octave transpositions of melodies as similar. The research capitalized on a clever paradigm that allowed the monkeys to express whether they perceived two stimuli as the same or different. In this paradigm, a monkey sits in a small booth with a speaker in the wall directly ahead of it, and a speaker in the wall to either side. A first sound is presented from the central speaker, followed by a second sound from both side speakers. If the first and second sounds are the same, then a touch to the right speaker elicits a food reward. If the sounds are different, a touch to the left speaker produces the reward.

Using this method, the researchers investigated octave equivalence. If a monkey perceives pitches separated by an octave as similar, they will be more likely to respond "same" to transpositions of an octave than to other transpositions. Wright et al. found that when Western tonal melodies were used as stimuli (e.g., from children's songs), the monkeys did indeed show evidence of octave equivalence, treating transpositions of 1 or 2 octaves as more similar to the original melody than transpositions of 1/2 octave or 1.5 octaves. This provided evidence for octave equivalence in monkeys, suggesting that the musical universal of octave equivalence has its roots in basic auditory processing mechanisms (cf. McKinney & Delgutte, 1999). (Interestingly, and in parallel to human studies, the monkeys did not show octave equivalence to isolated pitches.)

Wright et al. also conducted another experiment that has attracted a good deal of attention. The tested the monkeys for octave equivalence using novel tonal versus atonal melodies, and found that the monkeys did not show octave equivalence when atonal melodies were used.[18] To some, this might suggest that tonality is innately favored by the auditory system. However, close inspection of their data shows that the situation is not so clear cut. Octaves were treated as more similar than 1/2 octaves for *both* tonal and atonal melodies. Furthermore, in simple same-different discrimination trials in which melodies were not transposed, the monkeys showed superior discrimination for tonal melodies. These findings converge to suggest that the monkeys found atonal melodies harder to remember than tonal ones, which may in turn have been due to incidental exposure to music in captivity. Hauser and McDermott (2003) have noted that monkey facilities often have a TV, and in their own research they have shown that monkeys are adept at statistical learning, which is currently thought to be an important mechanism for tonality learning (Krumhansl, 1990, 2005). Thus the results of Wright et al. cannot be taken as evidence that Western tonality is somehow innately favored by the auditory system. For those interested in addressing this issue, it would be highly desirable to replicate the study of Wright et al. with monkeys (or other animals) whose acoustic environment was more tightly controlled.

An obvious question that arises from the Wright et al. study is whether monkeys would show a processing advantage for pitch patterns based on the perfect fifth, as young human infants do. If this is the case (especially for monkeys raised in acoustically controlled environments), this would provide evidence that the widespread use of the fifth in human music is based on basic auditory processing mechanisms rather than being a product of selection for music.

Wright et al.'s use of tonality as a variable in their research points the way to many studies one could do with animals with regard to the ease with which they learn tonal versus atonal sequences. For example, one set of animals could be trained to discriminate tonal sequences, whereas another set is trained to discriminate atonal sequences that have similar Gestalt properties (e.g., contour patterns and overall interval distributions). Number of trials to criterion could be studied (are tonal sequences easier to learn?), as could generalization to the

---

[18] The tonal and atonal melodies were 7-note sequences whose degree of tonality was quantified using the Maximum Key Profile Correlation (MKC) method of Takeuchi (1994), based on the work of Krumhansl and Kessler (1982). Atonal melodies had MKC values of less than 0.57, whereas tonal melodies had a value of 0.75 or above.

other type of sequence. At the risk of repeating myself once too often, I must reemphasize that the results of such studies will only be meaningful if the acoustic history of the animals is controlled from the time they first begin to hear (i.e., *before* birth), in order to control for effects of differential exposure. For example, animals could be raised hearing equal amounts of tonal versus atonal melodies.[19] In conducting such studies, it would be of great theoretical interest to expand the scope beyond Western music to ask about the pitch systems of other cultures. For example, are scales that follow Javanese conventions easier to learn than scales that the Javanese would regard as "ungrammatical"?

7.4 Music and Evolution: Neither Adaptation nor Frill

Let us step back and take stock. In the introduction, it was explained why the universality of human music and brain specialization for certain aspects of music do not provide any evidence that musical abilities have been the direct target of natural selection. In section 7.3.1, we saw that existing adaptationist conjectures about music are not very persuasive, and sections 7.3.2–7.3.5 showed that data from development, genetics, and animal studies provide (as yet) no compelling reasons to reject the null hypothesis that music has not been a direct target of natural selection. Thus based on current evidence, music does not seem to be a biological adaptation.

I hasten to add that the question is not yet settled, and that there is a little-explored area that will likely prove important for future research on the evolution of music, namely developmental studies of beat-based rhythm perception and synchronization. This area is the focus of the next section. Let us say for the sake of argument, however, that research in this (or any other) area does not provide evidence that human minds have been specifically shaped for music cognition. Does this force us to conclude that music is merely a frill, a hedonic diversion that tickles our senses and that could easily be dispensed with (Pinker, 1997)?

Not at all. I would like to suggest that the choice between adaptation and frill is a false dichotomy, and that music belongs in a different category. *Homo sapiens* is unique among all living organisms in terms of its ability to invent things that transform its own existence. Written language is a good example: This technology makes it possible to share complex thoughts across space and time and to accumulate knowledge in a way that transcends the limits of any single human mind. The invention of aircraft is another example: These machines have fundamentally changed the way ordinary humans experience their world, allowing large-scale movement between cultures. A final example is the

---

[19] One would not want to raise the animals in constant white noise, as this can lead to abnormal cortical auditory maps (Chang & Merzenich, 2003).

modern Internet, a technology that is changing the way people communicate, learn, and make communities. These are all examples of technologies invented by humans that have become intimately integrated into the fabric of our life, transforming the lives of individuals and groups. This never-ending cycle of invention, integration, and transformation is uniquely human (Clark, 2003), and has ancient roots. I believe music can be sensibly thought of in this framework, in other words, as something that we invented that transforms human life. Just as with other transformative technologies, once invented and experienced, it becomes virtually impossible to give it up.

This notion of music as a transformative technology helps to explain why music is universal in human culture. Music is universal because what it does for humans is universally valued. Music is like the making and control of fire in this respect. The control of fire is universal in human culture because it transforms our lives in ways we value deeply, for example, allowing us to cook food, keep warm, and see in dark places. Once a culture learns fire making, there is no going back, *even though we might be able to live without this ability.* Similarly, music is universal because it transforms our lives in ways we value deeply, for example, in terms of emotional and aesthetic experience and identity formation. Current archeological evidence suggests music has had this transformative power for a very long time: The oldest undisputed musical instrument is an approximately 36,000-year-old bone flute from Germany (Richter et al., 2000). It seems likely that even earlier instruments will be found, because human art is now known to have at least a 100,000-year-old history (the age of shell beads found in Israel and Algeria (Vanhaeren et al., 2006; cf. Henshilwood et al., 2004). (It will be particularly interesting to know if the most ancient musical instruments will also be found in Africa, because modern humans are thought to have evolved on that continent about 120,000 years ago, and to have emigrated from there about 45,000 years ago.)

Of course, there is one very important sense in which music is unlike other technologies such as fire making or the Internet. Music has the power to change the very structure of our brains, enlarging certain areas due to motor or perceptual experience (Elbert et al., 1995; Pantev et al., 1998, 2001; Münte et al., 2002; Pascual-Leone, 2003), or leading certain areas to specialize in music-specific knowledge (e.g., memories for melodies, as evidenced by selective amusias following brain damage; Peretz, 1996). However, music is not unique in this respect. The brain has a remarkable capacity to change due to experience, and numerous studies of animal and human brains have shown that motor or perceptual experience can change the relative size and organization of specific brain areas (Buonomano & Merzenich, 1998; Huttenlocher, 2002). Furthermore, the specialization of certain human brain regions for reading written orthography demonstrates that learning can lead to neural specialization during development. Thus the human process of invention, internalization, and transformation can change the very organ that makes this process possible (Clark, 2003).

7.5 Beat-Based Rhythm Processing as a Key Research Area

Thus far in this book, the final section of each chapter has outlined a promising area of research with regard to music-language relations. The current chapter is different. So far, it has been argued that there is (as yet) no evidence that seriously challenges the null hypothesis of no direct natural selection for musical abilities. To find such evidence, it will be necessary to demonstrate that there is a fundamental aspect of music cognition that is not a byproduct of cognitive mechanisms that also serve other, more clearly adaptive, domains (e.g., auditory scene analysis or language). Thus this section seeks an aspect of music cognition that *is not* related to language processing, to refine the evolutionary study of music.

A lack of relationship to language (or other structured cognitive domains) would establish the domain-specificity of the aspect of music cognition in question, which is one important criterion for evidence that the ability has been shaped by natural selection for music. It is not the only criterion, however, because domain-specificity can be a product of development (recall the discussion in section 7.1 of brain areas specialized for reading written text). To be of evolutionary relevance, this aspect of music cognition should develop in a manner that suggests the brain is specifically prepared to acquire this ability. That is, it should develop precociously and spontaneously (e.g., in contrast to learning to read, which is an effortful and slow process). Finally, it would be important to show that the aspect in question is unique to humans, and cannot be acquired by other animals. This last criterion is posited on the assertion that nonhuman animals do not naturally make music (cf. section 7.1 and McDermott & Hauser, 2005). If nonhuman animals can acquire a fundamental aspect of music cognition, then this aspect is latent in animal brains and does not require natural selection for music to explain its existence.

Is there any aspect of music cognition that has the potential to satisfy these three criteria (domain-specificity, innateness, and human-specificity)? Justus and Hutsler (2005) and McDermott and Hauser (2005) have argued that musical pitch processing does not satisfy these criteria (cf. section 7.3.3–7.3.5 above), but they leave the issue of musical rhythm largely unexplored. I believe there is one widespread aspect of musical rhythm that deserves attention in this regard, namely beat-based rhythm processing. In every culture, there is some form of music with a regular beat, a periodic pulse that affords temporal coordination between performers and elicits a synchronized motor response from listeners (McNeill, 1995; Nettl, 2000). Thus I would like to raise the following question: Might beat-based rhythm processing reflect evolutionary modifications to the brain for the purpose of music making?

In pursuing this question, we shall not concern ourselves with the issue of adaptation. If we have been specifically shaped by natural selection for beat-based processing, then presumably early humans who were able to perceive a musical beat (and synchronize their actions to it) had some selective advantage over those who did not have this ability. Hypotheses have been offered about the adaptive value of beat perception and synchronization in evolution (e.g., Merker, 2000), but these will not be the focus here because the prehistory of music will probably never be known with any certainty (as noted in section 7.3). Instead, the following sections focus on issues of development, domain-specificity, and human-specificity, because research on these issues has the potential to address evolutionary questions with empirical data. As we shall see, these are areas in which there are more questions than answers, with many open avenues for investigation (cf. Patel, 2006c).

7.5.1 Domain-Specificity

One important question about beat-based rhythm is its relationship to speech rhythm, because both music and language have richly structured rhythmic patterns. Although early theories of speech rhythm proposed an underlying isochronous pulse based on stresses or syllables, empirical data have not supported this idea, and contemporary studies of speech rhythm have largely abandoned the isochrony issue (cf. Chapter 3). However, a musical beat does have a more abstract connection to speech rhythm via the notion of meter. A musical beat typically occurs in the context of a meter, a hierarchical organization of beats in which some beats are perceived as stronger than others. Interestingly, speech also has a "metrical" hierarchy based on stress or prominence (Selkirk, 1984; Terken & Hermes, 2000), suggesting that a tendency to organize rhythmic sequences in terms of hierarchical prominence patterns may originate in language. Crucially, however, the "beats" of speech (stressed syllables) do not mark out a regular pulse. This difference has important cognitive consequences. In particular, the use of a perceptually isochronous pulse in music engages periodic temporal expectancies that play a basic role in music cognition (Jones 1976; Jones & Boltz, 1989), but that appear to play little or no role in ordinary speech perception (cf. Pitt & Samuel, 1990). Humans are able to extract periodicities from complex auditory stimuli, and can focus their expectancies on periodicities at different hierarchical levels in music (Drake, Jones, & Baruch, 2000). These periodic expectancies are the basis of motor synchronization to the beat on the part of listeners, as shown by the fact that listeners typically tap or move slightly *ahead* of the actual beat, indicating that synchronization is based on structured temporal anticipation (cf. Patel, Iversen, et al., 2005).

Turning from language to other cognitive abilities, one might sensibly ask if the periodic expectancies of beat-based processing are simply a byproduct of the brain's ability to do generic temporal anticipation, in other words, to gauge when exactly an event of interest is going to occur based on the timing of events in the immediate past. Human brains are adept at generic temporal anticipation. For example, each time we catch a ball or walk down a crowded sidewalk, we engage in this kind of temporal anticipation (e.g., in order to move a hand to the right position to catch the ball, or to step out of the way of an oncoming pedestrian before impact). Crucially, however, these are "ballistic" temporal expectancies based on anticipating a single event, rather than periodic expectancies based on a mental model of recurring time intervals. Informal observation suggests that some people who function perfectly well in everyday life have serious difficulties in musical beat-based processing, which would suggest that the ability to construct periodic expectancies is not a trivial byproduct of the ability to construct generic temporal expectancies.

Beat-based processing also appears to be distinct from the more generic ability to gauge the duration of time intervals, which is widespread among animals. Rabbits, for example, can be trained to learn the duration of a short time interval between a warning tone and a puff of air on the eye. After learning, once they hear the tone, they anticipate when in time the subsequent puff will occur, showing that their brain can do structured temporal anticipation. Neural research indicates that this sort of interval timing recruits a distributed neural network including the basal ganglia, cortex, and thalamus (Matell & Meck, 2000), a network that is probably quite similar across vertebrates. An important aspect of this network is its amodal nature: It is equally good at learning intervals between auditory events, visual events, and so forth. This stands in sharp contrast to beat-based rhythmic processing in music, which appears to have a special relationship to the auditory system, as evidenced by the fact that people have difficulty perceiving a beat in visual rhythmic sequences (Patel, Iversen, et al., 2005). Thus even if beat-based processing has its roots in brain circuits for interval timing, these circuits appear to have been modified in humans to create a special auditory-motor link. Such a modification may be one reason why no other animals besides humans have been reported to move in synchrony with a musical beat (a topic taken up at greater length in section 7.5.3. below).

From a neuropsychological standpoint, little is known about the domain-specificity of beat-based rhythmic processing. A key question here is whether brain damage that disrupts it also disrupts other basic nonmusical cognitive abilities. If so, this might suggest that beat-based processing is based on abilities recruited from other brain functions. The neuropsychological literature contains descriptions of individuals with musical rhythmic disturbance after brain damage, or "acquired arrhythmia" (cf. Chapter 3, section 3.5.3). Two notable findings from this literature are that rhythmic abilities can be selectively disrupted, leaving pitch processing skills relatively intact, and that there are dissociations between rhythmic tasks requiring simple discrimination of temporal patterns and those requiring the evaluation or production of periodic patterns. However, no neuropsychological studies to date have examined relations between deficits in beat-based processing and in other basic cognitive skills. One intriguing hint of a link between musical rhythm skills and language abilities comes from a study of a family in which some members have an inherited speech and language deficit (the KE family, discussed in sections 7.2.9 and 7.3.4 above). Individuals with this deficit—which influences both linguistic syntax and speech articulatory movements—also have difficulty discriminating and reproducing short musical rhythm patterns, in contrast with a relative facility with musical pitch patterns (Alcock et al., 2000b). Unfortunately, beat-based processing was not specifically investigated by Alcock et al., leaving open the question of how the disorder seen in the KE family relates to cognitive processing of periodic rhythmic patterns.

7.5.2 Development

One way to address the innateness of beat-based rhythm processing is via developmental studies, in order to explore whether the brain seems specifically prepared to acquire this ability. Specifically, it is of interest to know whether humans show precocious abilities when it comes to perceiving a musical beat, just as they show precocious abilities in language perception. As discussed in section 7.2.4, by 1 year of age, infants show impressive speech perception abilities. Is there evidence that infants younger than 12 months can perceive a beat in music, in other words, construct a mental framework of periodic temporal expectancies around an inferred pulse? The clearest evidence for this would be a demonstration that infants can synchronize their movements to the beat of music. In fact, young infants do not synchronize their movements to a musical beat (Longhi, 2003). In Western European cultures, the ability to synchronize with a beat does not appear to emerge till around age 4 (Drake, Jones, & Baruch, 2000; Eerola et al., 2006). This is striking given that there seems to be ample opportunity to learn synchronization skills early in life: Most children's songs have a very clearly marked beat that is emphasized in infant-directed singing (Trainor et al., 1997), nursery tunes have strong distributional cues to metrical structure (i.e., more frequent events on strong beats; Palmer & Pfordresher, 2003; cf. Palmer & Krumhansl, 1990), and infants are frequently rocked or bounced to music (Papousek, 1996). Yet despite these facts, and despite the fact that movement to a beat requires only relatively gross motor skills (e.g., clapping, bobbing up and down, or swaying side to side), synchronized movement to music appears to emerge relatively slowly in development.[20]

However, it is possible that beat perception skills precede motor synchronization abilities, just as children's understanding of speech is typically in advance of their own speech production skills. Perceptual studies can help determine

---

[20] We currently lack data on the youngest age at which children are capable of reliably synchronizing to a beat. Further developmental work is needed in this area. Experiments in cultures in which there is an active musical culture among children would be of particular interest here (Blacking, 1967).

whether the human brain is specifically prepared to construct periodic temporal expectancies from musical stimuli.

There is good evidence that infants are sensitive to basic rhythmic aspects of auditory sequences. For example, 2- to 4-month-olds can detect a change in the pattern of duration intervals, for example, a change from a short-long to a long-short pattern of intervals ([x-x---x] versus [x---x-x], in which each x marks a tone onset and each dash corresponds to approximately 100 ms of silence; Demany et al., 1977). At 7–9 months, infants can detect a change in the temporal pattern even when tempo varies. For example, when trained to detect a change from a short-long to a long-short pattern of intervals at one tempo, and then tested with stimuli at other tempi, they still show a response to the change in pattern (Trehub & Thorpe, 1989). This suggests that infants perceive grouping structure in rhythmic patterns, likely based on the patterning of duration ratios between successive events. A facility with grouping perception is also evident in 12-month-olds, who can discriminate rhythmic patterns that have the same duration and number of groups, but different numbers of events in each group (Morrongiello, 1984). Thus it appears that infants have a precocious facility with the perception of rhythmic grouping, which could stem from the importance of grouping in speech perception (cf. Chapter 3, section 3.2.3).

Is there evidence that infants are also adept at the perception of a beat in music? It is known that 2- to 4-month-old infants can detect a change in tempo (of 15%) in an isochronous sequence, when events have an approximately 600 ms IOI (Baruch & Drake, 1997), and by 6 months old, infants can detect a 10% change in durations of events in an isochronous sequence (Morrongiello & Trehub, 1987). However, the former finding could be explained via a sensitivity to the average rate of events over time, and the latter via sensitivity to the absolute durations of tones (cf. Morrongiello, 1984). Thus specific tests of sensitivity to beat-based rhythmic patterns are needed. Although there are a number of elegant studies of rhythm processing in infancy that might seem to indicate beat-based processing (e.g., Hannon & Trehub, 2005; Hannon & Johnson, 2005; Phillips-Silver & Trainor, 2005), closer examination suggests that caution is warranted (the interested reader may consult the chapter appendix for a detailed discussion). Here I focus on one study whose methodology seems promising for future work on periodic temporal expectancies in infants.

Bergeson and Trehub (2006) examined the ability of 9-month-old infants to detect a subtle temporal change in short rhythmic sequences of tones, in which all tones had the same pitch and intensity. Although the tones had no physical accents, according to the research of Povel and Okkerman (1981), some of the tones had "subjective accents" due to the position of events in groups (Figure 7.3). In three of these patterns, the subjective accents were consistent with a regular beat (one such pattern is shown in Figure 7.3a).

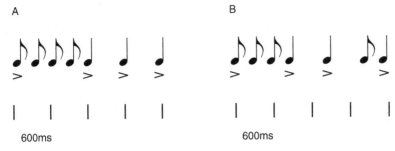

Figure 7.3 Two rhythm patterns used by Bergeson and Trehub (2006) to study infant perception of a beat. Tones bearing subjective accents are marked with a ">." Note how in pattern (A), accented tones tend to align with an isochronous beat with a period of 600 ms (marked by vertical lines below the rhythm pattern). In pattern (B), the accented tones do not align well with a regular beat. Subjective accents are assigned according to the rules of Povel and Okkerman (1981), in other words, on the first and last tones for groups with three or more tones, on the second tone for groups of two tones, and on isolated tones.

In a fourth sequence, however, the accents were not consistent with a regular beat (Figure 7.3b). (The reader may check this by listening to Sound Examples 7.2a and b, which correspond to the two rhythms in Figure 7.3a and b. It is relatively easy to tap a regular beat to Sound Example 7.2a, but harder for Sound Example 7.2b.) Research with adults has shown that rhythmic sequences with regular subjective accents are easier to learn and reproduce than those with irregular accents, presumably because they facilitate the perception of the pattern in terms of temporally predictable beats (Povel & Essens, 1985; cf. Patel, Iversen, et al., 2005). Using a conditioned head-turn procedure that rewarded detection of a change in a repeating pattern, Bergeson and Trehub found that the infants more easily detected a small duration decrement to a single note in patterns with regular accents. They interpret this to mean that the infants extracted the regularity of these accents and used it to induce a beat-based framework for perceiving the temporal pattern. The results are indeed consistent with this view, yet cannot be considered as definitive evidence for beat perception by infants, because they rely on just a single pattern with irregular accents.[21] More work is needed to show that the results generalize to other patterns with versus without regular subjective accents. The study is important, however, in introducing a useful method for testing beat perception by infants, together with suggestive evidence along these lines. If the results are upheld, this would stand as a challenge to the null hypothesis for the evolution of music. That is, a

[21] Furthermore, one of the patterns with regular accents did not show a processing advantage over the pattern with irregular accents, suggesting that other factors besides the regularity of subjective accents is at play in these results.

brain wired for beat perception from early in life would be suggestive of circuits shaped by natural selection for music.

7.5.3 Human-Specificity

Whereas the previous section focused on the perception of a musical beat, this section focuses on synchronized movement to a beat. It is an intriguing fact that that there are no reports of nonhuman animals spontaneously moving to the beat of music. This naturally leads to the question of whether synchronization to a beat involves cognitive and neural mechanisms that have been shaped by natural selection for musical abilities. One way to test this idea is to ask whether nonhuman animals (henceforth, animals) are capable of learning to move in synchrony with a musical beat. If so, this would show that natural selection for music is not necessary to account for this ability, because animal nervous systems have not been shaped by selection for music (cf. section 7.1 and McDermott & Hauser, 2005).

Recently, it has been shown that at least one species of animal (the Asian elephant, *Elephas maximus*) can learn to drum a steady beat on a musical instrument in the absence of ongoing timing cues from a human (Patel & Iversen, 2006). Indeed, using a mallet held in its trunk, an elephant can strike a drum with a rhythmic regularity that exceeds even humans drumming at the same tempo (Sound/Video Example 7.3).[22] However, the elephants studied (members of the Thai Elephant Orchestra) showed no evidence of synchronizing their drumming to a common beat when performing in an ensemble setting.

Of course, it is well known that animals can synchronize with each other in producing periodic signals, for example, the rhythmic chorusing of crickets, frogs, or fireflies in their courtship displays (cf. Gerhardt & Huber, 2002, Ch. 8). Superficially, this may seem equivalent to human synchronization with a beat. A closer examination of these communicative displays suggests otherwise. For example, research on crickets and katydids has revealed that group synchrony in chirping is likely to be an epiphenomenon of local competitive interactions between males all trying to call first. Males attempt to call ahead of other nearby males because females find "leading calls" attractive (Greenfield et al., 1997; Römer et al., 2002). Crucially, the mechanism used by males to adjust the rhythm of their calls (in order to try to call first) does not involve matching their call period to a periodic model, but rather is a cycle-by-cycle phase adjustment in response to the calls of other males. When multiple males

---

[22] Footage taken by the author in October 2006, in Lampang, Thailand, at the Thai Elephant Conservation Center, thanks to the kind hospitality of David Sulzer and Richard Lair. Note that the mahout (trainer), who is in blue and stands to the right and behind the elephant, is not giving any verbal, visual, or tactile timing cues. The elephant is a 13-year-old female named Pratida.

all use this strategy, episodes of synchrony emerge as an unintended byproduct. In other words, there is no evidence that rhythmic synchrony in crickets results from processes of structured temporal anticipation.

Interestingly, synchrony among fireflies may be a different story, involving changes to the period of rhythmic flashing in order to come into synchrony with neighbors (Buck, 1988; Greenfield, 2005). This sort of purposeful synchrony is more like human synchronization to a beat, but firefly flashing nevertheless differs in important ways from human movement to music. Notably, humans can synchronize across a wide tempo range, can synchronize with complex rhythmic stimuli (i.e., can move to the beat of complex acoustic patterns, including those with syncopation), and show cross-modal synchronization, with an auditory stimulus driving the motor system in periodic behavior that is not (necessarily) aimed at sound production. Firefly synchrony does not exhibit this these features: Fireflies synchronize within a very limited tempo range, show no evidence of synchronizing to the beat of complex rhythmic light patterns, and produce a response that is in the same modality as the input signal.

These differences argue against the view that human synchronization to a beat reflects widespread mechanisms of synchronization in biological systems. Instead, it appears that this behavior may reflect music-specific abilities. One way to test this idea is to see if nonhuman animals can be trained to move in synchrony with a musical beat. In this regard, it is a remarkable fact that despite decades of research in psychology and neuroscience in which animals have been trained to do elaborate tasks, there is not a single report of an animal being trained to tap, peck, or move in synchrony with an auditory beat. This is particularly surprising given the fact that there are many studies showing that animals have accurate neural mechanisms for interval timing (e.g., Moore et al., 1998).

One might object that moving to a beat is an unnatural behavior for an animal, but this misses the point. Monkeys, for example, are often trained to do highly ecologically unnatural tasks in neuroscience experiments for the purpose of research on neural mechanisms of perception or motor control (e.g., drawing figures with a cursor controlled by a handheld joystick; Schwartz et al., 2004). Thus the relevant question is whether an animal *could* learn to move to a beat. If so, then (as noted previously) this would indicate that natural selection for music is not necessary to account for this ability.

A question that immediately arises is which animals one should study. Chimps and bonobos may seem the obvious choice. Among the great apes, they are the most closely related to humans. They are also highly intelligent, as evidenced by research with language-trained apes such as Kanzi (Savage-Rumbaugh et al., 1998). Furthermore, chimps and bonobos produce short bouts of rhythmic "drumming" with their hands or feet as part of display or play behavior (Arcadi et al., 1998; Fitch, 2006; Kugler & Savage-Rumbaugh, 2002), meaning that they can voluntarily produce rhythmic movements on a timescale appropriate for synchronization to a beat.

Despite these facts, there are reasons to question whether apes (and non-human primates in general) are capable of moving in synchrony with a beat. These reasons pertain to the brain circuits that are involved in beat perception and motor control. Perceptual research on humans using fMRI indicates that rhythms that do (vs. do not) have a regular beat are associated with increased activity in the basal ganglia (Grahn & Brett, 2007). This deep brain structure is known to be an essential part of the distributed circuit (involving the cerebral cortex, basal ganglia, and thalamus) involved in interval timing, in other words, in gauging temporal intervals in the time range relevant to musical beat perception (Matell & Meck, 2000). Importantly, the basal ganglia are also involved in motor control and sequencing (cf. Janata & Grafton, 2003), meaning that a brain structure involved in perceptually "keeping the beat" is also involved in the coordination of patterned movement.

If synchronizing to a beat simply required that a common brain structure be involved in interval timing and motor control, then one would expect that chimps (and many other animals) would be capable of this behavior. This is because the basal ganglia subserve interval timing and motor control functions across a wide range of species, including primates and rodents (Buhusi & Meck, 2005). However, I suspect moving to a beat requires more than just a common brain structure that handles both of these functions. This is because synchronization to a beat involves a special relationship between *auditory* temporal intervals and patterned movement, as evidenced by the fact that visual rhythms poorly induce synchronized movement in humans (Patel, Iversen, et al., 2005). Yet the interval timing abilities of the basal ganglia are amodal, applying equally well to intervals defined by auditory versus visual events. This suggests that some additional force in human evolution modified the basal ganglia in a way that affords a tight coupling between auditory input and motor output.

One plausible candidate for this evolutionary force is vocal learning. Vocal learning involves learning to produce vocal signals based on auditory experience and sensory feedback. This ability seems commonplace to us, because every child exhibits it as part of learning to speak. An evolutionary perspective, however, reveals that vocal learning is an uncommon trait, having arisen in only a few groups of animals (including songbirds, parrots, cetaceans, and some pinnipeds; cf. Fitch, 2006; Merker, 2005, and section 7.2.3). Notably, humans are unique among primates in exhibiting complex vocal learning (Egnor & Hauser, 2004).

Vocal learning requires a tight coupling between auditory input and motor output in order to match vocal production to a desired model. This online integration of the auditory and motor system places special demands on the nervous system. Neurobiological research on birds indicates that vocal learning is associated with modifications to the basal ganglia, which play a key role in mediating a link between auditory input and motor output during learning

(Doupe et al., 2005). Because there are many anatomical parallels between basal ganglia anatomy in birds and mammals, it seems plausible to suggest that human basal ganglia have also been modified by natural selection for vocal learning (cf. Jarvis, 2004). The resulting tight coupling between auditory input and motor output may be a necessary foundation for synchronizing to a beat.

The foregoing observations can be condensed into a specific and testable hypothesis, namely that having the neural circuitry for complex vocal learning is a necessary prerequisite for the ability to synchronize with an auditory beat. This "vocal learning and rhythmic synchronization hypothesis" predicts that attempts to teach nonhuman primates to synchronize to a beat will not be successful.[23,24] Furthermore, it suggests that if primates do fail at synchronizing to a beat, it would be premature to conclude that this ability is unique to humans. It would be essential to test nonhuman vocal learners for this ability. In this regard, it is interesting to note that there are anecdotal reports of parrots moving rhythmically in response to music (Sound/Video Example 7.4; cf. Patel, 2006b).[25] If future research demonstrates that humans are unique in being able to learn to move in synchrony with a musical beat, this would be suggestive of circuits shaped by natural selection for music.

7.6 Conclusion

Whether human bodies and brains have been shaped by natural selection for music is a topic of vigorous debate. To address this question, this chapter

[23] There is an old report of a female white-handed gibbon (*Hylobates lar*) in a German zoo that followed the beats of a metronome with short calls (Ziegler & Knobloch, 1968, cited in Geissmann, 2000). However, Geissmann (personal communication) believes that the gibbon was likely calling in the intervals between the metronome ticks. This could be a stimulus-response pattern, as observed in certain frogs, rather than a behavior based on structured temporal anticipation (cf. Gerhardt & Huber, 2002, Ch. 8). As in studies of frogs, the critical test would be to manipulate the timing of the ticks so that they occurred at the same average tempo but with temporally irregular intervals. If the gibbon calls with short latency after each tick, this suggests a stimulus-response pattern because the animal cannot temporally anticipate when the ticks occur.

[24] Mithen (2005:153) also predicts that nonhuman primates will not able to synchronize to a musical beat, but for reasons different from those suggested here.

[25] Sound/Video Example 7.4 is an excerpt from the film *The Wild Parrots of Telegraph Hill* (reproduced with permission from Pelican Media), which describes the relationship between a flock of parrots that live wild in San Francisco and man who helps care for them (Mark Bittner). In this clip, Mark Bittner plays guitar while one of the parrots from the flock, named Mingus, moves rhythmically to the music. While Bittner himself moves rhythmically in this clip, raising the question of whether the parrot is imitating his own movements, he reports (personal communication) that he normally plays guitar while sitting still, and first noticed Mingus's rhythmic movements in that context.

has used language as a foil for music. In the case of language, there appears to be enough evidence to reject the null hypothesis that humans have not been directly shaped by natural selection for this ability. In the case of music, however, I do not think enough evidence has accumulated to reject the null hypothesis. I hasten to add, however, that this does not mean the question is settled. Further research is needed to address whether humans have been specifically shaped by evolution to acquire musical abilities. One line of research especially worth pursuing concerns beat-based rhythmic processing, and the extent to which this represents a domain-specific, innate, and uniquely human ability.

Whatever the outcome of this research, it should be kept in mind that the notion that something is either a product of biological adaptation or a frill is based on a false dichotomy (section 7.4). Music may be a human invention, but if so, it resembles the ability to make and control fire: It is something we invented that transforms human life. Indeed, it is more remarkable than fire making in some ways, because not only is it a product of our brain's mental capacities, it also has the power to change the brain. It is thus emblematic of our species' unique ability to change the nature of ourselves.

Appendix

This is an appendix to section 7.5.2.

Hannon and Trehub (2005) conducted an interesting study of musical meter perception. They familiarized adults and 6-month-old infants with two different kinds of musical excerpts that had a rich melodic and rhythmic structure. The first kind had a meter based on isochronous beats (as is typical in Western European music), whereas the second kind had a meter based on nonisochronous beats (specifically, the beats formed a repeating short-short-long pattern, common in Balkan music; cf. Chapter 3, section 3.2.1). The adults were asked to rate variations of each of these patterns for their rhythmic similarity to the original pattern. For each pattern (isochronous or nonisochronous meter), two variants were created by inserting a note into one of the measures of the pattern. In one variant, the insertion was made in a way that preserved the metrical pattern, whereas in the other variant, the insertion disrupted the meter (resulting in one measure with an extra 1/2 beat). These were called the "structure preserving" (SP) and "structure violating" (SV) patterns, respectively.

For North American adults, the key finding was that the SV pattern was rated less similar to the familiarization stimulus than the SP pattern for the isochronous meter condition, but not for the nonisochronous meter condition. In other words, adults seemed to find it easier to detect a rhythmic change that violated the prevailing meter when that meter was based on evenly timed beats than on unevenly timed beats. This suggests that the adults had difficulty extracting the unevenly timed beats from Balkan music and using them as a framework for the perception of temporal patterns. (This interpretation was supported by the fact that Balkan adults were also tested, and rated SV as worse than SP for both isochronous and nonisochronous meters.)

The infants in this study (all North American) were tested with a familiarization-preference procedure. After being familiarized with an excerpt in either the isochronous or nonisochronous meter, they were played the SV and SP variant of that same pattern in alternating trials, and their looking time to the two variants was quantified. A longer looking time to the SV variant was taken as an indication that they discriminated SV from SP. The main finding of interest was that the infants showed greater looking time to SV versus SP patterns for both the isochronous and nonisochronous meters (suggestive of a novelty preference). In other words, infants seemed to discriminate changes in isochronous and nonisochronous metrical patterns equally well. This finding is reminiscent of classic findings in speech perception development, showing that 6-month-olds can discriminate both native and nonnative phoneme contrasts, in contrast to adults, who have difficulty discriminating nonnative contrasts (cf. Chapter 2, section 2.3.4).

It is tempting to interpret this study as evidence that infants perceive a beat in music, in other words, that they form a mental framework of structured temporal anticipation based on the timing of beats in complex musical patterns, and that they are equally adept at doing this with isochronous and nonisochronous meters. However, there are other possible explanations of the results. Although it is reasonable to assume the adults extracted a beat whenever they could, it is possible that the infants did not extract regular beats and attended instead to nonperiodic duration ratio patterns between successive notes. Such patterns changed in both the SV and SP conditions in both meters, and could thus have served as a basis for the observed novelty preference. Thus the infants' responses do not necessarily indicate the perception of a regular beat in terms of a framework of periodic temporal anticipation.

One way to demonstrate true meter perception in infants would be to show that they extract meter as a feature from stimuli that vary along other dimensions. Hannon and Johnson (2005) conducted a relevant study in this regard. They used a habituation paradigm in which 7-month-old infants listened to complex rhythmic patterns that differed in their temporal structure, but that were all designed to yield a common sense of meter. Four different stimuli were used to evoke a duple meter (a perceived beat on every other event, with a strong beat every four events), whereas four other stimuli they used to evoke a triple meter (a perceived beat on every third event). The rhythmic patterns did not contain any physical accents: All tones were of the same intensity and frequency (C5, 523 Hz). Thus the only accents were "subjective accents" due to the position of events in groups, with the meter being created by the temporal structure of these subjective accent patterns (Povel & Essens, 1985). (Trained musicians confirmed that the first set of patterns fit better with a duple meter and the second set with a triple meter.)

Infants heard three of the patterns from one category repeatedly until they habituated (based on looking time) or a fixed number of trials elapsed. After this, they were presented with a test in which two novel rhythms alternated: one from the same metrical category and one from the other metrical category. The key question was whether infants would show some evidence of having extracted the meter of the habituation stimuli. Hannon and Johnson found that infants looked longer at the stimuli with the novel meter, and argued that this provides evidence for the extraction of metrical structure. They suggest that the precocious ability to extract meter may help the infant to learn other aspects of music such as tonality, because structurally important pitches tend to occur on metrically strong beats. They draw an analogy to the way that speech rhythm may help infants learn aspects of linguistic structure, such as the location of word boundaries in running speech (Cutler, 1994).[26]

This study is noteworthy because of its elegant design, clear results, and strong claims. However, once again there are some uncertainties about the interpretation of the results. Notably, there were differences in the grouping structure of patterns in duple and triple meters, so that the results could reflect a novelty preference based on grouping rather than meter (as noted by the authors). To control for this, the study included a second experiment with the same habituation stimuli but new test stimuli designed to eliminate this confound. Specifically, there were two test patterns: One had accents consistent with a duple meter but a grouping structure that resembled the triple meter patterns, whereas the other had accents consistent with a triple meter but a grouping structure resembling the duple meter patterns. As in the first experiment, infants were familiarized with either the duple or triple meter patterns and then given a preference test for the two novel patterns. Infants looked longer at the pattern with the novel meter. Although this seems like a straightforward confirmation of the findings in experiment 1, there is another possible interpretation of these results. As noted by the authors, creating test stimuli that had a novel meter but a familiar grouping structure resulted in patterns that did not have as strong cues to meter as did the habituation patterns. Thus recognizing a novel meter would be expected to be difficult.

This raises the concern that the observed asymmetry in looking time reflected a familiarity preference for the *old* grouping structure, rather than a novelty preference for the new meter. This explanation posits that infants in experiment 1 showed a novelty preference for a new grouping structure, whereas infants in experiment 2 showed a familiarity preference for an old grouping structure. At first glance, this may seem implausible, but the possibility of such

---

[26] Hannon and Johnson make no claim that speech rhythm is periodic, simply that organized patterns of timing and accent in both domains may help bootstrap learning of other aspects of structure.

a change in response pattern is raised by findings by Saffran and colleagues. These researchers familiarized infants with a tone sequence and then tested their ability to discriminate familiar versus unfamiliar fragments from this sequence (also using looking time as a dependent variable). Although infants showed a novelty preference in a first study (Saffran et al., 1999), they showed a familiarity preference in a second study that used a similar paradigm (Saffran et al., 2005). Hence flips between novelty and familiarity preference can occur between studies for reasons that are not well understood.

Thus more work is needed to resolve the issue of whether the infants in Hannon and Johnson's study reacted based on novelty or familiarity. Even if this question can be resolved and one can be confident that infants looked longer at novel metrical patterns, the question remains whether the cues that made these patterns novel were in fact metrical (e.g., periodic beats every three events instead of every two events), or if they were due to local cues (such as duration ratios and event density) that may have been confounded with the novel meter. This is worth asking because the use of local rhythmic cues would be consistent with past theorizing about infants' rhythm perception skills (Drake, 1998).

A different approach to infant meter perception was taken by Phillips-Silver and Trainor (2005). They played 7-month-old infants a rhythm consisting of a sequence of isochronous percussive sounds (about three per second) with no physical accents. The pattern used two different kinds of percussive sounds (snare drum and slapstick) arranged in a fashion that was meant to be ambiguous between a duple and a triple meter (an accent every second or every third event). During this familiarization phase, half the infants were bounced on every second sound, whereas the other half were bounced on every third sound. Immediately thereafter, infants were given a preference test based in which they heard two versions of the rhythm, one that had physical (intensity) accents on every other event, and one with accents on every third event. The infants controlled how long each version played by their direction of gaze, and showed a preference for hearing the version that matched their own movement experience. This shows a cross-modal integration of movement and audition in rhythm perception (which was the focus of the study). To some, it may also suggest that infants perceived meter, which entails beat perception based on periodic temporal expectancies. However, this need not be the case. The observed preference might be based on grouping rather than meter, because an accent every second versus third event creates chunks with two versus three elements. A critical question here is whether the regular timing of the events and accents is important to the cross-modal generalization, or whether what is being generalized is chunk size (in number of elements).

To summarize, studies of infant rhythm perception that aim to study beat perception need to demonstrate that infants are not simply responding on the basis of cues such as the absolute durations of events or of intervals between events, duration ratio patterns, grouping, or event density.

Afterword

This book has explored music-language relations from a variety of perspectives. These explorations indicate that music and language should be seen as complex constellations of subprocesses, some of which are shared, and others not. In many cases, the links are not obvious at first glance. Yet they are there, and they run deeper than has generally been believed. Exploring this network of relations, with due attention to both the similarities and the differences, can improve our understanding of how the mind assembles complex communicative abilities from elementary cognitive processes.

Indeed, a fundamental message that runs through this book can be summarized in two statements:

1. As cognitive and neural systems, music and language are closely related.
2. Comparing music and language provides a powerful way to study the mechanisms that the mind uses to make sense out of sound.

Music-language studies also suggest ways of bridging the current divide between the sciences and the humanities. Prominent minds on both sides of this divide are advocating for studies that bring these two frameworks of human knowledge together (e.g., Wilson, 1998; Becker, 2004; Edelman, 2006). The study of music-language relations is one area in which scientific and humanistic studies can meaningfully intertwine, and in which interactions across traditional boundaries can bear fruit in the form of new ideas and discoveries that neither side can accomplish alone. Studies that unify scientific and humanistic knowledge are still uncommon, yet to paraphrase the poet John Donne, they address that subtle knot which makes us human.

References

Abercrombie, D. (1967). *Elements of General Phonetics*. Chicago: Aldine.

Abraham, G. (1974). *The Tradition of Western Music*. Berkeley: University of California Press.

Acker, B. E., Pastore, R. E., & Hall, M. D. (1995). Within-category discrimination of musical chords: Perceptual magnet or anchor? *Perception and Psychophysics*, 57:863–874.

Adams, S. (1997). *Poetic Designs: An Introduction to Meters, Verse Forms, and Figures of Speech*. Peterborough, Ontario, Canada: Broadview Press.

Adolphs, R., Damasio, H., & Tranel, D. (2002). Neural systems or recognition of emotional prosody: A 3-D lesion study. *Emotion*, 2:23–51.

Agawu, K. (1991). *Playing With Signs: A Semiotic Interpretation of Classic Music*. Princeton, NJ: Princeton University Press.

Agawu, K. (1995). *African Rhythm: A Northern Ewe Perspective*. Cambridge, UK: Cambridge University Press.

Alcock, K. J., Passingham, R. E., Watkins, K. E., & Vargha-Khadem, F. (2000a). Oral dyspraxia in inherited speech and language impairment and acquired dysphasia. *Brain and Language*, 75:17–33.

Alcock, K. J., Passingham, R. E., Watkins, K., & Vargha-Khadem, F. (2000b). Pitch and timing abilities in inherited speech and language impairment. *Brain and Language*, 75:34–46.

Allen, G. (1878). Note-deafness. *Mind*, 3:157–167.

Allen, G. D., & Hawkins, S. (1978). The development of phonological rhythm. In: A. Bell & J. Hooper (Eds.), *Syllables and Segments* (pp. 173–175). Amsterdam: North-Holland.

Allen, R., Hill, E., & Heaton, P. (submitted). "Hath charms to soothe": An exploratory study of how high-functioning adults with ASD experience music.

Anderson, L. (1959). Ticuna vowels with special regard to the system of five tonemes (As vogais do tikuna com especial atenção ao sistema de cinco tonemas). *Série Lingüística Especial*, 1:76–119. Rio de Janeiro: Museu Nacional.

Anderson, S. R. (1978). Tone features. In: V. Fromkin (Ed.), *Tone: A Linguistic Survey* (pp. 133–176). New York: Academic Press.

Antinucci, F. (1980). The syntax of indicator particles in Somali. Part two: The construction of interrogative, negative and negative-interrogative clauses. *Studies in African Linguistics*, 11:1–37.

Anvari, S., Trainor, L. J., Woodside, J., & Levy, B. A. (2002). Relations among musical skills, phonological processing, and early reading ability in preschool children. *Journal of Experimental Child Psychology*, 83:111–130.

Arcadi, A. C., Robert, D., & Boesch, C. (1998). Buttress drumming by wild chimpanzees: Temporal patterning, phrase integration into loud calls, and preliminary evidence for individual distinctiveness. *Primates*, 39:503–516.

Areni, C. S., & Kim, D. (1993). The influence of background music on shopping behavior: Classical versus top-forty music in a wine store. *Advances in Consumer Research*, 20:336–340.

Arnold, K. M., & Jusczyk, P. W. (2002). Text-to-tune alignment in speech and song. In: B. Bell & I. Marlien (Eds.), *Proceedings of Speech Prosody, Aix-en-Provence*. Aix-en-Provence, France: Laboratoire Parole et Langage.

Arom, S., Léothaud, G., Voisin, F. (1997). Experimental ethnomusicology: An interactive approach to the study of musical scales. In: I. Deliège & J. Sloboda (Eds.), *Perception and Cognition of Music* (pp. 3–30). Hove, UK: Psychology Press.

Arvaniti, A. (1994). Acoustic features of Greek rhythmic structure. *Journal of Phonetics*, 22:239–268.

Arvaniti, A., & Garding, G. (in press). Dialectal variation in the rising accents of American English. In J. Hualde & Jo Cole (Eds.), *Papers in Laboratory Phonology 9*. Berlin, Germany: Mouton de Gruyter.

Arvaniti, A., Ladd, D. R., & Mennen, I. (1998). Stability of tonal alignment: The case of Greek prenuclear accents. *Journal of Phonetics*, 26:3–25.

Ashley, R. (2002). Do[n't] change a hair for me: The art of jazz rubato. *Music Perception*, 19:311–332.

Asu, E. L., & Nolan, F. (2006). Estonian and English rhythm: A two-dimensional quantification based on syllables and feet. *Proceedings of Speech Prosody 2006*, May 2–5, Dresden, Germany.

Atterer, M., & Ladd, D. R. (2004). On the phonetics and phonology of "segmental anchoring" of F0: Evidence from German. *Journal of Phonetics*, 32:177–197.

Au, T. K.-F., Knightly, L. M., Jun, S.-A., & Oh, J. S. (2002). Overhearing a language during childhood. *Psychological Science*, 13:238–243.

Ayari, M., & McAdams, S. (2003). Aural analysis of Arabic improvised instrumental music (taqsîm). *Music Perception*, 21:159–216.

Ayotte, J., Peretz, I., & Hyde, K. L. (2002). Congenital amusia: A group study of adults afflicted with a music-specific disorder. *Brain*, 125:238–251.

Ayotte, J., Peretz, I., Rousseau, I., Bard, C., & Bojanowski, M. (2000). Patterns of music agnosia associated with middle cerebral artery infarcts. *Brain*, 123:1926–1938.

Baharloo, S., Johnston, P. A., Service, S. K., Gitschier, J., & Freimer, N. B. (1998). Absolute pitch: An approach for identification of genetic and nongenetic components. *American Journal of Human Genetics*, 62:224–231.

Baharloo, S., Service, S. K., Risch, N., Gitschier, J., & Freimer, N. B. (2000). Familial aggregation of absolute pitch. *American Journal of Human Genetics*, 67:755–758.

Baker, M. (2001). *The Atoms of Language*. New York: Basic Books.

Balaban, E. (1988). Bird song syntax: Learned intraspecific variation is meaningful. *Proceedings of the National Academy of Sciences, USA*, 85:3657–3660.

Balaban, E. (2006). Cognitive developmental biology: History, process, and fortune's wheel. *Cognition*, 101:298–332.

Balaban, E., Teillet, M. A., & Le Douarin, N. (1988). Application of the quail-chick chimera system to the study of brain development and behavior. *Science*, 241:1339–42.

Balkwill, L. L., & Thompson, W. F. (1999). A cross-cultural investigation of the perception of emotion in music: Psychophysical and cultural cues. *Music Perception*, 17:43–64.

Balter, M. (2004). Seeking the key to music. *Science*, 306:1120–1122.

Balzano, G. J. (1980). The group-theoretic description of 12-fold and microtonal pitch systems. *Computer Music Journal*, 4:66–84.

Baptista, L. F., & Keister, R. A. (2005). Why birdsong is sometimes like music. *Perspectives in Biology and Medicine*, 48:426–43.

Barlow, H., & Morgenstern, S. (1983). *A Dictionary of Musical Themes, Revised Edition*. London: Faber and Faber.

Barnes, R., & Jones, M. R. (2000). Expectancy, attention, and time. *Cognitive Psychology*, 41:254–311.

Barrett, S. (1997). *Prototypes in Speech Perception*. Ph.D. dissertation, University of Cambridge, Cambridge, UK.

Barrett, S. (2000). The perceptual magnet effect is not specific to speech prototypes: New evidence from music categories. *Speech, Hearing and Language: Work in Progress*, 11:1–16.

Barry, W. J., Andreeva, B., Russo, M., Dimitrova, S., & Kostadinova, T. (2003). Do rhythm measures tell us anything about language type? *Proceedings of the 15th International Congress of Phonetic Sciences, Barcelona*, pp. 2693–2696.

Baruch, C., & Drake, C. (1997). Tempo discrimination in infants. *Infant Behavior and Development*, 20:573–577.

Bearth, T., & Zemp, H. (1967). The phonology of Dan (Santa). *Journal of African Languages*, 6:9–28.

Becker, A., & Becker, J. (1979). A grammar of the musical genre Srepegan. *Journal of Music Theory*, 23:1–43.

Becker, A., & Becker, J. (1983). Reflection on Srepegan: A reconsideration in the form of a dialogue. *Asian Music*, 14:9–16.

Becker, J. (1979). Time and tune in Java. In: A. L. Becker & A. A. Yengoyan (Eds.), *The Imagination of Reality: Essays in Southeast Asian Coherence Systems* (pp. 197–210). Norwood, NJ: Ablex.

Becker, J. (1986). Is Western art music superior? *Musical Quarterly*, 72:341–359.

Becker, J. (2001). Anthropological perspectives on music and emotion. In: P. N. Juslin & J. A. Sloboda (Eds.), *Music and Emotion: Theory and Research* (pp. 135–160). Oxford, UK: Oxford University Press.

Becker, J. (2004). *Deep Listeners: Music, Emotion, and Trancing*. Bloomington: Indiana University Press.

Becker, J., & Becker, A. (1981). A musical icon: Power and meaning in Javanese gamelan music. In: W. Steiner (Ed.), *The Sign in Music and Literature* (pp. 203–215). Austin: University of Texas Press.

Beckman, M. (1982). Segment duration and the "mora" in Japanese. *Phonetica*, 39:113–135.

Beckman, M. (1992). Evidence for speech rhythm across languages. In: Y. Tohkura et al. (Eds.), *Speech Perception, Production, and Linguistic Structure* (pp. 457–463). Tokyo: IOS Press.

Beckman, M. E., & Edwards, J., & Fletcher, J. (1992). Prosodic structure and tempo in a sonority model of articulatory dynamics. In: G. J. Docherty & D. R. Ladd (Eds.), *Papers in Laboratory Phonology II: Segment, Gesture, Prosody* (pp. 68–86). Cambridge, UK: Cambridge University Press.

Beckman, M. E., Hirschberg, J., & Shattuck-Hufnagel, S. (2005). The original ToBI system and the evolution of the ToBI framework. In: S. Jun (Ed.), *Prosodic Typology: The Phonology of Intonation and Phrasing* (pp. 9–54). Oxford, UK: Oxford University Press.

Beckman, M. E., & Pierrehumbert, J. B. (1986). Intonational structure in Japanese and English. *Phonology Yearbook,* 3:255–309.

Beeman, M. (1993). Semantic processing in the right hemisphere may contribute to drawing inferences during comprehension. *Brain and Language,* 44:80–120.

Beeman, M. (1998). Coarse semantic coding and discourse comprehension. In: M. Beeman & C. Chiarello (Eds.), *Getting It Right: The Cognitive Neuroscience of Right Hemisphere Language Comprehension* (pp. 225–284). Mahwah, NJ: Erlbaum.

Belin, P., Zatorre, R. J., Lafaille, P., Ahad, P., & Pike, B. (2000). Voice-selective areas in human auditory cortex. *Nature,* 403:309–12.

Belleville, S., Caza, N., & Peretz, I. (2003). A neuropsychological argument for a processing view of memory. *Journal of Memory and Language,* 48:686–703.

Bellugi, U., & St. George, M. (Eds.). (2001). *Journey From Cognition to Brain to Gene: Perspectives From Williams Syndrome.* Cambridge, MA: MIT Press.

Benamou, M. (2003). Comparing musical affect: Java and the West. *The World of Music,* 45:57–76.

Bengtsson, S. L., Nagy, Z., Skare, S., Forsman, L., Forssberg, H., & Ullén, F. (2005). Extensive piano practicing has regionally specific effects on white matter development. *Nature Neuroscience,* 8:1148–1150.

Bent, T., Bradlow, A. R., & Wright, B. A. (2006). The influence of linguistic experience on pitch perception in speech and non-speech sounds. *Journal of Experimental Psychology: Human Perception and Performance,* 32:97–103.

Bergeson, T. R., & Trehub, S. E. (2002). Absolute pitch and tempo in mothers' songs to infants. *Psychological Science,* 13:72–75.

Bergeson, T. R., & Trehub, S. E. (2006). Infants' perception of rhythmic patterns. *Music Perception,* 23: 345–360.

Berinstein, A. (1979). A cross-linguistic study on the perception of stress. *UCLA Working Papers in Phonetics,* 47:1–59.

Bernstein, L. (1959). *The Joy of Music.* New York: Simon & Schuster.

Bernstein, L. (1976). *The Unanswered Question.* Cambridge, MA: Harvard University Press.

Bertinetto, P. (1989). Reflections on the dichotomy "stress" vs. "syllable-timing." *Revue de Phonétique Appliquée,* 91–93:99–130.

Besson, M., & Faïta, F. (1995). An event-related potential (ERP) study of musical expectancy: Comparison of musicians with nonmusicians. *Journal of Experimental Psychology: Human Perception and Performance,* 21:1278–1296.

Besson, M., Faïta, F., Peretz, I., Bonnel, A.-M., & Requin, J. (1998). Singing in the brain: Independence of lyrics and tunes. *Psychological Science,* 9:494–498.

Besson, M., & Macar, F. (1987). An event-related potential analysis of incongruity in music and other non-linguistic contexts. *Psychophysiology,* 24:14–25.

Best, C. T. (1994). Learning to perceive the sound pattern of English. In: C. Rovee-Collier & L. Lipsitt (Eds.), *Advances in Infancy Research* (Vol. 9, pp. 217–304). Norwood, NJ: Ablex.

Best, C. T., & Avery, R. A. (1999). Left-hemisphere advantage for click consonants is determined by linguistic significance and experience. *Psychological Science,* 10:65–70.

Best, C. T., McRoberts, G. W., & Goodell, E. (2001). Discrimination of non-native consonant contrasts varying in perceptual assimilation to the listener's native phonological system. *Journal of the Acoustical Society of America,* 109:775–794.

Best, C. T., McRoberts, G. W., & Sithole, N. M. (1988). Examination of perceptual reorganization for nonnative speech contrasts: Zulu click discrimination by English-speaking adults and infants. *Journal of Experimental Psychology: Human Perception and Performance,* 14:345–360.

Bharucha, J. J. (1984a). Event hierarchies, tonal hierarchies and assimilation: A reply to Deutsch and Dowling. *Journal of Experimental Psychology, General,* 113:421–5.

Bharucha, J. J. (1984b). Anchoring effects in music—the resolution of dissonance. *Cognitive Psychology,* 16:485–518.

Bharucha, J. J. (1987). Music cognition and perceptual facilitation. *Music Perception,* 5:1–30.

Bharucha, J. J., & Stoeckig, K. (1986). Reaction time and musical expectancy. *Journal of Experimental Psychology: Human Perception and Performance,* 12:403–410.

Bharucha, J. J., & Stoeckig, K. (1987). Priming of chords: Spreading activation or overlapping frequency spectra? *Perception and Psychophysics,* 41:519–524.

Bickerton, D. (1984). The language bioprogram hypothesis. *Behavioral and Brain Sciences,* 7:173–188.

Bigand, E. (1997). Perceiving musical stability: The effect of tonal structure, rhythm and musical expertise. *Journal of Experimental Psychology: Human Perception and Performance,* 23, 808–812.

Bigand, E. (2003). More about the musical expertise of musically untrained listeners. *Annals of the New York Academy of Sciences,* 999:304–312.

Bigand, E., Madurell, F., Tillmann, B., & Pineau, M. (1999). Effect of global structure and temporal organization on chord processing. *Journal of Experimental Psychology: Human Perception and Performance,* 25:184–197.

Bigand, E., & Parncutt, R. (1999). Perceiving musical tension in long chord sequences. *Psychological Research,* 62:237–254.

Bigand, E., & Pineau, M. (1997). Context effects on musical expectancy. *Perception and Psychophysics,* 59:1098–1107.

Bigand, E., Poulin, B., Tillmann, B., Madurell, F., & D'Adamo, D. A. (2003). Sensory versus cognitive components in harmonic priming. *Journal of Experimental Psychology: Human Perception and Performance,* 29:159–171.

Bigand, E., & Poulin-Charronnat, B. (2006). Are we "experienced listeners"? A review of the musical capacities that do not depend on formal musical training. *Cognition,* 100:100–130.

Bigand, E., Tillmann, B., Poulin, B., D'Adamo, D., & Madurell, F. (2001). The effect of harmonic context on phoneme monitoring in vocal music. *Cognition,* 81:B11–B20.

Bigand, E., Tillmann, B., & Poulin-Charronnat, B. (2006). A module for syntactic processing in music? *Trends in Cognitive Sciences,* 10:195–196.

Bigand, E., Vieillard, S., Madurell, F., Marozeau, J., & Dacquet, A. (2005). Multidimensional scaling of emotional responses to music: The effect of musical expertise and of the duration of the excerpts. *Cognition and Emotion*, 19:1113–1139.

Blackburn, P. (1997). *Harry Partch*. St. Paul, MN: American Composer's Forum.

Blacking, J. (1967). *Venda Children's Songs: A Study in Ethnomusicological Analysis*. Johannesburg, South Africa: Witwatersrand University Press.

Blood, A. J., & Zatorre, R. J. (2001). Intensely pleasurable responses to music correlate with activity in brain regions implicated with reward and emotion. *Proceedings of the National Academy of Sciences, USA*, 98:11818–11823.

Blood, A. J., Zatorre, R. J., Bermudez, P., & Evans, A. C. (1999). Emotional responses to pleasant and unpleasant music correlate with activity in paralimbic brain regions. *Nature Neuroscience*, 2:382–387.

Boemio, A., Fromm, S., Braun, A., & Poeppel, D. (2005). Hierarchical and asymmetric temporal sensitivity in human auditory cortices. *Nature Neuroscience*, 8:389–395.

Bolinger, D. (1958). A theory of pitch accent in English. *Word*, 14:109–149.

Bolinger, D. (1981). *Two Kinds of Vowels, Two Kinds of Rhythm*. Bloomington, IN: Indiana University Linguistics Club.

Bolinger, D. (1985). *Intonation and Its Parts: Melody in Spoken English*. London: Edward Arnold.

Bolton, T. (1894). Rhythm. *American Journal of Psychology*, 6:145–238.

Boltz, M. G. (1989). Perceiving the end: Effects of tonal relationships on melodic completion. *Journal of Experimental Psychology: Human Perception and Performance*, 15:749–761.

Boltz, M. G. (1991). Some structural determinants of melody recall. *Memory and Cognition*, 19:239–251.

Boltz, M. G., & Jones, M. R. (1986). Does rule recursion make melodies easier to reproduce? If not, what does? *Cognitive Psychology*, 18:389–431.

Bonnel, A.-M., Faïta, F., Peretz, I., & Besson, M. (2001). Divided attention between lyrics and tunes of operatic songs: Evidence for independent processing. *Perception and Psychophysics*, 63:1201–1213.

Booth, J. R., Burman, D. D., Van Santen, F. W., Harasaki, Y., Gitelman, D. R., Parrish, T. B., et al. (2001). The development of specialized brain systems in reading an oral language. *Neuropsychology Development, and Cognition. Section C, Child Neuropsychology*, 7:119–141.

Bor, J. (Ed.). (1999). *The Raga Guide: A Survey of 74 Hindustani Ragas*. UK: Nimbus Records/Rotterdam Conservatory of Music. (NI 5536/9).

Bradlow, A. R., Nygaard, L. C., & Pisoni, D. B. (1999). Effects of talker, rate, and amplitude variation on recognition memory for spoken words. *Perception and Psychophysics*, 61:206–219.

Bramble, D. M., & Lieberman, D. E. (2004). Endurance running and the evolution of *Homo*. *Nature*, 432:345–352.

Brattico, E., Näätänen, R., & Tervaniemi, M. (2001). Context effects on pitch perception in musicians and nonmusicians: Evidence from event-related potential recordings. *Music Perception*, 19:199–222.

Bregman, A. (1990). *Auditory Scene Analysis: The Perceptual Organization of Sound*. Cambridge, MA: MIT Press.

Bretos, J., & Sundberg, J. (2003). Measurements of vibrato parameters in long sustained crescendo notes as sung by ten sopranos. *Journal of Voice*, 17:343–52.

Brinner, B. (1995). *Knowing Music, Making Music: Javanese Gamelan and the Theory of Musical Competence and Interaction.* Chicago: University of Chicago Press.

Brosch, M., Selezneva, E., Bucks, C., & Scheich, H. (2004). Macaque monkeys discriminate pitch relationships. *Cognition*, 91:259–272.

Brown, S., Martinez, M. J., & Parsons, L. M. (2006). Music and language side by side in the brain: A PET study of the generation of melodies and sentences. *European Journal of Neuroscience*, 23:2791–2803.

Brown, W. A., Cammuso, K., Sachs, H., Winklosky, B., Mullane, J., Bernier, R., et al. (2003). Autism-related language, personality, and cognition in people with absolute pitch: Results of a preliminary study. *Journal of Autism and Developmental Disorders*, 33:163–167.

Brownell, H. H., Potter, H. H., Bihrle, A. M., & Gardner, H. (1986). Inference deficits in right brain-damaged patients. *Brain and Language*, 29:310–321.

Bruce, G. (1977), *Swedish Word Accents in Sentence Perspective.* Lund, Sweden: Gleerup.

Bruce, G. (1981). Tonal and temporal interplay. In: T. Fretheim (Ed.), *Nordic Prosody II: Papers From a Symposium* (pp. 63–74). Lund, Sweden: Tapir.

Buchanan, T. W., Lutz, K., Mirzazade, S., Specht, K., Shah, N. J., Zilles, K., & Jancke, L. (2000). Recognition of emotional prosody and verbal components of spoken language: An fMRI study. *Cognitive Brain Research*, 9:227–238.

Buck, J. (1988). Synchronous rhythmic flashing in fireflies. II. *Quarterly Review of Biology*, 63:265–289.

Buhusi, C. V., & Meck, W. H. (2005). What makes us tick? Functional and neural mechanisms of interval timing. *Nature Reviews, Neuroscience*, 6:755–765.

Buonomano, D. V., & Merzenich, M. M. (1998). Cortical plasticity: From synapses to maps. *Annual Review of Neuroscience*, 21:149–186.

Burnham, D., Peretz, I., Stevens, K., Jones, C., Schwanhäusser, B., Tsukada, K., & Bollwerk, S. (2004, August). Do tone language speakers have perfect pitch? In: S. D. Lipscomb et al. (Eds.), *Proceedings of the 8th International Conference on Music Perception and Cognition, Evanston, IL* (p. 350). Adelaide, Australia: Causal Productions.

Burns, E. M. (1999). Intervals, scales, and tuning. In: D. Deutsch (Ed.), *The Psychology of Music,* (2nd ed., pp. 215–264). San Diego, CA: Academic Press.

Burns, E. M., & Ward, W. D. (1978). Categorical perception—phenomenon or epiphenomenon: Evidence from the perception of melodic musical intervals. *Journal of the Acoustical Society of America*, 63:456–468.

Busnel, R. G., & Classe, A. (1976). *Whistled Languages.* Berlin: Springer-Verlag.

Caclin, A., McAdams, S., Smith, B. K., & Winsberg, S. (2005). Acoustic correlates of timbre space dimensions: A confirmatory study using synthetic tones. *Journal of the Acoustic Society of America*, 118: 471–482.

Campbell, W. N. (1993). Automatic detection of prosodic boundaries in speech. *Speech Communication*, 13:343–354.

Caplan, D. (1992). *Language: Structure, Processing, and Disorders.* Cambridge, MA: MIT Press.

Caplan, D., Hildebrandt, N., & Makris, N. (1996). Location of lesions in stroke patients with deficits in syntactic processing in sentence comprehension. *Brain*, 119:933–949.

Caplan, D., & Waters, G. S. (1999). Verbal working memory and sentence comprehension. *Behavioral and Brain Sciences*, 22, 77–94.

Cariani, P. (2004). A temporal model for pitch multiplicity and tonal consonance. In: S. D. Lipscomb et al. (Eds.), *Proceedings of the 8th International Conference on Music Perception and Cognition, Evanston, IL, 2004* (pp. 310–314). Adelaide, Australia: Causal Productions.

Carlsen, J. C. (1981). Some factors which influence melodic expectancy. *Psychomusicology*, 1:12–29.

Carreiras, M., Lopez, J., Rivero, F., & Corina, D. (2005). Neural processing of a whistled language. *Nature*, 433:31–32.

Carrington, J. F. (1949a). *A Comparative Study of Some Central African Gong-Languages*. Brussels, Belgium: Falk G. van Campenhout.

Carrington, J. F. (1949b). *Talking Drums of Africa*. London: The Carey Kingsgate Press.

Carrington, J. F. (1971). The talking drums of Africa. *Scientific American*, 225:90–94.

Carroll, S. B. (2003). Genetics and the making of *Homo sapiens*. *Nature*, 422:849–857.

Casasanto, D. (in press). Space for thinking. In: V. Evans & P. Chilton (Eds.), *Language, Cognition, and Space: State of the Art and New Directions*. London: Equinox.

Castellano, M. A., Bharucha, J. J., & Krumhansl, C. L. (1984). Tonal hierarchies in the music of north India. *Journal of Experimental Psychology: General*, 113:394–412.

Catchpole, C. K., & Slater, P. J. B. (1995). *Bird Song: Biological Themes and Variations*. Cambridge, UK: Cambridge University Press.

Chafe, W. (1994). *Discourse, Consciousness, and Time*. Chicago: University of Chicago Press.

Chandola, A. (1988). *Music as Speech: An Ethnomusicolinguistic Study of India*. New Delhi, India: Narvang.

Chang, E. F., & Merzenich, M. M. (2003). Environmental noise retards auditory cortical development. *Science*, 300:498–502.

Charbonneau, S., Scherzer, B. P., Aspirot, D., & Cohen, H. (2002). Perception and production of facial and prosodic emotions by chronic CVA patients. *Neuropsychologia*, 41:605–613.

Chartrand, J.-P., & Belin, P. (2006). Superior voice timbre processing in musicians. *Neuroscience Letters*, 405:154–167.

Chela-Flores, B. (1994). On the acquisition of English rhythm: Theoretical and practical issue. *International Review of Applied Linguistics*, 32:232–242.

Cheney, D. L., & Seyfarth, R. M. (1982). Vervet alarm calls: Semantic communication in free ranging primates. *Animal Behaviour*, 28:1070–1266.

Chenoweth, V. (1980). *Melodic Perception and Analysis: A Manual on Ethnic Melody*. Ukarumpa, Papua New Guinea: Summer Institute of Linguistics.

Cheour, M., Ceponiene, R., Lehtokoski, A., Luuk, A., Allik, J., Alho, K., & Näätänen, R. (1998). Development of language-specific phoneme representations in the infant brain. *Nature Neuroscience*, 1:351–353.

Chin, C. S. (2003). The early development of absolute pitch: A theory concerning the roles of music training at an early developmental age and individual cognitive style. *Psychology of Music*, 31:155–171.

Cho, T., & Keating, P. (2001). Articulatory and acoustic studies on domain-initial strengthening in Korean. *Journal of Phonetics*, 29:155–190.

Chomsky, N. (1965). *Aspects of the Theory of Syntax*. Cambridge, MA: MIT Press.

Chomsky, N. (1972). *Language and Mind*. New York: Harcourt Brace Jovanovich.

Chomsky, N., & Halle, M. (1968). *The Sound Pattern of English*. New York: Harper & Row.

Christiansen, M. H., & Kirby, S. (Eds.). (2003a). *Language Evolution*. Oxford, UK: Oxford University Press.

Christiansen, M. H., & Kirby, S. (2003b). Language evolution: Consensus and controversies. *Trends in Cognitive Sciences*, 7:300–307.

Clark, A. (2003). *Natural Born Cyborgs*. Oxford, UK: Oxford University Press.

Clark, S., & Rehding, A. (2001). Introduction. In: S. Clark & A. Rehding (Eds.), *Music Theory and Natural Order From the Renaissance to the Early Twentieth Century* (pp. 1–13). Cambridge, UK: Cambridge University Press.

Clarke, E. (2001). Meaning and specification of motion in music. *Musicae Scientiae*, 5:213–234.

Clarke, E. (2005). *Ways of Listening: An Ecological Approach to the Perception of Musical Meaning*. Oxford, UK: Oxford University Press.

Clarke, E. F. (1987). Categorical rhythm perception: An ecological perspective. In: A. Gabrielsson (Ed.), *Action and Perception in Rhythm and Music* (pp. 19–34). Stockholm: Royal Swedish Academy of Music.

Clarke, E. F. (1993). Imitating and evaluating real and transformed musical performances. *Music Perception*, 10:317–343.

Clarke, E. F., & Krumhansl, C. L. (1990). Perceiving musical time. *Music Perception*, 7:213–251.

Cloarec-Heiss, F. (1999). From natural language to drum language: An economical encoding procedure in Banda-Linda (Central African Republic). In: C. Fuchs & S. Robert (Eds.), *Language Diversity and Cognitive Representations* (pp. 145–157). Amsterdam: John Benjamins.

Clough, J., Douthett, J., Ramanathan, N., & Rowell. L. (1993). Early Indian heptatonic scales and recent diatonic theory. *Music Theory Spectrum*, 15:36–58.

Clynes, M. (1977). *Sentics: The Touch of Emotions*. Garden City, New York: The Anchor Press.

Cogan, R. (1984). *New Images of Musical Sound*. Cambridge, MA: Harvard University Press.

Cogan, R., & Escot, P. (1976). *Sonic Design: The Nature of Sound and Music*. Englewood Cliffs, NJ: Prentice-Hall.

Cohen, A. J. (2000). Development of tonality induction: Plasticity, exposure, and training. *Music Perception*, 17:437–459.

Cohen, A. J. (2001). Music as a source of emotion in film. In: P. N. Juslin & J. A. Sloboda (Eds.), *Music and Emotion: Theory and Research* (pp. 249–272). Oxford, UK: Oxford University Press.

Cohen, A. J., Thorpe, L. A., & Trehub, S. E. (1987). Infants' perception of musical relations in short transposed tone sequences. *Canadian Journal of Psychology*, 41:33–47.

Cohen, D. (1971). Palestrina counterpoint: A musical expression of unexcited speech. *Journal of Music Theory*, 15:85–111.

Cohen, L. S., Lehericy, F., Chochon, F., Lemer, C., Rivaud, S., & Dehaene, S. (2002). Language-specific tuning of visual cortex? Functional properties of the visual word form area. *Brain*, 125:1054–1069.

Coker, W. (1972). *Music and Meaning: A Theoretical Introduction to Musical Aesthetics.* New York: Free Press.

Coleman, J. (1999). The nature of vocoids associated with syllabic consonants in Tash-lhiyt Berber. *Proceedings of the 14th International Congress of Phonetic Sciences, San Francisco,* pp. 735–738.

Collier, R. (1975). Physiological correlates of intonation patterns. *Journal of the Acoustical Society of America,* 58:249–255.

Collier, R. (1991). Multi-language intonation synthesis. *Journal of Phonetics,* 19:61–73.

Comrie, B., Matthews, S., & Polinsky, M. (Eds.). (1996). *The Atlas of Languages.* London: Quarto.

Cone, E. (1974). *The Composer's Voice.* Berkeley, CA: University of California Press.

Connell, B. (1999). Four tones and downtrend: A preliminary report of pitch realization in Mambila. In: P. F. A. Kotey (Ed.), *New Dimensions in African Linguistics and Languages (Trends in African Linguistics 3)* (pp. 74–88). Trenton, NJ: Africa World Press.

Connell, B. (2000). The perception of lexical tone in Mambila. *Language and Speech,* 43:163–182.

Conway, C. M., & Christiansen, M. H. (2001). Sequential learning in non-human primates. *Trends in Cognitive Sciences,* 5:539–546.

Cook, N. (1987a). *A Guide to Musical Analysis.* Oxford, UK: Oxford University Press.

Cook, N. (1987b). The perception of large-scale tonal closure. *Music Perception,* 5: 197–206.

Cook, N., & Dibben, N. (2001). Musicological approaches to emotion. In: P. N. Juslin & J. A. Sloboda (Eds.), *Music and Emotion: Theory and Research* (pp. 45–70). Oxford, UK: Oxford University Press.

Cook, N. D. (2002). *Tone of Voice and Mind.* Amsterdam: J. Benjamins.

Cook, N. D., & Fujisawa, T. X. (2006). The psychophysics of harmony perception: Harmony is a three-tone phenomenon. *Empirical Musicology Review,* 1:106–126.

Cooke, D. (1959). *The Language of Music.* Oxford, UK: Oxford University Press.

Cooke, P. (1992). Report on pitch perception experiments carried out in Buganda and Busoga (Uganda). *Journal of International Library of African Music,* 7:119–125.

Cooper, G. W., & Meyer, L. B. (1960). *The Rhythmic Structure of Music.* Chicago: University of Chicago Press.

Cooper, W. E., & Eady, S. J. (1986). Metrical phonology in speech production. *Journal of Memory and Language,* 25:369–384.

Cooper, W. E., & Sorensen, J. (1977). Fundamental frequency contours at syntactic boundaries. *Journal of the Acoustical Society of America,* 62:683–692.

Coppola, M. (2002). *The Emergence of Grammatical Categories in Homesign: Evidence From Family-Based Gesture Systems in Nicaragua.* Ph.D. dissertation, University of Rochester.

Costa-Giomi, E. (2003). Young children's harmonic perception. *Annals of the New York Academy of Sciences,* 999:477–484.

Courtney, D. (1998). *Fundamentals of Tabla* (3rd ed.). Houston, TX: Sur Sangeet Services.

Cowan, G. (1948). Mazateco whistle speech. *Language,* 24:280–286.

Croonen, W. J. M. (1994). *Memory for Melodic Patterns: An Investigation of Stimulus- and Subject-Related Characteristics*. Ph.D. dissertation, Technische Universiteit Eindhoven, The Netherlands.

Cross, I. (2001). Review of *The Origins of Music*. *Music Perception*, 18:513–521.

Cross, I. (2003). Music, cognition, culture, and evolution. In: N. L. Wallin, B. Merker, & S. Brown (Eds.), *The Origins of Music* (pp. 42–56). Cambridge, MA: MIT Press.

Cross, I. (submitted). Musicality and the human capacity for culture.

Cuddy, L. L., & Badertscher, B. (1987). Recovery of the tonal hierarchy: Some comparisons across age and levels of musical experience. *Perception and Psychophysics*, 41:609–20.

Cuddy, L. L., Balkwill, L.-L., Peretz, I., & Holden, R. R. (2005). A study of "tone deafness" among university students. *Annals of the New York Academy of Sciences*, 1060:311–324.

Cuddy, L. L., Cohen, A. J., & Mewhort, D. J. K. (1981). Perception of structure in short melodic sequences. *Journal of Experimental Psychology: Human Perception and Performance*, 7:869–883.

Cuddy, L. L, & Lunney, C. A. (1995). Expectancies generated by melodic intervals: Perceptual judgments and melodic continuity. *Perception and Psychophysics*, 57:451–462.

Cuddy, L. L., & Lyons, H. I. (1981). Musical pattern recognition: A comparison of listening to and studying tonal structure and tonal ambiguities. *Psychomusicology*, 1:15–33.

Cumming, N. (2000). *The Sonic Self: Musical Subjectivity and Signification*. Bloomington: Indiana University Press.

Cummins, F. (2002). Speech rhythm and rhythmic taxonomy. In: B. Bell & I. Marlien (Eds.), *Proceedings of Speech Prosody, Aix-en-Provence* (pp. 121–126). Aix-en-Provence, France: Laboratoire Parole et Langage.

Cummins, F., & Port, R. F. (1998). Rhythmic constraints on stress timing in English. *Journal of Phonetics*, 26:145–171.

Curtiss, S. (1977). *Genie: A Psycholinguistic Study of a Modern-Day "Wild Child."* New York: Academic Press.

Cutler, A. (1980). Syllable omission errors and isochrony. In: H. W. Dechert & M. Raupach (Eds.), *Temporal Variables in Speech* (pp. 183–190). The Hague, The Netherlands: Mouton.

Cutler, A. (1990). Exploiting prosodic probabilities in speech segmentation. In: G. Altmann (Ed.), *Cognitive Models of Speech Processing: Psycholinguistic and Computational Perspectives* (pp. 105–121). Cambridge, MA: MIT Press.

Cutler, A. (1994). Segmentation problems, rhythmic solutions. *Lingua*, 92:81–104.

Cutler, A. (2000). Listening to a second language through the ears of a first. *Interpreting*, 5:1–23.

Cutler, A., & Butterfield, S. (1992). Rhythmic cues to speech segmentation: Evidence from juncture misperception. *Journal of Memory and Language*, 31:218–236.

Cutler, A., & Carter, D. M. (1987). The predominance of strong initial syllables in the English vocabulary. *Computer Speech and Language*, 2:133–142.

Cutler, A., Dahan, D., & Van Donselaar, W. A. (1997). Prosody in the comprehension of spoken language: A literature review. *Language and Speech*, 40:141–202.

Cutler, A., & Darwin, C. J. (1981). Phoneme-monitoring reaction time and preceding prosody: Effects of stop closure duration and of fundamental frequency. *Perception and Psychophysics*, 29:217–224.

Cutler, A., & Foss, D. J. (1977). On the role of sentence stress in sentence processing. *Language and Speech*, 20:1–10.

Cutler, A., & Norris, D. G. (1988). The role of strong syllables in segmentation for lexical access. *Journal of Experimental Psychology: Human Perception and Performance*, 14:113–121.

d'Alessandro, C., & Castellengo, M. (1994). The pitch of short-duration vibrato tones. *Journal of the Acoustical Society of America*, 95:1617–1630.

d'Alessandro, C., & Mertens, P. (1995). Automatic pitch contour stylization using a model of tonal perception. *Computer Speech and Language*, 9:257–288.

Dahlhaus, C. (1990). *Studies on the Origin of Harmonic Tonality* (R. O. Gjerdingen, Trans.). Princeton, NJ: Princeton University Press.

Dainora, A. (2002). Does intonational meaning come from tones or tune? Evidence against a compositional approach. In: B. Bell & I. Marlien (Eds.), *Proceedings of Speech Prosody, Aix-en-Provence*. Aix-en-Provence, France: Laboratoire Parole et Langage.

Dalla Bella, S., Giguère, J.-F., & Peretz, I. (2007). Singing proficiency in the general population. *Journal of the Acoustical Society of America*, 121:1182–1189.

Dalla Bella, S., Palmer, C., & Jungers, M. (2003). Are musicians different speakers than nonmusicians? *Proceedings of the 2003 Meeting of the Society for Music Perception and Cognition, Las Vegas, NV* (p. 34).

Dalla Bella, S., & Peretz, I. (2003). Congenital amusia interferes with the ability to synchronize with music. *Annals of the New York Academy of Sciences*, 999:166–169.

Dalla Bella, S., Peretz, I., Rousseau, L., & Gosselin, N. (2001). A developmental study of the affective value of tempo and mode in music. *Cognition*, 80:B1–B10.

Damasio, A. (1994). *Descartes' Error: Emotion, Reason, and the Human Brain*. New York: Avon Books.

Damasio, A. (2003). *Looking for Spinoza: Joy, Sorrow, and the Feeling Brain*. Orlando, FL: Harcourt.

Daniele, J. R., & Patel, A. D. (2004). The interplay of linguistic and historical influences on musical rhythm in different cultures In: S. D. Lipscomb et al. (Eds.), *Proceedings of the 8th International Conference on Music Perception and Cognition, Evanston, IL, 2004* (pp. 759–762). Adelaide, Australia: Causal Productions.

Darwin, C. (1871). *The Descent of Man, and Selection in Relation to Sex*. London: John Murray.

Dasher, R., & Bolinger, D. (1982). On pre-accentual lengthening. *Journal of the International Phonetic Association*, 12:58–69.

Dauer, R. M. (1983). Stress-timing and syllable-timing reanalyzed. *Journal of Phonetics*, 11:51–62.

Dauer, R. M. (1987). Phonetic and phonological components of language rhythm. *Proceedings of the 11th International Congress of Phonetic Sciences, Tallinn*, 5:447–450.

Davidson, L., McKernon, P., & Gardner, H. (1981). The acquisition of song: A developmental approach. In: *Proceedings of the National Symposium on the Application of Psychology to the Teaching and Learning of Music*. Reston, VA: Music Educators National Conference.

Davies, S. (1980). The expression of emotion in music. *Mind*, 89:67–86.

Davies, S. (1994). *Musical Meaning and Expression*. Ithaca, New York: Cornell University Press.

Davies, S. (2002). Profundity in instrumental music. *British Journal of Aesthetics*, 42: 343–56.

Davies, S. (2003). *Themes in the Philosophy of Music*. Oxford, UK: Oxford University Press.

Davis, M. H., & Johnsrude, I. S. (2007). Hearing speech sounds: Top-down influences on the interface between audition and speech perception. *Hearing Research*, 29:229–237.

de Jong, K. J. (1995). The supraglottal articulation of prominence in English: Linguistic stress as localized hyperarticulation. *Journal of the Acoustical Society of America*, 97:491–504.

de Pijper, J. R. (1983). *Modeling British English Intonation*. Dordrecht, The Netherlands: Foris.

de Pijper, J. R., & Sanderman, A. A. (1994). On the perceptual strength of prosodic boundaries and its relation to suprasegmental cues. *Journal of the Acoustical Society of America*, 96:2037–2047.

Deacon, T. W. (1997). *The Symbolic Species: The Co-evolution of Language and the Brain*. New York: W. W. Norton.

Deacon, T. W. (2003). Universal grammar and semiotic constraints. In: M. H. Christiansen & S. Kirby (Eds.), *Language Evolution* (pp. 111–139). Oxford, UK: Oxford University Press.

DeCasper, A. J., & Fifer, W. P. (1980). of human bonding: Newborns prefer their mothers' voices. *Science*, 208:1174–1176.

DeCasper, A. J., Lecanuet, J.-P., Busnel, M.-C., Granier-Deferre, C., & Maugeais, R. (1994). Fetal reactions to recurrent maternal speech. *Infant Behavior and Development*, 17:159–164.

DeCasper, A. J., & Spence, M. J. (1986). Prenatal maternal speech influences newborns' perception of speech sounds. *Infant Behavior and Development*, 9:133–150.

Delattre, P. (1963). Comparing the prosodic features of English, German, Spanish and French. *International Review of Applied Linguistics*, 1:193–210.

Delattre, P. (1966). A comparison of syllable length conditioning among languages. *International Review of Applied Linguistics*, 4:183–198.

Deliège, I. (1987). Grouping conditions in listening to music: An approach to Lerdahl and Jackendoff's grouping preference rules. *Music Perception*, 4:325–360.

Deliège, I., Mélen, M., Stammers, D., & Cross, I. (1996). Musical schemata in real-time listening to a piece of music. *Music Perception*, 14:117–160.

Dell, F. (1989). Concordances rythmiques entre la musique et les paroles dans le chant. In: M. Dominicy (Ed.), *Le Souci des Apparences* (pp. 121–136). Brussels, Belgium: Éditions de l'Université de Bruxelles.

Dell, F., & Halle, J. (in press). Comparing musical textsetting in French and English songs. In: J.-L. Aroui (Ed.), *Proceedings of the Conference Typology of Poetic Forms*, April 2005, Paris.

Dellwo, V. (2004). The BonnTempo-Corpus & BonnTempo-Tools: A database for the study of speech rhythm and rate. In: *Proceedings of the 8th ICSLP, Jeju Island, Korea*.

DeLong, M. R. (2000). The basal ganglia. In: E. Kandel, J. H. Schwarz, and T. M. Jesseell (Eds.), *Principles of Neural Science* (4th ed., pp. 853–867). New York: McGraw-Hill.

Demany, L., & Armand, F. (1984). The perceptual reality of tone chroma in early infancy. *Journal of the Acoustical Society of America* 76:57–66.

Demany, L., & McAnally, K. I. (1994). The perception of frequency peaks and troughs in wide frequency modulations. *Journal of the Acoustical Society of America*, 96:706–715.

Demany, L., McKenzie, B., & Vurpillot, E. (1977). Rhythm perception in early infancy. *Nature*, 266:718–719.

Denora, T. (1999). Music as a technology of the self. *Poetics: Journal of Empirical Research on Literature, the Media, and the Arts*, 26:1–26.

Denora, T. (2001). Aesthetic agency and musical practice: New directions in the sociology of music and emotion. In: P. N. Juslin & J. A. Sloboda (Eds.), *Music and Emotion: Theory and Research* (pp. 161–180). Oxford, UK: Oxford University Press.

Desain, P. (1992). A(de)composable theory of rhythm perception. *Music Perception*, 9: 439–454.

Desain, P., & Honing, H. (1999). Computational models of beat induction: The rule-based approach. *Journal of New Music Research*, 28:29–42.

Deutsch, D. (1978). Delayed pitch comparisons and the principle of proximity. *Perception and Psychophysics*, 23:227–230.

Deutsch, D., & Feroe, J. (1981). The internal representation of pitch sequences in tonal music. *Psychological Review*, 88:503–522.

Deutsch, D., Henthorn, T., & Dolson, M. (2004). Absolute pitch, speech, and tone language: Some experiments and a proposed framework. *Music Perception*, 21:339–356.

Deutsch, D., Henthorn, T., Marvin, E., & Xu, H.-S. (2006). Absolute pitch among American and Chinese conservatory students: Prevalence differences, and evidence for a speech-related critical period. *Journal of the Acoustical Society of America*, 119:719–722.

Dewitt, L. A., & Crowder, R. G. (1986). Recognition of novel melodies after brief delays. *Music Perception*, 3:259–274.

Di Cristo, A. (1998). Intonation in French. In: D. Hirst & A. Di Cristo (Eds.)., *Intonation Systems: A Survey of Twenty Languages* (pp. 295–218). Cambridge, UK: Cambridge University Press.

Di Pietro, M., Laganaro, M., Leemann, B., Schnider, A. (2003). Amusia: Selective rhythm processing following left temporoparietal lesion in a professional musician with conduction aphasia. *Brain and Language*, 87:152–153.

Dibben, N. (2001). What do we hear, when we hear music? Music perception and musical material. *Musicae Scientiae*, 5:161–194.

Diehl, R. L., Lindblom, B., & Creeger, C. P. (2003). Increasing realism of auditory representations yields further insights into vowel phonetics. *Proceedings of the 15th International Congress of Phonetic Sciences, Barcelona*, pp. 1381–1384.

Diehl, R. L., Lotto, A. J., & Holt, L. L. (2004). Speech perception. *Annual Review of Psychology*, 55:149–179.

Dilley, L. (2005). *The Phonetics and Phonology of Tonal Systems*. Ph.D. dissertation, MIT.

Dilley, L., Shattuck-Hufnagel, S., & Ostendorf, M. (1996). Glottalization of word-initial vowels as a function of prosodic structure. *Journal of Phonetics*, 24, 423–444.

Dissanayake, E. (2000). Antecedents of the temporal arts in early mother-infant interaction. In: N. L. Wallin, B. Merker, & S. Brown (Eds.), *The Origins of Music* (pp. 389–410). Cambridge, MA: MIT Press.

Dloniak, S. M., & Deviche, P. (2001). Effects of testosterone and photoperiodic condition on song production and vocal control region volumes in adult male Dark-Eyed Juncos (*Junco hyemalis*). *Hormones and Behavior, 39*:95–105.

Docherty, G., & Foulkes, P. (1999). Instrumental phonetics and phonological variation: Case studies from Newcastle upon Tyne and Derby. In: P. Foulkes & G. Docherty (Eds.), *Urban Voices: Accent Studies in the British Isles* (pp. 47–71). London: Arnold.

Donovan, A., & Darwin, C. J. (1979). The perceived rhythm of speech. *Proceedings of the 9th International Congress of Phonetic Sciences, Copenhagen, 2*:268–274.

Douglas, K. M., & Bilkey, D. K. (2007). Amusia is associated with deficits in spatial processing. *Nature Neuroscience, 10*:915–921.

Doupe, A. J., & Kuhl, P. K. (1999). Birdsong and human speech: Common themes and mechanisms. *Annual Review of Neuroscience, 22*:567–631.

Doupe, A. J., Perkel, D. J., Reiner, A., & Stern, E. A. (2005). Birdbrains could teach basal ganglia research a new song. *Trends in Neurosciences, 28*:353–363.

Dowling, W. J. (1973). Rhythmic groups and subjective chunks in memory for melodies. *Perception and Psychophysics, 14*:37–40.

Dowling, W. J. (1978). Scale and contour: Two components of a theory of memory for melodies. *Psychological Review, 85*:341–354.

Dowling, W. J. (1986). Context effects on melody recognition: Scale-steps versus interval representations. *Music Perception, 3*:281–296.

Dowling, W. J. (1988). Tonal structure and children's early learning of music. In: J. A. Sloboda (Ed.), *Generative Processes in Music* (pp. 113–128). Oxford, UK: Oxford University Press.

Dowling, W. J. (2001). Perception of music: In: E. B. Goldstein (Ed.), *Blackwell Handbook of Perception* (pp. 469–498). Malden, MA: Blackwell.

Dowling, W. J., & Bartlett, J. C. (1981). The importance of interval information in long-term memory for melodies. *Psychomusicology 1*:30–49.

Dowling, W. J., & Harwood, D. L. (1986). *Music Cognition.* Orlando, FL: Academic Press.

Dowling, W. J., Kwak, S., & Andrews, M. W. (1995). The time course of recognition of novel melodies. *Perception and Psychophysics, 57*:136–149.

Drake, C. (1998). Psychological processes involved in the temporal organization of complex auditory sequences: Universal and acquired processes. *Music Perception, 16*:11–26.

Drake, C., & Ben El Heni, J. (2003). Synchronizing with music: Intercultural differences. *Annals of the New York Academy of Sciences, 999*:428–437.

Drake, C., & Botte, M. C. (1993). Tempo sensitivity in auditory sequences: Evidence for a multiple-look model. *Perception and Psychophysics, 54*:277–286.

Drake, C., Jones, M., & Baruch, C. (2000). The development of rhythmic attending in auditory sequence: Attunement, reference period, focal attending. *Cognition, 77*, 251–288.

Drake, C., Penel, A., & Bigand, E. (2000). Tapping in time with mechanically and expressively performed music. *Music Perception, 18*:1–24.

Drayna, D., Manichaikul, A., de Lange, M., Snieder, H., & Spector, T. (2001). Genetic correlates of musical pitch recognition in humans. *Science, 291*:1969–72.

Dunbar, R. I. (2003). The origin and subsequent evolution of language. In: M. H. Christiansen & S. Kirby (Eds.), *Language Evolution* (pp. 219–234). Oxford, UK: Oxford University Press.

Dupoux, E., Peperkamp, S., & Sebastián-Gallés, N. (2001). A robust method to study stress "deafness." *Journal of the Acoustical Society of America,* 110:1606–1618.

Eady, S. J. (1982). Differences in the F0 patterns of speech: Tone language versus stress language. *Language and Speech,* 25:29–42.

Earle, M. A. (1975). *An Acoustic Study of Northern Vietnamese Tones* (Monograph 11). Santa Barbara, CA: Speech Communications Research Laboratory.

Edelman, G. M. (2006). *Second Nature: Brain Science and Human Knowledge.* New Haven, CT: Yale University Press.

Edmondson, J. A., & Gregerson, K. J. (1992). On five-level tone systems. In: S. J. Hwang & W. R. Merrifield (Eds.), *Language in Context: Essays for Robert E. Longacre* (pp. 555–576). Dallas, TX: Summer Institute of Linguistics.

Edworthy, J. (1985a). Interval and contour in melody processing. *Music Perception,* 2:375–388.

Edworthy, J. (1985b). Melodic contour and musical structure. In: P. Howell, I. Cross, & R. West (Eds.), *Musical Structure and Cognition* (pp. 169–188). London: Academic Press.

Eerola, T., Luck, G., & Toiviainen, P. (2006). An investigation of pre-schoolers' corporeal synchronization with music. In: M. Baroni, A. R. Addessi, R. Caterina, M. Costa, *Proceedings of the 9th International Conference on Music Perception and Cognition (ICMPC9),* Bologna/Italy, pp. 472–476.

Egnor, S. E. R., & Hauser, M. D. (2004). A paradox in the evolution of primate vocal learning. *Trends in Neurosciences, 27,* 649–654.

Ehresman, D., & Wessel, D. (1978). Perception of timbral analogies. *Rapports Ircam,* 13/78.

Eimas, P. D., Siqueland, E. R., Jusczyk, P., & Vigorito, J. (1971). Speech perception by infants. *Science,* 171:303–306.

Eisler, H. (1976). Experiments on subjective duration 1868–1975: A collection of power function exponents. *Psychological Bulletin,* 83:1154–1171.

Ekman, P., Friesen, W., O'Sullivan, M., et al. (1987). Universals and cultural differences in the judgments of facial expressions of emotion. *Journal of Personality and Social Psychology,* 53:712–717.

Elbert, T., Pantev, C., Wienbruch, C., Rockstroh, B., & Taub, E. (1995). Increased use of the left hand in string players associated with increased cortical representation of the fingers. *Science,* 270:305–307.

Elbert, T., Ulrich, R., Rockstroh, B., & Lutzenberger, W. (1991). The processing of temporal intervals reflected by CNV-like brain potentials. *Psychophysiology,* 28:648–655.

Elfenbein, H. A., & Ambady, N. (2003). Universals and cultural differences in recognizing emotions. *Current Directions in Psychological Science,* 12:159–164.

Ellis, A. (1885). On the musical scales of various nations. *Journal of the Royal Society of Arts* 33:485–527.

Elman, J. (1999). The emergence of language: A conspiracy theory. In: B. MacWhinney (Ed.), *The Emergence of Language* (pp. 1–27). Mahwah, NJ: Erlbaum.

Elman, J. L., Bates, E. A., Johnson, M. H., Karmiloff-Smith, A., Parisi, D., & Plunkett, K. (1996). *Rethinking Innateness: A Connectionist Perspective on Development.* Cambridge, MA: MIT Press.

Emmorey, K. (2002). *Language, Cognition, and the Brain: Insights From Sign Language Research*. Mahwah, NJ: Lawrence Erlbaum.

Enard, W., Przeworski, M., Fisher, S. E., Lai, C. S. L., Wiebe, V., Kitano, T., et al. (2002). Molecular evolution of FOXP2, a gene involved in speech and language. *Nature*, 418:869–872.

Escoffier, N., & Tillmann, B. (2006). Tonal function modulates speed of visual processing. In: M. Baroni, A. R. Addessi, R. Caterina, & M. Costa (Eds.), *Proceedings of the 9th International Conference on Music Perception and Cognition (ICMPC9)*, Bologna/Italy, August 22–26, p. 1878.

Everett, D. L. (2005). Cultural constraints on grammar and cognition in Pirahã: Another look at the design features of human language. *Current Anthropology*, 46: 621–646.

Faber, D. (1986). Teaching the rhythms of English: A new theoretical base. *International Review of Applied Linguistics*, 24:205–216.

Falk, D. (2004a). Prelinguistic evolution in early hominins: Whence motherese? (Target article). *Behavioral and Brain Sciences*, 27:491–503.

Falk, D. (2004b). The "putting the baby down" hypothesis: Bipedalism, babbling, and baby slings (Response to commentaries). *Behavioral and Brain Sciences*, 27:526–534.

Fant, G., Kruckenberg, A., & Nord, L. (1991a). Durational correlates of stress in Swedish, French and English. *Journal of Phonetics*, 19, 351–365.

Fant, G., Kruckenberg, A., & Nord, L. (1991b). Stress patterns and rhythm in the reading of prose and poetry with analogies to music performance. In: J. Sundberg, L. Nord, & R. Carlson (Eds.), *Music, Language, Speech and Brain* (pp. 380–407). London: Macmillan.

Farnsworth, P. R. (1954). A study of the Hevner adjective list. *Journal of Aesthetics and Art Criticism*, 13:97–103.

Fassbender, C. (1996). Infant's auditory sensitivity toward acoustic parameters of speech and music. In: I. Deliège & J. Sloboda (Eds.), *Musical Beginnings* (pp. 56–87). Oxford, UK: Oxford University Press.

Fedorenko, E., Patel, A. D., Casasanto, D., Winawer, J., & Gibson, E. (2009). Structural integration in language and music: Evidence for a shared system. *Memory and Cognition*, 37:1–9.

Feld, S. (1974). Linguistic models in ethnomusicology. *Ethnomusicology*, 18:197–217.

Feld, S., & Fox, A. A. (1994). Music and language. *Annual Review of Anthropology*, 23:25–53.

Ferland, M. B., & Mendelson, M. J. (1989). Infant's categorization of melodic contour. *Infant Behavior and Development*, 12:341–355.

Fernald, A. (1985). Four-month-olds prefer to listen to motherese. *Infant Behavior and Development*, 8:181–195.

Fernald, A. (1992). Meaningful melodies in mothers' speech to infants. In: H. Papousek, U. Jurgens, & M. Papousek (Eds.), *Nonverbal Vocal Communication: Comparative and Developmental Aspects* (pp. 262–282). Cambridge, UK: Cambridge University Press.

Fernald, A., & Kuhl, P. (1987). Acoustic determinants of infant preference for motherese speech. *Infant Behavior and Development*, 10:279–293.

Fernald, A., Taeschner, T., Dunn, J., Papousek, M., Boysson-Bardies, B., & Fukui, I. (1989). A cross-language study of prosodic modifications in mothers' and fathers' speech to preverbal infants. *Journal of Child Language*, 16:477–501.

Ferreira, F. (1991). The creation of prosody during sentence production. *Psychological Review*, 100:233–253.

Filk, E. (1977). Tone glides and registers in five Dan dialects. *Linguistics* 201:5–59.

Fishman, Y. I., Volkov, I. O., Noh, M. D., Garell, P. C., Bakken, H., Arezzo, J. C., et al. (2001). Consonance and dissonance of musical chords: Neuronal in auditory cortex of monkeys and humans. *Journal of Neurophysiology,* 86:271–278.

Fitch, W. T. (2000). The evolution of speech: A comparative review. *Trends in Cognitive Sciences,* 4:258–267.

Fitch, W. T. (2006). The biology and evolution of music: A comparative perspective. *Cognition,* 100:173–215.

Fitch, W. T., & Giedd, J. (1999). Morphology and development of the human vocal tract: A study using magnetic resonance imaging. *Journal of the Acoustical Society of America,* 106:1511–1522.

Fitch, W. T., & Hauser, M. D. (2004). Computational constraints on syntactic processing in a nonhuman primate. *Science,* 303:377–380.

Floccia, C., Nazzi, T., & Bertoncini, J. (2000). Unfamiliar voice discrimination for short stimuli in newborns. *Developmental Science,* 3:333–343.

Fodor, J. A. (1983). *Modularity of Mind.* Cambridge, MA: MIT Press.

Foris, D. P. (2000). *A Grammar of Sochiapan Chinantec.* Dallas, TX: SIL International.

Fougeron, C., & Jun, S.-A. (1998). Rate effects on French intonation: Prosodic organization and phonetic realization. *Journal of Phonetics,* 26:45–69.

Fowler, C. A. (1986). An event approach to the study of speech perception from a direct realist perspective. *Journal of Phonetics,* 14:3–28.

Fowler, C. A., Brown, J., Sabadini, L., & Weihing, J. (2003). Rapid access to speech gestures in perception: Evidence from choice and simple response time tasks. *Journal of Memory and Language. 49,* 296–314.

Foxton, J. M., Dean, J. L., Gee, R., Peretz, I., & Griffiths, T. D. (2004). Characterisation of deficits in pitch perception underlying "tone deafness." *Brain,* 127:801–810.

Foxton, J. M., Nandy, R. K., & Griffiths, T. D. (2006). Rhythm deficits in "tone-deafness." *Brain and Cognition,* 62:24–29.

Foxton, J. M., Talcott, J. B., Witton, C., Brace, H., McIntyre, F., & Griffiths, T. D. (2003). Reading skills are related to global, but not local, acoustic pattern perception. *Nature Neuroscience,* 6:343–4.

Fraisse, P. (1982). Rhythm and tempo. In: D. Deutsch (Ed.), *The Psychology of Music* (pp. 149–180). New York: Academic Press.

Francès, R. (1988). *The Perception of Music* (W. J. Dowling, Trans.). Hillsdale, NJ: Erlbaum.

Francès, R., Lhermitte, F., & Verdy, M. (1973). Le déficit musical des aphasiques. *Revue Internationale de Psychologie Appliquée,* 22:117–135.

Francis, A. L., Ciocca, V., & Ng, B. K. C. (2003). On the (non)categorical perception of lexical tones. *Perception and Psychophysics,* 65:1029–1044.

Frankland, B. W., & Cohen, A. J. (2004). Parsing of melody: Quantification and testing of the local grouping rules of Lerdahl and Jackendoff's *A Generative Theory of Tonal Music. Music Perception,* 21: 499–543.

Friberg, A., & Sundberg, J. (1999). Does music performance allude to locomotion? A model of final ritardandi derived from measurements of stopping runners. *Journal of the Acoustical Society of America,* 105:1469–1484.

Friederici, A. D. (2002). Towards a neural basis of auditory sentence processing. *Trends in Cognitive Sciences*, 6:78–84.

Fries, W., & Swihart, A. A. (1990). Disturbance of rhythm sense following right hemisphere damage. *Neuropsychologia*, 28:1317–1323.

Fromkin, V. (Ed.). (1978). *Tone: A Linguistic Survey*. New York: Academic Press.

Frota, S., & Vigário, M. (2001). On the correlates of rhythmic distinctions: The European/Brazilian Portuguese case. *Probus*, 13:247–275.

Fry, D. B., Abramson, A. S., Eimas, P. D., & Liberman, A. M. (1962). Identification and discrimination of synthetic vowels. *Language and Speech*, 5:171–189.

Fujioka, T., Trainor, L. J., Ross, B., Kakigi, R., & Pantev, C. (2004). Musical training enhances automatic encoding of melodic contour and interval structure. *Journal of Cognitive Neuroscience*, 16:1010–1021.

Fussell, P. (1974). Meter. In: A. Priminger, (Ed.), *Princeton Encyclopedia of Poetry and Poetics* (pp. 496–500). Princeton, NJ: Princeton University Press.

Fussell, P. (1979). *Poetic Meter and Poetic Form* (Rev. ed.). New York: Random House.

Gabriel, C. (1978). An experimental study of Deryck Cooke's theory of music and meaning. *Psychology of Music*, 9:44–53.

Gabrielsson, A. (1973). Similarity ratings and dimension analyses of auditory rhythm patterns. I and II. *Scandinavian Journal of Psychology*, 14:138–160,161–175.

Gabrielsson, A. (1993). The complexities of rhythm. In: T. Tighe & W. J. Dowling (Eds.), *Psychology and Music: The Understanding of Melody and Rhythm*. Hillsdale, NJ: Erlbaum.

Gabrielsson, A., & Juslin, P. N. (1996). Emotional expression in music performance: Between the performer's intention and the listener's experience. *Psychology of Music*, 24:68–91.

Gabrielsson, A., & Lindström, E. (2001). The influence of musical structure on emotional expression. In: P. N. Juslin & J. A. Sloboda (Eds.), *Music and Emotion: Theory and Research* (pp. 223–248). Oxford, UK: Oxford University Press.

Gabrielsson, A., & Lindström Wik, S. (2003). Strong experiences related to music: A descriptive system. *Musicae Scientiae*, 7:157–217.

Galizio, M., & Hendrick, C. (1972). Effect of music accompaniment on attitude: The guitar as a prop for persuasion. *Journal of Applied Social Psychology*, 2:350–359.

Galves, A., Garcia, J., Duarte, D., & Galves, C. (2002). Sonority as a basis for rhythmic class discrimination. In: B. Bell & I. Marlien (Eds.), *Proceedings of Speech Prosody, Aix-en-Provence*. Aix-en-Provence, France: Laboratoire Parole et Langage.

Gandour, J., Wong, D., Hsieh, L., Weinzapfel, B., Van Lancker, D., & Hutchins, G. (2000). A crosslinguistic PET study of tone perception. *Journal of Cognitive Neuroscience*, 12:207–222.

Garfias, R. (1987). Thoughts on the process of language and music acquisition. In: F. R. Wilson & F. L. Roehmann (Eds.), *The Biology of Music Making: Music and Child Development* (pp. 100–105). St. Louis, MO: MMB Music.

Gaser, C., & Schlaug, G. (2003). Brain structures differ between musicians and non-musicians. *Journal of Neuroscience*, 23:9240–9245.

Gee, J. P., & Grosjean, F. (1983). Performance structures: A psycholinguistic and linguistic appraisal. *Cognitive Psychology*, 15:411–458.

Geissmann, T. (2000). Gibbon songs and human music from an evolutionary perspective. In: N. L. Wallin, B. Merker, & S. Brown (Eds.), *The Origins of Music* (pp. 102–123). Cambridge, MA: MIT Press.

Genter, D., & Goldin-Meadow, S. (Eds.). (2003). *Language in Mind.* Cambridge, MA: MIT Press.

Gentner, T., Fenn, K. M., Margoliash, D., & Nusbaum, H. C. (2006). Recursive syntactic pattern learning by songbirds. *Nature, 440:*1204–1207.

Gentner, T. Q., & Hulse, S. H. (1998). Perceptual mechanisms for individual recognition in European starlings (*Sturnus vulgaris*). *Animal Behaviour, 56:*579–594.

George, M. S., Parekh, P. I., Rosinsky, N., Ketter, T., Kimbrall, T. A., et al. (1996). Understanding emotional prosody activates right hemisphere regions. *Archives of Neurology, 53:*665–670.

Gerardi, G. M., & Gerken, L. (1995). The development of affective response to modality and melodic contour. *Music Perception, 12:*279–290.

Gerhardt, H. C., & Huber, F. (2002). *Acoustic Communication in Insects and Anurans.* Chicago: University of Chicago Press.

Gibson, E. (1998). Linguistic complexity: Locality of syntactic dependencies. *Cognition, 68:*1–76.

Gibson, E. (2000). The dependency locality theory: A distance-based theory of linguistic complexity. In: A. Marantz, Y. Miyashita, & W. O'Neil (Eds.), *Image, Language, Brain* (pp. 95–126). Cambridge, MA: MIT Press.

Gibson, J. J. (1979). *The Ecological Approach to Visual Perception.* Boston: Houghton Mifflin.

Giddings, R. (1984). *Musical Quotes and Anecdotes.* Burnt Mill, UK: Longman.

Giguère, J.-F., Dalla Bella, S., & Peretz, I. (2005). *Singing Abilities in Congenital Amusia.* Poster presented at the Cognitive Neuroscience Society meeting, New York, April 10–12.

Giles, H., Coupland, N., & Coupland, J. (Eds.). (1991). *Contexts of Accommodation: Developments in Applied Sociolinguistics.* Cambridge, UK: Cambridge University Press.

Gitschier, J., Athos, A., Levinson, B., Zemansky, J., Kistler, A., & Freimer, N. (2004). Absolute pitch: Genetics and perception. In: S. D. Lipscomb et al. (Ed.), *Proceedings of the 8th International Conference on Music Perception and Cognition, Evanston, IL* (pp. 351–352). Adelaide, Australia: Causal Productions.

Gjerdingen, R. O. (2007). *Music in the Galant Style.* New York: Oxford University Press.

Goldin-Meadow, S. (1982). The resilience of recursion: A study of a communication system developed without a conventional language model. In: E. Wanner & L. R. Gleitman (Eds.), *Language Acquisition: The State of the Art* (pp. 51–77). New York: Cambridge University Press.

Goldstein, A. (1980). Thrills in response to music and other stimuli. *Physiological Psychology, 8:*126–129.

Goldstein, M., King, A., & West, M. (2003). Social interaction shapes babbling: Testing parallels between birdsong and speech. *Proceedings of the National Academy of Sciences, USA, 100:*8030–8035.

Gopnik, M. (1990). Feature-blind grammar and dysphasia. *Nature, 244:*715.

Gopnik, M., & Crago, M. B. (1991). Familial aggregation of a developmental language disorder. *Cognition, 39:*1–50.

Gordon, J. W. (1987). The perceptual attack time of musical tones. *Journal of the Acoustical Society of America*, 82:88–105.

Gordon, P. C., Hendrick, R., & Johnson, M. (2001). Memory interference during language processing. *Journal of Experimental Psychology: Learning, Memory and Cognition*, 27:1411–1423.

Goto, H. (1971). Auditory perception by normal Japanese adults of the sounds "L" and "R." *Neuropsychologia*, 9:317–327.

Gouvea, A., Phillips, C., Kazanina, N., & Poeppel, D. (submitted). *The Linguistic Processes Underlying the P600*.

Grabe, E. (2002). Variation adds to prosodic typology. In: B. Bell & I. Marlien (Eds.), *Proceedings of Speech Prosody, Aix-en-Provence* (pp. 127–132). Aix-en-Provence, France: Laboratoire Parole et Langage.

Grabe, E., Gussenhoven, C., Haan, J., Post, B., & Marsi, E. (1997). Pre-accentual pitch and speaker attitudes in Dutch. *Language and Speech*, 41:63–85.

Grabe, E., & Low, E. L. (2002). Durational variability in speech and the rhythm class hypothesis. In C. Gussenhoven & N. Warner (Eds.), *Laboratory Phonology 7* (pp. 515–546). Berlin, Germany: Mouton de Gruyter.

Grabe, E., Post, B., & Watson, I. (1999). The acquisition of rhythmic patterns in English and French. *Proceedings of the 14th International Congress of Phonetic Sciences, San Francisco* (pp. 1201–1204).

Grabe, E., & Warren, P. (1995). Stress shift: Do speakers do it or do listeners use it? In: B. Connell & A. Arvaniti (Eds.), *Papers in Laboratory Phonology IV. Phonology and Phonetic Evidence* (pp. 95–110). Cambridge, UK: Cambridge University Press.

Grahn, J. A., & Brett, M. (2007). Rhythm and beat perception in motor areas of the brain. *Journal of Cognitive Neuroscience*, 19:893–906.

Greenberg, S. (1996). The switchboard transcription project. In: *Research Report #24, 1996 Large Vocabulary Continuous Speech Recognition Summer Workshop Technical Report Series*. Center for Language and Speech Processing, Johns Hopkins University, Baltimore, MD.

Greenberg, S. (2006). A multi-tier framework for understanding spoken language. In: S. Greenberg & W. A. Ainsworth (Eds.), *Listening to Speech: An Auditory Perspective* (pp. 411–433). Mahwah, NJ: Erlbaum.

Greenfield, M. D. (2005). Mechanisms and evolution of communal sexual displays in arthropods and anurans. *Advances in the Study of Behavior*, 35: 1–62.

Greenfield, M. D., Tourtellot, M. K., & Snedden, W. A. (1997). Precedence effects and the evolution of chorusing. *Proceedings of the Royal Society of London B*, 264:1355–1361.

Greenspan, R. (1995). Understanding the genetic construction of behavior. *Scientific American*, 272:72–78.

Greenspan, R. (2004). *E pluribus unum, ex uno plura*: Quantitative- and single-gene perspectives on the study of behavior. *Annual Review of Neuroscience*, 27:79–105.

Greenspan, R. J., & Tully, T. (1994). Group report: How do genes set up behavior? In: R. J. Greenspan & C. P. Kyriacou (Eds.), *Flexibility and Constraint in Behavioral Systems* (pp. 65–80). Chichester: John Wiley & Sons.

Gregersen, P. K., Kowalsky, E., Kohn, N., & Marvin, E. W. (1999). Absolute pitch: Prevalence, ethnic variation, and estimation of the genetic component. *American Journal of Medical Genetics*, 65:911–913.

Gregersen, P. K., Kowalsky, E., Kohn, N., & Marvin, E. W. (2000). Early childhood music education and predisposition to absolute pitch: Teasing apart genes and environment. *American Journal of Medical Genetics*, 98:280–282.

Gregory, A. H. (1995). Perception and identification of Wagner's Leitmotifs. Paper presented at the Society for Music Perception and Cognition conference, University of California, Berkeley.

Gregory, A. H. (1997). The roles of music in society: The ethnomusicological perspective. In: D. J. Hargreaves & A. C. North (Eds.), *The Social Psychology of Music* (pp. 123–140). Oxford, UK: Oxford University Press.

Gregory, A. H., & Varney, N. (1996). Cross-cultural comparisons in the affective response to music. *Psychology of Music*, 24:47–52.

Greig, J. (2003). *The Music of Language: A Comparison of the Rhythmic Properties of Music and Language in Spanish, French, Russian and English*. Unpublished bachelor's thesis, Guildhall School of Music and Drama, London.

Grey, J. (1977). Multidimensional perceptual scaling of musical timbres. *Journal of the Acoustical Society of America*, 61:1270–1277.

Griffiths, T. D. (2002). Central auditory processing disorders. *Current Opinion in Neurobiology*, 15:31–33.

Griffiths, T. D., Rees, A., Witton, C., Cross, P. M., Shakir, R. A., & Green, G. G. R. (1997). Spatial and temporal auditory processing deficits following right hemisphere infarction: A psychophysical study. *Brain*, 120:785–794.

Grodner, D. J., & Gibson, E. (2005). Consequences of the serial nature of linguistic input for sentential complexity. *Cognitive Science,29*, 261–291.

Gross, H. (Ed.). (1979). *The Structure of Verse* (2nd ed.). New York: Ecco Press.

Grout, D. J., & Palisca, C. V. (2000). A *History of Western Music* (6th ed.). New York: W. W. Norton.

Grover, C., Jamieson, D. G., & Dobrovolsky, M. B. (1987). Intonation in English, French, and German: Perception and production. *Language and Speech*, 30:277–296.

Guenther, F. H. (2000). An analytical error invalidates the "depolarization" of the perceptual magnet effect. *Journal of the Acoustical Society of America*, 107:3576–3580.

Guenther, F. H., & Gjaja, M. N. (1996). The perceptual magnet effect as an emergent property of neural map formation. *Journal of the Acoustical Society of America*, 100:1111–1121.

Guenther, F. H., Husain, F. T., Cohen, M. A., & Shinn-Cunningham, B. G. (1999). Effects of auditory categorization and discrimination training on auditory perceptual space. *Journal of the Acoustical Society of America*, 106:2900–2912.

Guenther, F. H., Nieto-Castanon, A., Ghosh, S. S., & Tourville, J. A. (2004). Representation of sound categories in auditory cortical maps. *Journal of Speech, Language, and Hearing Research*, 47:46–57.

Gunter, T. C., Friederici, A. D., & Schriefers, H. (2000). Syntactic gender and semantic expectancy: ERPs reveal early autonomy and late interaction. *Journal of Cognitive Neuroscience*, 12:556–568.

Gussenhoven, C., & Rietveld, A. C. M. (1991). An experimental evaluation of two nuclear tone taxonomies. *Linguistics*, 29:423–449.

Gussenhoven, C., & Rietveld, A. C. M. (1992). Intonation contours, prosodic structure and preboundary lengthening. *Journal of Phonetics*, 20:283–303.

Gut, U. (2005). Nigerian English prosody. *English World-Wide*, 26:153–177.

Haarmann, H. J., & Kolk, H. H. J. (1991). Syntactic priming in Broca's aphasics: Evidence for slow activation. *Aphasiology,* 5:247–263.

Hacohen, R., & Wagner, N. (1997). The communicative force of Wagner's leitmotifs: Complementary relationships between their connotations and denotations. *Music Perception,* 14:445–476.

Haeberli, J. (1979). Twelve Nasca panpipes: A study. *Ethnomusicology,* 23:57–74.

Haesler, S., Wada, K., Nshdejan, A., Morrisey, E. E., Lints, T., Jarvis, E. D., & Scharff, C. (2004). FoxP2 expression in avian vocal learners and non-learners. *Journal of Neuroscience,* 24:3164–75.

Hagoort, P., Brown, C. M., & Groothusen, J. (1993). The syntactic positive shift (SPS) as an ERP measure of syntactic processing. *Language and Cognitive Processes,* 8:439–483.

Hagoort, P., Brown, C. M., & Osterhout, L. (1999). The neurocognition of syntactic processing. In: C. M. Brown & P. Hagoort (Eds.), *The Neurocognition of Language* (pp. 273–316). Oxford, UK: Oxford University Press.

Hajda, J. A., Kendall, R. A., Carterette, E. C., & Harshberger, M. L. (1997). Methodological issues in timbre research. In: I. Deliège & J. A. Sloboda (Eds.), *Perception and Cognition of Music* (pp. 253–306). Hove, UK: Psychology Press.

Hale, J. (2001). A probabilistic Earley parser as a psycholinguistic model. *Proceedings of NAACL,* 2:159–166.

Hall, M. D., & Pastore, R. E. (1992). Musical duplex perception: Perception of figurally good chords with subliminal distinguishing tones. *Journal of Experimental Psychology: Human Perception and Performance,* 18:752–762.

Hall, R. A., Jr. (1953, June). Elgar and the intonation of British English. *The Gramophone,* pp. 6–7. Reprinted in D. Bolinger (Ed.). (1972). *Intonation: Selected Readings* (pp. 282–285). Harmondsworth: Penguin.

Halle, M., & Idsardi, W. (1996). General properties of stress and metrical structure. In: J. Goldsmith (Ed.), *The Handbook of Phonological Theory* (pp. 403–443). Cambridge, MA: Blackwell.

Halle, M., & Vergnaud, J.-R. (1987). *An Essay on Stress.* Cambridge, MA: MIT Press.

Halliday, M. A. K. (1970). *A Course in Spoken English: Intonation.* London: Oxford University Press.

Handel, S. (1989). *Listening: An Introduction to the Perception of Auditory Events.* Cambridge, MA: MIT Press.

Hannon, E. E., & Johnson, S. P. (2005). Infants use meter to categorize rhythms and melodies: Implications for musical structure learning. *Cognitive Psychology,* 50, 354–377.

Hannon, E. E., Snyder, J. S., Eerola, T., & Krumhansl, C. L. (2004). The role of melodic and temporal cues in perceiving musical meter. *Journal of Experimental Psychology: Human Perception and Performance,* 30:956–974.

Hannon, E. E., & Trehub, S. E. (2005). Metrical categories in infancy and adulthood. *Psychological Science,* 16:48–55.

Hanslick, E. (1854/1957). *The Beautiful in Music* (G. Cohen, Trans., 1885, 7th ed.). New York: Liberal Arts Press.

Harris, M. S., & Umeda, N. (1987). Difference limens for fundamental frequency contours in sentences. *Journal of the Acoustical Society of America,* 81:1139–1145.

Hart, B., & Risley, T. (1995). *Meaningful Differences in the Everyday Experiences of American Children.* Baltimore: P. H. Brooks.

Haspelmath, M., Dryer, M. W., Gil, D., & Comrie, B. (2005). *The World Atlas of Language Structures*. New York: Oxford University Press.

Hast, D. E., Cowdery, J. R., & Scott, S. (Eds.). (1999). *Exploring the World of Music*. Dubuque, IA: Kendall Hunt. (Quote from interview with Simon Shaheen in video program #6: Melody.)

Hatten, R. (2004). *Interpreting Musical Gestures, Topics, and Tropes: Mozart, Beethoven, Schubert*. Bloomington: Indiana University Press.

Hauser, M. D., Chomsky, N., & Fitch, W. T. (2002). The faculty of language: What is it, who has it, and how did it evolve? *Science*, 298:1569–1579.

Hauser, M. D., & Fowler, C. A. (1992). Fundamental frequency declination is not unique to human speech: Evidence from nonhuman primates. *Journal of the Acoustical Society of America*, 91:363–369.

Hauser, M. D., & McDermott, J. (2003). The evolution of the music faculty: A comparative perspective. *Nature Neuroscience*, 6:663–668.

Hauser, M. D., Newport, E. L., & Aslin, R. N. (2001). Segmentation of the speech stream in a nonhuman primate: Statistical learning in cotton-top tamarins. *Cognition, 78*: B53–B64.

Hawkins, S., & Barrett-Jones, S. (in preparation). On phonetic and phonemic categories: An experimental and theoretical appraisal of the perceptual magnet effect.

Hay, J. S. F., & Diehl, R. L. (2007). Perception of rhythmic grouping: Testing the iambic/trochaic law. *Perception and Psychophysics*, 69:113–122.

Hayes, B. (1989). The prosodic hierarchy in meter. In: P. Kiparsky & G. Youmans (Eds.), *Phonetics and Phonology, Vol. 1: Rhythm and Meter* (pp. 201–260). San Diego, CA: Academic Press.

Hayes, B. (1995a). *Two Japanese children's songs*. Unpublished manuscript.

Hayes, B. (1995b). *Metrical Stress Theory: Principle and Case Studies*. Chicago: University of Chicago Press.

Heaton, P., Allen, R., Williams, K., Cummins, O., & Happe, F. (in press). Do social and cognitive deficits curtail musical understanding? Evidence from Autism and Down syndrome. *British Journal of Developmental Psychology*.

Hébert, S., & Cuddy, L. L. (2006). Music-reading deficiencies and the brain. *Advances in Cognitive Psychology*, 2:199–206.

Helmholtz, H. von. (1954). *On the Sensations of Tone as a Physiological Basis for the Theory of Music* (2nd ed., A. J. Ellis, Trans.). New York: Dover. (Original work published 1885)

Henshilwood, C., d'Errico, F., Vanhaeren, M., van Niekerk, K., & Jacobs, Z. (2004). Middle Stone Age shell beads from South Africa. *Science*, 304:404.

Henthorn, T., & Deutsch, D. (2007). Ethnicity versus environment: Comment on 'Early childhood music education and predispositions to abosolute pitch: Teasing apart genes and environment' by Peter K. Gregersen, Elena Kowalsky, Nina Kohn, and Elizabeth West Marvin [2000]. *American Journal of Medical Genetics Part A,*143A:102–103.

Hepper, P. G. (1991). An examination of fetal learning before and after birth. *The Irish Journal of Psychology*, 12:95–107.

Herman, L. M., & Uyeyama, R. K. (1999). The dolphin's grammatical competency: Comments on Kako (1999). *Animal Learning and Behavior*, 27:18–23.

Hermerén, G. (1988). Representation, truth, and the languages of the arts. In: V. Rantala, L. Rowell, & E. Tarasti (Eds.), *Essays on the Philosophy of Music, Acta Philosophica Fennica* (Vol. 43, pp. 179–209). Helsinki: The Philosophical Society of Finland.

Hermes, D. (2006). Stylization of pitch contours. In: S. Sudhoff et al. (Eds.), *Methods in Empirical Prosody Research* (pp. 29–61). Berlin: Walter de Gruyter.

Hermes, D., & van Gestel, J. C. (1991). The frequency scale of speech intonation. *Journal of the Acoustical Society of America,* 90:97–102.

Herzog, G. (1926). Helen H. Roberts & Diamond Jenness, "Songs of the Copper Eskimo" (book review). *Journal of American Folklore,* 39:218–225.

Herzog, G. (1934). Speech-melody and primitive music. *The Musical Quarterly,* 20:452–466.

Herzog, G. (1945). Drum-signaling in a West African tribe. *Word,* 1:217–238.

Hevner, K. (1936). Experimental studies of the elements of expression in music. *American Journal of Psychology,* 48:246–268.

Hevner, K. (1937). The affective value of pitch and tempo in music. *American Journal of Psychology,* 49:621–630.

Hickok, G., & Poeppel, D. (2004). Dorsal and ventral streams: A framework for understanding aspects of the functional anatomy of language. *Cognition,* 92:67–99.

Hinton, L. (1984). *Havasupai Songs: A Linguistic Perspective.* Tübingen, Germany: Gunter Narr Verlag.

Hinton, L., Nichols, J., & Ohala, J. J. (Eds.). (1994). *Sound Symbolism.* Cambridge, UK: Cambridge University Press.

Hirsh-Pasek, K., Kemler Nelson, D. G., Jusczyk, P. W., Cassidy, K. W., Druss, B., & Kennedy, L. (1987). Clauses are perceptual units for young infants. *Cognition,* 26:269–286.

Hirst, D., & Di Cristo, A. (Eds.). (1998). *Intonation Systems: A Survey of Twenty Languages.* Cambridge, UK: Cambridge University Press.

Hobbs, J. R. (1985). *On the Coherence and Structure of Discourse.* CSLI Technical Report 85–37. Stanford, CA: CSLI.

Hobbs, J. R. (1990). *Literature and Cognition.* CLSI Lecture Notes 21: Stanford, CA: CSLI.

Hockett, C. A., & Altmann, S. (1968). A note on design features. In: T. A. Sebeok (Ed.), *Animal Communication: Techniques of Study and Results of Research* (pp. 61–72). Bloomington: Indiana University Press.

Hoequist, C. (1983). Durational correlates of linguistic rhythm categories. *Phonetica,* 40:19–31.

Hogan, J. T., & Manyeh, M. (1996). A study of Kono tone spacing. *Phonetica,* 53:221–229.

Hollander, J. (2001). *Rhyme's Reason: A Guide to English Verse* (3rd ed.). New Haven, CT: Yale University Press.

Holleran, S., Butler, D., & Jones, M. R. (1995). Perceiving implied harmony: The role of melodic and harmonic context. *Journal of Experimental Psychology:Learning, Memory and Cognition,* 21:737–753.

Holloway, C. (2001). *All Shook Up: Music, Passion, and Politics.* Dallas, TX: Spence.

Holm, J. (2000). *An Introduction to Pidgins and Creoles*. Cambridge, UK: Cambridge University Press.

Holst, I. (1962). *Tune*. London: Faber & Faber.

Holt, L. L., Lotto, A. J., & Diehl, R. L. (2004). Auditory discontinuities interact with categorization: Implications for speech perception. *Journal of the Acoustical Society of America*, 116:1763–1773.

Honey, J. (1989). *Does Accent Matter? The Pygmalion Factor*. London: Faber & Faber.

Honing, H. (2005). Is there a perception-based alternative to kinematic models of tempo rubato? *Music Perception*, 23:79–85.

Honorof, D. N., & Whalen, D. H. (2005). Perception of pitch location within a speaker's F0 range. *Journal of the Acoustical Society of America*, 117:2193–2200.

Horton, T. (2001). The compositionality of tonal structures: A generative approach to the notion of musical meaning. *Musicae Scientiae*, 5:131–160.

House, D. (1990). *Tonal Perception in Speech*. Lund, Sweden: Lund University Press.

Howard, D., Rosen, S., & Broad, V. (1992). Major/minor triad identification and discrimination by musically trained and untrained listeners. *Music Perception*, 10:205–220.

Howe, M. J. A., Davidson, J. W., & Sloboda, J. A. (1998). Innate talents: Reality or myth? *Behavioral and Brain Sciences*, 21:399–442.

Hudson, A., & Holbrook, A. (1982). Fundamental frequency characteristics of young black adults. Spontaneous speaking and oral reading. *Journal of Speech and Hearing Research*, 25:25–28.

Hughes, D. (2000). No nonsense: The logic and power of acoustic-iconic mnemonic systems. *British Journal of Ethnomusicology*, 9:95–122.

Hulse, S. H., Bernard, D. J., & Braaten, R. F. (1995). Auditory discrimination of chord-based spectral structures by European starlings (*Sturnus vulgaris*). *Journal of Experimental Psychology: General*, 124:409–423.

Hulse, S. H., Takeuchi, A. H., & Braaten, R. F. (1992). Perceptual invariances in the comparative psychology of music. *Music Perception*, 10:151–184.

Huron, D. (2003). Is music an evolutionary adaptation? In: N. L. Wallin, B. Merker, & S. Brown (Eds.), *The Origins of Music* (pp. 57–75). Cambridge, MA: MIT Press.

Huron, D. (2006). *Sweet Anticipation: Music and the Psychology of Expectation*. Cambridge, MA: MIT Press.

Huron, D., & Ollen, J. (2003). Agogic contrast in French and English themes: Further support for Patel and Daniele. *Music Perception*, 21:267–271.

Huron, D., & Parncutt, R. (1993). An improved model of tonality perception incorporating pitch salience and echoic memory. *Psychomusicology*, 12:154–171.

Huron, D., & Royal, M. (1996). What is melodic accent? Converging evidence from musical practice. *Music Perception*, 13:489–516.

Husain, F., Tagamets, M.-A., Fromm, S., Braun, A., & Horwitz, B. (2004). Relating neural dynamics for auditory object processing to neuroimaging activity: A computational modeling and fMRI study. *NeuroImage*, 21:1701–1720.

Hutchins, S. (2003). *Harmonic functional categorization*. Poster presented at the Society for Music Perception and Cognition conference, June 16–19, Las Vegas.

Huttenlocher, J., Haight, W., Bryk, A., Seltzer, M., et al. (1991). Early vocabulary growth: Relation to language input and gender. *Developmental Psychology*, 27:236–248.

Huttenlocher, P. (2002). *Neural Plasticity*. Cambridge, MA: Harvard University Press.

Hyde, K. L., & Peretz, I. (2004). Brains that are out of tune but in time. *Psychological Science*, 15:356–360.

Hyde, K. L., Peretz, I., & Cuvelier, H. (2004). Do possessors of absolute pitch have special pitch acuity? In: S. D. Lipscomb et al. (Eds.), *Proceedings of the 8th International Conference on Music Perception and Cognition, Evanston, IL, 2004* (pp. 741–742). Adelaide, Australia: Causal Productions.

Hyde, K. L., Zatorre, R., Griffiths, T. D., Lerch, J. P., & Peretz, I. (2006). Morphometry of the amusic brain: A two-site study. *Brain*, 129:2562–2570.

Hyman, L. M. (1973). The feature [Grave] in phonological theory. *Journal of Phonetics*, 1:329–337.

Hyman, L. M. (2001). Tone systems. In: M. Maspelmath et al. (Eds.), *Language Typology and Language Universals: An International Handbook* (pp. 1367–1380). Berlin, Germany: Walter de Gruyter.

Ilie, G., & Thompson, W. F. (2006). A comparison of acoustic cues in music and speech for three dimensions of affect. *Music Perception*, 23:319–330.

Imaizumi, S., Mori, K., Kirtani, S., Kwashima, R., Sugiura, M. et al. (1997). Vocal identification of speaker and emotion activates different brain regions. *NeuroReport*, 8:2809–2812.

Iversen, J. R., Patel, A. D., & Ohgushi, K. (2008). Perception of rhythmic grouping depends on auditory experience. *Journal of the Acoustical Society of America*, 124:2263–2271.

Iversen, J. R., Repp, B., & Patel, A. D. (2009). Top-down control of rhythm perception modulates early auditory responses. *Annals of the New York Academy of Sciences*, 1169:58–73.

Iverson, J., Rees, H., & Revlin, R. (1989). The effect of music on the personal relevance of lyrics. *Psychology: A Journal of Human Behaviour*, 26:15–22.

Iverson, P., & Kuhl, P. K. (2000). Perceptual magnet and phoneme boundary effects in speech perception: Do they arise from a common mechanism? *Perception and Psychophysics*, 62:874–86.

Iverson, P., Kuhl, P., Akahane-Yamada, R., Diesch, E., Tohkura, Y., Kettermann, A., & Siebert, C. (2003). A perceptual interference account of acquisition difficulties for non-native phonemes. *Cognition* 87:B47–B57.

Izumi, A. (2000). Japanese monkeys perceive sensory consonance of chords. *Journal of the Acoustical Society of America*, 108:3073–3078.

Jackendoff, R. (1977). Review of *The Unanswered Question* by Leonard Bernstein. *Language*, 53:883–894.

Jackendoff, R. (1989). A comparison of rhythmic structures in music and language. In: P. Kiparsky & G. Youmans (Eds.), *Phonetics and Phonology, Vol. 1: Rhythm and Meter* (pp. 15–44). San Diego, CA: Academic Press.

Jackendoff, R. (1991). Musical parsing and musical affect. *Music Perception*, 9:199–230.

Jackendoff, R. (2002). *Foundations of Language*. New York: Oxford University Press.

Jackendoff, R., & Lerdahl, F. (2006). The capacity for music: What is it, and what's special about it? *Cognition*, 100:33–72.

Jaeger, F., Fedorenko, E., & Gibson, E. (2005). *Dissociation Between Production and Comprehension Complexity*. Poster Presentation at the 18th CUNY Sentence Processing Conference, University of Arizona.

Jairazbhoy, N. A. (1995). *The Rags of North Indian Music* (Rev. ed.). Bombay, India: Popular Prakashan. (Original work published 1971)

Jairazbhoy, N. A., & Stone, A. W. (1963). Intonation in present-day North Indian classical music. *Bulletin of the School of Oriental and African Studies,* 26:110–132.

Jakobson, R. (1971). *Selected Writings* (Vol. 3, pp. 704–705). The Hague, The Netherlands: Mouton.

Jakobson, R., Fant, G., & Halle, M. (1952). *Preliminaries to Speech Analysis: The Distinctive Features and Their Correlates.* Acoustics Laboratory, MIT, Technical Report No. 13. Cambridge, MA: MIT.

Janata, P., Birk, J. L., Tillmann, B., & Bharucha, J. J. (2003). Online detection of tonal pop-out in modulating contexts. *Music Perception,* 20:283–305.

Janata, P., Birk, J. L., Van Horn, J. D., Leman, M., Tillmann, B., & Bharucha, J. J. (2002). The cortical topography of tonal structures underlying Western music. *Science,* 298:2167–2170.

Janata, P., & Grafton, S. T. (2003). Swinging in the brain: Shared neural substrates for behaviors related to sequencing and music. *Nature Neuroscience,* 6, 682–687.

Jarvis, E. D. (2004). Learned birdsong and the neurobiology of human language. *Annals of the New York Academy of Sciences,* 1016, 749–777.

Jaszczolt, K. M. (2002). *Semantics and Pragmatics: Meaning in Language and Discourse.* London: Longmans.

Johnson, J. S., & Newport, E. L. (1989). Critical period effects in second language learning: The influence of maturational state on the acquisition of English as a second language. *Cognitive Psychology,* 21:60–99.

Johnson, K. (1997). *Acoustic and Auditory Phonetics.* Cambridge, MA: Blackwell.

Johnsrude, I. S., Penhune, V. B., Zatorre, R. J. (2000). Functional specificity in the right human auditory cortex for perceiving pitch direction. *Brain,* 123:155–63.

Johnston, P. A. (1994). *Brain Physiology and Music Cognition.* Ph.D. dissertation, University of California, San Diego.

Johnstone, T., & Scherer, K. R. (1999). The effects of emotion on voice quality. *Proceedings of the 14th International Congress of Phonetic Sciences, San Francisco,* pp. 2029–2032.

Johnstone, T., & Scherer, K. R. (2000). Vocal communication of emotion. In: M. Lewis & J. M. Haviland-Jones (Eds.), *Handbook of Emotions* (2nd ed., pp. 220–235). New York: Guilford Press.

Jones, M. R. (1976). Time, our lost dimension: Toward a new theory of perception, attention, and memory. *Psychological Review,* 83:323–355.

Jones, M. R. (1987). Dynamic pattern structure in music: Recent theory and research. *Perception and Psychophysics,* 41:21–634.

Jones, M. R. (1993). Dynamics of musical patterns: How do melody and rhythm fit together? In: T. J. Tighe & W. J. Dowling (Eds.), *Psychology and Music: The Understanding of Melody and Rhythm* (pp. 67–92). Hillsdale, NJ: Lawrence Erlbaum.

Jones, M. R., & Boltz, M. (1989). Dynamic attending and responses to time. *Psychological Review,* 96:459–491.

Jones, M. R., & Pfordresher, P. Q. (1997). Tracking musical patterns using joint accent structure. *Canadian Journal of Experimental Psychology,* 51:271–290.

Jones, M. R., & Ralston, J. T. (1991). Some influences of accent structure on melody recognition. *Memory and Cognition,* 19:8–20.

Jones, S. (1995). *Folk Music of China*. New York: Oxford University Press.

Jongsma, M. L. A., Desain, P., & Honing, H. (2004). Rhythmic context influences the auditory evoked potentials of musicians and non-musicians. *Biological Psychology*, 66:129–152.

Jun, S.-A. (2003). Intonation. In: L. Nadel (Ed.), *Encyclopedia of Cognitive Science* (Vol. 2, pp. 618–624). London: Nature Group.

Jun, S.-A. (2005). Prosodic typology. In: S.-A. Jun (Ed.), *Prosodic Typology: The Phonology of Intonation and Phrasing* (pp. 430–458). Oxford, UK: Oxford University Press.

Jun, S.-A., & Fougeron, C. (2000). A phonological model of French intonation. In: A. Botinis (Ed.), *Intonation: Analysis, Modeling and Technology* (pp. 209–242). Dordrecht, The Netherlands: Kluwer Academic Publishers.

Jun, S.-A., & Fougeron, C. (2002). Realizations of accentual phrase in French intonation. *Probus*, 14:147–172.

Jungers, M., Palmer, C., & Speer, S. R. (2002). Time after time: The coordinating influence of tempo in music and speech. *Cognitive Processing*, 1–2:21–35.

Jurafsky, D. (2003). Probabilistic modeling in psycholinguistics: Linguistic comprehension and production. In: R. Bod, J. Hay, & S. Jannedy (Eds.), *Probabilistic Linguistics*. Cambridge, MA: MIT Press.

Jusczyk, P., & Krumhansl, C. (1993). Pitch and rhythmic patterns affecting infants' sensitivity to musical phrase structure. *Journal of Experimental Psychology: Human Perception and Performance*, 19:627–640.

Juslin, P. N., & Laukka, P. (2003). Communication of emotions in vocal expression and music performance: Different channels, same code? *Psychological Bulletin*, 129:770–814.

Juslin, P. N., & Laukka, P. (2004). Expression, perception, and induction of musical emotions: A review and questionnaire study of everyday listening. *Journal of New Music Research*, 33:217–238.

Juslin, P. N., & Sloboda, J. A. (Eds.). (2001). *Music and Emotion: Theory and Research*. Oxford, UK: Oxford University Press.

Justus, T., & Hutsler, J. J. (2005). Fundamental issues in the evolutionary psychology of music: Assessing innateness and domain-specificity. *Music Perception*, 23:1–27.

Justus, T. C., & Bharucha, J. J. (2001). Modularity in musical processing: The automaticity of harmonic priming *Journal of Experimental Psychology: Human Perception and Performance*, 27:1000–1011.

Kaan, E., Harris, T., Gibson, T., & Holcomb, P. J. (2000). The P600 as an index of syntactic integration difficulty. *Language and Cognitive Processes*, 15:159–201.

Kaan, E., & Swaab, T. Y. (2002). The brain circuitry of syntactic comprehension. *Trends in Cognitive Sciences*, 6:350–356.

Kalmus, H., & Fry, D. B. (1980). On tune deafness (dysmelodia): Frequency, development, genetics and musical background. *Annals of Human Genetics*, 43:369–382.

Kameoka, A., & Kuriyagawa, M. (1969a). Consonance theory part I: Consonance of dyads. *Journal of the Acoustical Society of America*, 45:1451–1459.

Kameoka, A., & Kuriyagawa, M. (1969b). Consonance theory part II: Consonance of complex tones and its calculation method. *Journal of the Acoustical Society of America*, 45:1460–1469.

Karmiloff-Smith, A. (1992). *Beyond Modularity: A Developmental Perspective on Cognitive Science*. Cambridge, MA: MIT Press.

Karmiloff-Smith, A., Brown, J. H., Grice, S., & Paterson, S. (2003). Dethroning the myth: Cognitive dissociations and innate modularity in Williams syndrome. *Developmental Neuropsychology*, 23:229–244.

Karno, M., & Konečni, V. J. (1992). The effects of structural intervention in the first movement of Mozart's Symphony in G-Minor, K. 550, on aesthetic preference. *Music Perception*, 10:63–72.

Karzon, R. G. (1985). Discrimination of polysyllabic sequences by one-to-four-month-old infants. *Journal of Experimental Child Psychology*, 39:326–342.

Kassler, J. C. (2005). Representing speech through musical notation. *Journal of Musicological Research*, 24: 227–239.

Kazanina, N., Phillips, C., & Idsardi, W. (2006). The influence of meaning on the perception of speech sounds. *Proceedings of the National Academy of Sciences USA*, 103:11381–11386.

Keane, E. (2006). Rhythmic characteristics of colloquial and formal Tamil. *Language and Speech*, 49:299–332.

Kehler, A. (2002). *Coherence, Reference, and the Theory of Grammar.* Stanford, CA: CLSI Publications.

Kehler, A. (2004). Discourse doherence. In: L. R. Horn & G. Ward (Eds.), *Handbook of Pragmatics* (pp. 241–265). Oxford, UK: Basil Blackwell.

Keiler, A. (1978). Bernstein's *The Unanswered Question* and the problem of musical competence. *The Musical Quarterly*, 64:195–222.

Kelly, M. H., & Bock, J. K. (1988). Stress in time. *Journal of Experimental Psychology: Human Perception and Performance*, 14:389–403.

Kendall, R., & Carterette, E. C. (1990). The communication of musical expression. *Music Perception*, 8:129–163.

Kessler, E. J., Hansen, C., & Shepard, R. (1984). Tonal schemata in the perception of music in Bali and the West. *Music Perception*, 2:131–165.

Kim, S. (2003). The role of post-lexical tonal contours in word segmentation. *Proceedings of the 15th International Congress of Phonetic Sciences, Barcelona*, pp. 495–498.

King, J., & Just, M. A. (1991). Individual differences in syntactic processing: The role of working memory. *Journal of Memory and Language*, 30:580–602.

Kippen, J. (1988). *The Tabla of Lucknow: A Cultural Analysis of a Musical Tradition.* Cambridge, UK: Cambridge University Press.

Kisilevsky, B. S., Hains, S. M. J., Lee, K., Xie, X., Huang, H., Ye, H. H., et al. (2003). Effects of experience on fetal voice recognition. *Psychological Science*, 14:220–224.

Kivy, P. (1980). *The Corded Shell: Reflections on Musical Expression.* Princeton, NJ: Princeton University Press.

Kivy, P. (1990). *Music Alone: Philosophical Reflections on the Purely Musical Experience.* Ithaca, New York: Cornell University Press.

Kivy, P. (2002). *Introduction to a Philosophy of Music.* Oxford, UK: Oxford University Press.

Klatt, D. (1976). Linguistic uses of segmental duration in English: Acoustic and perceptual evidence. *Journal of the Acoustical Society of America*, 59:1208–1221.

Klatt, D. (1979). Synthesis by rule of segmental durations in English sentences. In: B. Lindblom & S. Ohman (Eds.), *Frontiers of Speech Communication Research* (pp. 287–299). New York: Academic Press.

Klima, E., & Bellugi, U. (1979). *The Signs of Language.* Cambridge, MA: Harvard University Press.

Kluender, K. R., Diehl, R. L., & Killeen, P. R. (1987). Japanese quail can learn phonetic categories. *Science*, 237:1195–1197.

Kmetz, J., Finscher, L., Schubert, G., Schepping, W., & Bohlman, P. V. (2001). Germany. In: S. Sadie (Ed)., *The New Grove Dictionary of Music and Musicians* (Vol. 9, pp. 708–744). New York: Grove.

Knightly, L. M., Jun, S.-A., Oh, J. S., & Au, T. K.-F. (2003). Production benefits of childhood overhearing. *Journal of the Acoustical Society of America*, 114:465–474.

Knösche, T. R., Neuhaus, C., Haueisen, J., Alter, K., Maess, B., Witte, O. W., & Friederici, A. D. (2005). The perception of phrase structure in music. *Human Brain Mapping*, 24:259–273.

Koelsch, S., Grossmann, T., Gunter, T., Hahne, A., & Friederici, A. (2003). Children processing music: Electric brain responses reveal musical competence and gender differences. *Journal of Cognitive Neuroscience*,15:683–93.

Koelsch, S., Gunter, T. C., Friederici, A. D., & Schröger, E. (2000). Brain indices of music processing: "Non-musicians" are musical. *Journal of Cognitive Neuroscience*, 12:520–541.

Koelsch, S., Gunter, T. C., von Cramon, D. Y., Zysset, S., Lohmann, G., & Friederici, A. D. (2002). Bach speaks: A cortical "language-network" serves the processing of music. *NeuroImage*, 17:956–966.

Koelsch, S., Gunter, T. C., Wittforth, M., & Sammler, D. (2005). Interaction between syntax processing in language and music: An ERP study. *Journal of Cognitive Neuroscience*, 17:1565–1577.

Koelsch, S., Jentschke, S., Sammler, D., & Mietchen, D. (2007). Untangling syntactic and sensory processing: An ERP study of music perception. *Psychophysiology*, 44:476–490.

Koeslch, S., Kasper, E., Sammler, D., Schulze, K., Gunter, T., & Friederici, A. D. (2004). Music, language, and meaning: Brain signatures of semantic processing. *Nature Neuroscience*, 7:302–207.

Koelsch, S., & Mulder, J. (2002). Electric brain responses to inappropriate harmonies during listening to expressive music. *Clinical Neurophysiology*, 113:862–869.

Koelsch, S., & Siebel, W. A. (2005). Toward a neural basis of music perception. *Trends in Cognitive Sciences*, 9:578–584.

Kolk, H. H. (1998). Disorders of syntax in aphasia: Linguistic-descriptive and processing approaches. In: B. Stemmer & H. A. Whitaker (Eds.), *Handbook of Neurolinguistics* (pp. 249–260). San Diego, CA: Academic Press.

Kolk, H. H., & Friederici, A. D. (1985). Strategy and impairment in sentence understanding by Broca's and Wernicke's aphasics. *Cortex*, 21:47–67.

Konieczny, L. (2000). Locality and parsing complexity. *Journal of Psycholinguistic Research*, 29:627–645.

Koon, N. K. (1979). The five pentatonic modes in Chinese folk music. *Chinese Music*, 2:10–13.

Koopman, C., & Davies, S. (2001). Musical meaning in a broader perspective. *The Journal of Aesthetics and Art Criticism*, 59:261–273.

Kotz, S. A., Frisch, S., von Cramon, D. Y., & Friederici, A. D. (2003). Syntactic language processing: ERP lesion data on the role of the basal ganglia. *Journal of the International Neuropsychologcial Society*, 9:1053–1060.

Kraljic, T., & Samuel, A. (2005). Perceptual learning for speech: Is there a return to normal? *Cognitive Psychology*, 51:141–178.

Kramer, L. (2002). *Musical Meaning: Toward a Critical History.* Berkeley: University of California Press.

Kristofferson, A. B. (1980). A quantal step function in duration discrimination. *Perception and Psychophysics,* 27:300–6.

Kronman, U., & Sundberg, J. (1987). Is the musical retard an allusion to physical motion? In: A. Gabrielsson (Ed.), *Action and Perception in Rhythm and Music* (pp. 57–68). Stockholm: Royal Swedish Academy of Music.

Krumhansl, C. L. (1979). The psychological representation of musical pitch in a tonal context. *Cognitive Psychology,* 11:346–374.

Krumhansl, C. L. (1989). Why is musical timbre so hard to understand? In: S. Nielzén & O. Olsson (Eds.), *Structure and Perception of Electroacoustic Sound and Music* (pp. 43–54). New York: Excerpta Medica.

Krumhansl, C. L. (1990). *Cognitive Foundations of Musical Pitch.* New York: Oxford University Press.

Krumhansl, C. L. (1991). Melodic structure: Theoretical and empirical descriptions. In: J. Sundberg, L. Nord, & R. Carlson (Eds.), *Music, Language, Speech and Brain* (pp. 269–283). London: MacMillan.

Krumhansl, C. L. (1992). Internal representations for music perception and performance. In: M. R. Jones & S. Holleran (Eds.), *Cognitive Bases of Musical Communication* (pp. 197–211). Washington, DC: American Psychological Association.

Krumhansl, C. L. (1995a). Effects of musical context on similarity and expectancy. *Systematische Musikwissenschaft (Systematic Musicology),* 3:211–250.

Krumhansl, C. L. (1995b). Music psychology and music theory: Problems and prospects. *Music Theory Spectrum,* 17:53–90.

Krumhansl, C. L. (1996). A perceptual analysis of Mozart's Piano Sonata K. 282: Segmentation, tension, and musical ideas. *Music Perception,* 13:401–432.

Krumhansl, C. L. (1997). An exploratory study of musical emotions and psychophysiology. *Canadian Journal of Experimental Psychology,* 51:336–353.

Krumhansl, C. L. (1998). Topic in music: An empirical study of memorability, openness, and emotion in Mozart's String Quintet in C Major and Beethoven's String Quartet in A Minor. *Music Perception,*16:119–134.

Krumhansl, C. L. (2000). Tonality induction: A statistical approach applied cross-culturally. *Music Perception,* 17:461–479.

Krumhansl, C. L. (2005). The cognition of tonality—as we know it today. *Journal of New Music Research,* 33:253–268.

Krumhansl, C. L., Bharucha, J. J., & Kessler, E. J. (1982). Perceived harmonic structure of chords in thee related musical keys. *Journal of Experimental Psychology: Human Perception and Performance,* 8:24–36.

Krumhansl, C. L., & Jusczyk, P. (1990). Infants' perception of phrase structure in music. *Psychological Science,* 1:70–73.

Krumhansl, C. L., & Kessler, E. J. (1982). Tracing the dynamic changes in perceived tonal organization in a spatial representation of musical keys. *Psychological Review,* 89:334–368.

Krumhansl, C. L., Louhivouri, J., Toiviainen, P., Järvinen, T., & Eerola, T. (1999). Melodic expectancy in Finnish folk hymns: Convergence of behavioral, statistical, and computational approaches. *Music Perception,* 17:151–197.

Krumhansl, C. L., Toivanen, P., Eerola, T., Toiviainen, P, Järvinen, T., & Louhivuori, J. (2000). Cross-cultural music cognition: Cognitive methodology applied to North Sami yoiks. *Cognition, 76*:13–58.

Kugler, K., & Savage-Rumbaugh, S. (2002, June). Rhythmic drumming by Kanzi, an adult male bonobo (*Pan paniscus*) at the language research center. Paper presented at the 25th meeting of the American Society of Primatologists, Oklahoma University, Oklahoma.

Kuhl, P. K. (1979). Speech perception in early infancy: Perceptual constancy for spectrally dissimilar vowel categories. *Journal of the Acoustic Society of America, 66*:1668–1679.

Kuhl, P. K. (1983). Perception of auditory equivalence classes for speech in early infancy. *Infant Behavior and Development, 6*:263–285.

Kuhl, P. K. (1991). Human adults and human infants show a "perceptual magnet effect" for the prototypes of speech categories, monkeys do not. *Perception and Psychophysics 50*:93–107.

Kuhl, P. K. (1993). Innate predispositions and the effects of experience in speech perception: The native language magnet theory. In: J. Morton (Ed.), *Developmental Neurocognition: Speech and Face Processing in the First Year of Life* (pp. 259–274). Dordrecht, The Netherlands: Kluwer.

Kuhl, P. K. (2004). Early language acquisition: Cracking the speech code. *Nature Reviews (Neuroscience), 5*:831–843.

Kuhl, P. K., Andruski, J., Chistovich, I., Chistovich, L., Kozhevnikova, E., Ryskina, V., Stolyarova, E., Sundberg, U., & Lacerda, F. (1997). Cross-language analysis of phonetic units in language addressed to infants. *Science, 277*:684–686.

Kuhl, P. K., Conboy, B. T., Coffey-Corina, S., Padden, D., Rivera-Gaxiola, M., & Nelson, T. (in press). Phonetic learning as a pathway to language: New data and native language magnet theory expanded (NLM-e). *Philosophical Transactions of the Royal Society B.*

Kuhl, P. K., & Miller, J. D. (1975). Speech perception by the chinchilla: Voice–voiceless distinction in alveolar plosive consonants. *Science, 90*:69–72.

Kuhl, P. K., Tsao, F.-M., & Liu, H.-M. (2003). Foreign-language experience in infancy: Effects of short-term exposure and social interaction on phonetic learning. *Proceedings of the National Academy of Sciences, USA, 100*:9096–9101.

Kuhl, P. K., Williams, K. A., Lacerda, F., Stevens, K. N., & Lindblom, B. (1992). Linguistic experience alters phonetic perception in infants by 6 months of age. *Science, 255*:606–608.

Kuperberg, G. R., Lakshmanan, B. M., Caplan, D. N., & Holcomb, P. J. (2006). Making sense of discourse: An fMRI study of causal inferencing across sentences. *NeuroImage, 33*:343–361.

Kusumoto, K., & Moreton, E. (1997, December). Native language determines parsing of nonlinguistic rhythmic stimuli. Poster presented at the 134th meeting of the Acoustical Society of America, San Diego, CA.

Kutas, M., & Hillyard, S. A. (1984). Brain potentials during reading reflect word expectancy and semantic association. *Nature, 307*:161–163.

Labov, W. (1966). *The Social Stratification of English in New York City.* Washington, DC: Center for Applied Linguistics.

Ladd, D. R. (1986). Intonational phrasing: The case for recursive prosodic structure. *Phonology Yearbook,* 1:53–74.

Ladd, D. R. (1987). Review of Bolinger 1986. *Language,* 63:637–643.

Ladd, D. R. (1996). *Intonational Phonology.* Cambridge, UK: Cambridge University Press.

Ladd, D. R. (2001). Intonation. In: M. Haspelmath, E. König, W. Oesterreicher, & W. Raible (Eds.), *Language Typology and Language Universals* (Vol. 2, pp. 1380–1390). Berlin, Germany: Walter de Gruyter.

Ladd, D. R. (forthcoming). *Intonational Phonology* (2nd ed.). Cambridge, UK: Cambridge University Press.

Ladd, D. R., Faulkner, D., Faulkner, H., & Schepman, A. (1999). Constant "segmental anchoring" of F0 movements under changes in speech rate. *Journal of the Acoustical Society of America,* 106:1543–1554.

Ladd, D. R., & Morton, R. (1997). The perception of intonational emphasis: Continuous or categorical? *Journal of Phonetics,* 25:313–342.

Ladd, D. R., Silverman, K. E. A., Tolkmitt, F., Bergmann, G., & Scherer, K. R. (1985). Evidence for the independent function of intonation contour type, voice quality, and F0 range in signaling speaker affect. *Journal of the Acoustical Society of America,* 78:435–444.

Ladefoged, P. (1964). *A Phonetic Study of West African Languages.* London: Cambridge University Press.

Ladefoged, P. (1975). *A Course in Phonetics.* New York: Harcourt Brace Jovanovich.

Ladefoged, P. (2001). *Vowels and Consonants: An Introduction to the Sounds of Languages.* Malden, MA: Blackwell.

Ladefoged, P. (2006). *A Course in Phonetics* (5th Ed.). Boston: Thompson.

Ladefoged, P., & Maddieson, I. (1996).*The Sounds of the World's Languages.* Oxford, UK: Blackwell.

Lai, C. S. L., Gerrelli, D., Monaco, A. P., Fisher, S. E., & Copp, A. J. (2003). FOXP2 expression during brain development coincides with adult sites of pathology in a severe speech and language disorder. *Brain,* 126:2455–2462.

Lalitte, P., & Bigand, E. (2006) . Music in the moment: Revisiting the effect of large scale structure. *Perceptual and Motor Skills,* 103:811–828.

Lane, R., & Nadel, L. (Eds.). (2000). *Cognitive Neuroscience of Emotion.* New York: Oxford University Press.

Langacker, R. W. (1988). A view of linguistic semantics. In: B. Rudzka-Ostyn (Ed.), *Topics in Cognitive Linguistics* (pp. 49–60). Amsterdam/Philadelphia: J. Benjamins.

Langer, S. (1942). *Philosophy in a New Key: A Study in the Symbolism of Reason, Right, and Art.* Cambridge, MA: Harvard University Press.

Large, E. W. (2000). On synchronizing movements to music. *Human Movement Science,* 19:527–566.

Large, E. W., & Jones, M. R. (1999). The dynamics of attending: How we track time-varying events. *Psychological Review,* 106:119–159.

Large, E. W., & Palmer, C. (2002). Perceiving temporal regularity in music. *Cognitive Science,* 26:1–37.

Large, E. W., Palmer, C., & Pollack, J. B. (1995). Reduced memory representations for music. *Cognitive Science,* 19:53–96.

Lau, E., Stroud, C., Plesch, S., & Phillips, C. (2006). The role of structural prediction in rapid syntactic analysis. *Brain and Language*, 98:74–88.

Laukka, P., Juslin, P. N., & Bresin, R. (2005). A dimensional approach to vocal expression of emotion. *Cognition and Emotion*, 19:633–653.

Lecanuet, J. (1996). Prenatal auditory experience. In: I. Deliège & J. Sloboda (Eds.), *Musical Beginnings: Origins and Development of Musical Competence* (pp. 3–34). Oxford, UK: Oxford University Press.

Lecarme, J. (1991). Focus en somali: Syntaxe et interpretation. *Linguistique Africaine*, 7: 33–63.

LeDoux, J. (1996). *The Emotional Brain*. New York: Simon & Schuster.

Lee, C. S., & Todd, N. P. McA. (2004). Toward an auditory account of speech rhythm: Application of a model of the auditory "primal sketch" to two multi-language corpora. *Cognition*, 93:225–254.

Lehiste, I. (1977). Isochrony reconsidered. *Journal of Phonetics*, 5:253–263.

Lehiste, I. (1990). An acoustic analysis of the metrical structure of orally produced Lithuanian poetry. *Journal of Baltic Studies*, 21:145–155.

Lehiste, I. (1991). Speech research: An overview. In: J. Sundberg, L. Nord, & R. Carlson (Eds.), *Music, Language, Speech and Brain* (pp. 98–107). London: Macmillan.

Lehiste, I., & Fox, R. A. (1992). Perception of prominence by Estonian and English listeners. *Language and Speech*, 35:419–434.

Leman, M. (1995). *Music and Schema Theory*. Berlin, Germany: Springer.

Leman, M. (2000). An auditory model of the role of short-term memory in probe-tone ratings. *Music Perception*, 17:481–509.

Lennenberg, E. (1967). *Biological Foundations of Language*. New York: Wiley.

Lerdahl, F. (2001). *Tonal Pitch Space*. New York: Oxford University Press.

Lerdahl, F. (2003). The sounds of poetry viewed as music. In: I. Peretz & R. Zatorre (Eds.), *The Cognitive Neuroscience of Music* (pp. 413–429). New York: Oxford University Press.

Lerdahl, F., & Halle, J. (1991). Some lines of poetry viewed as music. In: J. Sundberg, L. Nord, & R. Carlson (Eds.), *Music, Language, Speech and Brain* (pp. 34–47). London: Macmillan.

Lerdahl, F., & Jackendoff, R. (1983). *A Generative Theory of Tonal Music*. Cambridge, MA: MIT Press.

Lerdahl, F., & Krumhansl, C. L. (2007). Modeling tonal tension. *Music Perception*, 24:329–366.

Levelt, W. J. M. (1989). *Speaking: From Intention to Articulation*. Cambridge, MA: MIT Press.

Levelt, W. J. M. (1999). Models of word production. *Trends in Cognitive Sciences*, 3:223–232.

Levinson, G. (1997). *Music in the Moment*. Ithaca, New York: Cornell University Press.

Lévi-Strauss, C. (1964/1969). *The Raw and the Cooked: Introduction to a Science of Mythology* (J. Weightman & D. Weightman, Trans.). New York: Harper and Row.

Levitin, D. J. (1994). Absolute memory for musical pitch: Evidence from the production of learned melodies. *Perception and Psychophysics*, 56:414–423.

Levitin, D. J., Cole, K., Chiles, M., Lai, Z., Lincoln, A., & Bellugi, U. (2004). Characterizing the musical phenotype in individuals with Williams Syndrome. *Child Neuropsychology,* 10:223–247.

Levitin, D. J., & Menon, V. (2003). Musical structure is processed in "language" areas of the brain: A possible role for Brodmann Area 47 in temporal coherence. *Neuro-Image,* 20:2141–2152.

Levitin, D. J., & Rogers, S. E. (2005). Absolute pitch: Perception, coding, and controversies. *Trends in Cognitive Sciences,* 9:26–33.

Levitin, D. J., & Zatorre, R. J. (2003). On the nature of early music training and absolute pitch: A reply to Brown, Sachs, Cammuso and Foldstein. *Music Perception,* 21:105–110.

Levy, M. (1982). *Intonation in North Indian Music: A Select Comparison of Theories With Contemporary Practice.* New Delhi, India: Biblia Impex.

Levy, R. (in press). Expectation-based syntactic comprehension. *Cognition.*

Lewis, R. L., Vasishth, S., & Van Dyke, J. A. (2006). Computational principles of working memory in sentence comprehension. *Trends in Cognitive Sciences,* 10:447–454.

Li, G. (2001). *Onomatopoeia and Beyond: A Study of the Luogu Jing of the Beijing Opera.* Ph.D. dissertation, University of California, Los Angeles.

Liberman, A. (1996). *Speech: A Special Code.* Cambridge, MA: MIT Press.

Liberman, A. M., Cooper, F. S., Shankweiler, D. P., & Studdert-Kennedy, M. (1967). Perception of the speech code. *Psychological Review,* 74:431–461.

Liberman, A. M., Harris, K. S., Hoffman, H., & B. Griffith. (1957). The discrimination of speech sounds within and across phoneme boundaries. *Journal of Experimental Psychology,* 54:358–368.

Liberman, M. (1975). *The Intonational System of English.* Ph.D. dissertation, Massachusetts Institute of Technology, Cambridge.

Liberman, M., & Pierrehumbert, J. (1984). Intonational invariance under changes in pitch range and length. In: M. Aronoff & R. Oerhle (Eds.), *Language Sound Structure* (pp. 157–233). Cambridge, MA: MIT Press.

Liberman, M., & Prince, A. (1977). On stress and linguistic rhythm. *Linguistic Inquiry,* 8:249–336.

Lieberman, P. (1967). *Intonation, Perception, and Language.* Cambridge, MA: MIT Press.

Lieberman, P. (1984). *The Biology and Evolution of Language.* Cambridge, MA: Harvard University Press.

Lieberman, P. (2000). *Human Language and Our Reptilian Brain: The Subcortical Bases of Speech, Syntax, and Thought.* Cambridge, MA: Harvard University Press.

Lieberman, P., Klatt, D. H., & Wilson, W. H. (1969). Vocal tract limitations on the vowel repertoires of rhesus monkeys and other nonhuman primates. *Science,* 164:1185–1187.

Liégeois, F., Baldeweg, T., Connelly, A., Gadian, D. G., Mishkin, M., & Vargha-Khadem, F. (2003). Language fMRI abnormalities associated with FOXP2 gene mutation. *Nature Neuroscience,* 6:1230–1237.

Liégeois-Chauvel, C., Peretz, I., Babaï, M., Laguitton, V., & Chauvel, P. (1998). Contribution of different cortical areas in the temporal lobes to music processing. *Brain,* 121:1853–1867.

Liljencrants, L., & Lindblom, B. (1972). Numerical simulations of vowel quality systems: The role of perceptual contrast, *Language,* 48: 839–862.

Lindblom, B. (1990). Explaining phonetic variation: A sketch of the H&H theory. In: W. J. Hardcastle & A. Marchal (Eds.), *Speech Production and Speech Modeling* (pp. 403–439). Dordrecht, The Netherlands: Kluwer.

Lively, S. E., & Pisoni, D. B. (1997). On prototypes and phonetic categories: A critical assessment of the perceptual magnet effect in speech perception. *Journal of Experimental Psychology: Human Perception and Performance*, 23:1665–79.

Lochy, A., Hyde, K. L., Parisel, S., Van Hyfte, S., & Peretz, I. (2004). *Discrimination of speech prosody in congenital amusia*. Poster presented at the 2004 meeting of the Cognitive Neuroscience Society, San Francisco.

Locke, D. (1982). Principles of offbeat timing and cross-rhythm in Southern Ewe dance drumming. *Ethnomusicology*, 26: 217–46.

Locke, D. (1990). *Drum Damba: Talking Drum Lessons*. Reno, NV: White Cliffs Media.

Locke, D., & Agbeli, G. K. (1980). A study of the drum language in Adzogbo. *Journal of the International Library of African Music*, 6:32–51.

Locke, J. L. (1993). *The Child's Path to Spoken Language*. Cambridge, MA: Harvard University Press.

Lockhead, G. R., & Byrd, R. (1981). Practically perfect pitch. *Journal of the Acoustical Society of America*, 70:387–389.

Löfqvist, A., Baer, T., McGarr, N. S., & Story, R. S. (1989). The cricothryroid muscle in voicing control. *Journal of the Acoustical Society of America*, 85:1314–1321.

London, J. (2002). Cognitive constraints on metric systems: Some observations and hypotheses. *Music Perception*, 19:529–550.

London, J. (2004). *Hearing in Time: Psychological Aspects of Musical Meter*. New York: Oxford University Press.

London, J. M. (1995). Some examples of complex meters and their implications for models of metric perception. *Music Perception*, 13:59–78.

Long, K. D., Kennedy, G., & Balaban, E. (2001). Transferring an inborn auditory perceptual predisposition with interspecies brain transplants. *Proceedings of the National Academy of Sciences, USA*, 98:5862–5867.

Long, K. D., Kennedy, G., Salbaum, M., & Balaban, E. (2002). Auditory stimulus-induced changes in immediate-early gene expression related to an inborn perceptual predisposition. *Journal of Comparative Physiology A: Sensory, Neural, and Behavioral Physiology*, 188:25–38.

Longacre, R. (1952). Five phonemic pitch levels in Trique. *Acta Linguistica* 7:62–82.

Longhi, E. (2003). *The Temporal Structure of Mother-Infant Interactions in Musical Contexts*. Ph.D. dissertation, University of Edinburgh, Scotland.

Lotto, A. J., Kluender, K. R., & Holt, L. L. (1998). Depolarizing the perceptual magnet effect. *Journal of the Acoustical Society of America*, 103:3648–3655.

Low, E. L., Grabe, E., & Nolan, F. (2000). Quantitative characterisations of speech rhythm: Syllable-timing in Singapore English. *Language and Speech*, 43:377–401.

Luce, P. A., & Lyons, E. A. (1998). Specificity of memory representations for spoken words. *Memory and Cognition*, 26:708–715.

Luce, P. A., & McLennan, C. T. (2005). Spoken word recognition: The challenge of variation. In: D. B. Pisoni & R. E. Remez (Eds.), *The Handbook of Speech Perception* (pp. 591–609). Malden, MA: Blackwell.

Luria, A. R., Tsvetkova, L. S., & Futer, D. S. (1965). Aphasia in a composer. *Journal of the Neurological Sciences*, 2:288–292.

Lynch, E. D., Lee, M. K., Morrow, J. E., Welcsh, P. L., Leon, P. E., & King, M. C. (1997). Nonsyndromic deafness DFNA1 associated with mutation of a human homolog of the *Drosophila* gene *diaphanous*. *Science*, 278:1315–1318.

Lynch, M. P., & Eilers, R. E. (1992). A study of perceptual development for musical tuning. *Perception and Psychophysics*, 52:599–608.

Lynch, M. P., Eilers, R. E., Oller, K., & Urbano, R. C. (1990). Innateness, experience, and music perception. *Psychological Science*, 1:272–276.

Lynch, M. P., Short, L. B., & Chua, R. (1995). Contributions of experience to the development of musical processing in infancy. *Developmental Psychobiology*, 28:377–398.

MacDonald, M. C., & Christiansen, M. H. (2002). Reassessing working memory: Comment on Just and Carpenter (1992) and Waters and Caplan (1996). *Psychological Review*, 109:35–54.

MacLarnon, A., & Hewitt, G. (1999). The evolution of human speech: The role of enhanced breathing control. *American Journal of Physical Anthropology*, 109:341–363.

Maddieson, I. (1978). Universals of tone. In: J. Greenberg (Ed.), *Universals of Language, Vol 2: Phonology* (pp. 335–365). Stanford, CA: Stanford University Press.

Maddieson, I. (1984). *Patterns of Sounds*. Cambridge, UK: Cambridge University Press.

Maddieson, I. (1991). Tone spacing. *York Papers in Linguistics*, 15:149–175.

Maddieson, I. (1999). In search of universals. *Proceedings of the14th International Congress of Phonetic Sciences, San Francisco*, pp. 2521–2528.

Maddieson, I. (2005). Tone. In: M. Haspelmath, M. S. Dryer, D. Gil, & B. Comrie (Eds.). *The World Atlas of Language Structures* (pp. 58–61). New York: Oxford University Press.

Maess, B., Koelsch, S., Gunter, T., & Friederici, A. D. (2001). Musical syntax is processed in Broca's area: An MEG study. *Nature Neuroscience*, 4:540–545.

Magne, C., Schön, D., & Besson, M. (2006). Musician children detect pitch violations in both music and language better than nonmusician children: Behavioral and electrophysiological approaches. *Journal of Cognitive Neuroscience*, 18:199–211.

Marcus, G. F., & Fisher, S. E. (2003). FOXP2 in focus: What can genes tell us about speech and language? *Trends in Cognitive Sciences*, 7:257–262.

Marcus, M., & Hindle, D. (1990). Description theory and intonational boundaries. In: G. T. M. Altmann, (Ed.). *Cognitive Models of Speech Processing* (pp. 483–512). Cambridge, MA: MIT Press.

Marin, O. S. M., & Perry, D. W. (1999). Neurological aspects of music perception and performance. In: D. Deutsch (Ed.), *The Psychology of Music* (2nd ed., pp. 653–724). San Diego, CA: Academic Press.

Marler, P. (1970). A comparative approach to vocal learning: Song development in white-crowned sparrows. *Journal of Comparative and Physiological Psychology*, 71:1–25.

Marler, P. (1991). Song-learning behavior: The interface with neuroethology. *Trends in Neurosciences*, 14:199–206.

Marler, P. (1997). Three models of song learning: Evidence from behavior. *Journal of Neurobiology*, 33:501–616.

Marler, P. (1999). On innateness: Are sparrow songs "learned" or "innate"? In: M. D. Hauser & M. Konishi (Eds.), *The Design of Animal Communication* (pp. 293–318). Cambridge, MA: MIT Press.

Marler, P. (2000). Origins of music and speech: Insights from animals. In: N. L. Wallin, B. Merker, & S.Brown, Eds. *The Origins of Music*. Cambridge, MA: MIT Press (pp. 31–48).

Marler, P., & Peters, S. (1977). Selective vocal learning in a sparrow. *Science*, 198:519–521.

Marslen-Wilson, W. (1975). Sentence perception as an interactive parallel process. *Science*, 189:382–386.

Martin, J. G. (1972). Rhythmic (hierarchical) versus serial structure in speech and other behavior. *Psychological Review*, 79:487–509.

Marvin, E., & Brinkman, A. (1999). The effect of modulation and formal manipulation on perception of tonal closure. *Music Perception*, 16:389–408.

Masataka, N. (1999). Preference for infant-directed singing in 2-day-old hearing infants of deaf parents. *Developmental Psychology*, 35:1001–1005.

Masataka, N. (2006). Preference for consonance over dissonance by hearing newborns of deaf parents and of hearing parents. *Developmental Science*, 9:46–50.

Mason, R. A., & Just, M. A. (2004). How the brain processes causal inferences in text. *Psychological Science*, 15:1–7.

Matell, M. S., & Meck, W. H. (2000). Neuropsychological mechanisms of interval timing behaviour. *BioEssays*, 22:94–103.

Mavlov, L. (1980). Amusia due to rhythm agnosia in a musician with left hemisphere damage: A non-auditory supramodal defect. *Cortex*, 16:331–338.

Mayberry, R. I., & Eichen, E. (1991). The long-lasting advantage of learning sign-language in childhood: Another look at the critical period for language acquisition. *Journal of Memory and Language*, 30:486–512.

Mayberry, R. I., & Lock, E. (2003). Age constraints on first versus second language acquisition: Evidence for linguistic plasticity and epigenesis. *Brain and Language*, 87:369–383.

Maye, J., & Weiss, D. J. (2003). Statistical cues facilitate infants' discrimination of difficult phonetic contrasts. In: B. Beachley et al. (Eds.), *BUCLD 27 Proceedings* (pp. 508–518). Somerville, MA: Cascadilla Press.

Maye, J., Weiss, D. J., & Aslin, R. (in press). Statistical phonetic learning in infants: Facilitation and feature generalization. *Developmental Science*.

Maye, J., Werker, J., & L. Gerken. (2002). Infant sensitivity to distributional information can affect phonetic discrimination. *Cognition*, 82:B101–B111.

McAdams, S. (1996). Audition: Cognitive psychology of music. In: R. Llinás & P. S. Churchland (Eds.), *The Mind-Brain Continuum: Sensory Processes* (pp. 251–279). Cambridge, MA: MIT Press.

McAdams, S., Beauchamp, J. M., & Meneguzzi, S. (1999). Discrimination of musical instrument sounds resynthesized with simplified spectrotemporal parameters. *Journal of the Acoustical Society of America*, 105:882–897.

McAdams, S., & Cunibile, J. C. (1992). Perception of timbral analogies. *Philosophical Transactions of the Royal Society, London, Series B*, 336:383–389.

McAdams, S., & Matzkin, D. (2001). Similarity, invariance, and musical variation. *Annals of the New York Academy of Sciences*, 930:62–76.

McAdams, S., Winsberg, S., Donnadieu, S., De Soete, G., & Krimphoff, J. (1995). Perceptual scaling of synthesized musical timbres: Common dimensions, specificities, and latent subject classes. *Psychological Research*, 58:177–192.

McDermott, J., & Hauser, M. (2004). Are consonant intervals music to their ears? Spontaneous acoustic preferences in a nonhuman primate. *Cognition,* 94:B11–B21.

McDermott, J., & Hauser, M. D. (2005). The origins of music: Innateness, development, and evolution. *Music Perception,* 23:29–59.

McKinney, M. F., & Delgutte, B. (1999). A possible neurophysiological basis of the octave enlargement effect. *Journal of the Acoustical Society of America,* 106:2679–92.

McLucas, A. (2001). Tune families. In: S. Sadie (Ed.), *The New Grove Dictionary of Music and Musicians* (Vol. 25, pp. 882–884). New York: Grove.

McMullen, E., & Saffran, J. R. (2004). Music and language: A developmental comparison. *Music Perception,* 21:289–311.

McNeill, W. H. (1995). *Keeping Together in Time: Dance and Drill in Human History.* Cambridge, MA: Harvard University Press.

McNellis, M. G., & Blumstein, S. E. (2001). Self-organizing dynamics of lexical access in normals and aphasics. *Journal of Cognitive Neuroscience,* 13:151–170.

McQueen, J. M., Norris, D., & Cutler, A. (2006). The dynamic nature of speech perception. *Language and Speech,* 49:101–112.

Mehler, J., Dommergues, J. Y., Frauenfelder, U., & Segui, J. (1981). The syllable's role in speech segmentation. *Journal of Verbal Learning and Verbal Behavior,* 20:298–305.

Mehler, J., Dupuox, E., Nazzi, T., & Dehaene-Lambertz, D. (1996). Coping with linguistic diversity: The infant's viewpoint. In: J. L. Morgan & D. Demuth (Eds.), *Signal to Syntax* (pp. 101–116). Mahwah, NJ: Lawrence Erlbaum.

Mehler, J., Jusczyk, P., Lambertz, G., Halsted, N., Bertoncini, J., & Amiel-Tison, C. (1988). A precursor to language acquisition in young infants. *Cognition,* 29:143–178.

Ménard, L., Schwartz, J.-L., & Boë, L.-J. (2004). Role of vocal tract morphology in speech development: Perceptual targets and sensorimotor maps for French synthesized vowels from birth to adulthood. *Journal of Speech, Language, and Hearing Research,* 47:1059–1080.

Menon, V., & Levitin, D. J. (2005). The rewards of music listening: Response and physiological connectivity of the mesolimbic system. *NeuroImage,* 28:175–184.

Menon, V., Levitin, D. J., Smith, B. K., Lembke, A., Krasnow, B. D., Glazer, D., Glover, G. H., & McAdams. S. (2002). Neural correlates of timbre change in harmonic sounds. *NeuroImage,* 17:1742–54.

Merker, B. (2000). Synchronous chorusing and human origins. In: N. L. Wallin, B. Merker, & S. Brown (Eds.), *The Origins of Music* (pp. 315–327). Cambridge, MA: MIT Press.

Merker, B. (2002). Music: The missing Humboldt system. *Musicae Scientiae,* 1:3–21.

Merker, B. (2005). The conformal motive in birdsong, music, and language: An introduction. *Annals of the New York Academy of Sciences,* 1060:17–28.

Mertens, P. (2004a). The prosogram: Semi-automatic transcription of prosody based on a tonal perception model. In: B. Bel & I. Marlien (Eds.), *Proceedings of Speech Prosody 2004, Nara (Japan), 23–26 March.*

Mertens, P. (2004b). Un outil pour la transcription de la prosodie dans les corpus oraux. *Traitement Automatique des Langues,* 45:109–130.

Meyer, J. (2004). Bioacoustics of human whistled languages: An alternative approach to the cognitive processes of language. *Anais da Academia Brasileira de Ciências* [Annals of the Brazilian Academy of Sciences], 76:405–412.

Meyer, L. B. (1956). *Emotion and Meaning in Music.* Chicago: University of Chicago Press.

Meyer, L. B. (1973). *Explaining Music: Essays and Explorations.* Berkeley: University of California Press.

Miller, G. (2000). Evolution of human music through sexual selection. In: N. L. Wallin, B. Merker, & S. Brown (Eds.), *The Origins of Music* (pp. 329–360). Cambridge, MA: MIT Press.

Miller, G. A. (1956). The magical number seven, plus or minus two: Some limits on our capacity for processing information. *Psychological Review,* 63:81–97.

Miller, L. K. (1989). *Musical Savants: Exceptional Skill in the Mentally Retarded.* Hillsdale, NJ: Erlbaum.

Miranda, R. A., & Ullman, M. T. (in press). Double dissociation between rules and memory in music: An event-related potential study. *NeuroImage.*

Mithen, S. (2005). *The Singing Neanderthals: The Origins of Music, Language, Mind and Body.* London: Weidenfeld & Nicolson.

Monelle, R. (2000). *The Sense of Music: Semiotic Essays.* Princeton, NJ: Princeton University Press.

Moon, C., Cooper, R. P., & Fifer, W. P. (1993). Two-day-olds prefer their native language. *Infant Behavior and Development,* 16:495–500.

Moore, B. C. J. (1997). Aspects of auditory processing related to speech perception. In: W. J. Hardcastle & J. Laver (Eds.), *The Handbook of Phonetic Sciences* (pp. 539–565). Oxford, UK: Blackwell.

Moore, B. C. J. (2001). Loudness, pitch, and timbre. In: E. B. Goldstein (Ed.), *Blackwell Handbook of Perception* (pp. 408–436). Malden, MA: Blackwell.

Moore, J. W., Choi, J.-S., & Brunzell, D. H. (1998). Predictive timing under temporal uncertainty: The time derivative model of the conditioned response. In: D. A. Rosenbaum & C. E. Collyer (Eds.), *Timing of Behavior: Neural, Psychological, and Computational Perspectives* (pp. 3–34). Cambridge, MA: MIT Press.

Morgan, J. L., Meier, R. P., & Newport, E. L. (1987). Structural packaging in the input to language learning: Contributions of prosodic and morphological marking of phrases in the acquisition of language. *Cognitive Psychology,* 19:498–550.

Morley, I. (2003). *The Evolutionary Origins and Archaeology of Music: An Investigation into the Prehistory of Human Musical Capacities and Behaviours.* Ph.D. dissertation, University of Cambridge.

Morrongiello, B. A. (1984). Auditory temporal pattern perception in 6- and 12-month-old infants. *Developmental Psychology,* 20:441–448.

Morrongiello, B. A., & Trehub, S. E. (1987). Age-related changes in auditory temporal perception. *Journal of Experimental Child Psychology,* 44:413–426.

Morton, D. (1974). Vocal tones in traditional Thai music. *Selected Reports of the Institute for Ethnomusicology,* 2:166–175.

Morton, J., Marcus, S., & Frankish, C. (1976). Perceptual centers (P centers). *Psychological Review,* 83:405–408.

Most, T., Amir, O., & Tobin, Y. (2000). The Hebrew vowels: Raw and normalized acoustic data. *Language and Speech,* 43:295–308.

Münte, T. F., Altenmüller, E., & Jäncke, L. (2002). The musician's brain as a model of neuroplasticity. *Nature Reviews (Neuroscience),* 3:473–478.

Myers, R. (1968). (Ed.). *Richard Strauss and Romain Rolland*. London: Calder & Boyars.

Näätänen, R. (1992). *Attention and Brain Function*. Hillsdale, NJ: Erlbaum.

Näätänen, R., Lehtokoksi, A., Lennes, M., et al. (1997). Language-specific phoneme representations revealed by electrical and magnetic brain responses. *Nature,* 385:432–434.

Näätänen, R., & Winker, I. (1999). The concept of auditory stimulus representation in cognitive neuroscience. *Psychological Bulletin,* 125:826–859.

Nadel, J., Carchon, I., Kervella, C., Marcelli, D., & Réserbat-Plantey, D. (1999). Expectancies for social contingency in 2-month-olds. *Developmental Science,* 2:164–173.

Nakata, T., & Trehub, S. E. (2004). Infants' responsiveness to maternal speech and singing. *Infant Behavior and Development,* 27:455–464.

Narayanan, S., & Jurafsky, D. (1998). Bayesian models of human sentence processing. In *Proceedings of the Twelfth Annual Meeting of the Cognitive Science Society.*

Narayanan, S., & Jurafsky, D. (2002). A Bayesian model predicts human parse preference and reading time in sentence processing. *Advances in Neural Information Processing Systems,* 14:59–65.

Narmour, E. (1990). *The Analysis and Cognition of Basic Melodic Structures: The Implication-Realization Model*. Chicago: University of Chicago Press.

Nattiez, J. J. (1990). *Music and Discourse: Toward a Semiology of Music* (C. Abate, Trans.). Princeton, NJ: Princeton University Press.

Nattiez, J. J. (2003). La signification comme parametre musical. In: J. J. Nattiez (Ed.)*Musique: Une Encyclopédie pour Le XXIe Siecle* (Vol. 2., pp. 256–289). Arles, France: Acte Sud/Cité de la Musique.

Nazzi, T., Bertoncini, J., & Mehler, J. (1998). Language discrimination in newborns: Toward an understanding of the role of rhythm. *Journal of Experimental Psychology: Human Perception and Performance,* 24:756–777.

Nazzi, T., Jusczyk, P. W., & Johnson, E. K. (2000). Language discrimination by English learning 5-month-olds: Effects of rhythm and familiarity. *Journal of Memory and Language,* 43:1–19.

Nearey, T. (1978). *Phonetic Features for Vowels*. Bloomington: Indiana University Linguistics Club.

Nespor, M. (1990). On the rhythm parameter in phonology. In: I. Rocca (Ed.), *Logical Issues in Language Acquisition* (pp. 157–175). Dordrecht, The Netherlands: Foris Publications.

Nespor, M., & Vogel, I. (1983). Prosodic structure above the word. In: A. Cutler & D. R. Ladd (Eds.), *Prosody: Models and Measurements*. Berlin, Germany: Springer-Verlag.

Nespor, M., & Vogel, I. (1989). On clashes and lapses. *Phonology,* 6:69–116.

Nettl, B. (1954). North American Indian musical styles. *Memoirs of the American Folklore Society* (Vol. 45). Philadelphia: American Folklore Society.

Nettl, B. (2000). An ethnomusicologist contemplates universals in musical sound and musical culture. In: N. L. Wallin, B. Merker, & S. Brown (Eds.), *The Origins of Music* (pp. 463–472). Cambridge, MA: MIT Press.

Neubauer, J. (1986). *The Emancipation of Music From Language: Departure From Mimesis in Eighteenth-Century Aesthetics*. New Haven, CT: Yale University Press.

Newport, E. (2002). Language development, critical periods in. In: L. Nadel (Ed.), *Encyclopedia of Cognitive Science* (pp. 737–740). London: MacMillan Publishers Ltd./Nature Group.

Newport, E. L., Hauser, M. D., Spaepen, G., & Aslin, R. N. (2004). Learning at a distance: II. Statistical learning of non-adjacent dependencies in a non-human primate. *Cognitive Psychology*, 49:85–117.

Nicholson, K. G., Baum, S., Kilgour, A., Koh, C. K., Munhall, K. G., & Cuddy, L. L. (2003). Impaired processing of prosodic and musical patterns after right hemisphere damage. *Brain and Cognition*, 52:382–389.

Nielzén, S., & Cesarec, Z. (1981). On the perception of emotional meaning in music. *Psychology of Music*, 9:17–31.

Nketia, K. J. H. (1974). *The Music of Africa*. New York: W. W. Norton.

Noad, M. J., Cato, D. H., Bryden, M. M., Jenner, M.-N., & Jenner, K. C. S. (2000). Cultural revolution in whale songs. *Nature*, 408:537.

Nolan, F. (2003). Intonational equivalence: An experimental evaluation of pitch scales. *Proceedings of the 15th International Congress of Phonetic Sciences, Barcelona*, pp. 771–774.

Nord, L., Krukenberg, A., & Fant, G. (1990). Some timing studies of prose, poetry and music. *Speech Communication*, 9:477–483.

North, A. C., Hargreaves, D. J., & McKendrick, J. (1999). The influence of in-store music on wine selections. *Journal of Applied Psychology*, 84:271–276.

North, A. C., Hargreaves, D. J., & O'Neill, S. A. (2000). The importance of music to adolescents. *British Journal of Educational Psychology*, 70:255–272.

Norton, A., Winner, E., Cronin, K., Overy, K., Lee, D. J., & Schlaug, G. (2005). Are there pre-existing neural, cognitive, or motoric markers for musical ability? *Brain and Cognition*, 59:124–134.

Nyklíček, I., Thayer, J. F., & van Doornen, L. J. P. (1997). Cardiorespiratory differentiation of musically-induced emotions. *Journal of Psychophysiology*, 11:304–321.

Ochs, E., & Schieffelin, B. (1984). Language acquisition and socialization. In: R. A. Shweder & R. A. Levine (Eds.), *Culture Theory: Essays on Mind, Self, and Emotion* (pp. 276–320). New York: Cambridge University Press.

Oh, J. S., Jun, S.-A., Knightly, L. M., & Au, T. K.-F. (2003). Holding on to childhood language memory. *Cognition*, 86:53–64.

Ohala, J. J. (1983). Cross-language use of pitch: An ethological view. *Phonetica*, 40:1–18.

Ohala, J. J. (1984). An ethological perspective on common cross-language utilization of F0 of voice. *Phonetica*, 41:1–16.

Ohala, J. J. (1994). The frequency code underlies the sound-symbolic use of voice pitch. In: L. Hinton, J. Nichols, & J. Ohala (Eds.), *Sound Symbolism* (pp. 325–347). Cambridge, UK: Cambridge University Press.

Ohgushi, K. (2002). Comparison of dotted rhythm expression between Japanese and Western pianists. In: C. Steven et al. (Eds.), *Proceedings of the 7th International Conference on Music Perception and Cognition, Sydney* (pp. 250–253). Adelaide, Australia: Causal Productions.

Ohl, F. W., Schulze, H., Scheich, H., & Freeman, W. J. (2000). Spatial representation of frequency-modulated tones in gerbil auditory cortex revealed by epidural electrocorticography. *Journal of Physiology–Paris*, 94:549–554.

Oller, K., & Eilers, R. E. (1988). The role of audition in infant babbling. *Child Development,* 59:441–466.

Oohashi, T., Kawai, N., Honda, M., Nakamura, S., Morimoto, M., Nishina, E., & Maekawa, T. (2002). Electroencephalographic measurement of possession trance in the field. *Clinical Neurophysiology,* 113:435–45.

Oram, N., & Cuddy, L. L. (1995). Responsiveness of Western adults to pitch-distributional information in melodic sequences. *Psychological Research,* 57:103–18.

Ortony, A., & Turner, T. J. (1990). What's basic about basic emotions? *Psychological Review,* 97:315–331.

Osterhout, L., & Holcomb, P. J. (1992). Event-related potentials elicited by syntactic anomaly. *Journal of Memory and Language,* 31:785–806.

Osterhout, L., & Holcomb, P. J. (1993). Event-related potential and syntactic anomaly: Evidence of anomaly detection during the perception of continuous speech. *Language and Cognitive Processes,* 8:413–437.

Otake, T., Hatano, G., Cutler, A., & Mehler, J. (1993). Mora or syllable? Speech segmentation in Japanese. *Journal of Memory and Language,* 32:258–278.

Overy, K. (2003). Dyslexia and music: From timing deficits to musical intervention. *Annals of the New York Academy of Sciences,* 999:497–505.

Paavilainen, P., Jaramillo, M., Näätänen, R., & Winkler, I. (1999). Neuronal populations in the human brain extracting invariant relationships from acoustic variance. *Neuroscience Letters* 265:179–182.

Pallier, C., Sebastian-Gallés, N., Felguera, T., Christophe, A., & Mehler, J. (1993). Attentional allocation within syllabic structure of spoken words. *Journal of Memory and Language,* 32:373–389.

Palmer, C. (1996). On the assignment of structure in music performance. *Music Perception,* 14:23–56.

Palmer, C. (1997). Music performance. *Annual Review of Psychology,* 48:115–138.

Palmer, C., Jungers, M., & Jusczyk, P. (2001). Episodic memory for musical prosody. *Journal of Memory and Language,* 45:526–545.

Palmer, C., & Kelly, M. H. (1992). Linguistic prosody and musical meter in song. *Journal of Memory and Language,* 31:525–542.

Palmer, C., & Krumhansl, C .L. (1990). Mental representations for musical meter. *Journal of Experimental Psychology: Human Perception and Performance,* 16:728–741.

Palmer, C., & Pfordresher, P. Q. (2003). Incremental planning in sequence production. *Psychological Review,* 110:683–712.

Panksepp, J. (1998). *Affective Neuroscience: The Foundations of Human and Animal Emotions.* New York: Oxford University Press.

Pannekamp, A., Toepel, U., Alter, K., Hahne, A., Friederici, A. D. (2005). Prosody driven sentence processing: An ERP study. *Journal of Cognitive Neuroscience,* 17:407–421.

Pantaleoni, H. (1985). *On the Nature of Music.* Oneonta, New York: Welkin Books.

Pantev, C., Oostenveld, R., Engelien, A., Ross, B., Roberts, L. E., & Hoke, M. (1998). Increased auditory cortical representation in musicians. *Nature,* 392:811–814.

Pantev, C., Roberts, L. E., Schulz, M., Engelien, A., & Ross, B. (2001). Timbre-specific enhancement of auditory cortical representations in musicians. *Neuroreport,* 12:169–174.

Papousek, M. (1996). Intuitive parenting: A hidden source of musical stimulation in infancy. In: I. Deliège & J. Sloboda (Eds.), *Musical Beginnings: Origins and Development of Musical Competence* (pp. 88–112). New York: Oxford University Press.

Papousek, M., Bornstein, M. H., Nuzzo, C., Papousek, H., & Symmes, D. (1990). Infant responses to prototypical melodic contours in parental speech. *Infant Behavior and Development*, 13:539–545.

Park, T., & Balaban, E. (1991). Relative salience of species maternal calls in neonatal gallinaceous birds: A direct comparison of Japanese quail (*Coturnix coturnix japonica*) and domestic chickens (*Gallus gallus domesticus*). *Journal of Comparative Psychology*, 105:45–54.

Parncutt, R. (1989). *Harmony: A Psychoacoustical Approach*. Berlin: Springer-Verlag.

Parncutt, R. (1994). A perceptual model of pulse salience and metrical accent in musical rhythms. *Music Perception*, 11:409–464.

Parncutt, R., & Bregman, A. (2000). Tone profiles following short chord progressions: Top-down or bottom up? *Music Perception*, 18:25–58.

Partch, H. (1974). *Genesis of a Music*. New York: Da Capo Press.

Partch, H. (1991). *Bitter Music*. (T. McGeary, Ed.). Urbana: University of Illinois Press.

Partee, B. (1995). Lexical semantics and compositionality. In: D. Osherson (Gen. Ed.), *An Invitation to Cognitive Science. Part I: Language* (2nd ed, pp. 311–360). Cambridge, MA: MIT Press.

Pascual-Leone, A. (2003). The brain that makes music and is changed by it. In: I. Peretz & R. Zatorre (Eds.), *The Cognitive Neuroscience of Music* (pp. 396–409). New York: Oxford University Press.

Pastore, R. E., Schmuckler, M. A., Rosenblum, L., & Szczesiul, R. (1983). Duplex perception with musical stimuli. *Perception and Psychophysics*, 33:469–474.

Patel, A. D. (2003a). A new approach to the cognitive neuroscience of melody. In: I. Peretz & R. Zatorre (Eds.), *The Cognitive Neursocience of Music* (pp. 325–345). Oxford, UK: Oxford University Press.

Patel, A. D. (2003b). Language, music, syntax, and the brain. *Nature Neuroscience*, 6:674–681.

Patel, A. D. (2005). The relationship of music to the melody of speech and to syntactic processing disorders in aphasia. *Annals of the New York Academy of Sciences*, 1060:59–70.

Patel, A. D. (2006a). An empirical method for comparing pitch patterns in spoken and musical melodies: A comment on J. G. S. Pearl's "Eavesdropping with a master: Leoš Janáček and the music of speech." *Empirical Musicology Review*, 1:166–169.

Patel, A. D. (2006b). *Music and the Mind*. Lecture given in the UCSD Grey Matters series. Available to view at: http://www.ucsd.tv/search-details.asp?showID=11189 or via YouTube.

Patel, A. D. (2006c). Musical rhythm, linguistic rhythm, and human evolution. *Music Perception*, 24:99–104.

Patel, A. D., & Balaban, E. (2000). Temporal patterns of human cortical activity reflect tone sequence structure. *Nature*, 404:80–84.

Patel, A. D., & Balaban, E. (2001). Human pitch perception is reflected in the timing of stimulus-related cortical activity. *Nature Neuroscience*, 4:839–844.

Patel, A. D., & Daniele, J. R. (2003a). An empirical comparison of rhythm in language and music. *Cognition*, 87:B35–B45.

Patel, A. D., & Daniele, J. R. (2003b). Stress-timed vs. syllable-timed music? A comment on Huron and Ollen (2003). *Music Perception*, 21:273–276.

Patel, A. D., Foxton, J. M., & Griffiths, T. D. (2005). Musically tone-deaf individuals have difficulty discriminating intonation contours extracted from speech. *Brain and Cognition*, 59:310–313.

Patel, A. D., Gibson, E., Ratner, J., Besson, M., & Holcomb, P. (1998). Processing syntactic relations in language and music: An event-related potential study. *Journal of Cognitive Neuroscience*, 10:717–733.

Patel, A. D., & Iversen, J. R. (2003). Acoustic and perceptual comparison of speech and drum sounds in the North Indian tabla tradition: An empirical study of sound symbolism. *Proceedings of the 15th International Congress of Phonetic Sciences, Barcelona*, pp. 925–928.

Patel, A. D., & Iversen, J. R. (2006). A non-human animal can drum a steady beat on a musical instrument. In: M. Baroni, A. R. Addessi, R. Caterina, M. Costa, *Proceedings of the 9th International Conference on Music Perception and Cognition (ICMPC9)*, Bologna/Italy, p. 477.

Patel, A. D., & Iversen, J. R. (2007). The linguistic benefits of musical abilities. *Trends in Cognitive Sciences*, 11:369–372.

Patel, A. D., Iversen, J. R., Chen, Y. C., & Repp, B. R. (2005). The influence of metricality and modality on synchronization with a beat. *Experimental Brain Research*, 163:226–238.

Patel, A. D., Iversen, J. R., & Rosenberg, J. C. (2006). Comparing the rhythm and melody of speech and music: The case of British English and French. *Journal of the Acoustical Society of America*, 119:3034–3047.

Patel, A. D., Iversen, J. R., Wassenaar, M., & Hagoort, P. (2008). Musical syntactic processing in agrammatic Broca's aphasia. *Aphasiology*, 22:776–780.

Patel, A. D., Löfqvist, A., & Naito, W. (1999). The acoustics and kinematics of regularly-timed speech: A database and method for the study of the P-center problem. *Proceedings of the 14th International Conference of Phonetic Sciences, 1999, San Francisco*, 1:405–408.

Patel, A. D., Peretz, I., Tramo, M., & Labrecque, R. (1998). Processing prosodic and musical patterns: A neuropsychological investigation. *Brain and Language*, 61:123–144.

Patel, A. D., Wong, M., Foxton, J., Lochy, A., & Peretz, I. (in press). Linguistic intonation perception deficits in musical tone deafness. *Music Perception*.

Payne, K. (2000). The progressively changing songs of humpback whales: A window on the creative process in a wild animal. In: N. L. Wallin, B. Merker, & S. Brown (Eds.), *The Origins of Music* (pp. 135–150). Cambridge, MA: MIT Press.

Pearl, J. (2006). Eavesdropping with a master: Leoš Janáček and the music of speech. *Empirical Musicology Review*, 1:131–165.

Penman, J., & Becker, J. (submitted). Religious ecstatics, "deep listeners," and musical emotion.

Pepperberg, I. M. (2002). *The Alex Studies: Cognitive and Communicative Abilities of Grey Parrots*. Cambridge, MA: Harvard University Press.

Peretz, I. (1989). Clustering in music: An appraisal of task factors. *International Journal of Psychology*, 24:157–178.

Peretz, I. (1990). Processing of local and global musical information by unilateral brain-damaged patients. *Brain*, 113:1185–1205.

Peretz, I. (1993). Auditory atonalia for melodies. *Cognitive Neuropsychology*, 10:21–56.

Peretz, I. (1996). Can we lose memory for music? A case of music agnosia in a nonmusician. *Journal of Cognitive Neuroscience*, 8:481–496.

Peretz, I. (2001). Listen to the brain: A biological perspective on musical emotions. In: P. N. Juslin & J. A. Sloboda (Eds.), *Music and Emotion: Theory and Research* (pp. 105–134). Oxford, UK: Oxford University Press.

Peretz, I. (2006). The nature of music from a biological perspective. *Cognition*, 100:1–32.

Peretz, I., Ayotte, J., Zatorre, R., Mehler, J., Ahad, P., Penhune, V., & Jutras, B. (2002). Congenital amusia: A disorder of fine-grained pitch discrimination. *Neuron*, 33:185–191.

Peretz, I., Brattico, E., & Tervaniemi, M. (2005). Abnormal electrical brain responses to pitch in congenital amusia. *Annals of Neurology*, 58:478–482.

Peretz, I., & Coltheart, M. (2003). Modularity of music processing. *Nature Neuroscience*, 6:688–691.

Peretz, I., Gagnon, L., & Bouchard, B. (1998). Music and emotion: Perceptual determinants, immediacy, and isolation after brain damage. *Cognition*, 68:111–141.

Peretz, I., Gagnon, L., Hébert, S., & Macoir, J. (2004). Singing in the brain: Insights from cognitive neuropsychology. *Music Perception*, 21:373–390.

Peretz, I., Gaudreau, D., & Bonnel, A.-M. (1998). Exposure effects on music preference and recognition. *Memory and Cognition*, 26:884–902.

Peretz, I., & Hyde, K. L. (2003). What is specific to music processing? Insights from congenital amusia. *Trends in Cognitive Sciences*, 7:362–367.

Peretz, I., Kolinsky, R., Tramo, M., Labrecque, R., Hublet, C., Demeurisse, G., & Belleville, S. (1994). Functional dissociations following bilateral lesions of auditory cortex. *Brain*, 117:1283–1302.

Perlman, M. (1997). The ethnomusicology of performer interaction in improvised ensemble music: A review of two recent studies. *Music Perception*, 15:99–118.

Perlman, M., & Krumhansl, C. L. (1996). An experimental study of internal interval standards in Javanese and Western musicians. *Music Perception*, 14:95–116.

Pesetsky, D. (2007). Music syntax is language syntax. Paper presented at "Language and Music as Cognitive Systems," May 11–13, Cambridge University, UK.

Peterson, G. E., & Barney, H. L. (1952). Control methods used in a study of the vowels. *Journal of the Acoustical Society of America*, 24:175–184.

Peterson, G. E., & Lehiste, I. (1960). Duration of syllable nuclei in English. *Journal of the Acoustical Society of America*, 32:693–703.

Petitto, L. A., Holowka, S., Sergio, L. E., Levy, B., & Ostry, D. J. (2004). Baby hands that move to the rhythm of language: Hearing babies acquiring sign language babble silently on the hands. *Cognition*, 93:43–73.

Petitto, L. A., Holowka, S., Sergio, L., & Ostry, D. (2001). Language rhythms in babies' hand movements. *Nature*, 413:35–36.

Petitto, L. A., & Marentette, P. (1991). Babbling in the manual mode: Evidence for the ontogeny of language. *Science*, 251:1483–1496.

Phillips, C., Pellathy, T., Marantz, A., Yellin, E., Wexler, K., Poeppel, D., McGinnis, M., & Roberts, T. P. L. (2000). Auditory cortex accesses phonological categories: An MEG mismatch study. *Journal of Cognitive Neuroscience*, 12:1038–1055.

Phillips-Silver, J., & Trainor, L. J. (2005). Feeling the beat in music: Movement influences rhythm perception in infants. *Science,* 308:1430.

Pierrehumbert, J. (1979). The perception of fundamental frequency declination. *Journal of the Acoustical Society of America,* 66:363–369.

Pierrehumbert, J. (1980). *The Phonetics and Phonology of English Intonation.* Ph.D. dissertation, Massachusetts Institute of Technology. [Reprinted by Indiana University Linguistics Club, 1987].

Pierrehumbert, J. (2000). Tonal elements and their alignment. In: M. Horne (Ed.), *Prosody: Theory and Experiment* (pp. 11–36). Dordrecht, The Netherlands: Kluwer.

Pierrehumbert, J., & Hirschberg, J. (1990). The meaning of intonational contours in the interpretation of discourse. In: P. Cohen, J. Morgan, & M. Pollack, (Eds.), *Intentions in Communication* (pp. 271–311). Cambridge, MA: MIT Press.

Pierrehumbert, J., & Steele, J. (1989). Categories of tonal alignment in English. *Phonetica,* 46:181–196.

Pike, K. N. (1945). *The Intonation of American English.* Ann Arbor: University of Michigan Press.

Pilon, R. (1981). Segmentation of speech in a foreign language. *Journal of Psycholinguistic Research,* 10:113–121.

Pinker, S. (1997). *How the Mind Works.* London: Allen Lane.

Pinker, S., & Jackendoff, R. (2005). The faculty of language: What's special about it? *Cognition,* 95:201–236.

Piske, T., MacKay, I., & Flege, J. (2001). Factors affecting degree of foreign accent in an L2: A review. *Journal of Phonetics,* 29:191–215.

Pisoni, D. B. (1977). Identification and discrimination of the relative onset time of two component tones: Implications for voicing perception in stops. *Journal of the Acoustic Society of America,* 61: 1352–1361.

Pisoni, D. B. (1997). Some thoughts on "normalization" in speech perception. In: K. Johnson & J. W. Mullennix (Eds.), *Talker Variability in Speech Processing* (pp. 9–32). San Diego, CA: Academic Press.

Piston, W. (1987). *Harmony* (5th ed., revised and expanded by M. DeVoto). New York: Norton.

Pitt, M. A., & Samuel, A. G. (1990). The use of rhythm in attending to speech. *Journal of Experimental Psychology: Human Perception and Performance,* 16:564–573.

Plack, C. J., Oxenham, A. J., Fay, R. R., & Popper, A. N. (Eds.). (2005). *Pitch: Neural Coding and Perception.* Berlin, Germany: Springer.

Plantinga, J., & Trainor, L. J. (2005). Memory for melody: Infants use a relative pitch code. *Cognition,* 98:1–11.

Plomp, R., & Levelt, W. J. M. (1965). Tonal consonance and critical bandwith. *Journal of the Acoustical Society of America* 38:548–560.

Poeppel, D. (2001). Pure word deafness and the bilateral processing of the speech code. *Cognitive Science,* 25:679–693.

Poeppel, D. (2003). The analysis of speech in different temporal integration windows: Cerebral lateralization as "asymmetric sampling in time." *Speech Communication,* 41:245–255.

Polka, L., Colantonio, C., & Sundara, M. (2001). A cross-language comparison of /d/~/D/ discrimination: Evidence for a new developmental pattern. *Journal of the Acoustical Society of America,* 109:2190–2201.

Poulin-Charronnat, B., Bigand, E., & Koelsch, S. (2006). Processing of musical syntax tonic versus subdominant: An event-related potential study. *Journal of Cognitive Neuroscience,* 18:1545–1554.

Poulin-Charronnat, B., Bigand, E., Madurell, F., & Peereman, R. (2005). Musical structure modulates semantic priming in vocal music. *Cognition,* 94:B67–78.

Pouthas, V. (1996). The development of the perception of time and temporal regulation of action in infants and children. In: I. Deliège & J. Sloboda (Eds.), *Musical Beginnings* (pp. 115–141). Oxford, UK: Oxford University Press.

Povel, D. J., & Essens, P. (1985). Perception of temporal patterns. *Music Perception,* 2:411–440.

Povel, D. J., & Jansen, E. (2001). Perceptual mechanisms in music processing. *Music Perception,* 19:169–197.

Povel, D. J., & Okkerman, H. (1981). Accents in equitone sequences. *Perception and Psychophysics,* 30:565–572.

Powers, H. S. (1980). Language models and music analysis. *Ethnomusicology,* 24:1–61.

Pressing, J. (2002). Black Atlantic rhythm: Its computational and transcultural foundations. *Music Perception,* 3:285–310.

Price, C. J., & Friston, K. J. (1997). Cognitive conjunction: A new approach to brain activation experiments. *NeuroImage,* 5:261–270.

Price, P., Ostendorf, M., Shattuck-Hufnagel, S., & Fong, C. (1991). The use of prosody in syntactic disambiguation. *Journal of the Acoustical Society of America,* 90:2956–2970.

Profita, J., & Bidder, T. G. (1988). Perfect pitch. *American Journal of Medical Genetics,* 29:763–71.

Provine, R. R. (1992). Contagious laughter: Laughter is a sufficient stimulus for laughs and smiles. *Bulletin of the Psychonomic Society,* 30:1–4.

Pullum, G. (1991). *The Great Eskimo Vocabulary Hoax, and Other Irreverent Essays on the Study of Language.* Chicago: University of Chicago Press.

Pyers, J. (2006). Constructing the social mind: Language and false-belief understanding. In: N. Enfield & S. C. Levinson (Eds.), *Roots of Human Sociality: Culture, Cognition, and Interaction.* Oxford: Berg.

Racette, A., Bard, C., & Peretz, I. (2006). Making non-fluent aphasics speak: Sing along! *Brain,* 129:2571–2584.

Raffman, D. (1993). *Language, Music, and Mind.* Cambridge, MA: MIT Press.

Rakowski, A. (1990). Intonation variants of musical intervals in isolation and in musical contexts. *Psychology of Music,* 18:60–72.

Rameau, J.-P. (1722/1971). *Treatise on Harmony* (P. Gossett, Trans.). New York: Dover.

Ramus, F. (2002a). Acoustic correlates of linguistic rhythm: Perspectives. In: B. Bell & I. Marlien (Eds.), *Proceedings of Speech Prosody, Aix-en-Provence* (pp. 115–120). Aix-en-Provence, France: Laboratoire Parole et Langage.

Ramus, F. (2002b). Language discrimination by newborns: Teasing apart phonotactic, rhythmic, and intonational cues. *Annual Review of Language Acquisition,* 2:85–115.

Ramus, F. (2003). Dyslexia: Specific phonological deficit or general sensorimotor dysfunction? *Current Opinion in Neurobiology,* 13:212–218.

Ramus, F. (2006). A neurological model of dyslexia and other domain-specific developmental disorders with an associated sensorimotor syndrome. In: G. D. Rosen

(Ed.), *The Dsylexic Brain: New Pathways in Neuroscience Discovery* (pp. 75–101). Mahwah, NJ: Lawrence Erlbaum.

Ramus, F., Dupoux, E., & Mehler, J. (2003). The psychological reality of rhythm classes: Perceptual studies. *Proceedings of the 15th International Congress of Phonetic Sciences, Barcelona*, pp. 337–342.

Ramus, F., Hauser, M. D., Miller, C., Morris, D., & Mehler, J. (2000). Language discrimination by human newborns and by cotton-top tamarin monkeys. *Science*, 288, 349–351.

Ramus, F., & Mehler, J. (1999). Language identification with suprasegmental cues: A study based on speech resynthesis. *Journal of the Acoustical Society of America*, 105:512–521.

Ramus, F., Nespor, M., & Mehler, J. (1999). Correlates of linguistic rhythm in the speech signal. *Cognition*, 73:265–292.

Randel, D. M. (1978). *Harvard Concise Dictionary of Music*. Cambridge, MA: Harvard University Press.

Rantala, V., Rowell, L., & Tarasti, E. (Eds.). (1988). *Essays on the Philosophy of Music, Acta Philosophica Fennica* (Vol. 43). Helsinki: The Philosophical Society of Finland.

Ratner, L. (1980). *Classic Music: Expression, Form, and Style*. New York: Schirmer Books.

Rauschecker, J. P. (1998a). Cortical processing of complex sounds. *Current Opinion in Neurobioliology*, 8:516–521.

Rauschecker, J. P. (1998b). Parallel processing in the auditory cortex of primates. *Audiology and Neuro-Otology*, 3:86– 103.

Reck, D. (1997). *Music of the Whole Earth*. New York: Da Capo Press.

Redi, L. (2003). Categorical effects in production of pitch contours in English. *Proceedings of the 15th International Congress of Phonetic Sciences, Barcelona*, pp. 2921–2924.

Regnault, P., Bigand, E., & Besson, M. (2001). Different brain mechanisms mediate sensitivity to sensory consonance and harmonic context: Evidence from auditory event related brain potentials. *Journal of Cognitive Neuroscience*, 13:241–255.

Remez, R. E., Rubin, P. E., Berns, S. M., Pardo, J. S., & Lang, J. M. (1994). On the perceptual organization of speech. *Psychological Review*, 101:129–156.

Remez, R. E., Rubin, P. E., Pisoni, D. B., & Carrell, T. D. (1981). Speech perception without traditional speech cues. *Science*, 212:947–950.

Repp, B. H. (1984). Categorical perception: Issues, methods, findings. In N. J. Lass (Ed.), *Speech and language: Advances in basic research and practice* (Vol. 10, pp. 243–335). New York: Academic Press.

Repp, B. H. (1992a). Probing the cognitive representation of musical time: Structural constraints on the perception of timing perturbations. *Cognition*, 44:241–281.

Repp, B. H. (1992b). Diversity and commonality in music performance: An analysis of timing microstructure in Schumann's "Träumerei." *Journal of the Acoustical Society of America*, 92:2546–2568.

Repp, B. H., & Williams, D. R. (1987). Categorical tendencies in imitating self-produced isolated vowels. *Speech Communication*, 6:1–14.

Rialland, A. (2003). A new perspective on Silbo Gomero. *Proceedings of the 15th International Congress of Phonetic Sciences, Barcelona*, pp. 2131–2134.

Rialland, A. (2005). Phonological and phonetic aspects of whistled languages. *Phonology*, 22:237–271.

Richard, P. (1972). A quantitative analysis of the relationship between language tone and melody in a Hausa song. *African Language Studies*, 13:137–161.

Richards, I. A. (1979). Rhythm and metre. In: H. Gross (Ed.), *The Structure of Verse* (2nd ed., pp. 68–76). New York: Ecco Press.

Richter, D., Waiblinger, J., Rink, W. J., & Wagner, G. A. (2000). Thermoluminescence, electron spin resonance and C-14-dating of the late middle and early upper palaeolithic site of Geissenklosterle Cave in southern Germany. *Journal of Archaeological Science*, 27:71–89.

Rimland, B., & Fein, D. (1988). Special talents of autistic savants. In: L. K.Obler & D. Fein (Eds.), *The Exceptional Brain: The Neuropsychology of Talent and Special Abilities* (pp. 474–492). New York: Guilford.

Ringer, A. L. (2001). Melody. In: S. Sadie (Ed.), *The New Grove Dictionary of Music and Musicians* (Vol. 16, pp. 363–373). New York: Grove.

Risset, J.-C. (1991). Speech and music combined: An overview. In: J. Sundberg, L. Nord, & R. Carlson (Eds.), *Music, Language, Speech and Brain* (pp. 368–379). London: Macmillan.

Risset, J.-C., & Wessel, D. (1999). Exploration of timbre by analysis and synthesis. In: D. Deutsch (Ed.), *The Psychology of Music* (2nd ed., pp. 113–169). San Diego.CA: Academic Press.

Rivenez, M., Gorea, A., Pressnitzer, D., & Drake, C. (2003). The tolerance window for sequences of musical, environmental, and artificial sounds. *Proceedings of the 7th International Conference on Music Perception and Cognition, Sydney*, pp. 560–563.

Roach, P. (1982). On the distinction between "stress-timed" and "syllable-timed" languages. In: D. Crystal (Ed.), *Linguistic Controversies: Essays in Linguistic Theory and Practice in Honour of F. R. Palmer* (pp. 73–79). London: Edward Arnold.

Rohrmeier, M. (2007). A generative approach to diatonic harmonic structure. In: *Proceedings of the 4th Sound and Music Computing Conference, Lefkada, Greece*, pp. 97–100.

Römer, H., Hedwig, B., & Ott, S. R. (2002). Contralateral inhibition as a sensory bias: The neural basis for a female preference in a synchronously calling bushcricket, *Mecopoda elongata. European Journal of Neuroscience*, 15:1655–1662.

Rosch, E. (1973). Natural categories. *Cognitive Psychology*, 4:328–350.

Rosch, E. (1975). Cognitive reference points. *Cognitive Psychology*, 7:532–547.

Rosen, S. (2003). Auditory processing in dyslexia and specific language impairment: Is there a deficit? What is its nature? Does it explain anything? *Journal of Phonetics*, 31:509–527.

Rosen, S., & Howell, P. (1991). *Signals and Systems for Speech and Hearing*. San Diego, CA: Academic Press.

Ross, D. A., Olson, I. R., & Gore, J. C. (2003). Absolute pitch does not depend on early musical training. *Annals of the New York Academy of Sciences*, 999:522–526.

Ross, E. (1981). The aprosodias: Functional-anatomic organization of the affective components of language in the right hemisphere. *Archives of Neurology*, 38:561–569.

Ross, E. (2000). Affective prosody and the aprosodias. In: M.-M. Mesulaum (Ed.), *Principles of Behavioral and Cognitive Neurology*, (pp. 316–331). Oxford, UK: Oxford University Press.

Ross, J. (1989). A study of timing in an Estonian runic song. *Journal of the Acoustical Society of America*, 86:1671–1677.

Ross, J., & Lehiste, I. (2001). *The Temporal Structure of Estonian Runic Songs*. Berlin, Germany: Mouton de Gruyter.

Ross, J. M., & Lehiste, I. (1998). Timing in Estonian folksongs as interaction between speech prosody, metre, and musical rhythm. *Music Perception*, 15:319–333.

Rossi, M. (1971). Le seuil de glissando ou seuil de perception des variations tonales pour la parole. *Phonetica*, 23:1–33.

Rossi, M. (1978a). La perception des glissandos descendants dans les contours prosodiques. *Phonetica*, 35:11–40.

Rossi, M. (1978b). Interactions of intensity glides and frequency glissandos. *Language and Speech*, 21:384–396.

Rothstein, E. (1996). *Emblems of Mind: The Inner Life of Music and Mathematics*. New York: Avon Books.

Russell, J. A. (1989). Measures of emotion. In: R. Plutchik & H. Kellerman (Eds.), *Emotion: Theory Research and Experience* (Vol. 4, pp. 81–111). New York: Academic Press.

Russolo, L. (1986). *The Art of Noises*. New York: Pendragon Press.

Rymer, R. (1993). *Genie: A Scientific Tragedy*. New York: Harper Perennial.

Sacks, O. (1984). *A Leg to Stand On*. New York: Summit Books.

Sacks, O. (2007). *Musicophilia: Tales of Music and the Brain*. New York: Knopf.

Sadakata, M., Ohgushi, K., & Desain, P. (2004). A cross-cultural comparison study of the production of simple rhythmic patterns. *Psychology of Music*, 32:389–403.

Saffran, J. R. (2003). Absolute pitch in infancy and adulthood: The role of tonal structure. *Developmental Science*, 6:37–45.

Saffran, J. R., Aslin, R. N., & Newport, E. L. (1996). Statistical learning by 8-month old infants. *Science*, 274:1926–1928.

Saffran, J. R., & Griepentrog, G. J. (2001). Absolute pitch in infant auditory learning: Evidence for developmental reorganization. *Developmental Psychology*, 37:74–85.

Saffran, J. R., Johnson, E. K., Aslin, R. N., & Newport, E. L. (1999). Statistical learning of tone sequences by human infants and adults. *Cognition*, 70:27–52.

Saffran, J. R., Reeck, K., Niebuhr, A., & Wilson, D. (2005). Changing the tune: The structure of the input affects infants' use of absolute and relative pitch. *Developmental Science*, 8:1–7.

Sandler, W., Meir, I., Padden, C., & Aronoff, M. (2005). The emergence of grammar: Systematic structure in a new language. *Proceedings of the National Academy of Sciences, USA*, 102:2661–2665.

Savage-Rumbaugh, S., Shanker, S. G., & Taylor, T. J. (1998). *Apes, Language, and the Human Mind*. New York: Oxford.

Schaefer, R., Murre, J., & Bod, R. (2004). Limits to universality in segmentation of simple melodies. In: S. D. Lipscomb et al. (Eds.), *Proceedings of the 8th International Conference on Music Perception and Cognition, Evanston, IL* (pp. 247–250). Adelaide, Australia: Causal Productions.

Schafer, A. J., Carter, J., Clifton, C., & Frazier, L. (1996). Focus in relative clause construal. *Language and Cognitive Processes*, 11:135–163.

Schaffrath, H. (1995). *The Essen Folksong Collection in the Humdrum Kern Format*, D. Huron (Ed.). Menlo Park, CA: Center for Computer Assisted Research in the Humanities.

Schegloff, E. A. (1982). Discourse as an interactional achievement: Some uses of "uh huh" and other things that come between sentences. In: D. Tannen (Ed.), *Georgetown University Round Table on Linguistics 1981. Analysing Discourse:Text and Talk* (pp. 71–93). Washington, DC: Georgetown University Press.

Scheirer, E., & Slaney, M. (1997). Construction and evaluation of a robust multifeature speech/music discriminator, *Proceedings of ICASSP-97, Munich, Germany* (Vol. 2; pp. 1331–1334).

Schellenberg, E. G. (1996). Expectancy in melody: Tests of the implication-realization model. *Cognition*, 58:75–125.

Schellenberg, E. G. (1997). Simplifying the implication-realization model of melodic expectancy. *Music Perception*, 14:295–318.

Schellenberg, E. G., Adachi, M., Purdy, K. T., & McKinnon, M. C. (2002). Expectancy in melody: Tests of children and adults. *Journal of Experimental Psychology: General*, 131:511–537.

Schellenberg, E. G., & Trehub, S. E. (1996). Natural music intervals: Evidence from infant listeners. *Psychological Science*, 7:272–277.

Schellenberg, E. G., & Trehub, S. E. (1999). Redundancy, conventionality, and the discrimination of tone sequences: A developmental perspective. *Journal of Experimental Child Psychology*, 74:107–127.

Schellenberg, E. G., & Trehub, S. E. (2003). Good pitch memory is widespread. *Psychological Science*, 14:262–266.

Schenker, H. (1969). *Five Graphic Music Analyses*. New York: Dover.

Schenker, H. (1979). *Free Composition*. New York: Longmans.

Scherer, K. R. (1986). Vocal affect expression: A review and a model for future research. *Psychological Bulletin*, 99:143–165.

Scherer, K. R. (1995). Expression of emotion in voice and music. *Journal of Voice*, 9:235–248.

Scherer, K. R. (2004). Which emotions can be induced by music? What are the underlying mechanisms? And how can we measure them? *Journal of New Music Research*, 33:239–251.

Scherer, K. R., Banse, R., & Wallbott, H. G. (2001). Emotional inferences from vocal expression correlate across languages and cultures. *Journal of Cross-Cultural Psychology*, 32:76–92.

Schieffelin, B. (1985). The acquisition of Kaluli. In: D. Slobin (Ed.), *The Crosslinguistic Study of Language Acquisition* (pp. 525–594). Hillsdale, NJ: Erlbaum.

Schlaug, G., Jancke, L., Huang, Y., Staiger, J. F., & Steinmetz, H. (1995). Increased corpus callosum size in musicians. *Neuropsychologia*, 33:1047–55.

Schmidt, L. A., & Trainor, L. J. (2001). Frontal brain electrical activity (EEG) distinguishes valence and intensity of musical emotions. *Cognition and Emotion*, 15:487–500.

Schmuckler, M. A. (1989). Expectation in music: Investigation of melodic and harmonic processes. *Music Perception*, 7:109–150.

Schmuckler, M. A. (1999). Testing models of melodic contour similarity. *Music Perception,* 16:295–326.

Schoenberg, A. (1911). *Harmonielehre.* Leipzig, Germany: Universal Edition.

Schulkind, M., Posner, R. J., & Rubin, D. C. (2003). Musical features that facilitate melody identification: How do you know its "your" song when they finally play it? *Music Perception,* 21:217–249.

Schulze, H.-H. (1989). Categorical perception of rhythmic patterns. *Psychological Research,* 51:10–15.

Schuppert, M., Münte, T. F., Wieringa, B. M., & Altenmüller, E. (2000). Receptive amusia: Evidence for cross-hemispheric neural networks underlying music processing strategies. *Brain,* 123, 546–559.

Schwartz, A. B., Moran, D. W., & Reina, A. (2004). Differential representation of perception and action in the frontal cortex. *Science,* 303:380–383.

Schwartz, D. A., Howe, C. Q., & Purves, D. (2003). The statistical structure of human speech sounds predicts musical universals. *Journal of Neuroscience,* 23:7160–7168.

Scott, D. R. (1982). Duration as a cue to the perception of a phrase boundary. *Journal of the Acoustical Society of America,* 71:996–1007.

Scott, D. R., Isard, S. D., & Boysson-Bardies, B. de. (1985). Perceptual isochrony in English and French. *Journal of Phonetics,* 13:155–162.

Scott, S. K., & Johnsrude, I. S. (2003). The neuroanatomical and functional organization of speech perception. *Trends in Neurosciences,* 26:100–107.

Seashore, C. (1938). *Psychology of Music.* New York: McGraw-Hill.

Sebeok, T. A., & Umiker-Sebeok, D. J. (Eds.). (1976). *Speech Surrogates: Drum and Whistle Systems* (2 Vols.). The Hague, The Netherlands: Mouton.

Seeger, A. (1987). *Why Suya Sing: A Musical Anthropology of an Amazonian People.* Cambridge, UK: Cambridge University Press.

Seifritz, E., Neuhoff, J. G., Bilecen, D., Scheffler, D., Mustovic, H., Schächinger, H., Elefante, R., & Di Salle, F. (2002). Neural processing of auditory "looming" in the human brain. *Current Biology,* 12:2147–2151.

Selfridge-Feld, E. (1995). *The Essen Musical Data Package.* CCARH (Center for Computer Assisted Research in the Humanities), Technical Report No. 1. Menlo Park, CA: CCARCH.

Selkirk, E. O. (1981). On the nature of phonological representation. In: J. Anderson, J. Laver, & T. Myers (Eds.), *The Cognitive Representation of Speech.* Amsterdam: North Holland.

Selkirk, E. O. (1984). *Phonology and Syntax: The Relation Between Sound and Structure.* Cambridge, MA: MIT Press.

Semal, C., Demany, L., Ueda, K., & Halle, P. A. (1996). Speech versus nonspeech in pitch memory. *Journal of the Acoustical Society of America,* 100:1132–40.

Semendeferi, K., Lu, A., Schenker, N., & Damasio, H. (2002). Humans and great apes share a large frontal cortex. *Nature Neuroscience* 5:272–276.

Senghas, A., & Coppola, M. (2001). Children creating language: How Nicaraguan Sign Language acquired a spatial grammar. *Psychological Science,* 12:323–328.

Senghas, A., Kita, S., & Özyürek, A. (2004). Children creating core properties of language: Evidence from an emerging sign language in Nicaragua. *Science,* 305:1779–1782.

Sethares, W. A. (1999). *Tuning, Timbre, Spectrum, Scale.* London: Springer.

Shamma, S., & Klein, D. (2000). The case of the missing pitch templates: How harmonic templates emerge in the early auditory system. *Journal of the Acoustical Society of America,* 107:2631–2644.

Shamma, S. A., Fleshman, J. W., Wiser, P. R., Versnel, H. (1993). Organization of response areas in ferret primary auditory cortex. *Journal of Neurophysiology,* 69:367–383.

Shattuck-Hufnagel, S., Ostendorf, M., & Ross, K. (1994). Stress shift and early pitch accent placement in lexical items in American English. *Journal of Phonetics,* 22:357–388.

Shattuck-Hufnagel, S., & Turk, A. E. (1996). A prosody tutorial for investigators of auditory sentence processing. *Journal of Psycholinguistic Research,* 25:193–247.

Shenfield, T., Trehub, S. E., & Nakata, T. (2003). Maternal singing modulates infants arousal. *Psychology of Music,* 31:365–375.

Shepard, R. N. (1982). Structural representations of musical pitch. In: D. Deutsch (Ed.), *The Psychology of Music* (pp. 343–390). Orlando, FL: Academic Press.

Shepard, R. N., & Jordan, D. S. (1984). Auditory illusions demonstrating that tones are assimilated to an internalized musical scale. *Science,* 226:1333–1334.

Shields, J. L., McHugh, A., & Martin, J. G. (1974). Reaction time to phoneme targets as a function of rhythmic cues in continuous speech. *Journal of Experimental Psychology,* 102:250–255.

Shriberg, E., Ladd, D. R., Terken, J., & Stolcke, A. (2002). Modeling pitch range variation within and across speakers: Predicting F0 targets when "speaking up." In: B. Bell & I. Marlien (Eds.), *Proceedings of Speech Prosody, Aix-en-Provence.* Aix-en-Provence, France: Laboratoire Parole et Langage.

Silk, J. B., Alberts, S. C., & Altmann, J. (2003). Social bonds of female baboons enhance infant survival. *Science,* 302:1231–1234.

Singer, A. (1974). The metrical structure of Macedonian dance. *Ethnomusicology,* 18:379–404.

Singh, L., Morgan, J. L., & Best, C. T. (2002). Infants' listening preferences: Baby talk or happy talk? *Infancy,* 3:365–394.

Slater, P. J. B. (2000). Birdsong repertoires: Their origins and use. In: N. L. Wallin, B. Merker, & S. Brown (Eds.), *The Origins of Music* (pp. 49–63). Cambridge, MA: MIT Press.

Slevc, L. R., & Miyake, A. (2006). Individual differences in second language proficiency: Does musical ability matter? *Psychological Science,* 17:675–681.

Slevc, L. R., Rosenberg, J. C., & Patel, A. D. (2009). Making psycholinguistics musical: Self-paced reading time evidence for shared processing of linguistic and musical syntax. *Psychonomic Bulletin and Review,* 16:374–381.

Sloboda, J. (1983). The communication of musical metre in piano performance. *Quarterly Journal of Experimental Psychology,* 35A:377–396.

Sloboda, J. (1985). *The Musical Mind.* Oxford, UK: Oxford University Press.

Sloboda, J. A. (1991). Music structure and emotional response: Some empirical findings. *Psychology of Music,* 19:110–120.

Sloboda, J. A. (1998). Does music mean anything? *Musicae Scientiae,* 2:21–31.

Sloboda, J. A., & Gregory, A. H. (1980). The psychological reality of musical segments. *Canadian Journal of Psychology/Revue Canadienne de Psychologie,* 34:274–280.

Sloboda, J. A., & Juslin, P. N. (2001). Music and emotion: Commentary. In: P. N. Juslin & J. A. Sloboda (Eds.), *Music and Emotion: Theory and Research* (pp. 453–462). Oxford, UK: Oxford University Press.

Sloboda, J. A., & O'Neill, S. A. (2001). Emotions in everyday listening to music. In: P. N. Juslin & J. A. Sloboda (Eds.), *Music and Emotion: Theory and Research* (pp. 415–429). Oxford, UK: Oxford University Press.

Sloboda, J. A., O'Neill, S. A., & Ivaldi, A. (2001). Functions of music in everyday life: An exploratory study using the experience sampling methodology. *Musicae Scientiae*, 5:9–32.

Sloboda, J. A., & Parker, D. H. H. (1985). Immediate recall of melodies. In: P. Howell, I. Cross, & R. West (Eds.), *Musical Structure and Cognition* (pp. 143–167). London: Academic Press.

Sloboda, J. A., Wise, K. J., & Peretz, I. (2005). Quantifying tone deafness in the general population. *Annals of the New York Academy of Sciences*, 1060: 255–261.

Sluijter, A. J. M., & van Heuven, V. J. (1996). Spectral balance as an acoustic correlate of linguistic stress. *Journal of the Acoustical Society of America*, 100:2471–2485.

Sluijter, A. J. M., van Heuven, V. J., & Pacilly, J. J. A. (1997). Spectral balance as a cue in the perception of linguistic stress. *Journal of the Acoustical Society of America*, 101:503–513.

Smiljanic, R., & Bradlow, A. R. (2005). Production and perception of clear speech in Croatian and English. *Journal of the Acoustical Society of America*, 118:1677–1688.

Smith, J. D. (1997). The place of musical novices in music science. *Music Perception*, 14:227–262.

Smith, J. D., Kelmer Nelson, D. G., Grohskopf, L. A., & Appleton, T. (1994). What child is this? What interval was that? Familiar tunes and music perception in novice listeners. *Cognition*, 52:23–54.

Smith, J. D., & Melara, R. J. (1990). Aesthetic preference and syntactic prototypicality in music: 'Tis the gift to be simple. *Cognition*, 34:279–298.

Smith, N., & Cuddy, L. L. (2003). Perceptions of musical dimensions in Beethoven's *Waldstein* sonata: An application of Tonal Pitch Space theory. *Musicae Scientiae*, 7:7–34.

Snyder, J., & Krumhansl, C. L. (2001). Tapping to ragtime: Cues to pulse finding. *Music Perception*, 18:455–489.

Snyder, J. S., & Large, E. W. (2005). Gamma-band activity reflects the metric structure of rhythmic tone sequences. *Cognitive Brain Research*, 24:117–126.

Sober, E. (1984). *The Nature of Selection: Evolutionary Theory in Philosophical Focus*. Cambridge, MA: MIT Press.

Soto-Faraco, S., Sebastián-Gallés, N., & Cutler, A. (2001). Segmental and suprasegmental mismatch in lexical access. *Journal of Memory and Language*, 45:412–432.

Speer, S. R., Warren, P., & Schafer, A. J. (2003, August 3–9). Intonation and sentence processing. *Proceedings of the Fifteenth International Congress of Phonetic Sciences*, Barcelona.

Spencer, H. (1857). The origin and function of music. *Fraser's Magazine*, 56:396–408.

Steele, J. (1779). *Prosodia Rationalis: Or, An Essay Toward Establishing the Melody and Measure of Speech, to Be Expressed and Perpetuated by Peculiar Symbols* (2nd ed.). London: J. Nichols. (Reprinted by Georg Olms Verlag, Hildesheim, 1971)

Steinbeis, N., & Koelsch, S. (in press). Shared neural resources between music and language indicate semantic processing of musical tension-resolution patterns. *Cerebral Cortex*.

Steinbeis, N., Koelsch, S., & Sloboda, J. A. (2006). The role of harmonic expectancy violations in musical emotions: Evidence from subjective, physiological, and neural responses. *Journal of Cognitive Neuroscience*, 18:1380–1393.

Steinhauer, K., Alter, K., & Friederici, A. D. (1999). Brain potentials indicate immediate use of prosodic cues in natural speech processing. *Nature Neuroscience*, 2:191–196.

Steinhauer, K., & Friederici, A. D. (2001). Prosodic boundaries, comma rules, and brain responses: The closure positive shift in ERPs as a universal marker for prosodic phrasing in listeners and readers. *Journal of Psycholinguistic Research*, 30:267–295.

Steinke, W. R., Cuddy, L. L., & Holden, R. R. (1997). Dissociation of musical tonality and pitch memory from nonmusical cognitive abilities. *Canadian Journal of Experimental Psychology*, 51:316–334.

Steinschneider, M., Volkov, I. O., Fishman, Y. I., Oya, H., Arezzo, J. C., & Howard, M. A. (2005). Intracortical responses in human and monkey primary auditory cortex support a temporal processing mechanism for encoding of the voice onset time phonetic parameter. *Cerebral Cortex*, 15:170–186.

Stern, T. (1957). Drum and whistle "languages": An analysis of speech surrogates. *American Anthropologist*, 59:487–506.

Stetson, R. H. (1951). *Motor Phonetics, a Study of Speech Movements in Action.* Amsterdam: North Holland.

Stevens, J. (2002). *The Songs of John Lennon: The Beatles Years.* Boston: Berklee Press.

Stevens, K. N. (1997). Articulatory-acoustic-auditory relationships. In: W. J. Hardcastle & J. Laver (Eds.), *The Handbook of Phonetic Sciences* (pp. 463–506). Oxford, UK: Blackwell.

Stevens, K. N. (1989). On the quantal nature of speech. *Journal of Phonetics*, 17:3–45.

Stevens, K. N. (1998). *Acoustic Phonetics.* Cambridge, MA: MIT Press.

Stevens, K. N., Liberman, A. M., Studdert-Kennedy, M., & Öhman, S. E. G. (1969). Crosslanguage study of vowel perception. *Language and Speech*, 12:1–23.

Stewart, L., Henson, R., Kampe, K., Walsh, V., Turner, R., & Frith, U. (2003). Becoming a pianist: Brain changes associated with learning to read and play music. *NeuroImage*, 20:71–83.

Stewart, L., von Kriegstein, K., Warren, J. D., & Griffiths, T. D. (2006). Music and the brain: Disorders of musical listening. *Brain*, 129:2533–2553.

Stobart, H., & Cross, I. (2000). The Andean anacrusis? rhythmic structure and perception in Easter songs of Northern Potosí, Bolivia. *British Journal of Ethnomusicology*, 9:63–94.

Stoffer, T. H. (1985). Representation of phrase structure in the perception of music. *Music Perception*, 3:191–220.

Stokes, M. (Ed.). (1994). *Ethnicity, Identity, and Music: The Musical Construction of Place.* Oxford, UK: Berg.

Stone, R. M. (1982). *Let the Inside Be Sweet: The Interpretation of Music Event Among the Kpelle of Liberia.* Bloomington: Indiana University Press.

Stratton, V. N., & Zalanowski, A. H. (1994). Affective impact of music vs. lyrics. *Empirical Studies of the Arts*, 12:173–184.

Streeter, L. A. (1978). Acoustic determinants of phrase boundary perception. *Journal of the Acoustical Society of America*, 64:1582–1592.

Strogatz, S. (2003). *Sync: The Emerging Science of Spontaneous Order.* New York: Hyperion.

Stumpf, C. (1883). *Tonpsychologie* (Vol. 1). Leipzig, Germany: S. Hirzel.

Sundberg, J. (1982). Speech, song, and emotions. In: M. Clynes (Ed.), *Music, Mind and Brain: The Neuropsychology of Music* (pp. 137–149). New York: Plenum Press.

Sundberg, J. (1987). *The Science of the Singing Voice.* DeKalb, IL: Northern Illinois University Press.

Sundberg, J. (1994). Musical significance of musicians' syllable choice in improvised nonsense text singing: A preliminary study. *Phonetica,* 54:132–145.

Sundberg, J., & Lindblom, B. (1976). Generative theories in language and music descriptions. *Cognition,* 4:99–122.

Sutton, R. A. (2001). Asia/Indonesia. In: J. T. Titon (Gen. Ed.), *Worlds of Music: An Introduction to the Music of the World's Peoples (Shorter Version)* (pp. 179–209). Belmont, CA: Thompson Learning.

Swaab, T. Y., Brown, C. M., & Hagoort, P. (1998). Understanding ambiguous words in sentence contexts: Electrophysiological evidence for delayed contextual selection in Broca's aphasia. *Neuropsychologia,* 36:737–761.

Swain, J. (1997). *Musical Languages.* New York: Norton.

't Hart, J. (1976). Psychoacoustic backgrounds of pitch contour stylization. *I.P.O. Annual Progress Report,* 11:11–19.

't Hart, J., & Collier, R. (1975). Integrating different levels of intonation analysis. *Journal of Phonetics,* 3:235–255.

't Hart, J., Collier, R., & Cohen, A. (1990). *A Perceptual Study of Intonation: An Experimental-Phonetic Approach to Speech Melody.* Cambridge, UK: Cambridge University Press.

Tagg, P., & Clarida, B. (2003). *Ten Little Tunes.* New York and Montreal: The Mass Media Music Scholar's Press.

Takayama, Y., et. al. (1993). A case of foreign accent syndrome without aphasia caused by a lesion of the left precentral gyrus. *Neurology,* 43:1361–1363.

Takeuchi, A. H. (1994). Maximum key-profile correlation (MKC) as a measure of tonal structure in music. *Perception and Psychophysics,* 56:335–346.

Takeuchi, A., & Hulse, S. (1993). Absolute pitch. *Psychological Bulletin,* 113:345–61.

Tallal, P., & Gaab, N. (2006). Dynamic auditory processing, musical experience and language development. *Trends in Neurosciences,* 29:382–370.

Tan, N., Aiello, R., & Bever, T. G. (1981). Harmonic structure as a determinant of melodic organization. *Memory and Cognition,* 9:533–539.

Tan, S.-L., & Kelly, M. E. (2004). Graphic representations of short musical compositions. *Psychology of Music,* 32:191–212.

Tan, S.-L., & Spackman, M. P. (2005). Listener's judgments of musical unity of structurally altered and intact musical compositions. *Psychology of Music,* 33:133–153.

Taylor, D. S. (1981). Non-native speakers and the rhythm of English. *International Review of Applied Linguistics,* 19:219–226.

Tekman, H. G., & Bharucha, J. J. (1998). Implicit knowledge versus psychoacoustic similarity in priming of chords. *Journal of Experimental Psychology: Human Perception and Performance,* 24:252–260.

Temperley, D. (1999). Syncopation in rock: A perceptual perspective. *Popular Music,* 18:19–40.

Temperley, D. (2000). Meter and grouping in African music: A view from music theory. *Ethnomusicology,* 44:65–96.

Temperley, D. (2004). Communicative pressure and the evolution of musical styles. *Music Perception,* 21:313–37.

Temperley, D., & Bartlette, C. (2002). Parallelism as a factor in metrical analysis. *Music Perception,* 20:117–149.

Teramitsu, I., Kudo, L. C., London, S. E., Geschwind, D. H., & White, S. A. (2004). Parallel FoxP1 and FoxP2 expression in songbird and human brain predicts functional interaction. *Journal of Neuroscience,* 24:3152–3163.

Terhardt, E. (1984). The concept of musical consonance: A link between music and psychoacoustics. *Music Perception* 1:276–295.

Terken, J. (1991). Fundamental frequency and perceived prominence of accented syllables. *Journal of the Acoustical Society of America,* 89:1768–1776.

Terken, J., & Hermes, D. J. (2000). The perception of prosodic prominence. In: M. Horne (Ed.), *Prosody: Theory and Experiment, Studies Presented to Gösta Bruce* (pp. 89–127). Dordrecht, The Netherlands: Kluwer Academic Publishers.

Tervaniemi, M., Kujala, A., Alho, K., Virtanen, J., Ilmoniemi, R. J., & Näätänen, R. (1999). Functional specialization of the human auditory cortex in processing phonetic and musical sounds: A magnetoencephalographic (MEG) study. *NeuroImage,* 9:330–336.

Tervaniemi, M., Medvedev, S. V., Alho, K., Pakhomov, S. V., Roudas, M. S., van Zuijen, T. L., & Näätänen, R. (2000). Lateralized automatic auditory processing of phonetic versus musical information: A PET study. *Human Brain Mapping,* 10:74–79.

Tervaniemi, M., Szameitat, A. J., Kruck, S., Schröger, E., Alter, K., De Baene, W., & Friederici, A. (2006). From air oscillations to music and speech: fMRI evidence for fine-tuned neural networks in audition. *Journal of Neuroscience,* 26:8647–8652.

Thaut, M. H., Kenyon, G. P., Schauer, M. L., & McIntosh, G. C. (1999). The connection between rhythmicity and brain function: Implications for therapy of movement disorders. *IEEE Transactions on Engineering Biology and Medicine,* 18:101–108.

Thierry, E. (2002). *Les langages sifflés.* Unpublished dissertation, Ecole Pratique des Hautes Etudes IV, Paris.

Thomassen, J. M. (1983). Melodic accent: Experiments and a tentative model. *Journal of the Acoustical Society of America,* 71:1596–1605.

Thompson, A. D., Jr., & Bakery, M. C. (1993). Song dialect recognition by male white-crowned sparrows: Effects of manipulated song components. *The Condor,* 95:414–421.

Thompson, W. F., & Balkwill, L.-L. (2006). Decoding speech prosody in five languages. *Semiotica,* 158–1/4:407–424.

Thompson, W. F., & Cuddy, L. L. (1992). Perceived key movement in four-voice harmony and single voices. *Music Perception,* 9, 427–438.

Thompson, W. F., & Russo, F. A. (2004). The attribution of meaning and emotion to song lyrics. *Polskie Forum Psychologiczne,* 9, 51–62.

Thompson, W. F., Schellenberg, E. G., & Husain, G. (2004). Decoding speech prosody: Do music lessons help? *Emotion,* 4:46–64.

Thorsen, N. (1980). A study of the perception of sentence intonation: Evidence from Danish. *Journal of the Acoustical Society of America*, 67:1014–1030.

Tillmann, B. (2005). Implicit investigations of tonal knowledge in nonmusician listeners. *Annals of the New York Academy of Sciences*, 1060:100–110.

Tillmann, B., Bharucha, J. J., & Bigand, E. (2000). Implicit learning of tonality: A self-organizing approach. *Psychological Review*, 107:885–913.

Tillmann, B., & Bigand, E. (1996). Does formal musical structure affect perception of musical expressiveness? *Psychology of Music*, 24: 3–17.

Tillmann, B., & Bigand, E. (2001). Global context effects in normal and scrambled musical sequences. *Journal of Experimental Psychology: Human Perception and Performance*, 27:1185–1196.

Tillmann, B., Bigand, E., & Pineau, M. (1998). Effect of local and global contexts on harmonic expectancy, *Music Perception*, 16:99–118.

Tillmann, B., Janata, P., & Bharucha, J. J. (2003). Activation of the inferior frontal cortex in musical priming. *Cognitive Brain Research*, 16:145–161.

Titon, J. T. (Ed.). (1996). *Worlds of Music: An Introduction to the Music of the World's Peoples* (3rd ed.). New York: Schirmer.

Todd, N. P. McA. (1985). A model of expressive timing in tonal music. *Music Perception*, 3:33–58.

Todd, N. P. Mc-A. (1999). Motion in music: A neurobiological perspective. *Music Perception*, 17:115–126.

Todd, N. P. McA., O'Boyle, D. J., & Lee, C. S. (1999). A sensory-motor theory of rhythm, time perception and beat induction. *Journal of New Music Research*, 28:5–28.

Toga, A. W., Thompson, P. M., & Sowell, E. R. (2006). Mapping brain maturation. *Trends in Neurosciences*, 29, 148–159.

Toiviainen, P., & Eerola, T. (2003). Where is the beat? Comparison of Finnish and South African listeners. In: R. Kopiez, A. C. Lehmann, I. Wolther, & C. Wolf (Eds.), *Proceedings of the 5th Triennial Escom Conference* (pp. 501–504). Hanover, Germany: Hanover University of Music and Drama.

Toiviainen, P., & Krumhansl, C. L. (2003). Measuring and modeling real-time responses to music: The dynamics of tonality induction. *Perception*, 32:741–766.

Toiviainen, P., & Snyder, J. S. (2003). Tapping to Bach: Resonance-based modeling of pulse. *Music Perception*, 21:43–80.

Tojo, S., Oka, Y., & Nishida, M. (2006). Analysis of chord progression by HPSG. In: *Proceedings of the 24th IASTED International Multi-Conference (Artificial Intelligence and Applications)*, pp. 305–310. Innsbruck, Austria.

Tomasello, M. (1995). Language is not an instinct. *Cognitive Development*, 10:131–156.

Tomasello, M. (2003). On the different origins of symbols and grammar. In: M. H. Christiansen & S. Kirby (Eds.), *Language Evolution* (pp. 94–110). Oxford, UK: Oxford University Press.

Tomasello, M., Carpenter, M., Call, J., Behne, T., & Moll, H. (2005). Understanding and sharing intentions: The origins of cultural cognition. *Behavioral and Brain Sciences*, 28: 675–691.

Trail, A. (1994). *A !Xóõ Dictionary*. Cologne, Germany: Rüdiger Köppe.

Trainor, L. J. (2005). Are there critical periods for music development? *Developmental Psychobiology*, 46: 262–278.

Trainor, L. J., & Adams, B. (2000). Infants' and adults' use of duration and intensity cues in the segmentation of tone patterns. *Perception and Psychophysics*, 62:333–340.

Trainor, L. J., Austin, C. M., & Desjardins, R. N. (2000). Is infant-directed speech prosody a result of the vocal expression of emotion? *Psychological Science*, 11:188–195.

Trainor, L. J., Clark, E. D., Huntley, A., & Adams, B. A. (1997). The acoustic basis of preferences for infant-directed singing. *Infant Behavior and Development*, 20:383–396.

Trainor, L. J., & Heinmiller, B. M. (1998). The development of evaluative responses to music: Infants prefer to listen to consonance over dissonance. *Infant Behavior and Development*, 21:77–88.

Trainor, L. J., McDonald, K. L., & Alain, C. (2002). Automatic and controlled processing of melodic contour and interval information measured by electrical brain activity. *Journal of Cognitive Neuroscience*, 14:430–442.

Trainor, L. J., McFadden, M., Hodgson, L., Darragh, L., Barlow, J., et al. (2003). Changes in auditory cortex and the development of mismatch negativity between 2 and 6 months of age. *International Journal of Psychophysiology*, 51:5–15.

Trainor, L. J., & Schmidt, L. A. (2003). Processing Emotions Induced by Music. In: I. Peretz & R. Zatorre, (Eds.), *The Cognitive Neuroscience of Music* (pp. 310–324). Oxford, UK: Oxford University Press.

Trainor, L. J., & Trehub, S. E. (1992). A comparison of infants' and adults' sensitivity to Western musical structure. *Journal of Experimental Psychology: Human Perception and Performance*, 18:394–402.

Trainor, L. J., & Trehub, S. E. (1993). Musical context effects in infants and adults: Key distance. *Journal of Experimental Psychology: Human Perception and Performance*, 19:615–26.

Trainor, L. J., & Trehub, S. E. (1994). Key membership and implied harmony in Western tonal music: Developmental perspectives. *Perception and Psychophysics*, 56:125–132.

Trainor, L. J., Tsang, C. D., & Cheung, V. H. W. (2002). Preference for consonance in 2-month-old infants. *Music Perception*, 20:185–192.

Tramo, M. J., Bharucha, J. J., & Musiek, F. E. (1990). Music perception and cognition following bilateral lesions of auditory cortex. *Journal of Cognitive Neuroscience*, 2:195–212.

Tramo, M. J., Cariani, P. A., Delgutte, B., & Braida, L. D. (2003). Neurobiology of harmony perception. In: I. Peretz & R. Zatorre (Eds.), *The Cognitive Neuroscience of Music* (pp. 127–151). New York: Oxford.

Trehub, S. E. (2000). Human processing predispositions and musical universals. In: N. L. Wallin, B. Merker, & S. Brown (Eds.), *The Origins of Music* (pp. 427–448). Cambridge, MA: MIT Press.

Trehub, S. E. (2003a). The developmental origins of musicality. *Nature Neuroscience*, 6:669–673.

Trehub, S. E. (2003b). Musical predispositions in infancy: An update. In: I. Peretz & R. Zatorre (Eds.), *The Cognitive Neuroscience of Music* (pp. 3–20). New York: Oxford University Press.

Trehub, S. E., Bull, D., & Thorpe, L. A. (1984). Infants' perception of melodies: The role of melodic contour. *Child Development*, 55:821–830.

Trehub, S. E., & Hannon, E. E. (2006). Infant music perception: Domain-general or domain-specific mechanisms? *Cognition*,100:73–99.

Trehub, S. E., Morrongiello, B. A., & Thorpe, L. A. (1985). Children's perception of familiar melodies: The role of intervals, contour, and key. *Psychomusicology*, 5:39–48.

Trehub, S. E., Schellenberg, E. G., & Hill, D. (1997). The origins of music perception and cognition: A developmental perspective. In: I. Deliège & J. A. Sloboda (Eds.), *Perception and Cognition of Music* (pp. 103–128). Hove, UK: Psychology Press.

Trehub, S. E., Schellenberg, E. G., & Kamenetsky, S. B. (1999). Infants' and adults' perception of scale structure. *Journal of Experimental Psychology: Human Perception and Performance*, 25:965–975.

Trehub, S. E., & Thorpe, L. A. (1989). Infant's perception of rhythm: Categorization of auditory sequences by temporal structure. *Canadian Journal of Psychology*, 43:217–229.

Trehub, S. E., Thorpe, L. A., & Morrongiello, B. A. (1987). Organizational processes in infants' perception of auditory patterns. *Child Development*, 58:741–9.

Trehub, S. E., & Trainor, L. J. (1998). Singing to infants: Lullabies and playsongs. *Advances in Infancy Research*, 12:43–77.

Trehub, S. E., Unyk, A. M., Kamenetsky, S. B., Hill, D. S., Trainor, L. J., Henderson, J. L., et al. (1997). Mothers' and fathers' singing to infants. *Developmental Psychology*, 33:500–507.

Trehub, S. E., Unyk, A. M., & Trainor, L. J. (1993). Maternal singing in cross-cultural perspective. *Infant Behavior and Development*, 16:285–95.

Trevarthen, C. (1999). Musicality and the intrinsic motivic pulse: Evidence from human psychobiology and infant communication [Special issue 1999–2000]. *Musicae Scientiae*, 155–215.

Tronick, E. Z., Als, H., Adamson, L., Wise, S., & Brazelton, T. B. (1978). The infant's response to entrapment between contradictory messages in face-to-face interaction. *Journal of the American Academy of Child Psychiatry*, 17:1–13.

Trout, J. D. (2003). Biological specializations for speech: What can animals tell us? *Current Directions in Psychological Science*, 12:155–159.

Tsukada, K. (1997). Drumming, onomatopoeia and sound symbolism among the Luvale of Zambia. In: J. Kawada (Ed.), *Cultures Sonores D'Afrique* (pp. 349–393). Tokyo: Institute for the Study of Languages and Cultures of Asia and Africa (IL-CAA).

Tyack, P. L., & Clark, C. W. (2000). Communication and acoustic behavior in whales and dolphins. In: W. W. L. Au, A. N. Popper, & R. R. Fay (Eds.), *Hearing by Whales and Dolphins* (pp. 156–224). New York: Springer.

Tzortzis, C., Goldblum, M.-C. , Dang, M., Forette, F., & Boller, F. (2000). Absence of amusia and preserved naming of musical instruments in an aphasic composer. *Cortex*, 36:227–242.

Ulanovsky, N., Las, L., & Nelken, I. (2003). Processing of low-probability sounds by cortical neurons. *Nature Neuroscience*, 6:391–398.

Ullman, M. T. (2001). A neurocognitive perspective on language: The declarative/procedural model. *Nature Reviews (Neuroscience)*, 2:717–726.

Umeda, N. (1982). F0 declination is situation dependent. *Journal of Phonetics,* 20:279–290.

Unyk, A. M., Trehub, S. E., Trainor, L. J., & Schellenberg, E. G. (1992). Lullabies and simplicity: A cross-cultural perspective. *Psychology of Music,* 20:15–28.

Vaissiere, J. (1983). Language-independent prosodic features. In: A. Cutler & D. R. Ladd (Eds.), *Prosody: Models and Measurements* (pp. 53–66). Berlin, Germany: Springer.

van de Weijer, J. (1998). *Language Input for Word Discovery.* Nijmegen: Max Planck Institute for Psycholinguistics.

van Gulik, R. H. (1940). *The lore of the Chinese lute: An essay in ch'in ideology.* Tokyo: Sophia University.

Van Khê, T. (1977). Is the pentatonic universal? A few reflections on pentatonism. *The World of Music,* 19:76–91.

van Noorden, L., & Moelants, D. (1999). Resonance in the perception of musical pulse. *Journal of New Music Research, 28,* 43–66.

van Ooyen, B., Bertoncini, J., Sansavini, A., & Mehler, J. (1997). Do weak syllables count for newborns? *Journal of the Acoustical Society of America,* 102:3735–3741.

Van Valin, R. D. (2001). *An Introduction to Syntax.* Cambridge, UK: Cambridge University Press.

Vanhaeren, M., d'Errico, F., Stringer, C., James, S. L., Todd, J. A., & Mienis, H. K. (2006). Middle Paleolithic shell beads in Israel and Algeria. *Science,* 312:1785–1788.

Vargha-Khadem, F., Watkins, K., Alcock, K., Fletcher, P., & Passingham, R. (1995). Praxic and nonverbal cognitive deficits in a large family with a genetically transmitted speech and language disorder. *Proceedings of the National Academy of Sciences, USA,* 92:930–933.

Vargha-Khadem, F., Watkins, K. E., Price, C. J., Ashburner, J., Alcock, K. J., Connely, A., et al. (1998). Neural basis of an inherited speech and language disorder. *Proceedings of the National Academy of Sciences, USA,* 95:12695–12700.

Vasishth, S., & Lewis, R. L. (2006). Argument-head distance and processing complexity: Explaining both locality and anti-locality effects. *Language,* 82:767–794.

Vassilakis, P. (2005). Auditory roughness as means of musical expression. *Selected Reports in Ethnomusicology,* 12:119–144.

Voisin, F. (1994). Musical scales in central Africa and Java: Modeling by synthesis. *Leonardo Music Journal,* 4:85–90.

von Hippel, P., & Huron, D. (2000). Why do skips precede reversals? The effect of tessitura on melodic structure. *Music Perception,* 18:59–85.

von Steinbüchel, N. (1998). Temporal ranges of central nervous processing: Clinical evidence. *Experimental Brain Research,* 123:220–233.

Vos, P. G., & Troost, J. M. (1989). Ascending and descending melodic intervals: Statistical findings and their perceptual relevance. *Music Perception,* 6:383–396.

Vouloumanos, A., & Werker, J. F. (2004). Tuned to the signal: The privileged status of speech for young infants. *Developmental Science,* 7:270–276.

Wagner, P. S., & Dellwo, V. (2004). Introducing YARD (Yet Another Rhythm Determination) and re-introducing isochrony to rhythm research. *Proceedings of Speech Prosody 2004, Nara, Japan.*

Walker, R. (1990). *Musical Beliefs*. New York: Teachers College Press.

Wallin, N. L., Merker, B., & Brown, S. (Eds.). (2000). *The Origins of Music*. Cambridge, MA: MIT Press.

Ward, W. D. (1999). Absolute pitch. In: D. Deutsch (Ed.), *The Psychology of Music* (2nd ed., pp. 265–298). San Diego, CA: Academic Press.

Warren, T., & Gibson, E. (2002). The influence of referential processing on sentence complexity. *Cognition, 85*, 79–112.

Watanabe, S., & Nemoto, M. (1998). Reinforcing property of music in Java sparrows (*Padda oryzivora*). *Behavioural Processes*, 43:211–218.

Watkins, K. E., Dronkers, N. F., & Vargha-Khadem, F. (2002). Behavioural analysis of an inherited speech and language disorder: Comparison with acquired aphasia. *Brain*, 125:452–464.

Watson, D., & Gibson, E. (2004). The relationship between intonational phrasing and syntactic structure in language production. *Language and Cognitive Processes*, 19:713–755.

Watt, R. J., & Ash, R. L. (1998). A psychological investigation of meaning in music. *Musicae Scientiae*, 2:33–53.

Webb, D. M., & Zhang, J. (2005). *FoxP2* in song-learning birds and vocal-learning mammals. *Journal of Heredity*, 96:212–216.

Wedekind, K. (1983). A six-tone language in Ethiopia. *Journal of Ethopian Studies*, 16:129–156.

Wedekind, K. (1985). Thoughts when drawing a map of tone languages. *Afrikanistische Arbeitspapiere*, 1:105–124.

Weisman, R. G., Njegovan, M. G., Williams, M. T., Cohen, J. S., & Sturdy, C. B. (2004). A behavior analysis of absolute pitch: Sex, experience, and species. *Behavioural Processes*, 66:289–307.

Welmers, W. E. (1973). *African Language Structures*. Berkeley: University of California Press.

Wenk, B. J. (1987). Just in time: On speech rhythms in music. *Linguistics*, 25:969–981.

Wenk, B. J., & Wioland, F. (1982). Is French really syllable-timed? *Journal of Phonetics*,10:193–216.

Wennerstrom, A. (2001). *The Music of Everyday Speech: Prosody and Discourse Analysis*. Oxford, UK: Oxford University Press.

Werker, J. F., & Curtin, S. (2005). PRIMIR: A developmental framework of infant speech processing. *Language, Learning and Development*, 1:197–234.

Werker, J. F., Gilbert, J. V. H., Humphrey, K., & Tees, R. C. (1981). Developmental aspects of cross-language speech perception. *Child Development*, 52:349–355.

Werker, J. F., & Tees, R. C. (1984). Cross-language speech perception: Evidence for perceptual reorganization during the first year of life. *Infant Behavior and Development*, 7:49–63.

Werker, J. F., & Tees, R. C. (1999). Influences on infant speech processing: Toward a new synthesis. *Annual Review of Psychology, 50*:509–535.

Wetzel, W., Wagner, T., Ohl, F. W., & Scheich, H. (1998). Right auditory cortex lesion in Mongolian gerbils impairs discrimination of rising and falling frequency-modulated tones. *Neuroscience Letters*, 252:115–118.

Whalen, D. H., & Levitt, A. G. (1995). The universality of intrinsic F0 of vowels. *Journal of Phonetics*, 23:349–366.

Whalen, D. H., Levitt, A. G., & Wang, Q. (1991). Intonational differences between the reduplicative babbling of French- and English-learning infants. *Journal of Child Language,* 18:501–516.

Whalen, D. H., & Xu, Y. (1992). Information for Mandarin tones in the amplitude contour and in brief segments. *Phonetica,* 49:25–47.

Whaling, C. S. (2000). What's behind a song? The neural basis of song learning in birds. In: N. L. Wallin, B. Merker, & S. Brown (Eds.), *The Origins of Music* (pp. 65–76). Cambridge, MA: MIT Press.

Whaling, C. S., Solis, M. M., Doupe, A. J., Soha, J. A., & Marler, P. (1997). Acoustic and neural bases for innate recognition of song. *Proceedings of the National Academy of Sciences, USA,* 94:12694–12698.

White, L. S., & Mattys, S. L. (2007). Rhythmic typology and variation in first and second languages. In: P. Prieto, J. Mascaró, & M.-J. Solé (Eds.)., *Segmental and Prosodic Issues in Romance Phonology* (pp. 237–257). Current Issues in Linguistic Theory Series. Amsterdam: John Benjamins.

Wightman, C. W., Shattuck-Hufnagel, S., Ostendorf, M., & Price, P. J. (1992). Segmental durations in the vicinity of prosodic boundaries. *Journal of the Acoustical Society of America,* 91:1707–1717.

Will, U., & Ellis, C. (1994). Evidence for linear transposition in Australian Western Desert vocal music. *Musicology Australia,* 17:2–12.

Will, U., & Ellis, C. (1996). A re-analyzed Australian Western desert song: Frequency performance and interval structure. *Ethnomusicology,* 40:187–222.

Willems, N. (1982). *English Intonation From a Dutch Point of View.* Dordrecht, The Netherlands: Foris.

Williams, B., & Hiller, S. M. (1994). The question of randomness in English foot timing: A control experiment. *Journal of Phonetics,* 22:423–439.

Willmes, K., & Poeck, K. (1993). To what extent can aphasic syndromes be localized? *Brain,* 116:1527–1540.

Wilson, E. O. (1998). *Consilience: The Unity of Knowledge.* New York: Knopf.

Wilson, R. J. (1985). *Introduction to Graph Theory* (3rd ed.). Harlow, UK: Longman.

Wilson, S. J., Pressing, J. L., &Wales, R. J. (2002). Modelling rhythmic function in a musician post-stroke. *Neuropsychologia,* 40:1494–1505.

Windsor, W. L. (2000). Through and around the acousmatic: The interpretation of electroacoustic sounds. In: S. Emmerson (Ed.), *Music, Electronic Media and Culture* (pp. 7–35). Aldershot, UK: Ashgate Press.

Wingfield, P. (Ed.). (1999). *Janáček Studies.* Cambridge, UK: Cambridge University Press.

Winner, E. (1998). Talent: Don't confuse necessity with sufficiency, or science with policy. *Behavioral and Brain Sciences,* 21:430–431.

Wolf, F., & Gibson, E. (2005). Representing discourse coherence: A corpus-based study. *Computational Linguistics,* 31:249–287.

Wong, P. C. M., & Diehl, R. L. (2002). How can the lyrics of a song in a tone language be understood? *Psychology of Music,* 30:202–209.

Wong, P. C. M., & Diehl, R. L. (2003). Perceptual normalization of inter- and intra-talker variation in Cantonese level tones. *Journal of Speech, Language, and Hearing Research,* 46:413–421.

Wong, P. C. M., Parsons, L. M., Martinez, M., & Diehl, R. L. (2004). The role of the insula cortex in pitch pattern perception: The effect of linguistic contexts. *Journal of Neuroscience*, 24:9153–60.

Wong, P. C. M., Skoe, E., Russon, N. M., Dees, T., & Kraus. N. (2007). Musical experience shapes human brainstem encoding of linguistic pitch patterns. *Nature Neuroscience*, 10:420–422.

Woodrow, H. A. (1909). A quantitative study of rhythm: The effect of variations in intensity, rate and duration. *Archives of Psychology*, 14:1–66.

Wright, A. A., Rivera, J. J., Hulse, S. H., Shyan, M., & Neiworth, J. J. (2000). Music perception and octave generalization in rhesus monkeys. *Journal of Experimental Psychology: General*, 129:291–307.

Xu, Y. (1994). Production and perception of coarticulated tones. *Journal of the Acoustical Society of America*, 95: 2240–2253.

Xu, Y. (1999). Effects of tone and focus on the formation and alignment of F0 contours. *Journal of Phonetics*, 27:55–105.

Xu, Y. (2006). Tone in connected discourse. In K. Brown (Ed.), *Encyclopedia of Language and Linguistics* (2nd ed., Vol. 12, pp. 742–750). Oxford, UK: Elsevier.

Xu, Y., & Sun, X. (2002). Maximum speed of pitch change and how it may relate to speech. *Journal of the Acoustical Society of America*, 111:1399–1413.

Xu, Y., & Xu, C. X. (2005). Phonetic realization of focus in English declarative intonation. *Journal of Phonetics*, 33:159–197.

Yamomoto, F. (1996). English speech rhythm studied in connection with British traditional music and dance. *Journal of Himeji Dokkyo University Gaikokugogakubo*, 9:224–243.

Youens, S. (1991). *Retracing a Winter's Journey: Schubert's Winterreise*. Ithaca, New York: Cornell University Press.

Yung, B. (1991). The relationship of text and tune in Chinese opea. In: J. Sundberg, L. Nord & R. Carlson (Eds.), *Music, Language, Speech and Brain* (pp. 408–418). London: MacMillan.

Zanto, T. P, Snyder, J. S., & Large, E. W. (2006). Neural correlates of rhythmic expectancy. *Advances in Cognitive Psychology*, 2:221–231.

Zatorre, R. J. (2003). Absolute pitch: A model for understanding the influence of genes and development on neural and cognitive function. *Nature Neuroscience*, 6:692–695.

Zatorre, R. J., Belin, P., & Penhune, V. B. (2002). Structure and function of auditory cortex: Music and speech. *Trends in Cognitive Sciences*, 6:37–46.

Zattore, R. J., Evans, A. C., & Meyer, E. (1994). Neural mechanisms underlying melodic perception and memory for pitch. *Journal of Neuroscience*, 14:1908–1919.

Zatorre, R. J., & Halpern, A. R. (1979). Identification, discrimination, and selective adaptation of simultaneous musical intervals. *Perception and Psychophysics*, 26:384–395.

Zatorre, R. J., Meyer, E., Gjedde, A., & Evans, A. C. (1996). PET studies of phonetic processing of speech: Review, replication, and reanalysis. *Cerebral Cortex*, 6:21–30.

Zbikowski, L. M. (1999). The blossoms of "Trockne Blumen": Music and text in the early nineteenth century. *Music Analysis*, 18:307–345.

Zbikowski, L. M. (2002). *Conceptualizing Music: Cognitive Structure, Theory, and Analysis*. New York: Oxford University Press.

Zeigler, H. P., & Marler, P. (2004). (Eds.). Behavioral Neurobiology of Bird Song. *Annals of the New York Academy of Sciences*, 1016.

Zellner Keller, B. (2002). Revisiting the status of speech rhythm. In: B. Bell & I. Marlien (Eds.), *Proceedings of Speech Prosody, Aix-en-Provence*. Aix-en-Provence, France: Laboratoire Parole et Langage.

Zemp, H. (1981). Melanesian solo polyphonic panpipe music. *Ethnomusicology*, 25:383–418.

Zetterholm, E. (2002). Intonation pattern and duration differences in imitated speech. In: B. Bell & I. Marlien (Eds.), *Proceedings of Speech Prosody, Aix-en-Provence*. Aix-en-Provence, France: Laboratoire Parole et Langage.

Zipf, G. K. (1949). *Human Behavior and the Principle of Least Effort*. Cambridge, MA: Addison-Wesley.

Zohar, E., & Granot, R. (2006). How music moves: Musical parameters and listeners images of motion. *Music Perception*, 23:221–248.

Sound Examples

The following sound and sound/video examples, referenced in this book on the pages listed, can be found at www.oup.com/us/patel

Sound Example 2.1: Four short tone sequences, corresponding to Figure 2.3, panels A–D (p. 23)

Sound Example 2.2: A short piano passage, followed by the same passage with the acoustic signal time-reversed (p. 29)

Sound Example 2.3: Eight tabla drum sounds, corresponding to Table 2.1 (cf. Sound Example 2.7 for corresponding vocables) (pp. 35, 36, 63)

Sound/Video Example 2.4: Movie of a professional tabla player uttering a sequence of tabla vocables, then playing the corresponding drum sequence (p. 37)

Sound Example 2.5: A short passage in Jukun, a discrete level tone language from Nigeria (p. 46)

Sound Example 2.6: A sentence of British English, corresponding to Figures 2.21a, 2.21b, and 2.21c (pp. 61, 62, 63)

Sound Example 2.7: Examples of eight tabla drum vocables (cf. Sound Example 2.3 for the corresponding drum sounds) (p. 63)

Sound Example 2.8: A sentence of sine wave speech and the original sentence from which it was created (p. 76)

Sound Example 3.1: A simple Western European folk melody (K0016), corresponding to Figure 3.1 (p. 99)

Sound Example 3.2: K0016 played twice, with two different indications of the beat (p. 100)

Sound Example 3.3: A strongly metrical rhythmic pattern (p. 101)

Sound Example 3.4: A weakly metrical (syncopated) rhythmic pattern, with frequent "silent beats" containing no events (p. 101)

Sound Example 3.5: A sentence of British English and a sentence of continental French, corresponding to Figures 3.8a and 3.8b (pp. 130, 131)

Sound Example 3.6: An English sentence transformed from its original version into an increasingly abstract temporal pattern of vowels and consonants (p. 136)

Sound Example 3.7: A Japanese sentence transformed from its original version into an increasingly abstract temporal pattern of vowels and consonants (p. 136)

Sound Example 3.8: A sentence of British English and a sentence of continental French, corresponding to Figure 3.15 (pp. 162, 163)

Sound Example 3.9: Easter song from the Bolivian Andes, played on a small guitar (charango) (p. 169)

Sound Example 3.10: Examples of tone sequences in which tones alternate in amplitude or duration (p. 170)

Sound Example 4.1: A sentence of British English, corresponding to Figures 4.2, 4.3, and 4.4 (pp. 186, 187, 188, 189)

Sound Example 4.2: A sentence of British English, corresponding to Figure 4.5 (p. 191)

Sound Example 4.3: A sentence of continental French, corresponding to Figure 4.6 (pp. 192, 193)

Sound Example 4.4: A synthesized sentence of English, with either English or French intonation (p. 192)

Sound Example 4.5: Two short melodies illustrating the influence of tonality relations on the perception of a tone's stability (p. 201)

Sound Example 4.6: K0016 with a sour note (p. 201)

Sound Example 4.7: K0016 with a chordal accompaniment (p. 202)

Sound Example 4.8: A sentence of continental French, corresponding to Figure 4.9 (pp. 203, 204)

Sound Example 4.9: A pair of sentences and a corresponding pair of tone analogs (p. 227)

Sound Example 4.10: A pair of sentences, a corresponding pair of discrete-tone analogs, and a corresponding pair of gliding-pitch analogs (p. 231)

Sound Example 5.1: A musical phrase from J. S. Bach, corresponding to Figure 5.10 (p. 257)

Sound Example 5.2: Two chord progressions in which the final two chords are physically identical but have different harmonic functions (p. 260)

Sound Example 5.3: Musical chord sequences, corresponding to Figure 5.12 (p. 274)

Sound Example 7.1: A Mozart minuet in its original and dissonant versions (p. 380)

Sound Example 7.2: Short rhythmic sequences, corresponding to Figure 7.3 (p. 407)

Sound/Video Example 7.3: Movie of a female Asian elephant (*Elephas maximus*) in the Thai Elephant Orchestra, drumming on two Thai temple drums (p. 408)

Sound/Video Example 7.4: Movie of a red-masked parakeet or "cherry-headed conure" (*Aratinga erythrogenys*) moving to music (p. 411)

Credits

Figure 2.1: From Roger Shepard, "Structural representations of musical pitch," in Diana Deutsch (Ed.), *The Psychology of Music* (pp. 343–390). © 1982 by Academic Press. Used by permission.

Figure 2.2b: From *Worlds of Music: An Introduction to Music of the World's Peoples*, Shorter Ed., 1st ed. by Titon, 2001. Reprinted with permission of Wadsworth, a division of Thomson Learning: www.thomsonrights.com. Fax 800-730-2215.

Figure 2.3: From W. J. Dowling, S. Kwak, & M. W. Andrews, "The time course of recognition of novel melodies," *Perception and Psychophysics*, 57:136–149. © 1995 by the Psychonomic Society. Used by permission.

Figure 2.8: From Rodolfo R. Llinás & Patricia Smith Churchland, *Mind-Brain Continuum: Sensory Processes*, figure 12.9, page 267. © 1996 by the Massachusetts Institute of Technology. Used by permission of MIT Press.

Figure 2.11: From B. Connell, "The perception of lexical tone in Mambila," *Language and Speech*, 43:163–182. © 2000 by Kingston Press. Used by permission.

Figure 2.12: From J. A. Edmondson & K. J. Gregerson, "On five-level tone systems," in S. J. Hwang & W. R. Merrifield (Eds.), *Language in Context: Essays for Robert E. Longacre* (pp. 555–576). Dallas, TX: Summer Institute of Linguistics. © 1992 by SIL International. Used by permission.

Figure 2.13: From K. Wedekind, "Thoughts when drawing a map of tone languages," *Afrikanistische Arbeitspapiere*, 1:105–124. © 1985 by Klaus Wedekind. Used by permission.

Figure 2.16: From Peter Ladefoged & Ian Maddieson, *The Sounds of the World's Languages*. © 1996 by Blackwell Publishing. Used by permission.

Figure 2.18: Reprinted with permission from G. E. Peterson & H. L. Barney, "Control methods used in the study of vowels," *Journal of the Acoustical Society of America*, 24:175–184. © 1952 by the American Institute of Physics. Used by permission.

Figure 3.18: From A. D. Patel & J. R. Daniele, "Stress-timed vs. syllable-timed music? A comment on Huron and Ollen (2003)," *Music Perception*, 21:273–276. © 2003 by the University of California Press. Used by permission.

Figure 4.1: From J. Terken, "Fundamental frequency and perceived prominence of accented syllables," *Journal of the Acoustical Society of America*, 89:1768–1776. © 1991 by the American Institute of Physics. Used by permission.

Figure 4.7: From A. D. Patel, "A new approach to the cognitive neuroscience of melody," in I. Peretz & R. Zatorre (Eds.), *The Cognitive Neuroscience of Music*. © 2003 by Oxford University Press. Used by permission.

Figure 4.8: From C. L. Krumhansl & E. J. Kessler, "Tracing the dynamic changes in perceived tonal organization in a spatial representation of musical keys," *Psychological Review*, 89:334–368. © 1982 by the American Psychological Association. Used by permission.

Figure 4.10: From J. 't Hart, R. Collier, & A. Cohen, *A Perceptual Study of Intonation: An Experimental-Phonetic Approach to Speech Melody*. Cambridge, UK: Cambridge University Press. © 1990 by Cambridge University Press. Used by permission.

Figure 4.11: From J. 't Hart, R. Collier, & A. Cohen, *A Perceptual Study of Intonation: An Experimental-Phonetic Approach to Speech Melody*. Cambridge, UK: Cambridge University Press. © 1990 by Cambridge University Press. Used by permission.

Figure 4.13: From P. G. Vos & J. M. Troost, "Ascending and descending melodic intervals: Statistical findings and their perceptual relevance," *Music Perception*, 6:383–396. © 1989 by the University of California Press. Used by permission.

Figure 4.15: From A. D. Patel, J. R. Iversen, & J. Rosenberg, "Comparing the rhythm and melody of speech and music: The case of British English and French," *Journal of the Acoustical Society of America*, 119:3034–3047. © 2006 by the American Institute of Physics. Used by permission.

Figure 4.17: From A. D. Patel, I. Peretz, M. Tramo, & R. Labrecque, "Processing prosodic and musical patterns: A neuropsychological investigation," *Brain and Language*, 61:123–144. © 1998 by Elsevier. Used by permission.

Figure 4.18: From A. D. Patel, J. M. Foxton, & T. D. Griffiths, "Musically tone-deaf individuals have difficulty discriminating intonation contours extracted from speech," *Brain and Cognition*, 59:310–313. © 2005 by Elsevier. Used by permission.

Figure 5.1: From E. Balaban, "Bird song syntax: Learned intraspecific variation is meaningful," *Proceedings of the National Academy of Sciences, USA*, 85:3657–3660. © 1988 by the National Academy of Sciences, USA. Used by permission.

Figure 5.2: From L. L. Cuddy, A. J. Cohen, & D. J. K. Mewhort, "Perception of structure in short melodic sequences," *Journal of Experimental Psychology: Human Perception*

Figure 5.15: From F. Lerdahl, *Tonal Pitch Space*, 32. © 2001 by Oxford University Press. Used by permission.

Figure 5.17: From A. D. Patel, "The relationship of music to the melody of speech and to syntactic processing disorders in aphasia," *Annals of the New York Academy of Sciences*, 1060:59–70. © 2005 by Blackwell Publishing. Used by permission.

Figure 5.20: From A. D. Patel, "The relationship of music to the melody of speech and to syntactic processing disorders in aphasia," *Annals of the New York Academy of Sciences*, 1060:59–70. © 2005 by Blackwell Publishing. Used by permission.

Figure 6.1: From A. Gabrielsson & E. Lindström, "The influence of musical structure on emotional expression," in P. N. Juslin & J. A. Sloboda (Eds.), *Music and Emotion: Theory and Research* (pp. 223–248). © 2001 by Oxford University Press. Used by permission.

Figure 6.2: From C. L. Krumhansl, "Topic in music: An empirical study of memorability, openness, and emotion in Mozart's String Quintet in C Major and Beethoven's String Quartet in A Minor," *Music Perception*, 16:119–134. © 1998 by the University of California Press. Used by permission.

Table 6.2: From P. N. Juslin & P. Laukka, "Communication of emotions in vocal expression and music performance: Different channels, same code?" *Psychological Bulletin*, 129:770–814. © 2003 by the American Psychological Association. Used by permission.

Figure 6.3: From R. Hacohen & N. Wagner, "The communicative force of Wagner's leitmotifs: Complementary relationships between their connotations and denotations," *Music Perception*, 14:445–476. © 1997 by the University of California Press. Used by permission.

Figure 6.4: From R. Hacohen & N. Wagner, "The communicative force of Wagner's leitmotifs: Complementary relationships between their connotations and denotations," *Music Perception*, 14:445–476. © 1997 by the University of California Press. Used by permission.

Figure 6.5: From S. Koeslch, E. Kasper, D. Sammler, K. Schulze, T. Gunter, & A. D. Friederici, "Music, language, and meaning: Brain signatures of semantic processing," *Nature Neuroscience*, 7:302–307. © 2004 by Macmillan Publishers Ltd., *Nature Neuroscience*. Used by permission.

Figure 6.6: From F. Wolf & E. Gibson, "Representing discourse coherence: A corpus-based study," *Computational Linguistics*, 31:249–287. © 2005 by the Massachusetts Institute of Technology. Used by permission of MIT Press.

Figure 7.2: From R. J. Greenspan & T. Tully, "Group report: How do genes set up behavior?" in R. J. Greenspan & C. P. Kyriacou (Eds.), *Flexibility and Constraint in*

Author Index

Subject Index

CPSIA information can be obtained
at www.ICGtesting.com
Printed in the USA
BVHW040349051221
623253BV00002B/5

9 780199 755301